Biochemical Actions of Hormones

VOLUME I

CONTRIBUTORS

JULIUS AXELROD

IRA B. BLACK

J. E. DUMONT

ISIDORE S. EDELMAN

DARRELL D. FANESTIL

EARL FRIEDEN

ALLAN L. GOLDSTEIN

OLGA GREENGARD

JOHN J. JUST

K. L. MANCHESTER

CARLOS O. MILLER

HOWARD RASMUSSEN

THOMAS R. RIGGS

E. SCHELL-FREDERICK

J. R. TATA

ALAN TENENHOUSE

ULRICH WESTPHAL

ABRAHAM WHITE

Biochemical Actions of Hormones

Edited by GERALD LITWACK

Fels Research Institute
Temple University
School of Medicine
Philadelphia, Pennsylvania

VOLUME I

QP571
B56
v.1
1970

1970

ACADEMIC PRESS   New York   San Francisco   London

A Subsidiary of Harcourt Brace Jovanovich, Publishers

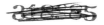

ACADEMIC PRESS, INC.
111 Fifth Avenue, New York, New York 10003

United Kingdom Edition published by
ACADEMIC PRESS, INC. (LONDON) LTD.
24/28 Oval Road, London NW1

LIBRARY OF CONGRESS CATALOG CARD NUMBER: 70-107567

PRINTED IN THE UNITED STATES OF AMERICA

Contents

1.   **Hormonal Responses in Amphibian Metamorphosis**

         Earl Frieden and John J. Just

2.   **The Developmental Formation of Enzymes in Rat Liver**

         Olga Greengard

8. Mineralocorticoids

Isidore S. Edelman and Darrell D. Fanestil

9. Parathyroid Hormone and Calcitonin

Howard Rasmussen and Alan Tenenhouse

10. Mechanism of Action of Thyrotropin

E. Schell-Frederick and J. E. Dumont

11. The Thymus as an Endocrine Gland: Hormones and Their Actions

Allan L. Goldstein and Abraham White

12. Plant Hormones

Carlos O. Miller

List of Contributors

Numbers in parentheses indicate the pages on which the authors' contributions begin.

Julius Axelrod (135), Laboratory of Clinical Sciences, National Institute of Mental Health, Bethesda, Maryland

Ira B. Black (135), Laboratory of Clinical Sciences, National Institute of Mental Health, Bethesda, Maryland

J. E. Dumont (415), Laboratory of Nuclear Medicine, School of Medicine, University of Brussels, and Biology Department, Euratom, Brussels, Belgium

Isidore S. Edelman (321), Department of Medicine, University of California, San Francisco, California

Darrell D. Fanestil (321), Department of Internal Medicine, University of Kansas, School of Medicine, Kansas City, Kansas

Earl Frieden (1), Department of Chemistry, Institute of Molecular Biophysics, Florida State University, Tallahassee, Florida

Allan L. Goldstein (465), Department of Biochemistry, Albert Einstein College of Medicine, The Bronx, New York

Olga Greengard (53), Department of Biological Chemistry, Harvard Medical School, Boston, Massachusetts

John J. Just (1), Department of Chemistry, Institute of Molecular Biophysics, Florida State University, Tallahassee, Florida

K. L. Manchester (267), Department of Biochemistry, University College London, London, England

Carlos O. Miller (503), Botany Department, Indiana University, Bloomington, Indiana

Howard Rasmussen (365), Department of Biochemistry, University of Pennsylvania, Philadelphia, Pennsylvania

Thomas R. Riggs (157), Department of Biological Chemistry, University of Michigan, Ann Arbor, Michigan

E. Schell-Frederick (415), Laboratory of Nuclear Medicine, School of Medicine, University of Brussels, and Biology Department, Euratom, Brussels, Belgium

J. R. Tata* (89), National Institute for Medical Research, Mill Hill, London, England

Alan Tenenhouse (365), Department of Pharmacology, McGill University, Montreal, Canada

Ulrich Westphal (209), Biochemistry Department, University of Louisville, School of Medicine, Louisville, Kentucky

Abraham White (465), Department of Biochemistry, Albert Einstein College of Medicine, The Bronx, New York

* Present address: Department of Biochemistry, University of California, Berkeley, California.

Preface

This collection of papers by researchers in the field of hormone action surveys the significant developments in our progress toward understanding the primary effects of hormones in cellular receptors at the molecular level. During the last six years, there have been enormous developments in this field. The extent of progress is reflected in the size of this two-volume work. An advantage in having two volumes is the prompt publication in Volume I of those manuscripts completed at an early date, an important consideration in a rapidly expanding area of research.

Some informational overlap between contributions was unavoidable, but, hopefully, has been held to a minimum. It seemed more sensible to tolerate a small degree of redundancy than to tamper with cohesiveness. There are certain areas in which relatively little progress has been made. Accordingly, a few gaps in coverage will be evident, such as the absence of a contribution on intestinal hormones.

The coverage is broad enough to make this work useful as a modern reference text for the endocrinologist. In many cases, new data from the contributors' laboratories are presented. Thus, the purpose of these two volumes is to provide in one source an up-to-date survey of molecular and biochemical approaches bearing on the problem of hormone mechanism.

Biochemical Actions of Hormones

VOLUME I

CHAPTER 1

Hormonal Responses in Amphibian Metamorphosis

Earl Frieden and John J. Just

I. INTRODUCTION[1]

Amphibian metamorphosis is a postembryonic developmental process in which nonreproductive structures and organ systems of the amphibian larva change drastically to an adult form during a relatively brief and discrete period. The dramatic nature of the morphological transformations during this transition has excited biologists since the beginning of this century. The basic hormonal controls of this process were established by Gudernatsch, Allen, and others in the period 1912 to 1930. Our knowledge of the chemical and molecular changes associated with the biological transitions of amphibian metamorphosis is of a much more recent vintage. The process of metamorphosis is one of the classic examples of differentiation and of comparative and developmental biochemistry. In many of the amphibians there is a remarkable physiological adaptation during the transformation of an aquatic larva to a terrestrial adult. It also illustrates one of the most dramatic effects of the thyroid hormone, or any hormone for that matter. The rapid changes in function and in some cell types frequently have been compared to changes occurring in tumor cells. Much of our current knowledge in this field has been summarized in two recent volumes, one devoted principally to amphibians, edited by Moore (1964) and a second devoted to metamorphosis, edited by Etkin and Gilbert (1968). Numerous additional

[1] In addition to the standard abbreviations used for amino acids, nucleotides, and polynucleotides, the following more specialized abbreviations are used in this review: A. A., amino acid; Act D, actinomycin D; CM, carboxymethyl; GC ratio, guanylic acid to cytidylic acid ratio; Hb(s), hemoglobin(s); i-T_2, L-3'-isopropyl-3,5-diiodo-thyronine; LMC, lateral motor column; M-cells, Mauthner's cells; M-V, mesencephalic V nucleus; mRNA, messenger RNA; MSH, melanocyte-stimulating hormone; ppb, parts per billion; RBC(s), red blood cell(s); rRNA, ribosomal RNA; T_3, triiodo-thyronine; T_4, thyronine; TRH, thyrotropin-releasing hormone; tRNA, transfer RNA; TSH, thyroid-stimulating hormone.

reviews have appeared during the last decade (Bennett and Frieden, 1962; P. P. Cohen, 1966; Frieden, 1967; Weber, 1967a,b). Thus a significant literature characterizing the biological and biochemical aspects of this developmental phenomenon has accumulated in recent years.

Our objective in this chapter is to survey the metamorphic process in Amphibia using several recent reviews (Frieden, 1967, 1968; Weber, 1967a,b), as a point of reference. We attempted to include tissues that have been shown to respond directly to thyroid hormones or, conversely, which may not be under the sole control of the thyroid hormone, and finally, to bring up to date several of the very active areas of research, e.g., developmental changes in the liver, tail, etc.

In order to use various phases of the metamorphic process as points of reference in our discussion, the key morphological events are summarized in Fig. 1. Leg growth and tail regression are correlated with the stages of development and other significant structural changes. This description appears to fit *Rana pipiens* (leopard frog) and *Rana catesbeiana* (bullfrog) specifically and is probably representative of many anuran species. A comprehensive survey of the variation in amphibian life histories was published by Dent (1968). There are four distinct periods in the life history of amphibians: embryonic, larval, juvenile, and adult forms. In our treatment of hormonal responses during metamorphosis, we arbitrarily accept for discussion all changes that occur in the larval period, although we recognize that this inclusion may eventually prove to be too broad. Because of the availability of useful data principally on anuran metamorphosis, most of the discussion in this chapter necessarily emphasizes research on this group of amphibians.

A major source of interest in amphibian metamorphosis stems from its use as a model system for studying the mechanism of thyroid hormone action. Although there is no doubt that thyroid hormones play a dominant role in amphibian metamorphosis, it is likely that as for most vertebrates, amphibian larvae have an intricate system of endocrine interplay. Caution should be exercised in interpreting current data because few typical glandular ablative experiments combined with hormone replacement have been reported using amphibian larvae. Until such experiments, or adequate perfusion or tissue culture experiments are performed, it is not certain that the observed responses are indeed direct effects or are indirect effects triggered by the thyroid hormone.

Localized morphological changes associated with thyroid hormone implants were first reported 30 years ago, strongly suggesting a direct effect of thyroid hormone on certain anatomical responses (Hartwig, 1940; Kollros, 1942). These early observations have been extended to other morphological systems (see review of Kaltenbach, 1968). It should

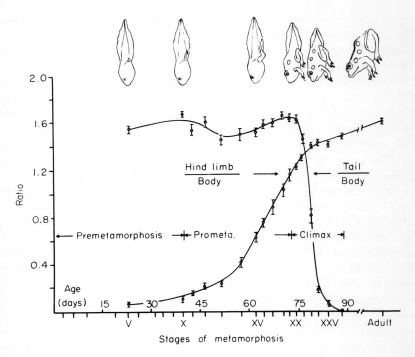

Fɪɢ. 1. Morphological events during spontaneous metamorphosis of *R. pipiens* larvae. The ages and stages are taken directly from A. C. Taylor and Kollros (1946). The illustrations depict several striking anatomical changes correlated with appropriate stages. The ratios represent the means of ten or more tadpoles at $19 \pm 1°$ with the standard error indicated (Just, 1968). Pre-, prometamorphosis, and climax are as defined by Etkin (1964).

be emphasized that only a few of the biochemical changes that have been associated with metamorphosis have been shown to be directly affected by thyroid hormone.

II. INTERRELATIONSHIPS OF HORMONES DURING ANURAN METAMORPHOSIS

Although the major purpose of this chapter is to review the peripheral responses associated with amphibian metamorphosis, we will comment briefly on the endocrine relationships involved. Most of the previous work was concerned with demonstrating that the hypothalamus–pituitary–

thyroid axis was necessary for metamorphosis (see review by Etkin, 1968). Confirmation of this hypothesis by Etkin (1964) and Voitkevich (1962) led to further examination of the role of other hormones in the control of metamorphosis. The contributions of Bern, Etkin, and their co-workers implicated other pituitary hormones in amphibian development, an idea that had been inferred earlier from the effects of pituitary transplants. Berman *et al.* (1964) first demonstrated that prolactin promoted tadpole growth and retarded metamorphosis, and Bern *et al.* (1967) have summarized their view on endocrine relationships in the peripheral tissues. Numerous recent papers have established the following facts.

1. Mammalian prolactin and growth hormones accelerated growth rates in normal (Berman *et al.*, 1964; Remy and Bounhiol, 1965, 1966; Etkin and Gona, 1967) and in hypophysectomized tadpoles (Etkin and Gona, 1967; Just and Kollros, 1969).

2. Hypophysectomized tadpoles attain normal or larger than normal size, indicating that pituitary hormones are not essential for larval growth (Hanaoka, 1967; Just and Kollros, 1968).

3. Prolactin and growth hormone counteracted tail reduction (Bern *et al.*, 1967; Etkin and Gona, 1967) and inhibited urea excretion stimulated by thyroid hormones (Medda and Frieden, 1970). Prolactin did not inhibit the thyroxine-stimulated appearance of carbamyl phosphate synthetase, a liver urea cycle enzyme (Blatt *et al.*, 1969).

4. Prolactin also inhibits thyroid gland function in tadpoles (Gona, 1968).

Although these data suggest a possible role for prolactin and growth hormone in delaying the initiation of metamorphosis, it must be emphasized that neither hormone has been demonstrated in the tadpole pituitary or blood. The amounts of mammalian prolactin and growth hormone frequently used to produce the foregoing effects appear to be massive and nonphysiological. Furthermore, these hormones usually are administered to intact animals, and the observed effects could be caused by numerous hormonal interactions. Clearly, many decisive experiments remain to be done.

A hypothesis to account for the endocrine control of amphibian metamorphosis has been proposed by Etkin (1963). The postulated interaction of endocrine factors in determining the time and pattern of anuran metamorphosis is illustrated in Fig. 2. We quote from Etkin's most recent review in 1968:

"In the early premetamorphic period the thyroxine level is very low and remains so until just before prometamorphosis begins. At

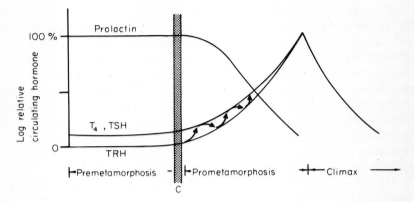

FIG. 2. Diagram of the relationships between the thyroid, pituitary, and hypothalamic hormones as proposed by Etkin (1968). C refers to the stage when the
hypothalamus acquires capability for a response to thyroxine. TRH—thyrotrophin-
releasing hormone; TSH—thyroid-stimulating hormone; T₄—thyroxine.

this time, the hypothalamic TRH mechanism becomes sensitive to
positive thyroxine feedback, thereby initiating prometamorphosis.
The increase in the TRH provoked by the action of the initial
thyroxine level upon the hypothalamus stimulates increased TSH
release, which acts back to raise the thyroxine level. This leads to a
spiraling action which raises the thyroxine level and thereby induces
prometamorphosis with its characteristic sequence of changes. The
positive feedback cycle leads to maximal activation of the pituitary–
thyroid axis, thereby bringing on metamorphic climax. During early
premetamorphosis, prolactin is produced at a high rate. With the
activation of the hypothalamus, the production of prolactin drops
under the inhibitory influence of hypothalamic activity. As the level
of TSH rises during prometamorphosis, that of prolactin decreases.
The growth rate of the animal therefore falls, and the metamor-
phosis-restraining activity of prolactin diminishes. Thus the premetamorphic period in which growth is active and metamorphosis
is inhibited is characterized by the predominance of prolactin over
TSH. The reverse holds during metamorphosis. The time of shift
in hormone balance is determined by the initiation of positive thyroid
feedback to the hypothalamus. This varies greatly between species.
The pattern of change during metamorphosis is regulated by the
pattern of the feedback buildup and is much the same in most
anurans."

This highly speculative proposal lacks confirmation at a number of key points as follows: (1) circulating levels of thyroid hormones in the tad-pole do not increase as described (Just, 1968); (2) the presence of prolactin and TRH in their respective glands or in the blood have not been demonstrated; and (3) TSH has not been identified in larval blood.

Evidence that appears inconsistent with Etkin's hypothesis includes (1) the lack of a requirement of the hypothalamus for metamorphosis in one species, *X. laevis* (Guardabassi, 1961); (2) the failure of mam-malian TRH to induce metamorphosis (Etkin and Gona, 1968); and (3) the large difference in the half-lives in mammals of blood TSH (< 2 hours) and blood T_4 (20 hours) would probably not account for the correspondence of blood TSH and T_4 levels (Pittman and Shimizu, 1966; Odell *et al.*, 1967). Although this hypothesis or some modified form (Just, 1968) is valuable in that it serves as a basis for experimental design, we emphasize that it should not be accepted without further confirmation.

III. CHANGES IN BLOOD

A. Immune Response

The demonstration of immune responses by skin rejection has been made in numerous anurans (see Bovbjerg, 1966, for earlier references) and urodeles (N. Cohen, 1966; Charlemagne and Houillon, 1968), and many early investigators demonstrated allograft destruction of various tissues in larval amphibians. The immunological basis for graft rejection was shown by Hildemann and Haas (1959), who reported a significantly earlier rejection of second-set grafts, compared with first grafts.

There are indications that very young larvae do not have a fully developed immune response (Harris, 1941; Eakin and Harris, 1945; Hildemann, 1966; Bovbjerg, 1966). During the critical period of immune response maturation, the numbers of small lymphocytes have been found to be increased as much as tenfold (Hildemann and Haas, 1962). Anti-body production in response to a variety of antigens has been demon-strated in larvae (Cooper *et al.*, 1964; Cooper and Hildemann, 1965a), and recently it was shown that lymphocytes and histocytes produce antibodies in amphibians (Du Pasquier, 1967).

Although little work has been done on the role of the thymus in the immune response in larval amphibians, the development of the thymus

(Fabrizio and Charipper, 1941; Rossini, 1965; Fox, 1967; Cooper, 1967a) and several other lymphoid organs (reviewed by Cooper, 1967b; Baculi and Cooper, 1967) has been described. Thymectomy was found to increase the survival of skin grafts in larval amphibians (Cooper and Hildemann, 1965b; N. Cohen, 1966; DeLanney and Prahlad, 1966; Charlemagne and Houillon, 1968), and following thymectomy larvae showed weakened antibody production (Cooper *et al.*, 1964). Thymectomy influenced graft survival only in very young animals rather than older *R. catesbeiana* larvae (Cooper and Hildemann, 1965b). This may be one factor in the lack of effect of thymectomy on eye transplantation in *Bufo* (Guardabassi and Lattes, 1965). In adult toads the lymph nodes are involved in antibody production (Diener and Nossal, 1966). A recent study in bullfrog tadpoles showed that after lymph node removal, antibodies to bovine serum albumin were not synthesized, yet the normal rejection of skin allografts occurred (Cooper, 1968).

At the present time it is not known whether there is a major shift in the organs responsible for immune response during metamorphosis; a partial shift away from the thymus is indicated in *R. catesbeiana* larvae oper, 1968). Whether a single cell line is involved in the immune response of larvae and adult amphibians is also undetermined. Bovbjerg (1966) demonstrated that neither hypophysectomy nor thyroxine treatment of larvae affected the rate of homograft rejection. If similar experiments were performed after various lymphatic organs were removed, the endocrine influences in immune response could be investigated.

B. Alterations in Serum Proteins

It is now well documented that serum proteins are drastically modified during metamorphosis (Frieden *et al.*, 1957; Herner and Frieden, 1960; Hahn, 1962; Manwell, 1966; Richmond, 1968; Just, 1968). Whereas the data suggested extensive shifts in the globulin patterns, the most striking observation was a huge increase in albumin from values of less than 0.10 gm/100 ml in the tadpole to over 1.00 gm/100 ml in the postmetamorphic frog (Herner and Frieden, 1960). Evidence has recently been obtained confirming earlier assumptions that the biosynthesis of a protein corresponding to albumin occurred in the liver of *R. catesbeiana* tadpoles and increased during metamorphosis (Ledford and Frieden, 1969).

Another serum protein that undergoes an even greater stimulation than albumin during metamorphosis is ceruloplasmin. The catalytic activity of this copper protein in tadpole serum increases 50–100-fold during metamorphosis (Inaba and Frieden, 1967). The rise in ceruloplasmin precedes significant changes in hemoglobin biosynthesis and may reflect the role of this copper protein in iron utilization as proposed by Osaki *et al.* (1966). Levels of other serum globulins, e.g., transferrin, carbonic anhydrase, are also elevated during metamorphosis (Francis and Frieden, 1964).

Numerous serum proteins with unique immunochemical properties appear during metamorphosis in the urodele *Triturus alpestris* (Charlemagne, 1967), in *Pleurodeles waltlii* (Chalumeau-Le Foulgac, 1967), and in *R. catesbeiana* (Wise, 1970), but the significance of these observations has not been determined.

C. Red Cell and Hemoglobin Transitions

Since it was first suggested that hormones effect mRNA production (Karlson, 1963), numerous investigations on the mechanism of hormone action have been performed, attempting to substantiate or refute this hypothesis. Because the usual endocrine response is a modulation of protein synthesis rather than a complete shift in patterns of protein synthesis, direct evidence for this mechanism has been difficult to obtain. The amphibian erythropoietic system offers several advantages for studying the role of hormones in gene expression. These are (1) the cell type, the erythrocyte, is well defined; (2) the major protein component, hemoglobin (Hb), is well characterized; and (3) there is a change in Hb from tadpole to adult form. Finally, a recent observation that anuran (Flores and Frieden, 1968) and urodele (Grasso and Shephard, 1968) larvae can be made totally anemic, and yet survive, may prove a powerful tool in the investigation of the Hb transition.

1. Larval and Adult Hemoglobins

The numerous differences between the larval and adult Hb molecules are summarized in Table I. These biochemical differences reside exclusively in the globin portion of the molecule. There is general agreement that tadpole and adult Hb do not share a common polypeptide chain (see review by Frieden, 1968; Moss and Ingram, 1968a; Aggarwal and Riggs, 1969; Wise, 1970), although one claim has been made that a common α-chain is present in both adult and larval Hb (Hamada and Shukuya,1966). A rapid shift from the larval to the adult type of Hb's occurs during tail regression. Because larval Hb does not have SH groups but adult Hb does, the appearance of SH groups has been used to demonstrate the Hb transition (Hamada *et al.*, 1966; Ashley and Frieden, 1967). Carboxymethyl cellulose columns (Hamada *et al.*, 1966) and disk electrophoresis (Moss and Ingram, 1968b) have demonstrated a complete Hb

TABLE I

COMPARISON OF THE PROPERTIES OF TADPOLE AND ADULT BULLFROG HEMOGLOBINS

Property	Tadpole	Adult	Reference no.[c]
pO_2 for 50% saturation	4 mm	14 mm	1
Bohr effect[a]	None	Typical	1
Heme spectrum	Same	Same	2
Methemoglobin formation	Resistant	Less resistant	3
Alkali denaturation	Resistant	Less resistant	3
Electrophoretic mobility (on paper, starch block, gel, etc.)	Fast	Slower	3,4,5
Number of protein components	4	5	5
Average molecular weight	68,000	68,000	4, 6
Dimerizable	0	80%	4
Protein chains	$\alpha_2^T\beta_2^T$	$\alpha_2^F\beta_2^F$	5, 7, 8
N-Termini	Val	Gly	5
	N-Acetylgly	N-Acetylgly	5
C-Termini	his, ala	his, glu	9
Amino acid analysis			
Residues of acidic A.A. in 65,000 g	104	98	4
Residues of basic A.A. in 65,000 g^b	52	62	4
½ Cystine	0	8	4

[a] A typical Bohr effect refers to the decrease in oxygen binding affinity as the pH is decreased.

[b] Histidine is omitted from this calculation because it is assumed to be essentially uncharged at the electrophoretic pH, 8.6.

[c] Key to references: 1. Riggs (1951); 2. Trader *et al.* (1963); 3. Herner and Frieden (1961); 4. Trader and Frieden (1966); 5. Moss and Ingram (1968a); 6. Riggs *et al.* (1964); 7. Stratton and Frieden (1967); 8. Riggs and Aggarwal (1968); 9. Hamada and Shukuya (1966).

transition at metamorphic climax (Fig. 3). Using paper electrophoresis, Theil (1967) detected adult Hb in tadpoles at stages XXIV and XXV. However, in a recent abstract (Benbasset, 1969), the shift from larval to adult Hb was reported to require several weeks after metamorphic climax.

2. Red Cell Differentiation

This repression and induction of specific Hb proteins and/or cell types has led to speculation as to their origin. During normal metamorphosis there are several possible ways for thyroid hormone or some other factor to cause this differentiation.

1. An effect on the maturation of the stem cells; erythropoietic sites would continue to produce RBC's, but the maturation process would result in production of adult Hb.

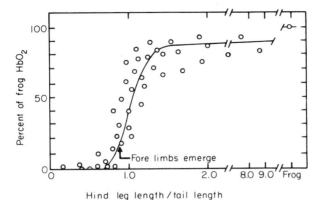

Hind leg length / tail length

F ig. 3. The transition from tadpole to frog hemoglobin during the spontaneous metamorphosis of *R. catesbeiana*. The switch is rapid; fewer than 10 days are required for a change in the length of hind leg to tail ratio of 0.6 to 2.0. The frog hemoglobins were determined after separation by CM-cellulose column chromatography. Data from Hamada *et al.* (1966).

2. A change in the erythropoietic centers. In the new centers, new stem cells would be activated while the old stem cells at the former site(s) would be suppressed. Stimulation of the old stem cells to migrate to new erythropoietic sites, where adult Hb is produced in response to the new environment.

3. Alternation of the Hb production in the circulating RBC's.

4. Alteration in Hb resulting from some combination of the previous possibilities.

Hollyfield (1966a) has reviewed the limited literature on the existence of several erythropoietic centers in amphibians. The important early paper by Jordan and Speidel (1923) reported that the site of erythropoietic activity shifted from the kidney to the spleen and bone marrow during induced metamorphosis, but they used few specimens and were able to induce complete metamorphosis in only one case. Furthermore, their criteria for the identification of the erythrocyte stem cell probably is not valid. Hollyfield (1966a) transplanted hemopoietic anlagen between embryos of different ploidy and concluded that blood islands do not act as stem cells for RBC's produced in other areas. Transplants of nephric anlagen demonstrate that stem cells in the intertubular spaces of these structures develop *in situ*. Hollyfield (1966b) demonstrated a histological change in the RBC's of tadpoles induced to metamorphose, and suggested that these erythrocytes may originate in the spleen. But he did not transplant spleen anlagen and thus there is no certainty that different stem cells are involved at metamorphosis.

In mammals and birds it is generally assumed that a differentiated

RBC stops synthesis of Hb and the development of a new stem cell is required for biosynthesis of different Hb's (see review by Wilt, 1967). In amphibian metamorphosis it has been proposed that a differentiated RBC stops synthesis of tadpole Hb, and stem cells must be stimulated to produce adult Hb (Moss and Ingram, 1965, 1968b). The complete change in Hb types that occurs during metamorphosis takes place in less than 20 days. Yet the average life span of adult anuran RBC's of different species has been reported to be 24 days in *R. catesbeiana* (Baca Saravia, 1961), 200 days in *R. pipiens* (Cline and Waldmann, 1962), and between 700 and 1400 days in *B. marinus* (Atland and Brace, 1962). To account for the rapid replacement of Hb types one would have to postulate a relatively short life span of tadpole RBC's, as in adult *R. catesbeiana*, or, alternatively, an acceleration of the aging process at metamorphic climax. Shukuya (1966) has claimed that both tadpole and frog Hb are present in a single cell, suggesting an alteration in Hb production within the circulating RBC's.

3. Protein and RNA Biosynthesis in Amphibian Red Blood Cells

Changes in protein synthesis of RBC's *in vitro* are observed in tadpoles induced to metamorphose by thyroid hormones (Moss and Ingram, 1965, 1968b; Theil and Frieden, 1966; Theil, 1967). Under *in vitro* conditions it was demonstrated that 3–8 days after thyroid hormone administration amino acid incorporation was depressed. Beyond this time the incorporation levels returned to prestimulation levels. Moss and Ingram (1965, 1968b) reported a depression of incorporation during the early time period in the larval Hb. When incorporation returned to prestimulation levels, and only if adult Hb carrier was added, the amino acids could be detected in adult Hb (Moss and Ingram, 1965, 1968b). Histologically, a new cell type appeared at this time (De Witt, 1968). It should be emphasized that the RBC's from thyroxine-treated animals did not develop the electrophoretic patterns of adult Hb, and adult electrophoretic patterns could be demonstrated only when the new cell type was concentrated (De Witt, 1968).

After thyroxine treatment, McMahon and De Witt (1968) demonstrated changes in incorporation of uridine after labeling for 24 hours. These authors show a depression of incorporation during the first 11 days of thyroxine administration, and a concomitant decrease in discrete ribosomal RNA peaks. At 14 and 22 days after hormone treatment there is an increase in incorporation as well as a reappearance of ribosomal RNA. They concluded that old cells producing larval Hb were repressed, and new cells that synthesize frog Hb were stimulated.

In a recent study of amino acid incorporation into RBC's *in vivo*, Just and Atkinson (1969) did not observe a statistically significant depression of incorporation after T_3 injection. In fact, from 8–12 days after hormone injection there was a stimulation of amino acid incorporation above the pretreated levels. As in the *in vitro* incorporation studies, the electrophoretic patterns were not changed even 16 days following hormone treatment. Because during the course of normal metamorphosis, larval Hb does disappear and adult Hb appears, Just and Atkinson (1969) propose that induction with T_3 does not completely mimic normal metamorphosis, an idea that will be explored later.

Shukuya and co-workers (Hirayama, 1967) also demonstrated changes in amino acid incorporation by blood cells *in vivo* during normal and induced metamorphosis. Less radioactivity is incorporated in normal cells by premetamorphic animals than during climax. When premetamorphic animals were treated with T_4 to induce metamorphosis, the rate of amino acid incorporation was found to increase (Hirayama, 1967).

The Hb transition in amphibians represents one of the most promising systems to study differentiation and hormone action. Much additional information is needed; e.g., are there two or more cell lines? What is (are) the site(s) of origin and maturation of cell line(s)? Are these sites identical? Answers to these questions are essential in understanding the mechanism of differentiation and hormone action in this transition.

IV. THE DEVELOPMENT OF THE NERVOUS SYSTEM

The developing amphibian nervous system offers an excellent vehicle for the investigation of the hormonal alteration of nervous function. Following the first reported modification of neural development by alteration of thyroid function (Allen, 1918), numerous studies have emphasized specific regions of the brain or spinal cord. Ablative experiments (hypophysectomy or thyroidectomy) and additive experiments (direct implantations of thyroid hormone into the nervous system, or whole animal immersion in thyroid hormone) have demonstrated that many aspects of the amphibian nervous system development are under the influence of the thyroid hormone.

The corneal reflex (ability of the eyeball to retract into the orbit upon stimulation of the cornea) develops at late larval stages in anuran development. Kollros (1942) induced this ability with thyroxine–agar implants into the fourth ventricle. Because the peripheral components of the reflex are present before neural maturation, this modified behavioral ability is considered a direct result of the response of the neuronal center to thyroid hormone. Later, Kollros (1958) treated hypophysectomized tadpoles with T_4 in concentrations approximately capable of bringing about forelimb emergence. After prolonged treatment, he was able to separate the onset of the corneal reflex and the emergence of the forelimbs beyond the average value of 4 days to over 100 days, indicating the independence of these two different responses to T_4.

The cells of the mesencephalic nucleus of the trigeminal nerve in *R. pipiens* remain small during most of the larval period and grow rapidly during metamorphic climax (Kollros and McMurray, 1955). Thyroxine–cholesterol pellets, imbedded adjacent to the midbrain, increased the size of cells nearest the hormone source (Kollros and McMurray, 1956). This stimulatory effect could not be demonstrated during the earliest part of larval life in *R. pipiens* (Kollros and McMurray, 1956).

The lateral motor column (LMC) cells provide the motor innervation to the limb and the girdle. These cells are formed from the adjacent gray matter and little differentiation occurs until the early midlarval period. During and after the midlarval period over half of the cells die and the surviving cells increase in size. Thyroxine promotes the earlier appearance of LMC cells in *R. pipiens* (Reynolds, 1963). In cells that appear similar histologically, both degeneration and growth have simultaneously been stimulated by thyroxine implantation in this area (Beaudoin, 1956; Race, 1961). Presumably, cells that have made peripheral connection grow and differentiate, whereas those that have not connected degenerate. In the tree frog, *Eleutherodactylus martinicensis,* unlike *R. pipiens,* the cell number of the LMC is not altered by thyroidectomy or hypophysectomy (Hughes, 1966), although axon growth is altered.

The hindbrain of tadpoles contains a pair of giant neurons, Mauthner's cells (M-cells), with large axons descending into the trunk and tail. The M-cells normally atrophy after metamorphic climax. Thyroxine treatment of these cells by implantation leads to precocious atrophy (Weiss and Rossetti, 1951; Pesetsky and Kollros, 1956). Thyroidectomized tadpoles have smaller M-cells (Pesetsky, 1966a; Fox and Moulton, 1968) but, unexpectedly, the M-cells grow larger than normal (Pesetsky, 1962; Fox and Moulton, 1968) when the tadpoles are immersed in high concentrations of thyroxine. A recent cytological study demonstrated that changes in rough endoplasmic reticulum and in RNase-sensitive–pyronine-positive material occur during the growth and atrophy phenomena in M-cells (Moulton *et al.,* 1968). These findings led Pesetsky (1962) to suggest that the growth of M-cells is stimulated by thyroxine and that the hormone is required for the further growth and maintenance of these cells. The atrophy seen in implantation studies may be caused by a depletion of hormone concentration in the pellet.

These examples (see review of Kollros, 1968) illustrate the varied responses to thyroxine. Thyroxine can cause premature differentiation of specific nerve cells, death, and growth of other cells, and may be required for the maintenance of some cells. Species differences exist in comparing the same cell. Little histochemical and enzymic data are available concerning changes induced by thyroid hormones in the nervous system of amphibians (Janosky and Wenger, 1956; Pesetsky, 1965, 1966b; Kim *et al.*, 1966; Manwell, 1966; Moulton *et al.*, 1968). New microtechniques for protein and RNA synthesis (i.e., Felgenhauer, 1968; Hydén, 1968; Egyhazi *et al.*, 1968) should yield more precise biochemical information.

V. RESPONSES OF THE SKIN

The skin of anurans during the first third of larval life consists of two or three layers of epithelial cells; a thin basement membrane; a thick basement lamella (a series of orthogonally arranged collagen fibrils embedded in a viscous ground substance); and layers of connective tissue cells (i.e., mesenchymal cells, pigment cells, and fibroblasts) beneath the lamella. After the midlarval period, collagen begins to break down and the basement lamella is invaded by mesenchymal cells. Connective tissue cells migrate and serous and mucous epidermal glands grow into the space created by the breakdown process.

A. COLLAGEN BREAKDOWN

Gross and co-workers have studied the degradation of collagen in the skin of tadpoles. They have developed *in vitro* assays for a collagenase (Gross and Lapiere, 1962) and hyaluronidase (Silbert *et al.*, 1965). Using cultured epithelial and mesenchymal cells it was demonstrated that these cells produce collagenase and hyaluronidase respectively (Eisen and Gross, 1965). By freeze-thawing isolated cells and by using puromycin, an inhibitor of protein synthesis, it was shown that epithelial cells store little active collagenase and require protein synthesis to produce the functional enzyme, whereas mesenchymal cells store hyaluronidase and release active enzyme irrespective of protein synthesis (Eisen and Gross, 1965). Electron-microscope studies indicate that T_4 promoted the breakdown of collagen fibers and stimulated movement of mesenchymal cells into the collagen fibers of the tail and back skin (Kemp, 1963; Usuku and Gross, 1965). Neither pretreatment of larvae with T_4 nor addition of T_4 to cultured skin and tail tissue showed an increase in collagenase activity (Nagai *et al.*, 1966). Because the EM studies clearly indicate a decrease in collagen of the skin, this suggests that either the rate of collagen synthesis is decreased by T_4 or the type of collagenase changes during metamorphosis.

B. Skin Glands

Adult amphibians usually have two types of subepidermal skin glands: serous and mucous. The serous glands have large granule-filled lumina; the mucous glands are usually smaller than the serous. The gland rudiments enlarge by cell division, and maturation into the adult gland occurs gradually during the rest of the metamorphic period (Bovbjerg, 1963; Vanable, 1964). Electron-microscope studies indicate two cell types present in the serous gland, namely the secretory cell itself, and the so-called ersatzzelle containing poorly developed endoplasmic reticulum and Golgi apparatus (Pflugfelder and Schubert, 1965). It is not known whether T_4 stimulation of gland development affects this presumed ersatzzelle. The development of these glands is dependent on the thyroid hormones. Hypophysectomized animals do not have skin glands (Bovbjerg, 1963), and chemical inhibition of the biosynthesis of thyroid hormone prevents skin gland formation in anurans (Pflugfelder and Schubert, 1965) and, perhaps, in urodeles (Pflugfelder, 1967). Thyroxine pellets placed under *R. pipiens* skin cause local maturation of these glands (Kollros and Kaltenbach, 1952; Kaltenbach, 1953a). The effect of a single concentration of T_4 *in vitro* on skin gland development in *X. laevis* depends on the degree of maturation of the skin at the time of explantation (Vanable and Mortensen, 1966).

Serotonin (5-hydroxytryptamine) is considered a product of the serous glands because granules of the serous glands gave histochemical reactions predicted for serotonin, and 50% of the serotonin from *X. laevis* was in a sedimentable fraction of skin. As increasing numbers of serous rudiments mature, this compound increased more than seventyfold (Vanable, 1964). The decarboxylase that converts 5-hydroxytryptophan to 5-hydroxytryptamine increased approximately tenfold, but at a slightly earlier time than serotonin. Skin fragments of postclimax, but not of preclimax animals, cultured in a medium with ^{14}C-tryptophan produced labeled serotonin (Vanable, 1966). This suggests either a shift in the amount of the enzyme hydroxylating tryptophan or removal of an inhibitor during metamorphosis. An EM study indicates that the secretory cells of the serous glands contain highly developed endoplasmic reticulum and Golgi apparatus. The cell membrane of the secretory cell is broken at the lumen of this gland and numerous highly complex granules are seen in the lumen of the gland. The complexity of these granules suggests that serotonin is not the sole product of the gland, and may not be the major product. A thorough study of the particulate fractions of the skin should give much additional information about serous gland development.

C. PIGMENT CELLS

Although numerous studies exist describing pigment cell differentiation (see review of Wilde, 1961), little information is available concerning the hormones involved in the process (see review of Bagnara, 1966). The four major pigment cells and associated pigments in amphibians are melanophores containing melanin; iridophores with purine; and xanthophores and erythrophores with pteridines, carotenes, and flavins. These chromophores are intimately related spatially in the so-called "dermal-chromatophore unit," which probably integrates the total pigment response to hormones in the animal (Bagnara *et al.*, 1968).

It has long been known that removal of the pituitary causes a bleaching of tadpole skin. The bleaching is due to changes in two cell populations: (1) in hypophysectomized tadpoles the melanophores are contracted and decreased in number (Blount, 1945; Burch, 1938; Eakin, 1939; Bagnara and Neidleman, 1958); (2) the iridophores are dispersed and increased in number (Bagnara and Neidleman, 1958). In 1958 Bagnara indicated that a lack of MSH resulted in the bleaching of hypophysectomized tadpoles. He found that MSH injection caused both an iridophore contraction and a melanophore expansion, and later demonstrated that the same peptide fragment of the MSH molecule caused both responses (Bagnara, 1964a).

The increase in melanophore number seen during metamorphosis was attributed to both division of old melanocytes and differentiation of melanocytes from unpigmented cells (Pehlemann, 1967). It was concluded that the rate of division of melanocytes was dependent upon pituitary MSH, and new pigment cell formation was dependent upon the population density of melanophores.

The pathway of pteridine biosynthesis is currently under investigation in larval aphibians (Ziegler-Gunder *et al.*, 1956; Levy, 1964; Stackhouse, 1966; Sugiura and Goto, 1968). After MSH injection into hypophysectomized tadpoles, an increase in pteridines is seen, while certain purines, possible precursors of pteridines, are decreased (Bagnara, 1961; Stackhouse, 1966). This decline in purines also is associated with a decrease in iridophore numbers (Bagnara and Neidleman, 1958; Stack-house, 1966). The types and amounts of pteridine present show developmental changes in certain amphibian species (Bagnara, 1961; Hama, 1963). Whether this represents two populations of chromophores or a change in the pathway of pteridine biosynthesis in the same chromophore is not known. In adult *R. japonica,* organelles called pterinosomes have been isolated and biochemical analysis indicated that they contain most of the skin pteridine (Obika and Matsumoto, 1968). These authors suggested that xanthophores and erythrophores are interconvertible. Thus shifts in biosynthesis of pteridine need not imply two different cell lines.

It would appear that MSH can cause dispersion, division, and possibly differentiation in melanophores, contraction and decrease in number of iridophores, and a stimulation of pteridine biosynthesis in xanthophores. The mechanisms for these alterations by MSH are unknown. However, thyroid hormones may play some role in pigment cell development, because thyroxine pellets implanted into the skin can change pteridine content (Bagnara, 1964b), and cause local maturation (Kollros and Kaltenbach, 1952). Finally, hypophysectomized *R. pipiens* treated with thyroid hormones develop adult pigment patterns, albeit paler than the normal in respect to background colors and the intensity of the black pigment (Kollros, 1969).

D. Other Skin Effects

During metamorphosis there is a change in active sodium ion transport as measured by the quantity of external current required to reduce the potential difference to zero between serousal and epidermal surfaces of the skin. Sodium transport is absent in young bullfrog tadpoles and develops after forelimb emergence. T_4 can accelerate the appearance of the sodium pump (R. E. Taylor and Barker, 1965a,b). In adult amphibians the adrenals and the pituitary are the major regulatory glands of water balance. Hypophysectomized tadpoles were not used in this study, and therefore it is not certain whether the stimulation of sodium transport is a direct result of thyroid hormones on the skin, or is an effect of pituitary hormones on sodium transport due to T_4-stimulated maturation of the median eminence (Etkin, 1966).

Dowling and Razevska (1966) reported that in adult amphibians the epidermis of the skin can deiodinate thyroxine and that this activity increases during metamorphosis.

Although increases in total body oxygen consumption during spontaneous metamorphosis have not been demonstrated (see review of

Frieden, 1967; Funkhouser and Mills, 1969a), Barch (1953) found a two-fold increase in the metabolic rate of whole skin pieces during normal and induced metamorphosis.

VI. INTESTINAL DEVELOPMENT

Striking changes occur in the intestine during metamorphosis. At metamorphic climax there is an overall shortening and rearrangement of the coils of the intestine. Various morphological techniques have been utilized to observe cell degeneration and regeneration (see references in Griffiths, 1961; Bonneville, 1963). Although older literature refers to the stomach of anuran larvae, the digestive tract of anuran larvae probably does not contain the functional equivalent of a stomach (Griffiths, 1961; Ueck, 1967, 1968). The foregut, the ciliated portion of the intestine, shows tryptic activity until metamorphic climax, then loses its tryptic activity and develops pepsinlike activity, more typical of a functional stomach (Griffiths, 1961).

Several enzymatic changes have been detected histochemically in the intestine (Lipson and Kaltenbach, 1965; Botte, 1966; Manwell, 1966; Lipson, 1967). Thyroxine deiodinase activity of the viscera is low before the onset of metamorphic climax, rises at climax, then as suddenly decreases (Yamamoto, 1964). Because of their classical temporal relationship in differentiation, phosphatases have received the most attention (Chieffi and Carfagna, 1959a,b, 1960; Kaltenbach and Lipson, 1962; Botte and Buonanno, 1962; Botte, 1966; Lipson, 1967; Brodsky, 1968). In both anurans and urodeles there is no alkaline phosphatase activity in the foregut or the large intestinal epithelium, but there is strong activity in the anterior regions of the small intestinal epithelia (Lipson, 1967). Although changes in alkaline phosphatase activity can be induced by T_4 (Kaltenbach and Lipson, 1962; Lipson and Kaltenbach, 1965; Lipson, 1967) the adrenals may also be involved in these changes. The fall in alkaline phosphatase of the intestine seen at metamorphic climax is claimed to be a result of a decrease in adrenal hormone output (Chieffi and Carfagna, 1959a,b, 1960; Botte and Buonanno, 1962). The *in vitro* or *in vivo* addition of adrenal hormones prevents the decrease in alkaline phosphatase seen at climax (Chieffi and Carfagna, 1959a, 1960). Steroid production also seems to decrease at metamorphic climax (Dale, 1962; Rapola, 1963), consistent with the hypothesis that steroid hormones influence alkaline phosphatase levels in the developing digestive system of amphibian larvae. In other developmental systems, namely the chick and mouse, the role of the adrenal–pituitary axis in regulating intestinal alkaline phosphatase is now well documented (see review of Moog and Grey, 1966).

VII. REGRESSION OF THE PANCREAS

A. Acinar Cells

During spontaneous metamorphosis the pancreas undergoes a great reduction in size, and after metamorphosis the gland again increases in size (see references in Janes, 1937). The reduction in size can be stimulated by thyroid hormones (Kaywin, 1936; Janes, 1937; Race et al., 1966). In normal metamorphosis, the major weight loss of the pancreas may be attributed to dehydration (Race et al., 1966) or necrosis of acinar cells, collecting ducts, capillaries, and other connective elements (Kaywin, 1936; Janes, 1937).

Slickers and Kim (1969) have observed a gradual loss of both tRNA and rRNA (Fig. 4) as the earliest detectable effect after T_4 immersion

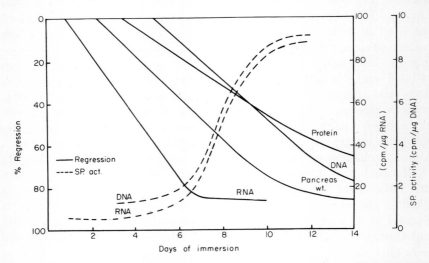

Fig. 4. Changes in macromolecules and their turnover in *R. catesbeiana* tadpole pancreas after immersion in $2.6 \times 10^{-8} M$ T_4. The percent regressions were calculated on the basis of the amount of RNA, pancreas weight, DNA, and soluble protein, compared to control animals. The specific activity of RNA and DNA were determined after a 3-hour pulse label of uridine and thymidine, respectively. Data from Slickers and Kim (1969).

of whole animals. This was followed by reduction in weight, protein, and DNA from the fourth to the tenth day. The weight loss in induced metamorphosis is caused by cell death rather than dehydration. Using 3-hour labels of tritiated thymidine or uridine these authors noted a stimulation of isotope incorporation into DNA and RNA on the eighth day after T_4 treatment.

In comparing the pancreatic proteins of tadpoles and frogs, a unique tadpole esterase, extensive tadpole amylase activity, and numerous differences in soluble proteins were found (Manwell, 1966). In the pancreas there is an increase in acid phosphatase activity during induced regression, followed by the appearance of a distinct α-amylase isozyme (Slickers and Kim, 1969).

B. ISLET CELLS

Although several different cell types occur in islet tissue of adult amphibian pancreas (see review of Epple, 1968), only the β-cells have received attention in amphibian development. Embryologically, the pancreas arises from two to three rudiments. In amphibians that have been thoroughly investigated, the dorsal rudiment is the only source of β-cells (Wolf-Heidegger, 1937; Frye, 1958; 1962). Complete removal of the pancreas is fatal to larvae of *R. clamitans* (Frye, 1964), but there is no evidence that the β-cells of the pancreas are essential for growth or metamorphosis of amphibian larvae (Frye, 1962, 1964). At all stages of tadpole development, insulin has been observed histochemically in the pancreas, and its secretion can be stimulated when stressed by exogenous glucose (Frye, 1964). Between stages XIX–XXII the amount of insulin increases markedly (Frye, 1964). Pancreatic regulation of normal glucose levels is initiated after stage V, appears to be lost at stage XIX, and is regained at stage XXII. Frye (1964, 1965) has tentatively concluded that maturational changes that occur in the β-cells are not caused by a direct action of thyroxine on these cells.

VIII. DEVELOPMENTAL CHANGES IN THE LIVER

During metamorphosis the amphibian liver undergoes a metabolic reorganization in the direction of increased protein and RNA biosynthesis. Except for the limbs, the bones, certain facial muscles, and perhaps the tongue and the nictitating membrane, no other tissue seems to be undergoing a comparable anabolic thrust in response to thyroid hormones.

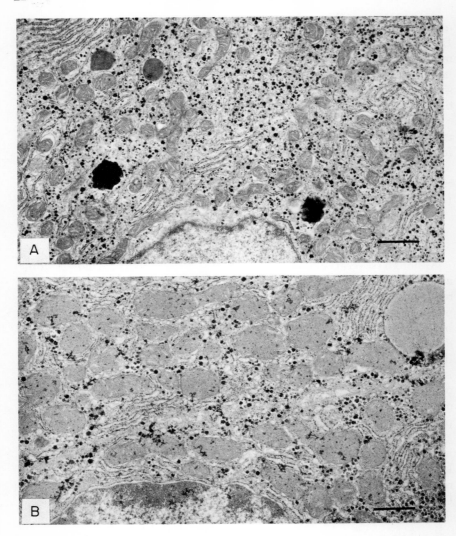

Fɪɢ. 5. Electron micrograph showing the difference in cytoplasmic fine structure, particularly the mitochondria, of the liver cells of *R. catesbeiana* tadpole, stage XI (A) and frog (B). Magnification line shows 1.0 μ. Figure from Bennett and Glynn (1969).

Historically, the demonstration of increased protein synthesis preceded the recognition of greater RNA synthesis. Only in the last decade has evidence accumulated confirming extensive changes in the RNA of tadpole liver after thyroid hormone administrations. Electron microscopy also has revealed changes in the ultrastructure of tadpole liver cells which reflect extensive development of RNA and protein biosynthetic machinery. Bennett and Glynn (1969) have observed significant increases in the prominence and fine structure of mitochondria and the proportion of cytoplasmic space that they occupy during spontaneous metamorphosis (Fig. 5). Marked redistribution of ribosomal populations coinciding with the appearance of newly formed ribosomes and membranes of the endoplasmic reticulum has also been observed in the later stages of induced metamorphosis (Tata, 1968a; Bennett and Glynn, 1969).

A. The Shift from Ammonotelism to Ureotelism

The evolution from aquatic to terrestrial habitat of many amphibians has resulted in a drastic shift in the principal nitrogenous excretory products. This transition from ammonotelism to ureotelism has become a classical example of comparative biochemistry. It reflects one of the major metabolic activities of the liver. An extensive exploration of urea excretion in the bullfrog tadpole was recently reported by Ashley *et al.* (1968). As shown in Fig. 6, urea remains relatively low until Taylor-

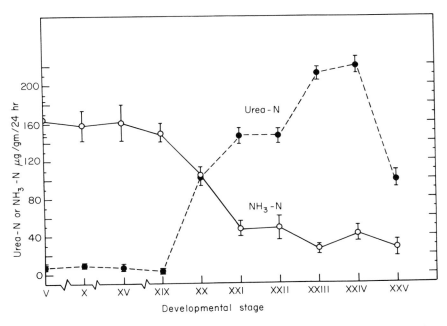

Fig. 6. Changes in nitrogen excretion during spontaneous metamorphosis of *R. catesbeiana* tadpoles at 25°. Urea-N and ammonia-N were determined for larvae at various stages as defined by A. C. Taylor and Kollros (1946). Data from Ashley *et al.* (1968).

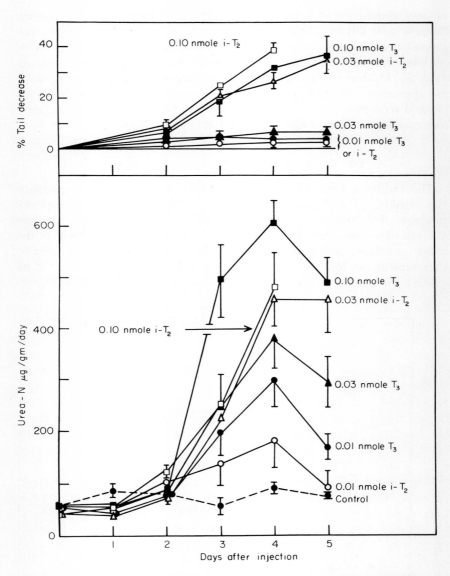

FIG. 7. The effect of L-triiodothyronine (T₃) and L-3′-isopropyl-3,5-diiodothyronine (i-T₂) on the percent tail decrease and urea-N excretion of *R. grylio* tadpoles under fasting conditions at 25°. A single indicated dose of T₃ or i-T₂ expressed in nmole/gm was injected at day zero. Data from Ashley *et al.* (1968).

Kollros stage XIX, after which there is a rapid increase until urea comprises 80–90% of the total nitrogen excreted. The ammonia output also falls at stage XIX. The sharp drop in urea excretion at stage XXIV–XXV may be due to the impact of metabolic changes or, less likely, to a cessation of thyroid hormone secretion at this final stage of metamorphosis. Hsu and Wu (1964) showed that thyroidectomized tadpoles after T_4 treatment produce a nitrogen excretory pattern similar to that of spontaneously metamorphosed animals. In the new froglet, 48 hours after total hepatectomy, urea-N decreases to 10% of the normal value, indicating that the liver is the major site of urea production (Atkinson and Just, 1969).

An even larger than normal increase in urea output can be induced by thyroid hormones. The data in Fig. 7 indicate a 25–30-fold increase after the injection of a single dose of 10^{-10} mole (65 ng) T_3 per gram body weight. For urea excretion comparable to that obtained with T_3, two or three times the dose of T_4 is required. The new analog, 3′-isopropyl-3,5-diiodothyronine (i-T_2) is more active than T_3 in evoking a tail resorption and a urea response (Fig. 7). The induction of tail resorption and of urea excretion by thyroid hormone is arrested for over 3 months when bullfrog tadpoles are kept at 5°. Nutritional and other parameters were shown to affect urea excretion (Ashley *et al.*, 1968).

B. Changing Patterns of Enzyme Activity and Protein Synthesis

Extensive alteration of the patterns of protein synthesis in the liver during metamorphosis was strongly suggested by the marked shifts in the electrophoretic profile of serum proteins believed to originate in the liver, particularly the manyfold increase in serum albumin and ceruloplasmin described earlier.

The most complete studies of protein changes in the liver are those involving the enzymes associated with the development of the ornithine–urea cycle. Preparatory for the ureogenesis accompanying metamorphosis, all the enzymes of the urea cycle, especially carbamyl phosphate synthetase and arginine synthetase, increase significantly as shown in Table II. Extensive reports by P. P. Cohen and associates (1966) have established carbamyl phosphate synthetase as a useful model system for the study of hormonal induction of protein synthesis. Several of the transaminases and dehydrogenases that might be expected to be involved in ammonia production appear to decrease except for the two enzymes associated with glutamate deamination. Galton *et al.* (1965) have found a 15–25-fold increase in liver catalase activity. This results in

TABLE II

RELATIVE ACTIVITIES OF LIVER ENZYMES
IN TADPOLES AND ADULT BULLFROGS[a]

Enzymes	Metamorphic: premetamorphic		Adult: premeta- morphic[d]	Reference no.[e]
	Thyroxine[b]	Spontan.[c]		
Urea biosynthesis				
Carbamyl phosphate synthetase	14	15	30	1
Ornithine transcarbamylase	2	2.5	8	1
Argininosuccinate synthetase	—	15	35	1
Argininosuccinase	—	—	20	1
Arginase	8	8	30	2
Transaminases				
Glutamate-oxalacetate	2	3	5	3
Glutamate-pyruvate	1	1	0.5	3
Tyrosine-α-ketoglutarate	0.5	0.2	0.2	3
Ornithine-α-ketoglutarate	0.6	0.7	0.5	4
Dehydrogenases				
Glutamate	6	6	10	5
Lactate	0.6	0.6	0.4	5
Glucose-6-PO$_4$	0.8	0.8	0.5	5
Malate	—	1.2	1.4	5
Glycerate-3-PO$_4$	—	0.5	< .1	6
D-Glycerate	—	2	3–4	6
Phosphatases				
Pyrophosphatase	1.2	—	2.2	7
ATPase	2.5	4	—	8
Glucose-6-phosphatase	1.6	4.4	—	8
Acid phosphatase	2.5	—	—	9
Alkaline phosphatase	2.3	—	—	9
Other enzymes				
Amino acid activating enzymes	1	—	2	7
Tryptophan pyrrolase	0.2	0.2	0.2	10
Uridine kinase	1	1	1	11
Uridine phosphorylase	2.2	2.3	0.2	11
Catalase	—	5–10	15	12
Pyrogallol peroxidase	—	2	5	12

[a] The data apply mostly to *Rana catesbeiana* but some data on *R. grylio* are included.

[b] Ratio of enzymic activities in tadpole liver: thyroxine induced metamorphosis to premetamorphic stages.

[c] Ratio of enzymic activities in liver: spontaneous metamorphosis to premetamorphic stages.

[d] Ratio of enzymic activities in liver: adult frogs to premetamorphic stages.

[e] Key to references: 1. Brown *et al.* (1959); 2. Dolphin and Frieden (1955); 3. Chan and Cohen (1964); 4. Nakagawa and Cohen (1968); 5. DeGroot and Cohen (1962a); 6. Sallach and Kmiotek (1968); 7. DeGroot and Cohen (1962b); 8. Frieden and Mathews (1958); 9. Yanagisawa (1954); 10. Spiegel and Spiegel (1964); 11. Akamatsu *et al.* (1964); 12. Galton *et al.* (1965).

a reduced H_2O_2 content of homogenates of frog liver and a consequent decrease in deiodination of T_4. It was further postulated that in the anurans the transition from larva to adult is associated with a decrease or a loss of the ability both to deiodinate the thyroid hormones and to respond to them metabolically (Galton and Ingbar, 1962). Manwell (1966) has reported numerous differences in the mobility on starch gel electrophoresis of many tadpole and frog enzymes and proteins in several tissues including liver malate dehydrogenase and other unidentified liver proteins. Details of many of these enzymatic changes recently have been summarized by P. P. Cohen (1966), Frieden (1967), and Weber (1967a,b). None of the other liver enzymes studied seem to play a significant role in metamorphosis.

C. Mode of Action of Thyroid Hormone on Tadpole Liver Metabolism

The recognition that thyroid hormones unleash a plethora of protein changes in the tadpole liver has inspired several research groups to explore the underlying mechanisms of this effect. The normal size of the amphibian chromosome does not lend itself to experiments similar to those with dipterans. Furthermore, DNA biosynthesis in the liver as measured by $^{32}PO_4$ incorporation is low and unresponsive to thyroid hormone (Finamore and Frieden, 1960; Paik *et al.*, 1961). Experimental efforts of the past decade have concentrated on the transcriptional and translational phases of protein biosynthesis, and have led to the conclusion that T_3 and T_4 are deeply involved in both RNA biosynthesis and in the protein synthetic machinery of the tadpole liver. Recent experimental efforts on these biosyntheses have been summarized in several recent reviews (P. P. Cohen, 1966; Frieden, 1965, 1967, 1968; Kim and Cohen, 1968; Tata, 1964, 1968a).

1. Transcriptional Effects

Finamore and Frieden (1960) first reported an increase in RNA biosynthesis 24–48 hours after T_3 injection, with no change in RNA base composition. The details of this process have been further explored by Tata (1965), Nakagawa *et al.* (1967), and Eaton and Frieden (1968). A mysterious but reproducible cyclical variation of RNA biosynthesis was reported in two of these papers. There is even a small but significant change in the amount of both RNA and nucleotide pools (Eaton and Frieden, 1968). Several additional long-term effects of T_4 on RNA metabolism have been reported (Kim and Cohen, 1966, 1968; Wyatt and Tata, 1968). Five to seven days after immersion in 2.6×10^{-8} M T_4, there is about a 50% increase in RNA polymerase activity in tadpole liver

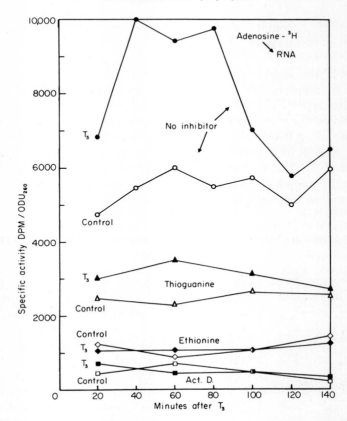

Fɪɢ. 8. The early effect of T₃ on RNA biosynthesis using a 20-minute pulse label of ³H-adenosine. The specific activity of RNA was determined after injection of 0.30 nmole T₃ per gram of *R. catesbeiana* tadpoles at 25°. The inhibitors were injected 4 hours prior to T₃ treatment at the following doses; ethionine and thioguanine 200 μg/gm; actinomycin D, 2 μg/gm. Data from Eaton and Frieden (1969b).

nuclei. A modest increase in the template efficiency of chromatin was also noted 7 days after T_4 treatment (Kim and Cohen, 1966).

While all previous effects on RNA metabolism were reported after 24–48 hours, Eaton and Frieden (1968) detected the stimulation of RNA biosynthesis (as measured by labeled adenosine incorporation) within 30 minutes to 3 hours after injection of T_3; that is, during the so-called lag period usually associated with thyroid hormone action. This effect appears to be maximal at 3×10^{-10} mole/gm tadpole, significantly slower at 3×10^{-11} mole/gm, and barely detectable at 3×10^{-12} mole/gm. When tadpoles are immersed in 2.0×10^{-8} M T_4, there is a 2–3-hour delay in the increase in uridine incorporation into RNA (Eaton and Frieden, 1969c), but the effect precedes by many hours those reported by Nakagawa *et al.* (1967).

This early stimulation of RNA synthesis can be blocked by a spectrum of protein and RNA biosynthetic inhibitors. As shown in Fig. 8, when no inhibitor is present, T_3 doubles the incorporation of ^{3}H-adenosine into RNA after the first 40 minutes. Actinomycin D and ethionine inhibit incorporation both in the control and T_3 groups, whereas thioguanine shows a small but significant increase after 60 minutes (Eaton and Frieden, 1969b).

2. Induced RNA Biosynthesis

Because it is agreed that there is no significant change in overall base composition in induced metamorphosis, the rate of biosynthesis of RNA has been studied. Using density gradient centrifugal separation, Nakagawa and Cohen (1967) reported that 48 hours exposure to T_4 stimulated the biosynthesis of tRNA, rRNA, and mRNA. The rapidly labeled RNA, presumably mostly mRNA, had a higher concentration of UMP compared to bulk liver RNA. The most rapid RNA labeling response was reported by Eaton and Frieden (1968) using a $^{32}PO_4$ RNA labeling technique. Three hours after T_3 injection, a labeling pattern different from the 24–48-hour distribution was observed. After 3 and 12 hours of hormone treatment, the GC content of the RNA was 51%, compared with 61% for controls. At later times the $^{32}PO_4$ labeling pattern approaches the ribosomal and bulk RNA compositions. These values fit the data of tadpole DNA (50% GC) and ribosomal RNA (61% GC) reported by Nakagawa and Cohen (1967). In the RNA from T_3-treated animals, there is appreciable replacement of GMP by AMP with 3–5 times more isotope in the adenine-containing positions but not in the guanine positions. There were higher levels of labeling found in the nucleotides derived from the initiating positions of the RNA chains. Overall it was concluded that new RNA chains with a base composition differing from controls were synthesized as a result of T_3 action (Eaton and Frieden, 1969b).

That thyroid hormone effects are accompanied by an eventual shift in the kind of RNA produced in tadpole liver is also shown by several recent studies on RNA hybridization. Wyatt and Tata (1968) found that in whole *Xenopus* larvae there was a stimulation of the synthesis of RNA that did not hybridize with DNA. This was interpreted as reflecting preferential synthesis of ribosomal RNA in response to thyroid hormone. In *R. catesbeiana* tadpole liver 2 or 6 days after T_3, the production of nonhybridizing RNA is stimulated to an even greater extent. Kim and Cohen (1968) also mentioned that partially melted liver chromatin DNA hybridizes more efficiently with pulse-labeled RNA from T_4-treated tadpoles.

3. Translational Effects

Though an experimental distinction between transcriptional and translational events in protein synthesis is undoubtedly arbitrary, it will be convenient to discuss these separately. An early effect on labeled amino acid incorporation into liver protein was noted by Eaton and Frieden (1969b). Within 1–2 hours after T_3, glycine uptake into tadpole liver protein was accelerated. This early effect of T_3 may be a reflection of a transport phenomenon (Eaton and Frieden, 1969a). The variety of proteins whose synthesis is greatly increased or whose degradation is reduced during metamorphosis may reflect a higher overall translational activity. It is not certain that a translational step is the rate limiting step. For example, the effect of metamorphosis on amino acid activating enzymes is probably not important (Table II), but the acceleration of amino-acyl tRNA transferase activity reported by Unsworth and Cohen (1968) may be significant in affecting the overall rate of protein synthesis. A crucial step in translation affecting protein synthesis may be the rate of formation of tRNA. Several developmental phenomena have already been shown to depend on tRNA levels, e.g., chick oviduct differentiation (O'Malley et al., 1968), and pupation in insects (Ilan, 1968).

Tonoue et al. (1969) found that T_3 altered the chromatographic profiles of ^3H- and ^{14}C-leucyl-tRNA charged in vivo in the liver, kidney, tail, and gills of bullfrog tadpoles. Though the chromatographic profiles differed from tissue to tissue, two main leucyl-tRNA components were observed for each tissue. Twenty-four hours after T_3 injection the proportion of the rapidly eluted tRNA was reduced and the more slowly eluted tRNA component was increased. A similar shift in leucyl-tRNA was observed in liver and kidney slices from spontaneously metamorphosing tadpoles.

Tata (1968a) has ascribed the long-term thyroid hormone induced changes in liver protein biosynthesis to the coordinated proliferation of ribosomes and microsomal membranes. Microsomal preparations were progressively enriched with labeled uridine in newly made polysomes and residual membrane phospholipids. Electron microscopy of tadpole liver slices confirmed the topographical redistribution of the ribosomal population coinciding with the appearance of newly formed ribosomes and membranes of the endoplasmic reticulum.

4. Summary

In summary we have outlined the present status of the information about the mechanism of action of the thyroid hormone on tadpole liver

(Eaton and Frieden, 1968, 1969a,b; Kim and Cohen, 1968). The sequence of early events in the tadpole liver cell after T_3 treatment has been discussed in detail recently (Eaton and Frieden, 1969a,b). Thyroid hormones act early on systems involved in the mobilization and/or the *de novo* biosynthesis of nucleotides and, soon after, by an increased and specific RNA and protein biosynthesis. This rapid burst of selective RNA and protein synthesis eventually leads to a major reorganization of many intracellular structures, particularly those involved in the transcriptional and translational aspects of protein biosynthesis.

IX. TAIL RESORPTION

The versatility of the metamorphosing tadpole as a model for the study of differentiation and development arises not only from the presence of numerous anabolic tissues such as liver and limbs but also from the variety of tissues such as tail, gut, and gills in which ultimately numerous catabolic reactions predominate. The possibility that tail resorption is a controlled expression of activity of intracellular catabolic enzymes has long been entertained. There are numerous examples of controlled cell death in developing biological systems. The unique feature of amphibian metamorphosis is that the triggering agent is known and comparable effects can be produced with exogenous T_3 or T_4. An extensive review of the background and history of this subject has recently been published by Weber (1967a,b).

The surviving tail fin has been utilized for an *in vitro* quantitative analysis of the response of tadpole tissue to T_4 (Derby, 1968). This is a useful confirmation of localized T_4 pellet effects reported earlier (Hartwig, 1940; Kaltenbach, 1959). Dorsal tail fin discs of *R. pipiens* shrink to 10–30% of their original area when cultured in 3–27 parts per billion T_4 ($4 \times 10^{-9} M$). A quantitative relationship was shown between resorption in the range of 3–27 ppb T_4. The response was specific in that comparable concentrations of iodide, diiodotyrosine and thyronine were ineffective. Response of tail discs depended upon the continuous presence of T_4 and increased in their sensitivity to T_4 as metamorphosis proceeded. Amphibian pituitary implants have been shown to inhibit the shrinkage effect of T_4 on *R. pipiens* tail discs (Derby and Etkin, 1968).

A. TISSUE ACIDITY AND TAIL HYDROLASES

The dramatic nature of tail resorption led to experimental work on its mechanism more than 40 years ago. Alterations in the tissue acidity of tadpole tail have long been associated with the demolitive changes in the tail triggered by the thyroid hormone. Heightened metabolic processes in the tadpole tail could increase the production of acidic metabolites such as CO_2, lactic acid, and pyruvic acid. The resulting increased acidity from pH 7.1 to 6.6 during tail resorption might activate acid proteases or modify certain intracellular structures to release degradative enzymes. During tail resorption there is also a conspicuous increase in amino acid and polypeptide nitrogen in tail tissue, reflecting an increase in protein hydrolysis. The transport of these acidic products contributes to a decrease in blood pH from 7.5 to 7.2 during metamorphosis. These autolytic and pH changes and other studies of enzymic hydrolysis have been reviewed (Frieden, 1961, 1964, 1965, 1967; Weber, 1967a,b).

Numerous experiments later suggested a dominant role of the hydro-

TABLE III

CHANGES IN TADPOLE TAIL ENZYMES DURING SPONTANEOUS METAMORPHOSIS

| Enzyme[b] | Metamorphic climax[a] | | |
| | Premetamorphic tadpoles | | |
	Specific activity	Total activity	Reference no.[c]
β-Glucuronidase	34	3–4	1
	12–50	2–3	2
Deoxyribonuclease (acid)	50	2–3	7
	3	—	3
Ribonuclease (acid)	20	1	2
Cathepsin	22	2	4
	50	2–3	2
Phosphatase (acid)	5–20	1–1.5	2, 5
Phosphatase (alkaline)	1.5–2.8	—	6
Collagenase	10	—	7
Proteinases (acid)	9.2	—	8
Dipeptidases, tripeptidases	3–7	—	8
Catalase	6	—	2
ATPase (Mg^{++})	0.5	—	9
Aldolase	0.2	—	2

[a] Where possible, data are based on enzyme measurements performed on tadpole tails that were reduced to 10% of their original weight.

[b] Enzymes that have been reported not to change or to decrease in activity ratio include alkaline proteinases, alkaline RNase, amylase, lipase, glutamic and succinic dehydrogenase.

[c] Key to references: 1. Kubler and Frieden (1964); 2. Eeckhout (1965); 3. Coleman (1962); 4. Weber (1957); 5. Weber and Niehus (1961); 6. Yanagisawa (1954); 7. Lapiere and Gross (1963); 8. Urbani (1957); 9. Frieden and Mathews (1958).

lytic enzymes present in the tail itself (Eeckhout, 1965; Kubler and Frieden, 1964; Salzmann and Weber, 1963; Weber, 1957, 1963a). A major contribution has emerged from the work of Weber and his associates (Weber, 1963a, 1967a,b) in establishing the significance of alterations in cathepsins and phosphatase activity during tail resorption. Thus evidence accumulated that there was a generalized increase in most hydrolytic enzymes as summarized in Table III.

B. THE LYSOSOMAL HYPOTHESIS

The numerous mechanisms proposed for the control and regulation of the degradative action of the intracellular hydrolases have been discussed by Frieden (1964). A recent hypothesis was that of deDuve, who earlier had proposed the existence of an intracellular entity, the lysosome, which contained numerous lytic enzymes. The controlled disintegration of this subcellular particle could produce cytolysis and tissue disappearance. Support for this idea came from observations in which lysosomolytic agents such as vitamin A either promoted tail resorption or otherwise enhanced the thyroid hormone effect (Weissman, 1961). Salzmann and Weber (1963) found some evidence to support the existence of hydrolase-rich "phagosomes" among the macrophages of the subepidermal connective tissue. During metamorphosis, a progressive activation of these cells begins in the connective tissue of the tail fin and spreads to the tail muscle. Weber (1967a) recently proposed that the increase in the activity of acid hydrolases might reflect the transition of histocytes into active macrophages.

C. STIMULATION OF SELECTED PROTEIN SYNTHESIS

In the absence of definitive cytological evidence for the presence or modifications of typical lysosomes in the tadpole tail during metamorphosis, Weber (1963a,b) and Frieden (1964) and their associates tested this hypothesis at the biochemical level using several lysosomal enzymes—cathepsin, β-glucuronidase, and phosphatase—as indicator enzymes. Both groups reached essentially similar conclusions.

1. The distribution of and the changes in these enzymes did not correspond to the prediction of the "lysosomal hypothesis." The enzymes were almost uniformly distributed throughout the mitochondrial–lysosomal, microsomal, and supernatant fractions. Tail β-glucuronidase from premetamorphic tadpoles was even less "releasable" than the corresponding enzyme of froglet tail stump.

2. An unexpected observation in this regressing tissue was the demon-

stration of an increase in the synthesis of these enzymes. For example, Kubler and Frieden (1964) found that while the tail was decreasing to one tenth of its original weight and protein content, the specific activity of β-glucuronidase was increasing by a factor of 34-fold. Weber (1963b) reported a twofold increase in cathepsin and phosphatase activities. Typical tests precluded the role of activators or other modifiers of these enzymes' activity; a careful comparison of several key kinetic properties of partially purified β-glucuronidase revealed no difference in the tadpole and froglet enzymes (Price and Frieden, 1963). Thus, an initial synthesis of certain tail enzymes appeared to precede the dissolution of tail tissue.

D. Prevention of Tail Regression by Protein Synthesis Inhibitors

Support for this idea has now come from several sources. A comprehensive study of tail metamorphosis was reported by Eeckhout (1965). Eeckhout confirmed the increase in several hydrolases: cathepsin, β-glucuronidase, phosphatase, RNase, and DNase and concluded that protein synthesis was a prelude to tail resorption. To test this further, Eeckhout employed an organ culture of tadpole tail pieces as suggested by Shaffer (1963) and Weber (1962). He observed that actinomycin D, an inhibitor of RNA biosynthesis, puromycin, which suppresses both protein and nuclear RNA synthesis, and ethionine, which blocks protein biosynthesis, blocked the tail shrinkage induced by thyroxine. Weber (1962, 1965) also showed that actinomycin D prevented tail atrophy in isolated tails or in intact *Xenopus* larvae during metamorphosis.

The extreme usefulness of the tadpole tail system was further illustrated by the elegant studies of Gross and co-workers on collagen metabolism during metamorphosis. Increased degradation of collagen in the tail fin proceeds during resorption in contrast to the metabolic stability of the collagen in the back skin (Gross and Lapiere, 1962). It was possible to isolate, for the first time, an animal collagenase from the epithelial cells of tail cultures undergoing metamorphosis. Tadpole collagenase appears earlier but in about the same amount after T_4 stimulation (Nagai *et al.*, 1966). The products of tadpole collagenase action have also been analyzed by Kang *et al.* (1966). A hyaluronidase has been detected in the mesenchymal cells of the tail fin (Silbert *et al.*, 1965).

A comprehensive study of selected enzymes related to energy metabolism (mostly glycolytic and Krebs cycle enzymes) in tail tissue during the metamorphosis of *Xenopus* larvae has been reported by Marty and Weber (1968). Most of these enzymes decreased in total activity by 50–70% on a dry weight basis during late stages of tail regression, except for glutamate–pyruvate transaminase and glutamate dehydrogenase, which remain unchanged. Many of these enzymes maintained constant proportions and their intracellular distribution pattern was not modified during regression. Marty and Weber (1968) concluded that the involution of the tail tissue is not correlated with a drastic change in the intracellular organization of energy metabolism.

E. Requirement of RNA and Protein Synthesis

Using surviving tail pieces, Tata (1966) explored the requirement for RNA and protein synthesis during tail resorption. He confirmed the fact that protein synthesis blocking agents, cycloheximide, actinomycin D, and puromycin interfered with tail regression and hydrolase production induced by T_3. Tata also found that T_3 added to the medium increased the rate of total protein and RNA biosynthesis prior to visible resorption. The incorporation of ^{14}C-amino acids into protein increased before ^{3}H-uridine incorporation into RNA. This sequence of events was not that predicted if the new RNA was serving as the messenger for additional protein synthesis. Tata also reported that puromycin and cycloheximide prevented the ^{14}C-amino acid uptake, whereas actinomycin D and cycloheximide inhibited the ^{3}H-uridine incorporation.

Thus it appeared that an increase in overall protein and RNA biosynthesis preceded tail regression. However, the necessity for caution in accepting data from isolated systems as representative of what happens *in vivo* has been emphasized in some recent data of Tonoue and Frieden (1970). When ^{3}H-leucine uptake into tadpole tail proteins was studied *in vivo*, T_3 produced only decreases in radioactivity at time periods studied: 16% at 3 hours, 37% at 24 hours, and 60% at 48 hours. This decrease was not the result of any significant change in the labeled leucine of the pool. It was concluded that there is a generalized decrease in leucine incorporation *in vivo* after T_3 injection during the preregression period when tail pieces *in vitro* showed an increase in protein and RNA biosynthesis. Several explanations could account for this discrepancy. In the tail-piece experiments the culture medium contained numerous antibiotics (penicillin, streptomycin, terramycin, mycostatin) which might have affected the response to T_3. Tata (1966) had to use huge doses of T_3 ($1-2 \times 10^{-6}\ M$) in the culture medium to obtain significant effects. This excessive T_3 concentration could produce an artifactual stimulation of protein synthesis, an unusual role for the thyroid hormone because at high doses in mammals T_3 usually stimulates protein catabolism. Finally, it is conceivable that in surviving tail pieces, amino acid incorporation occurs in a limited number of cells, whereas the remainder are relatively inert in both T_3 and control experiments.

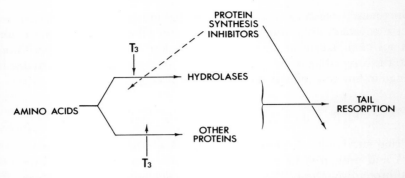

Fɪɢ. 9. Summary of effects of thyroid hormone and protein synthesis inhibitors on the proposed mechanism of resorption of the tadpole tail. T_3 stimulates hydrolase synthesis but blocks the incorporation of amino acids into overall tail proteins. The protein biosynthesis inhibitors block tail resorption but their specific site of action is not known.

F. Summary of Biochemical Changes in the Tail

It is now well documented that a remarkable increase in a wide spectrum of hydrolytic enzymes accompanies tail resorption during either induced or spontaneous metamorphosis. This is probably a selective and directed stimulation of protein biosynthesis. The process is sensitive to *in vivo* and *in vitro* RNA and protein synthesis inhibitors. *In vivo* there is early evidence of a generalized decrease in amino acid uptake into protein in contrast to an early *in vitro* increased amino acid and nucleotide incorporation. There may be at least two types of cells in the tail relative to response to thyroid hormones: one type is stimulated to make more hydrolytic enzymes; a second, larger group undergoes a depression of protein synthesis. The entire process, diagrammed in Fig. 9, can be arrested by low temperature (Frieden *et al.*, 1965; Ashley *et al.*, 1968). Thus the mechanism of tail resorption reflects the ability of the thyroid hormone to produce a controlled stimulation of enzyme synthesis and also a regulated triggering of protein degradative reactions leading to tail resorption.

X. CHANGES IN CALCIUM AND BONE METABOLISM

In adult amphibians calcium metabolism is influenced by parathyroids (see review of Cortelyou and McWhinnie, 1967) and the ultimobranchial bodies (see references in Robertson, 1968), but little is known about the function of these organs during larval life, although their development has been described. Stores of calcium have been reported in the skin and endolymphatic sac of larval amphibians (see R. E. Taylor *et al.,* 1966; Pilkington and Simkiss, 1966). Although probably no changes occur in skin calcium (R. E. Taylor *et al.,* 1966), evidence is available suggesting that the calcium of the endolymphatic sacs is resorbed during metamorphic climax and used for skeletal ossification (Guardabassi, 1959; Pilkington and Simkiss, 1966). No reports are available on the effect of calcitonin in larvae. Parathyroid hormone reduces the calcium level of the endolymphatic sacs, but effects on osteoclasts are in doubt (Belanger and Drouin, 1966; Guardabassi and Lattes, 1968).

In 1918 Terry observed that thyroidectomy of anuran larvae prevented both ossification and growth of bones. More recent investigators have shown that thyroxine administration to normal animals stimulated bone ossification (Keller, 1946; Kuhn and Hammer, 1956; Kemp and Hoyt, 1969a,b). Maturation of the skeleton is known to be promoted by thyroid hormone in mammals and birds (see review by Tata, 1964). Tissue culture of embryonic chick bones (Fell and Mellanby, 1955, 1956; Lengemann, 1962; Lawson, 1963) and local thyroid hormone implants in anuran larvae (Kaltenbach, 1953a; Kuhn and Hammer, 1956) demonstrate the direct effect of thyroid hormone on bone ossification. A relevant recent observation by Adamson and Ingbar (1967a,b) indicates that thyroid hormones stimulate the transport of certain amino acids into embryonic chick cartilage. Further investigation on the mechanism of bone ossification would provide a valuable insight into this aspect of thyroid hormone action.

XI. MISCELLANEOUS EFFECTS

There are two visual pigments, porphyropsin (opsin and vitamin A_2 aldehyde) and rhodopsin (opsin and vitamin A_1 aldehyde). The distribution of these two visual pigments may or may not vary between the larvae and adult, depending upon species (see review of Weber, 1967a). In *Rana catesbeiana* Wilt and co-workers (Wilt, 1959a,b; Ohtsu *et al.,* 1964) have demonstrated that porphyropsin is the principal visual pigment in larvae, whereas rhodopsin predominates in adults. These workers concluded that thyroid hormone decreases vitamin A_2 aldehyde production and therefore permits an increase in vitamin A_1 production.

Anatomical and probably functional changes occur in the pronephros and mesonephros during larval life (see review of Fox, 1963; Deyrup, 1964). Chemical inhibition of the thyroid prevents pronephros degener-

ation; thyroid hormone administration stimulates pronephric degeneration (Hurley, 1958). Recently Tonoue and Frieden (1970) have shown
a decrease in labeled leucine incorporation into kidney protein after T_3
injection.

Hypophysectomized or thyroidectomized larvae show little limb growth
or differentiation unless animals are treated with thyroid hormone.
Holmes (1966) has shown that 48 hours after T_4 administration the
specific activity (using ^{14}C-leucine and ^{3}H-uridine) of muscle tissue
increases drastically. Sucrose density gradients of low-speed pellets from
muscle of treated animals also indicate changes in the type of RNA
produced. Bern et al. (1967) recently suggested that growth hormone
preferentially stimulates leg growth. Just and Kollros (1968), however,
have suggested that these observations may be accounted for by TSH
contamination of growth hormone because other morphological changes
are induced by growth hormone.

Hypophysectomy and thyroidectomy may or may not have an effect on
larval sexual differentiation, depending upon the species (see reviews of
Iwasawa, 1961; Witschi, 1967). The initiation of steroid hormone production has recently been reviewed (Chieffi, 1965; Witschi, 1967). Breed-
ing experiments indicate that administration of estrogens and/or androgens during larval life can cause a complete sex reversal in some
amphibian species (see review of Gallien, 1965; Witschi, 1967). Recently
Vannini and Stagni (1967, 1968) have shown that this induced sex
reversal is inhibited by puromycin and actinomycin D. The phonomenon
of sex reversal might be a useful system to further explore basic mechanisms of hormone action.

A unique difference in the effect of catecholamines on amphibian
erythrocytes during metamorphosis has been reported by Rosen and
Rosen (1968). Isopropylarterenol (0.1 to 2.5 μg/mg) greatly stimulated
cyclic-3',5'-AMP formation in R. pipiens adult red cell hemolysates but
did not affect the adenyl cyclase activity in tadpole hemolysates. A similar
but smaller difference was observed in R. catesbeiana tadpole and frog
hemolysates. The acquisition of sensitivity of the red cell adenyl cyclase
system to catecholamines may indicate an alteration in the enzyme and/
or the erythrocyte membrane during metamorphosis.

XII. SOME GENERAL COMMENTS AND CONCLUSIONS
ABOUT ANURAN METAMORPHOSIS

In the preceding sections we have attempted to describe the most
significant changes reported to occur during metamorphosis. These many

transitions and their role in metamorphosis have been summarized in Tables IV and IVA, first in terms of well-documented biochemical modifications and next in the more general terms of anatomical, histological, and other changes. In our discussions we have also emphasized the effect of thyroid hormones on the various tissue responses during metamorphosis. This may have created the impression that these responses depend solely on the presence or absence of thyroid hormones. Although this may hold for most adult tissues that respond to particular hormones, developing systems are influenced by numerous factors that may modify a direct adultlike response.

TABLE IV

BIOCHEMICAL SYSTEMS KNOWN TO BE EXTENSIVELY MODIFIED
DURING ANURAN METAMORPHOSIS

Tissue, organ	Biochemical system	Effect	Role in metamorphosis
Respiration	Whole animal	No increase; decrease in some species	Calorigenic response not associated with metamorphosis
Liver	RNA and protein biosynthesis	Increased and different	Thyroxine-mediated genetic expression via DNA
	Urea production	Increase in urea cycle enzymes	Transition from ammonotelism to ureotelism
Tail	Hydrolytic enzymes of lysosomal type	Stimulation of the biosynthesis of cathepsin, phosphatase, RNase, DNase, β-glucuronidase, etc.	Accounts for tail resorption, adaptation to rapid movement
Blood	Erythrocytes: hemoglobin (Hb)	Repression of tadpole Hb, induction of frog Hb synthesis (increased adenyl cyclase)	Adaptive oxygen capture
	Serum protein biosynthesis (in liver)	Increase in serum albumin, ceruloplasmin, etc.	Improved homeostasis
Pancreas			Greater enzyme and hormone secretion
Acinar cells	DNA, RNA, proteins	Regression, then regrowth; increase in acid phosphatase, a new α-amylase	
Islet cells	Insulin	Stimulation of insulin secretion	
Eye	Light-sensitive pigments	Shift to rhodopsin	Repression of porphyropsin synthesis

TABLE IVA

OTHER SYSTEMS MODIFIED DURING ANURAN METAMORPHOSIS

Tissues, organ	Effect	Role in metamorphosis
Intestine	Extensive shortening; relocation, development of hydrolytic enzymes	Accommodation to diet
Limb buds	Development and growth of tissues (muscles, nerve, etc.)	Locomotion on land
Skin	Collagenolysis; development of sérous mucous glands; increased serotonin, melanophores, Na transport	Protective coloration, etc.
Nervous system	LM cells enlarged but fewer; initiation of corneal reflex; atrophy of Mauthnor cells	Innervation of new structures
Reticuloendothelial system	Increase in lymphocytes and immune response	Improved immune mechanism
Bone	Stimulation of Ca transport and ossification	Formation of juvenile frog skeleton
Gills, kidney, spleen, etc.	Gills atrophy; other changes	Preparation for land

A. ACQUISITION OF TISSUE SENSITIVITY

The capacity of various tissues to respond to thyroid hormones is known to appear late in embryonic life (e.g., Geigy, 1941; Etkin, 1950; Ferguson, 1966), but the time of sensitivity of tissues to other hormones has received little attention. It seems certain now that various organs acquire this sensitivity at different times (Moser, 1950). The M-V cells do not begin to become sensitive to thyroid hormones until stage III or IV and they do not show complete response until after stage V (Kollros and McMurray, 1956). Etkin (1966) showed that the median eminence is not competent to respond to thyroid hormone until one-third of larval life has passed. Finally, several urodele tissues also show differences in the time of acquisition of sensitivity (Prahlad and DeLanney, 1965).

The various times of acquisition of tissue sensitivity make it difficult to interpret any biochemical data when whole animals are studied (Tata, 1968b). Only if the various tissues have identical mechanisms for acquiring sensitivity can intact animals be used to study the acquisition of sensitivity. Most biochemical investigations (i.e., liver and Hb transitions) have been based on the assumption that organ systems are completely responsive at the time of hormone administration. If this assumption is incorrect, tremendous variability will result, and this is already a common complaint of workers in this area. To eliminate this major source of potential variation, it is important to be well past the period of the acquisition of tissue sensitivity.

The acquisition of tissue sensitivity to hormones is not unique to amphibian metamorphosis. For example, enzymic differentiation (glucose-6-phosphatase, NADP dehydrogenase) in rat liver is promoted by T_4 only in the late stages of fetal life (Greengard, 1969). In the chick embryo, glucose transport into heart muscle becomes sensitive to insulin after one-third of its embryonic life (Foa and Guidotti, 1966). A permanent alteration in the neural regulation of ovulation can be achieved by androgen administration to neonatal rats but only during a limited period in post-natal life (see review of Gorski, 1968). In order to account for the acquisition of sensitivity, it is assumed that receptor sites for hormones develop or are altered, and/or that other biochemical changes occur which finally make cells sensitive to hormone.

B. SPECIFICITY OF RESPONSES

Although tissue specific responses are known in adult mammals (e.g., cortisone effects on thymus and liver), few hormonal responses are more striking in their specificity than the stimulation of leg growth and tail regression observed in anuran metamorphosis. The most convincing proof for specific responses came from organ transplantation studies (see review of Needham, 1942). Eye-cup transplants or hindlimb-bud transplants onto the tail survived while the tail regressed. The reverse experiment, transplanting a tail into back muscle, showed that the ability of the tail to regress was retained. Although not as obvious as organ responses, this selective response also operates at the individual cell level. After thyroxine-pellet implantations into tadpole medulla, some nerve cell bodies enlarged while the giant Mauthner cells regressed (Weiss and Rossetti, 1951; Pesetsky and Kollros, 1956). Skin cells that histologically appear identical, reacted differently after thyroid hormone treatment. A dual response was also seen in resorption of opercular skin and maturation of adjacent body skin (Kaltenbach, 1953b).

It is apparent that developmental changes of either organs or cells are controlled by the intrinsic capacity of the tissue, but little is known about the molecular basis of this specificity. Differences in molecular responses at the organ level have been demonstrated (Tonoue and Frieden, 1970). The embryological time at which organ or cell specificity is achieved is not understood. We know that the fate of many organs is determined during embryonic life and also that there are inductive inter-reactions for many of these organs. However, it is not known whether the hormonal response patterns are established at the time of embryological determination.

C. Sequence of Metamorphic Events

The sequence of early metamorphic events has been attributed to gradual increases in the level of thyroid hormones and to either stoichiometric (Etkin, 1955, 1964, 1968) or threshold relationships (Kollros, 1959, 1961) in the responding tissues. In the stoichiometric view each tissue requires a unique total amount of thyroid hormone to undergo the metamorphic process. This amount can be achieved either by high concentrations of hormone acting over a short time, or low concentrations acting for a longer period. This relationship held true for concentrations (10^{-8} M T_4 or higher) used by Etkin (1935, 1964). In the threshold idea, metamorphosis is accounted for by the hypothesis that each tissue has a certain minimum hormone requirement for response. Kollros (1959, 1961) has shown that at extremely low doses of T_4 (10^{-12} to 10^{-9} M T_4) for extended periods of time, different metamorphic events have different minimum hormone requirements, irrespective of duration (up to a year) of treatment. Although thresholds have been demonstrated in induced metamorphosis, the synchrony and coordination of normal metamorphosis may well involve both stoichiometric and threshold relationships.

D. Induced versus Spontaneous Metamorphosis

The literature repeatedly asserts that thyroid hormones produce effects comparable to spontaneous metamorphosis. This certainly appears to be true for certain external morphological criteria where the animals are exposed to increasing concentrations of hormone (Etkin, 1935). However, both Etkin (1935, 1964) and Kollros (1959, 1961) have demonstrated that a single concentration of thyroid hormones is not sufficient to reproduce the morphological changes observed in normal metamorphosis.

When changes in certain organs are examined, it becomes apparent that administration of a single dose of thyroid hormone does not mimic normal metamorphosis. In the pancreas, the weight loss during normal metamorphosis is about 80%; yet when the animals are immersed in a single high concentration of thyroxine, there is a 99.5% weight loss (Race *et al.*, 1966). Kuntz (1924) has reported an 80% reduction in liver weight during normal metamorphosis in *R. pipiens*. Atkinson and Just (1969) have observed that livers of normal young froglets weigh less and appear more lobulated than do premetamorphic tadpoles. These observations may indicate that cell death occurs during normal metamorphosis. Yet the often cited study of Kaywin (1936) reported no cell death in the liver during induced metamorphosis.

At the ultrastructural level, Bonneville (1962) reported that immersion in 1 μg/ml T_4 resulted in an intestinal epithelium of only one cell layer thick. No indications of mitotic figures are seen. During normal metamorphosis, numerous mitotic figures are seen and the intestine is more than one cell layer thick. Bonneville concluded that high dosages of T_4 inhibited cell division, but not differentiation. In a recent EM study of tadpole liver, Bennett and Glynn (1969) have reported differences between induced and normal metamorphosis at the ultrastructural level.

Differences between induced and spontaneous metamorphosis have also been observed at the biochemical level. No one has yet succeeded in inducing a complete Hb transition in larval amphibians. During normal metamorphosis, there is either no increase, or an actual decrease in the oxygen consumption of the total animal. In induced metamorphosis, when high doses of hormone are given, there is an increase in the respiration rate (see review by Frieden, 1968; Funkhouser and Mills, 1969b). Kubler and Frieden (1964) found that during induced metamorphosis, soluble β-glucuronidase activity is only one-third of the increase noted in spontaneous metamorphosis for the equivalent tail resorption. These authors also found that with induction, soluble protein of the tail is twice as high as that found in normal metamorphosis.

A careful examination of the timing of key events during spontaneous metamorphosis may offer an important clue as to the reason for the lack of correspondence between spontaneous and induced metamorphosis. As shown in Table V, numerous abrupt biochemical and morphological changes occur between stages XX and XXIII, a period of rapid development usually requiring only 5 days in most species, including the bullfrog. Because these changes follow the rather abrupt increase in circulating levels of thyroid hormone (Just, 1968), it is obvious that at stage XIX the tissues showing the drastic changes are completely competent to respond (Table V). Apparently during the earlier larval stages, competence for these rapid changes steadily accumulates, preparing tadpole tissues and organs for explosive development after stage XIX. Therefore, it might be expected that when a tadpole younger than stage XII is exposed to T_3 or T_4, uncoordinated responses are frequently observed. The various tadpole tissues do not have sufficient time to develop full competence in preparation for the metamorphic climax beginning at stage XX. It should be noted that several responses are more gradual, requiring

TABLE V

MORPHOLOGICAL AND BIOCHEMICAL SYSTEMS CHANGING RAPIDLY
AT THE METAMORPHIC CLIMAX

System	Type of change	Stage(s)[a]	Reference no.[b]
Blood			
Protein-bound iodine	80% Decrease	XIX–XXIII	1
Erythrocyte	Change in cell population	XX–XXIII	2
Hemoglobin	Switch from larval to adult Hb	XXI–XXIII	3
		XX–XXV	4
SH groups of red cells	Appearance of 4 or 8 SH groups	XXIII–XXV	5
		XXI–XXIII	6
Skin			
5-Hydroxytryptophan decarboxylase	10 × Increase	XX–XXIII	7
Serotonin	30 × Increase	XXI–XXV	7
Na pump	Initiated	XXI	8
Foregut	Appearance of peptic activity	XXII	9
Liver			
NH_3 Excretion	75% Decrease	XIX–XXI	10
Urea excretion	15 × Increase	XIX–XXI	11
Urea cycle enzymes	2–5 × Increase	XX–XXIV	12
Tail			
Morphological	90% Reduction	XX–XXIII	13
Many enzymes	2–35 × Increase	XXI–XXIII	14
Bones			
Cranial, visceral	Initiation of ossification	XX	15

[a] Taylor-Kollros (1946) stages during which a rapid change is observed.

[b] Key to references: 1. Just (1968); 2. Hollyfield (1966b); 3. Hamada et al. (1966); 4. Moss and Ingram (1968b); 5. Ashley and Frieden (1967); 6. Hamada et al. (1966); 7. Vanable (1964); 8. R. E. Taylor and Barker (1965a,b); 9. Griffiths (1961); 10. Ashley et al. (1968); 11. See Fig. 6; 12. See Table II; 13. See Fig. 1; 14. See Table III; 15. Kemp and Hoyt (1969a).

eight to ten stages extending over a much longer time period, e.g., limb growth, lateral motor cell development, and serum albumin or ceruloplasmin changes.

Another rationale for these morphological, cellular, and biochemical discrepancies during induced and normal metamorphosis, may lie in the dosage effects of thyroid hormone. The dosage may have been too high or too low, or an ever-changing level of available hormone might be required to mimic normal metamorphosis. We should not overlook the possibility that other hormonal or metabolic responses may occur in normal metamorphosis, which have not been matched in induced metamorphosis.

E. Adaptive and Nonadaptive Features of Amphibian Metamorphosis

In an earlier review (Bennett and Frieden, 1962) the adaptive significance of the many anatomical and chemical changes that occur in the tadpole during metamorphosis was emphasized. The adaptive nature of these changes supercedes the many useful descriptions of metamorphosis as an extended embryological process paralleling fetal to adult changes. Listed here are several of the most impressive changes accompanying anuran metamorphosis, which especially contribute to adaptation to land:

1. Tail regression and limb development leading to more powerful locomotion on land.

2. The shift from ammonotelism to ureotelism reflecting the change in environmental water availability.

3. Change in the hemoglobins reflecting the greater availability of oxygen to the frog.

4. Increase in serum proteins, particularly serum albumin, reflecting homeostasis and maintenance of the circulatory volume.

5. Changes in digestive enzymes and in intestinal design reflecting the necessary adjustment to a significant alteration of the diet.

These transitions are perhaps only the most obvious examples of metamorphic events that have an apparent direct adaptive value or serve as a basis for morphological or other changes that lead to improved adaptation.

In considering the many biochemical and morphological events of metamorphosis, Dr. Alan Kent has pointed out that many of these changes may be related to effects of thyroid hormones on developing vertebrates, e.g., the maturation of the nervous system in mammals; epiphysis closure in birds and mammals; effects on feathers, a skin derivative in birds; and even certain enzyme inductions in fetal and neonatal mammals. On the other hand, there are a group of events unique to metamorphosis and apparently controlled by the thyroid. Many of these changes appear to have adaptive value. In amphibian evolution, useful, adaptive changes came under the influence of the thyroid hormone, and these are superimposed on other more general responses to the thyroid hormone. Thus the metamorphic transition in amphibians stands out as one of the major contributions of a hormone to biological evolution.

ACKNOWLEDGMENTS

We are grateful to J. J. Kollros, B. Atkinson, J. Eaton, and A. Kent for critically reviewing this manuscript during its preparation. We are indebted to K. H. Kim, N.

Kemp, and T. P. Bennett for providing manuscripts in advance of publication. We are also grateful to Janet Schene, Lenore Haggard, and Jeanne Just for help in preparing the manuscript for publication and to Sharon Stuckey for the illustrations. This work was supported by an NIH postdoctoral fellowship No. HE-40,126 to John J. Just and by Grant No. HD-01236 from the National Institute of Health Paper #36 in a series from this laboratory on the biochemistry of metamorphosis.

REFERENCES

Adamson, L. F., and Ingbar, S. H. (1967a). *Endocrinology* **81**, 1362.
Adamson, L. F., and Ingbar, S. H. (1967b). *Endocrinology* **81**, 1372.
Aggarwal, S. J., and Riggs, A. (1969). *J. Biol. Chem.* **244**, 2372.
Akamatsu, N., Lindsay, R. H., and Cohen, P. P. (1964). *J. Biol. Chem.* **239**, 2246.
Allen, B. M. (1918). *J. Exptl. Zool.* **24**, 499.
Ashley, H., and Frieden, E. (1967). Cited in Frieden (1967).
Ashley, H., Katti, P., and Frieden, E. (1968). *Develop. Biol.* **17**, 293.
Atkinson, B., and Just, J. J. (1969). Unpublished observations.
Atland, D. D., and Brace, K. C. (1962). *Am. J. Physiol.* **203**, 1188.
Baca Saravia, R. (1961). *Haematol. Latina* (*Milan*) **6**, 107.
Baculi, B. S., and Cooper, E. L. (1967). *J. Morphol.* **123**, 463.
Bagnara, J. T. (1958). *J. Exptl. Zool.* **137**, 265.
Bagnara, J. T. (1961). *Gen. Comp. Endocrinol.* **1**, 124.
Bagnara, J. T. (1964a). *Gen. Comp. Endocrinol.* **4**, 290.
Bagnara, J. T. (1964b). *Compt. Rend.* **285**, 5969.
Bagnara, J. T. (1966). *Intern. Rev. Cytol.* **20**, 173–205.
Bagnara, J. T., and Neidleman, S. (1958). *Proc. Soc. Exptl. Biol. Med.* **97**, 671.
Bagnara, J. T., Taylor, J. D., and Hadley, M. E. (1968). *J. Cell. Biol.* **38**, 29.
Barch, S. H. (1953). *Physiol. Zool.* **26**, 223.
Beaudoin, A. R. (1956). *Anat. Record* **125**, 247.
Bélanger, L. F., and Drouin, P. (1966). *Can. J. Physiol. Pharmacol.* **44**, 919.
Benbasset, J. (1969). *Federation Proc.* **28**, 836.
Bennett, T. P., and Frieden, E. (1962). *Comp. Biochem.* **4**, 483–556.
Bennett, T. P., and Glynn, J. (1969). Unpublished observations.
Berman, R., Bern, H. A., Nicoll, C. S., and Strohman, R. C. (1964). *J. Exptl. Zool.* **156**, 353.
Bern, H. A., Nicoll, C. S., and Strohman, R. C. (1967). *Proc. Soc. Exptl. Biol. Med.* **126**, 518.
Blatt, L., Slickers, K. A., and Kim, K. H. (1969). Personal communications.
Blount, R. F. (1945). *J. Exptl. Zool.* **100**, 79.
Bonneville, M. A. (1962). *Proc. 5th Intern. Congr. Electron Microscopy, Philadelphia, 1962* Art. SS-15. Academic Press, New York.
Bonneville, M. A. (1963). *J. Cell Biol.* **18**, 579.
Botte, V. (1966). *Riv. Biol.* (*Perugia*) **59**, 209.
Botte, V., and Buonanno, C. (1962). *Boll. Zool.* **29**, 471.
Bovbjerg, A. M. (1963). *J. Morphol.* **113**, 231.
Bovbjerg, A. M. (1966). *J. Exptl. Zool.* **162**, 69.

Brodsky, R. A. (1968). *J. Gen. Biol.* **29**, 731.

Brown, G. W., Brown, W. R., and Cohen, P. P. (1959). *J. Biol. Chem.* **234**, 1775.

Burch, A. B. (1938). *Proc. Soc. Exptl. Biol. Med.* **38**, 608.

Chalumeau-Le Foulgoc, M. (1967). *Compt. Rend.* **265**, 1508.

Chan, S. K., and Cohen, P. P. (1964). *Arch. Biochem. Biophys.* **104**, 325.

Charlemagne, J. (1967). *Bull. Soc. Zool. France* **92**, 153.

Charlemagne, J., and Houillon, C. (1968). *Compt. Rend.* **267**, 253.

Chieffi, G. (1965). *In* "Organogenesis" (R. L. DeHaan and H. Ursprung, eds.), pp. 653–671. Holt, New York.

Chieffi, G., and Carfagna, M. (1959a). *Atti. Accad. Nazl. Lincei, Mem., Classe Sci. Fis., Mat. Nat., Sez. III.[a]* [7] **26**, 94.

Chieffi, G., and Carfagna, M. (1959b). *Acta Embryol. Morphol. Exptl.* **2**, 317.

Chieffi, G., and Carfagna, M. (1960). *Acta Embryol. Morphol. Exptl.* **3**, 213.

Cline, M. J., and Waldmann, T. A. (1962). *Am. J. Physiol.* **203**, 401.

Cohen, N. (1966). *Am. Zoologist* **6**, 608.

Cohen, P. P. (1966). *Harvey Lectures* **60**, 119.

Coleman, J. R. (1962). *Develop. Biol.* **5**, 232.

Cooper, E. L. (1967a). *In* "Ontogeny of Immunity" (R. T. Smith, R. A. Good, and P. A. Miescher, eds.), pp. 87–101. Univ. of Florida Press, Gainesville, Florida.

Cooper, E. L. (1967b). *J. Morphol.* **122**, 381.

Cooper, E. L. (1968). *Anat. Record* **162**, 453.

Cooper, E. L., and Hildemann, W. H. (1965a). *Ann. Acad. Sci.* **126**, 647.

Cooper, E. L., and Hildemann, W. H. (1965b). *Transplantation* **3**, 446.

Cooper, E. L., Pinkerton, W., and Hildemann, W. H. (1964). *Biol. Bull.* **127**, 232.

Cortelyou, J. R., and McWhinnie, D. J. (1967). *Am. Zoologist* **7**, 843.

Dale, E. (1962). *Gen. Comp. Endocrinol.* **2**, 171.

DeGroot, N., and Cohen, P. P. (1962a). *Biochim. Biophys. Acta* **59**, 588.

DeGroot, N., and Cohen, P. P. (1962b). *Biochim. Biophys. Acta* **59**, 595.

DeLanney, L. E., and Prahlad, K. V. (1966). *Am. Zoologist* **6**, 580.

Dent, J. N. (1968). *In* "Metamorphosis" (W. Etkin and L. I. Gilbert, eds.), pp. 271–311. Appleton, New York.

Derby, A. (1968). *J. Exptl. Zool.* **168**, 147.

Derby, A., and Etkin, W. (1968). *J. Exptl. Zool.* **169**, 1.

De Witt, W. (1968). *J. Mol. Biol.* **32**, 502.

Deyrup, I. J. (1964). *In* "Physiology of the Amphibia" (J. A. Moore, ed.), pp. 251–328. Academic Press, New York.

Diener, E., and Nossal, G. J. V. (1966). *Immunology* **10**, 535.

Dolphin, J., and Frieden, E. (1955). *J. Biol. Chem.* **217**, 735.

Dowling, J. T., and Razevska, D. (1966). *Gen. Comp. Endocrinol.* **6**, 162.

Du Pasquier, L. (1967). *Compt. Rend. Soc. Biol.* **161**, 1974.

Eakin, R. M. (1939). *Growth* **3**, 373.

Eakin, R. M., and Harris, M. (1945). *J. Exptl. Zool.* **98**, 35.

Eaton, J. E., and Frieden, E. (1968). *Gunma Symp. Endocrinol.* **5**, 43.

Eaton, J. E., and Frieden, E. (1969a). *Gen. Comp. Endocrinol. Suppl.* **2**, 398.

Eaton, J. E., and Frieden, E. (1969b). *Proc. Nottingham Conf.* (in press).

Eaton, J. E., and Frieden, E. (1969c). Unpublished data.

Eeckhout, Y. (1965). Docteur en Sciences Thesis, Universite Catholique de Louvain Faculte des Sciences.

Egyhazi, E., Ringborg, U., Daneholt, B., and Lambert, B. (1968). *Nature* **220**, 1036.

Eisen, A. Z., and Gross, J. (1965). *Develop. Biol.* **12**, 408.

Epple, A. (1968). *Endocrinol. Japon.* **15**, 107.

Etkin, W. (1935). *J. Exptl. Zool.* **71**, 317.

Etkin, W. (1950). *Anat. Record* **108**, 541.

Etkin, W. (1955). In "Analysis of Development" (B. H. Willier, P. A. Weiss, and V. Hamburger, eds.), pp. 631–663. Saunders, Philadelphia, Pennsylvania.

Etkin, W. (1963). *Science* **139**, 810.

Etkin, W. (1964). In "Physiology of the Amphibia" (J. A. Moore, ed.), pp. 427–468. Academic Press, New York.

Etkin, W. (1966). *Neuroendocrinology* (*N. Y.*) **1**, 293.

Etkin, W. (1968). In "Metamorphosis" (W. Etkin and L. I. Gilbert, eds.), pp. 313–348. Appleton, New York.

Etkin, W., and Gilbert, L. I., eds. (1968). "Metamorphosis." Appleton, New York.

Etkin, W., and Gona, A. G. (1967). *J. Exptl. Zool.* **165**, 249.

Etkin, W., and Gona, A. G. (1968). *Endocrinology* **82**, 1067.

Fabrizio, M., and Charipper, H. A. (1941). *J. Morphol.* **68**, 179.

Felgenhauer, K. (1968). *Biochim. Biophys. Acta* (*London*) **160**, 267.

Fell, H. B., and Mellanby, E. (1955). *J. Physiol.* (*London*) **127**, 427.

Fell, H. B., and Mellanby, E. (1956). *J. Physiol.* (*London*) **133**, 89.

Ferguson, T. (1966). *Gen. Comp. Endocrinol.* **7**, 74.

Finamore, F. J., and Frieden, E. (1960). *J. Biol. Chem.* **235**, 1751.

Flores, G., and Frieden, E. (1968). *Science* **159**, 101.

Foà, P. P., and Guidotti, G. G. (1966). *Am. J. Physiol.* **211**, 981.

Fox, H. (1963). *Quart. Rev. Biol.* **38**, 1.

Fox, H. (1967). *Arch. Biol.* (*Liege*) **78**, 595.

Fox, H., and Moulton, J. M. (1968). *Arch. Anat. Microscop. Morphol. Exptl.* **57**, 107.

Francis, A., and Frieden, E. (1964). Unpublished observations.

Frieden, E. (1961). *Am. Zoologist* **1**, 115.

Frieden, E. (1964). *Proc. 2nd Intern. Congr. Congenital Malformations,* p. 191. Intern. Med. Congr., New York.

Frieden, E. (1965). *Proc. 2nd Intern. Congr. Endocrinol., London, 1964* p. 34. Excerpta Med. Found., Amsterdam.

Frieden, E. (1967). *Recent Prog. Hormone Res.* **23**, 139–194.

Frieden, E. (1968). In "Metamorphosis" (W. Etkin and L. I. Gilbert, eds.), pp. 349–398. Appleton, New York.

Frieden, E., and Mathews, H. (1958). *Arch. Biochem. Biophys.* **73**, 107.

Frieden, E. Herner, A., Fish, L., and Lewis, E. (1957). *Science* **126**, 559.

Frieden, E., Wahlborg, A., and Howard, E. (1965). *Nature* **205**, 1173.

Frye, B. E. (1958). *Am. J. Anat.* **102**, 117.

Frye, B. E. (1962). *Anat. Record* **144**, 97.

Frye, B. E. (1964). *J. Exptl. Zool.* **155**, 215.

Frye, B. E. (1965). *J. Exptl. Zool.* **158**, 133.

Funkhouser, A., and Mills, K. S. (1969a). *Physiol. Zool.* **42**, 14.

Funkhouser, A., and Mills, K. S. (1969b). *Physiol. Zool.* **42**, 22.

Gallien, L. G. (1965). In "Organogenesis" (R. L. DeHaan and H. Ursprung, eds.), pp. 583–610. Holt, New York.

Galton, V. A., and Ingbar, S. H. (1962). *Endocrinology* **70**, 622.

Galton, V. A., Ingbar, S. H., and von der Heyde, S. (1965). *Endocrinology* **76**, 479.

Geigy, R. (1941). *Verhandl. Schweiz. Naturforsch. Ges.* **121**, 161.

Gona, A. G. (1968). *Gen. Comp. Endocrinol.* **11,** 278.

Gorski, R. A. (1968). *Endocrinology* **82,** 1001.

Grasso, J. A., and Shephard, D. C. (1968). *Nature* **218,** 1274.

Greengard, O. (1969). *Science* **163,** 891.

Griffiths, I. (1961). *Proc. Zool. Soc. London* **137,** 249.

Gross, J., and Lapiere, C. M. (1962). *Proc. Natl. Acad. Sci. U. S.* **48,** 1014.

Guardabassi, A. (1959). *Monitore Zool. Ital.* **66,** 1.

Guardabassi, A. (1961). *Gen. Comp. Endocrinol.* **1,** 348.

Guardabassi, A., and Lattes, M. G. (1965). *Arch. Zool. Ital.* **50,** 315.

Guardabassi, A., and Lattes, M. G. (1968). *Arch. Zool. Ital.* **51,** 697.

Hahn, E. W. (1962). *Comp. Biochem. Physiol.* **7,** 55.

Hama, T. (1963). *Ann. N. Y. Acad. Sci.* **100,** 977.

Hamada, K., and Shukuya, R. (1966). *J. Biochem. (Tokyo)* **59,** 397.

Hamada, K., Sakai, Y., Tsushima, K., and Shukuya, R. (1966). *J. Biochem. (Tokyo)* **60,** 37.

Hanaoka, Y. (1967). *Gen. Comp. Endocrinol.* **8,** 417.

Harris, M. (1941). *J. Exptl. Zool.* **88,** 373.

Hartwig, H. (1940). *Biol. Zentr.* **60,** 473.

Herner, A. E., and Frieden, E. (1960). *J. Biol. Chem.* **235,** 2845.

Herner, A. E., and Frieden, E. (1961). *Arch. Biochem. Biophys.* **95,** 25.

Hildemann, W. H. (1966). *In* "Phylogeny of Immunity" (R. T. Smith, P. A. Miescher and R. A. Good, eds.), pp. 236–242. Univ. of Florida Press, Gainesville, Florida.

Hildemann, W. H., and Haas, R. (1959). *J. Immunol.* **83,** 478.

Hildemann, W. H., and Haas, R. (1962). *In* "Mechanisms of Immunological Tolerance," p. 35. Ized Acad. Sci., Prague.

Hirayama, T. (1967). *Nichidai Igaku Zasshi* **34,** 391.

Hollyfield, J. G. (1966a). *Develop. Biol.* **14,** 461.

Hollyfield, J. G. (1966b). *J. Morphol.* **119,** 1.

Holmes, D. W. (1966). *Dissertation Abstr.* **26,** 4902.

Hsu, C. Y., and Wu, W. L. (1964). *Chinese J. Physiol.* **19,** 155.

Hughes, A. (1966). *J. Embryol. Exptl. Morphol.* **16,** 401.

Hurley, M. P. (1958). *Growth* **22,** 125.

Hydén, H. (1968). *Currents Mod. Biol.* **2,** 57.

Ilan, J. (1968). *J. Biol. Chem.* **243,** 5859.

Inaba, T., and Frieden, E. (1967). *J. Biol. Chem.* **242,** 218.

Iwasawa, H. (1961). *Japan. J. Zool.* **13,** 69.

Janes, R. G. (1937). *J. Morphol.* **61,** 581.

Janosky, I. D., and Wenger, B. S. (1956). *J. Comp. Neurol.* **105,** 127.

Jordan, H. E., and Speidel, C. C. (1923). *J. Exptl. Med.* **38,** 529.

Just, J. J. (1968). Ph.D. Thesis, University of Iowa, Iowa City, Iowa.

Just, J. J., and Atkinson, B. (1969). Unpublished observations.

Just, J. J., and Kollros, J. J. (1968). *Am. Zoologist* **8,** 762.

Just, J. J., and Kollros, J. J. (1969). Unpublished observations.

Kaltenbach, J. C. (1953a). *J. Exptl. Zool.* **122,** 21.

Kaltenbach, J. C. (1953b). *J. Exptl. Zool.* **122,** 449.

Kaltenbach, J. C. (1959). *J. Exptl. Zool.* **140,** 1.

Kaltenbach, J. C. (1968). *In* "Metamorphosis" (W. Etkin and L. I. Gilbert, eds.), pp. 399–411. Appleton, New York.

Kaltenbach, J. C., and Lipson, M. J. S. (1962). *Am. Zoologist* **2,** 418.

Kang, A. H., Nagai, Y., Piez, K. A., and Gross, J. (1966). *Biochemistry* **5**, 509.
Karlson, P. (1963). *Perspectives Biol. Med.* **6**, 203.
Kaywin, L. (1936). *Anat. Record* **64**, 413.
Keller, R. (1946). *Rev. Suisse Zool.* **53**, 329.
Kemp, N. E. (1963). *Develop. Biol.* **7**, 244.
Kemp, N. E., and Hoyt, J. A. (1969a). *J. Morphol.* **129**, 415.
Kemp, N. E., and Hoyt, J. A. (1969b). *Develop. Biol.* **20**, 387.
Kim, H. C., D'Iorio, A., and Paik, W. K. (1966). *Can. J. Biochem.* **44**, 303.
Kim, K. H., and Cohen, P. P. (1966). *Proc. Natl. Acad. Sci. U. S.* **55**, 1251.
Kim, K. H., and Cohen, P. P. (1968). *Am. Zoologist* **8**, 243.
Kollros, J. J. (1942). *J. Exptl. Zool.* **89**, 37.
Kollros, J. J. (1958). *Science* **128**, 1505.
Kollros, J. J. (1959). *In* "Symposium on Comparative Endocrinology" (A. Gorbman, ed.), pp. 340–350. Wiley, New York.
Kollros, J. J. (1961). *Am. Zoologist* **1**, 107.
Kollros, J. J. (1968). *Ciba Found. Symp., Growth Nervous System* pp. 179–192.
Kollros, J. J. (1969). Personal communication.
Kollros, J. J., and Kaltenbach, J. C. (1952). *Physiol. Zool.* **25**, 163.
Kollros, J. J., and McMurray, V. M. (1955). *J. Comp. Neurol.* **102**, 47.
Kollros, J. J., and McMurray, V. M. (1956). *J. Exptl. Zool.* **131**, 1.
Kubler, H., and Frieden, E. (1964). *Biochim. Biophys. Acta* **93**, 635.
Kuhn, O., and Hammer, H. O. (1956). *Experientia* **12**, 231.
Kuntz, A. (1924). *J. Morphol.* **38**, 581.
Lapiere, C. M., and Gross, J. (1963). *In* "Mechanisms of Hard Tissue Destruction," Publ. No. 75, pp. 663–694. Am. Assoc. Advance. Sci., Washington, D. C.
Lawson, K. (1963). *J. Embryol. Exptl. Morphol.* **11**, 383.
Ledford, B. E., and Frieden, E. (1969). Unpublished observations.
Lengemann, F. W. (1962). *Endocrinology* **70**, 774.
Levy, C. C. (1964). *J. Biol. Chem.* **239**, 560.
Lipson, M. J. S. (1967). *Dissertation Abst.* **28**, 1730.
Lipson, M. J. S., and Kaltenbach, J. C. (1965). *Am. Zoologist* **5**, 212.
McMahon, E. M., and De Witt, W. (1968). *Biochem. Biophys. Res. Commun.* **31**, 176.
Manwell, C. (1966). *Comp. Biochem. Physiol.* **17**, 805.
Marty, A., and Weber, R. (1968). *Helv. Physiol. Pharmacol. Acta* **26**, 62.
Medda, A. K., and Frieden, E. (1970). *Endocrinol.* (in press).
Moog, F., and Grey, R. D. (1966). *Biol. Neonatorum* [N. S.] **9**, 10.
Moore, J. A., ed. (1964). "Physiology of the Amphibia." Academic Press, New York.
Moser, H. (1950). *Rev. Suisse Zool.* **57**, 1.
Moss, B., and Ingram, V. M. (1965). *Proc. Natl. Acad. Sci. U. S.* **54**, 967.
Moss, B., and Ingram, V. M. (1968a). *J. Mol. Biol.* **32**, 481.
Moss, B., and Ingram, V. M. (1968b). *J. Mol. Biol.* **32**, 493.
Moulton, J. M., Jurand, A., and Fox, H. (1968). *J. Embryol. Exptl. Morphol.* **19**, 415.
Nagai, Y., Lapiere, C. M., and Gross, J. (1966). *Biochemistry* **5**, 3123.
Nakagawa, H., and Cohen, P. P. (1967). *J. Biol. Chem.* **242**, 642.
Nakagawa, H., and Cohen, P. P. (1968). Unpublished observations (cited in Kim and Cohen, 1968).
Nakagawa, H., Kim, K. H., and Cohen, P. P. (1967). *J. Biol. Chem.* **242**, 635.
Needham, J. (1942). "Biochemistry and Morphogenesis." Cambridge Univ. Press, London and New York.

Obika, M., and Matsumoto, J. (1968). *Exptl. Cell. Res.* **52**, 646.
Odell, W. D., Wilbert, J. F., and Utiger, R. D. (1967). *Recent Progr. Hormone Res.* **23**, 47.
Ohtsu, K., Naito, K., and Wilt, F. H. (1964). *Develop. Biol.* **10**, 216.
O'Malley, B. W., Aronow, A., Peacock, A. C., and Dingman, C. W. (1968). *Science* **162**, 567.
Osaki, S., Johnson, D. A., and Frieden, E. (1966). *J. Biol. Chem.* **241**, 2746.
Paik, W. K., Metzenberg, R. L., and Cohen, P. P. (1961). *J. Biol. Chem.* **236**, 536.
Pehlemann, F. W. (1967). *Z. Zellforsch. Mikroskop. Anat.* **78**, 484.
Pesetsky, I. (1962). *Gen. Comp. Endocrinol.* **2**, 229.
Pesetsky, I. (1965). *Gen. Comp. Endocrinol.* **5**, 411.
Pesetsky, I. (1966a). *Z. Zellforsch. Mikroskop. Anat.* **75**, 138.
Pesetsky, I. (1966b). *Anat. Record* **154**, 401.
Pesetsky, I., and Kollros, J. J. (1956). *Exptl. Cell Res.* **11**, 477.
Pflugfelder, O. (1967). *Arch. Entwicklungsmech. Organ.* **159**, 433.
Pflugfelder, O., and Schubert, G. (1965). *Z. Zellforsch. Mikroskop. Anat.* **67**, 96.
Pilkington, J. B., and Simkiss, K. (1966). *J. Exptl. Biol.* **45**, 329.
Pittman, C. S., and Shimizu, C. (1966). *Endocrinology* **79**, 1109.
Prahlad, K. V., and DeLanney, L. E. (1965). *J. Exptl. Zool.* **160**, 137.
Price, S., and Frieden, E. (1963). *Comp. Biochem. Physiol.* **10**, 245.
Race, J. (1961). *Gen. Comp. Endocrinol.* **1**, 322.
Race, J., Robinson, C., and Terry, R. J. (1966). *J. Exptl. Zool.* **162**, 181.
Rapola, J. (1963). *Gen. Comp. Endocrinol.* **3**, 412.
Remy, C., and Bounhiol, J. J. (1965). *Compt. Rend. Soc. Biol.* **159**, 1532.
Remy, C., and Bounhiol, J. J. (1966). *Ann. Endocrinol.* (*Paris*) **27**, 377.
Reynolds, W. A. (1963). *J. Exptl. Zool.* **153**, 237.
Richmond, J. E. (1968). *Comp. Biochem. Physiol.* **24**, 991.
Riggs, A. (1951). *J. Gen. Physiol.* **35**, 23.
Riggs, A., and Aggarwal, S. J. (1968). *Proc. 7th Intern. Congr. Biochem., Tokyo, 1967.* p. 595. Sci. Council Japan, Tokyo.
Riggs, A., Sullivan, B., and Agee, J. R. (1964). *Proc. Natl. Acad. Sci. U. S.* **51**, 1127.
Robertson, D. R. (1968). *Z. Zellforsch. Mikroskop. Anat.* **90**, 273.
Rosen, O. M., and Rosen, S. M. (1968). *Biochem. Biophys. Res. Commun.* **31**, 82.
Rossini, M. C. (1965). *Arch. Zool. Ital.* **50**, 145.
Sallach, H. J., and Kmiotek, E. H. (1968). *Comp. Biochem. Physiol.* **27**, 213.
Salzmann, R., and Weber, R. (1963). *Experientia* **19**, 352.
Shaffer, B. M. (1963). *J. Embryol. Exptl. Morphol.* **11**, 77.
Shukuya, R. (1966). *Protein, Nucleic Acid, Enzyme* **11**, 228.
Silbert, J. E., Nagai, Y., and Gross, J. (1965). *J. Biol. Chem.* **240**, 1509.
Slickers, K. A., and Kim, K. H. (1969). *Proc. Nottingham Conf.* (in press).
Spiegel, M., and Spiegel, E. S. (1964). *Biol. Bull.* **126**, 307.
Stackhouse, H. L. (1966). *Comp. Biochem. Physiol.* **17**, 219.
Stratton, L. P., and Frieden, E. (1967). *Nature* **216**, 932.
Sugiura, K., and Goto, M. (1968). *J. Biochem.* (*Tokyo*) **64**, 657.
Tata, J. R. (1964). *Nature* **204**, 939.
Tata, J. R. (1965). *Nature* **207**, 378.
Tata, J. R. (1966). *Develop. Biol.* **13**, 77.
Tata, J. R. (1968a). *Nature* **219**, 331.
Tata, J. R. (1968b). *Develop. Biol.* **18**, 415.
Taylor, A. C., and Kollros, J. J. (1946). *Anat. Record* **94**, 7.
Taylor, R. E., and Barker, S. B. (1965a). *J. Endocrinol.* **31**, 175.

Taylor, R. E., and Barker, S. B. (1965b). *Science* **148**, 1612.
Taylor, R. E., Taylor, H. C., and Barker, S. B. (1966). *J. Exptl. Zool.* **161**, 271.
Terry, G. (1918). *J. Exptl. Zool.* **24**, 567.
Theil, E. C. (1967). *Biochem. Biophys. Acta* **138**, 175.
Theil, E. C., and Frieden, E. (1966). *Federation Proc.* **25**, 3548.
Tonoue, T., and Frieden, E. (1970). *J. Biol. Chem.* (in press).
Tonoue, T., Eaton, J. E., and Frieden, E. (1969). *Biochem. Biophys. Res. Commun.* **37**, 81.
Trader, C. D., and Frieden, E. (1966). *J. Biol. Chem.* **241**, 357.
Trader, C. D., Wortham, J. S., and Frieden, E. (1963). *Science* **139**, 918.
Ueck, M. (1967). *Z. Wiss. Zool.* **176**, 173.
Ueck, M. (1968). *Zool. Anz. Suppl.* **31**, 192.
Unsworth, B., and Cohen, P. P. (1968). *Biochemistry* **7**, 2581.
Urbani, E. (1957). *Rend. Ist. Lombardo Sci. Lettere* **B92**, 69.
Usuku, G., and Gross, J. (1965). *Develop. Biol.* **11**, 352.
Vanable, J. W. (1964). *Develop. Biol.* **10**, 331.
Vanable, J. W. (1966). *Am. Zoologist* **6**, 523.
Vanable, J. W., and Mortensen, R. D. (1966). *Exptl. Cell Res.* **44**, 436.
Vannini, E., and Stagni, A. (1967). *Exptl. Cell Res.* **46**, 460.
Vannini, E., and Stagni, A. (1968). *Exptl. Cell Res.* **50**, 683.
Voitkevich, A. A. (1962). *Gen. Comp. Endocrinol.* Suppl. 1, 133.
Weber, R. (1957). *Rev. Suisse Zool.* **64**, 326.
Weber, R. (1962). *Experientia* **18**, 84.
Weber, R. (1963a). *Ciba Found. Symp., Lysosomes* pp. 282–305.
Weber, R. (1963b). *Helv. Physiol. Pharmacol. Acta* **21**, 277.
Weber, R. (1965). *Experientia* **21**, 665.
Weber, R. (1967a). *In* "The Biochemistry of Animal Development" (R. Weber, ed.), Vol. 2 pp. 227–301. Academic Press, New York.
Weber, R. (1967b). *In* "Comprehensive Biochemistry" (M. Florkin and E. Stotz, eds.), Vol. 28, pp. 145–198. Elsevier, Amsterdam.
Weber, R., and Niehus, B. (1961). *Helv. Physiol. Pharmacol. Acta* **19**, 103.
Weiss, P., and Rossetti, R. (1951). *Proc. Natl. Acad. Sci. U. S.* **37**, 546.
Weissmann, G. (1961). *J. Exptl. Med.* **114**, 581.
Wilde, C. E. (1961). *Advan. Morphogenesis* **1**, 267–300.
Wilt, F. H. (1959a). *Develop. Biol.* **1**, 199.
Wilt, F. H. (1959b). *J. Embryol. Exptl. Morphol.* **7**, 556.
Wilt, F. H. (1967). *Advan. Morphogenesis* **6**, 89–125.
Wise, R. (1970). *Comp. Biochem. Physiol.* **32**, 89.
Witschi, E. (1967). *In* "The Biochemistry of Animal Development" (R. Weber, ed.), Vol. 2, pp. 193–225. Academic Press, New York.
Wolf-Heidegger, G. (1937). *Arch. Entwicklungsmech. Organ.* **135**, 114.
Wyatt, G. R., and Tata, J. R. (1968). *Biochem. J.* **109**, 253.
Yamamoto, K. (1964). *Gen. Comp. Endocrinol.* **4**, 360.
Yanagisawa, T. (1954). *Rept. Liberal Arts Sci. Fac. Shizuoka Univ., Nat. Sci.* **5**, 33.
Ziegler-Gunder, I., Simon, H., and Wacker, A. (1956). *Z. Naturforsch.* **11b**, 82.

CHAPTER 2

The Developmental Formation of Enzymes in Rat Liver

Olga Greengard

I. INTRODUCTION

The general concern of this account is the mechanisms underlying the transformation of the quantitative pattern of enzymes of fetal liver to that of adult liver. This process of enzymic differentiation involves both positive changes, the appearance or sudden rise in the amount of some enzymes, and negative changes, the diminution in the amount of other enzymes. I shall concentrate on the more extensively studied positive changes, many of which are associated with the development of specific

53

metabolic potentialities characteristic of mammalian liver, such as the ability to accumulate glycogen, to utilize glycogen, to synthesize glucose or lipids, and to catabolize amino acids.

Quantitative studies of recent years established good correlations between the function of these pathways and the amounts of enzymes that catalyze the reactions involved. Metabolic regulations by possible alteration of the *activity* of enzymes will not be considered here; only those studies where efforts were made to use assay conditions in which the *amount* of the enzyme alone was limiting will be discussed. Most of those studies excluded changes *in vivo* in the concentration of activators or inhibitors as possible reasons for rises in activity during development. The use of inhibitors of protein or RNA synthesis *in vivo* often provided additional evidence that the observed rises in the activity of various enzymes during development reflected increases in the amounts of protein moiety of the enzyme systems. However, the possibility of error cannot be completely eliminated. In some cases, inactive or unstable precursors of an enzyme may have appeared in the course of development before they could be detected. In other cases, inadequate control of unknown endogenous cofactors might have rendered the measurement of the rate of accumulation of an enzyme inaccurate. For each single enzyme there are different analytical problems that vex the investigator attempting to quantify *amount*. Sometimes these technical questions of detail are exaggerated into doubts as to whether differentiation involves changes in the amount or the activity of enzymes. There is no justification for posing such a general question. In the fertilized egg there is neither a miniature organism nor a preformed mixture of all enzymes of the future organism. Thus, enzymic differentiation is essentially a problem of enzyme synthesis; regulation of the catalytic efficiency of the enzyme molecule is an important, superimposed, secondary mechanism.

The primary role of hormones in biochemical differentiation will be considered here as one of regulating gene expression. Two major reasons for concentrating on hormones as specific stimuli for the developmental formation of liver enzymes are: (1) several hormones are known to induce the synthesis of specific enzymes in adult liver (Knox *et al.*, 1956; Greengard, 1967), and (2) major changes in the enzymic pattern of late fetal and young postnatal liver coincide with major changes in endocrine functions (Gorbman and Evans, 1943; Jost, 1953; Kitchell and Wells, 1952; Feldman *et al.*, 1961; Levine and Mullins, 1966; Roos, 1967). In addition to these considerations, as will be seen, there is now some direct evidence for the evocation of specific enzymes by appropriate hormones.

II. CRITICAL STAGES OF ENZYMIC DIFFERENTIATION IN THE LIVER

A large number of enzymes characteristic of adult liver have been reported to be essentially absent at some stage of development, often at a single, ill-defined fetal or early postnatal stage. For the present purposes, only those studies are useful that provide several intermediate points sufficient to establish accurately the time at which the enzyme begins to rise as well as the time at which it reaches the adult level. Enzymes that require several weeks to accumulate will be neglected in favor of those whose rise is much more rapid than the gradual increase in body weight or the increase in size and protein content of the liver. Such rapid changes in enzyme amount are then equally significant whether expressed per gram liver, per total liver, or per unit amount of liver protein. Also, the stimuli that initiate the rapid rises are more accessible for experimental identification than the conditions that promote enzyme accumulations progressing for many weeks during which a large number of parameters change in the developing animal.

A comprehensive survey of the developmental formations of enzymes in rat liver or in any mammalian organ is not available although there are broad reviews containing examples of interesting enzyme changes in various developing tissues of different species (Herrmann and Tootle, 1964; Moog, 1965). In surveying the data pertaining to rat liver, scattered in the literature, one gets an impression of the discontinuous nature of enzymic differentation: some distinct developmental stages are associated with a multiplicity of enzymic changes whereas other periods are relatively uneventful. Because of this tendency for the enzyme changes to cluster in time, the enzymes to be discussed here will be grouped into clusters *a*, *b*, and *c* according to the three stages in development at which they first appear, irrespective of their catalytic role, although each cluster may include some functionally related enzymes. Additional clusters, or subdivisions of these, may be necessary to accommodate new findings. For example, liver enzymes formed when the gonads mature may constitute such a subgroup.

The three stages of development that appear to be associated with the sudden accumulation of a significant number of enzymes in rat liver are (a) the sixteenth to twentieth days of gestation (total = 22 days), or late fetal period (Table I); (b) the first day after birth, also referred to as the early postnatal or neonatal period (Table II); and (c) the third week of postnatal life, or the late suckling period (Table III).

The groups of enzymes that exhibit sudden rises in amount at stages (a), (b) and (c) will be referred to as cluster *a* (Table I), *b* (Table II), and *c* (Table III), respectively. Sections III, IV, and V will deal with the three clusters separately but will not discuss individually all enzymes listed in the tables. Thus, by inspecting the tables per se, the reader may notice important relationships between enzymic, metabolic, and endocrine events that have been neglected by this writer.

Each enzyme in Fig. 1 is typical of one of the three clusters: *a*, ketose-*l*-phosphate aldolase, like some others in this group, will be considered to reach a maximum just before birth, since the adult level is only about 20% higher and will be reached in the course of several weeks; *b*, phosphoenolpyruvate carboxylase (PEP carboxylase) begins to rise immediately after birth and, like most others in this cluster, temporarily overshoots the adult level; and *c*, tryptophan oxygenase appears in the third week of postnatal life. Others in this cluster may appear a few days later and some may temporarily overshoot the adult level. The times, given in days before or after birth, at which the different enzymes of clusters *a*, *b*, and *c* (Tables I to III) begin to rise or reach a maximum are approximate, since they are sometimes based on insufficiently detailed time curves or estimated as the most probable value discernible from reports of different laboratories.

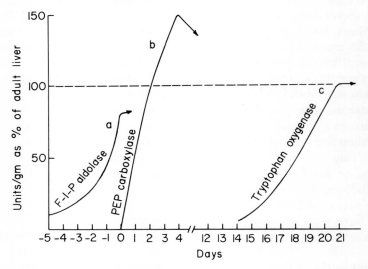

FIG. 1. Examples of the rate of enzyme accumulation at the late fetal, early postnatal, and late suckling stage. Levels for enzymes *a*, *b*, and *c* are based on data by Burch *et al.* (1963), Yeung *et al.* (1967), and Franz and Knox (1967), respectively.

Several enzymes undergo more than one abrupt rise in the course of development; they may appear during the fetal stage and mount again together with the early postnatal cluster or at the late suckling period. It is important to recognize each of these rises in the history of an enzyme in order to elucidate eventually the different sequential stimuli that contribute to its developmental formation. Therefore, glucose-6-phosphatase, for example, has been listed in both Tables I and II. On the other hand, NADP and NAD dehydrogenases are mentioned in Table I only because their second phase of accumulation, around the age of weaning, has not been studied in detail. Conversely, xanthine oxidase is listed only in Table III because the earlier stage of development during which it attains a finite level (from which it then rises during the late suckling period) has not been determined.

The explanation for the clustering of the enzymic changes at these particular times can be sought in terms of the stimuli that may promote appearance of several enzymes at once. Each of the three stages described is associated with major physiological events: (a) the late fetal stage is the time at which the pituitary, the thyroid, the adrenal cortex, and the β-cells of the pancreas begin to function; (b) at the early postnatal stage, the α-cells of the pancreas develop and at this time there must be complex modifications of endocrine control associated with the separation of the organism from the intrauterine environment and adjustment to its new aerobic existence; and (c) at the late suckling stage the full functioning of the pituitary–adrenal axis is established, and, presumably, additional endocrine regulatory circuits, related to the new diet, begin to function. This classification into three clusters of enzymes and the three physiological corollaries is an oversimplification, but it introduces some order into the random enumeration of developmental enzyme changes often seen in reviews. Clearly, with more precise timing of endocrine events and coincident steps of enzymic differentiation, the aforementioned clusters will be resolved to meaningful microclusters and their specific hormonal stimuli.

III. THE LATE FETAL STAGE

The enzymes, cluster a, listed in Table I appear in significant amounts during the last few days of gestation. Some of these begin to exert essential functions as soon as they appear; others seem to be formed in preparation for the needs of the newborn. Thus, UDPG-glycogen gluco-

Olga Greengard

TABLE I
Enzyme Formations in Rat Liver—Late Fetal Period[*]

Enzyme	E.C. Number (IUB, 1965)	Beginning of Rise Day before birth, − after birth, +	Maximum Reached Relative to Adult (A)	Increase inhibited by:	Premature rise caused by an injection of:	Treatments without effect	Remarks
UDPG-glycogen glucosyltransferase	2.4.1.11	−5[a,b,c]	>A	Fetal decapitation[b]	—	—	Premature deposition of glycogen upon hydrocortisone injection (Fig. 3)
UDPG-Pyrophosphorylase	2.7.7.9	−4[a,b,d]	>A	Fetal decapitation[b]	—	—	—
Phosphoglucomutase	2.7.5.1	−5[a,b]	>A	Fetal decapitation[b]	—	—	—
Glycogen phosphorylase	2.4.1.1	−3[a,b,e,f]	=A	—	—	—	—
Ketose-1-phosphate aldolase	4.1.2.7	−5[f]	=A	—	—	—	—
Glycerolphosphate dehydrogenase	1.1.99.5	−3[f]	>A	—	—	—	—
Glucose-6-phosphatase (see also Table II)	3.1.3.9	−4[f,g,h]	>A	Fetal decapitation,[b] Hydrocortisone[g,i]	Glucagon,[i] Thyroxine,[j] Epinephrine, cAMP[k]	Fetal injection of insulin, growth hormone[j]	Prematurely induced rises are prevented by actinomycin (Fig. 4)
Fructose-1,6-diphosphatase (see also Table II)	3.1.3.11	−1 or 0[a,h,m,n]	>A	—	—	Fetal injection of cyclic AMP[a]	—

Enzyme	EC		Day	Sign			Premature/mature delivery	Remarks
Pyruvate carboxylase	6.4.1.1	−3[o,o]	+2 to +7	>A	—	—	—	—
Carbamyl phosphate synthetase	2.7.2.2	−4	+1	<A	—	—	—	—
Ornithine transcarbamylase	2.1.3.3	−4	0	<A	—	—	—	—
Argininosuccinate synthetase	(6.3.4.5)	−2 }[p,q,r]	+1	<A	Adrenalectomy at birth[p]	Triamcinolone at birth[p]	Premature or post-mature delivery[p]	—
Arginosuccinase	4.3.2.1	−4	+1	<A	—	—	—	Second rapid rise in third week[q]
Arginase	3.5.3.1	−4	+1	<A	—	Thyroxine[s] (see Fig. 5)	—	—
Histidine pyruvate aminotransferase	none	−4[t]	+1	=A	—	—	—	—
Phenylalanine pyruvate aminotransferase	none	−1[u]	+1	>A	—	—	—	—
NADPH-dehydrogenase	1.6.99.2	−3[i,v]	0	<A	Actinomycin and puromycin[v]	Thyroxine[j]	—	Second rapid rise in third postnatal week[v]
Malate dehydrogenase (NAD)	1.1.1.37	−4[h,x]	−1	=A	—	—	—	—
Isocitrate dehydrogenase (NADP)	1.1.1.42	−4[h,x]	−1	=A	—	—	—	—
Flavokinase	2.7.1.26	−2 } or earlier[y]	0	=A	—	—	—	{Transient 30% drop after birth
FAD-Pyrophosphorylase	2.7.7.2	−2 }	0	=A	—	—	—	
NADH-Dehydrogenase	1.6.99.3	−3[o,z]	−1 or 0	<A	—	—	—	Second rapid rise on third postnatal week[o,z]

* The text refers to these enzymes as cluster a. Signs >A and <A indicate that after reaching the maximum on the indicated day, the levels will decrease and increase, respectively, towards the adult value; further information under "Remarks"; =A indicates that the further change, if any, is insignificant or very slow in comparison to the dramatic rise during early development. Superscripts a through z refer to the following publications: [a] Ballard and Oliver (1963); [b] Jacquot and Kretchmer (1964); [c] Burch (1965–1966); [d] Isselbacher (1957); [e] Coquoin-Carnot and Roux (1962); [f] Burch et al. (1963); [g] Yeung et al. (1967); [h] Vernon and Walker (1968a); [i] Greengard and Dewey (1968); [j] Greengard (1969a); [k] Greengard (1969c); [m] Ballard and Oliver (1962); [n] Yeung and Oliver (1968b); [o] Ballard and Hanson (1967b); [p] Räihä and Suihkonen (1968); [q] Charbonneau et al. (1967); [r] Kennan and Cohen (1959); [s] Greengard (1969b); [t] Makoff and Baldridge (1964); [u] Auerbach and Waisman (1959); [v] Lang (1965); [w] Dallner et al. (1965); [x] Ballard and Hanson (1967a); [y] Rivlin (1969); [z] Dawkins (1959).

syl-transferase, UDPG pyrophosphorylase, and phosphoglucomutase are necessary for the formation of glycogen in fetal liver. Phosphorylase and glucose-6-phosphatase will be essential for the release of free glucose after birth when, for a short period, the stored liver glycogen provides the only source of glucose. Similarly, the urea cycle enzymes will become essential at birth; up to that time the elimination and detoxification of nitrogenous waste products is probably effected by the maternal metabolism. Table I lists several enzymes whose physiological role is equivocal and thus a teleological explanation for their appearance during late fetal life cannot be attempted.

Changes in the cell population of an organ may constitute a reason for the alteration in enzymic pattern. In the case of fetal and neonatal liver this possibility has often been erroneously overemphasized. The concentration of hematopoietic cells in the liver decreases from 50 to 25% during the last 5 days of gestation and becomes insignificant on the fifth postnatal day (Oliver *et al.*, 1963). The corresponding increase in the number of hepatocytes is too small to account for any of the normal or experimentally enhanced changes in enzyme levels (usually well over 100% increases per gram liver in 5 to 48 hours) discussed here and in Section IV.

It should be noted that in Table I several subcellular compartments are represented, which include soluble, mitochondrial, and microsomal enzymes. Thus, one cannot designate the eighteenth to nineteenth day of gestation as being the specific time for major changes in the composition of one of these fractions in preference to the others.

The pituitary, the adrenal cortex (Kitchell and Wells, 1952; Jost, 1953; Roos, 1967), the thyroid (Jost, 1953; Gorbman and Evans, 1943), and the β-cells of the pancreas (Willier, 1955) are known to start to function just before or around the time at which the enzymes listed in Table I begin to accumulate. [131]I uptake into fetal rat thyroid increases rapidly between the seventeenth and twentieth days of gestation and there is some evidence that the fetus secretes thyroid hormone (Feldman *et al.*, 1961). However it is difficult to time exactly the beginning of this function. It may start earlier than suggested by these observations because there is evidence for the presence of fetal thyroid hormone before there is measurable iodine uptake or storage of colloid (Jost, 1954). Adrenal organogenesis occurs in the rat between the twelfth and sixteenth days of gestation; on the fourteenth day the tissue can make corticosterone (Roos, 1967). But on the sixteenth day this capacity appears to be diminished even though the growth of the gland progresses. This pause in secretion corresponds to the beginning of dependence on ACTH, whereas before the seventeenth day the absence of the pituitary does not cause adrenal atrophy. Prior to these recent studies by Roos, Jost (1953) suggested that in mice, too, only during the very last stages of gestation does the pituitary control adrenal differentiation. Similarly, according to Jost (1954) the hypophysis is not necessary for the early development of the thyroid gland. Only later does the pituitary control the intensity of thyroid function. Thus, initially, the "spontaneous" secretion of thyroxine and corticosterone, determined by the synthetic capacity of the gland may influence differentiation. The thyroid gland then becomes subject to trophic control, serving as a part of the centrally regulated endocrine system ready to serve the needs of extrauterine life.

The accumulation of epinephrine in the fetal adrenal gland is apparently controlled by the pituitary. Decapitation of rat fetuses depletes whereas ACTH or cortisol restores both the level of epinephrine and the rise of the activity of phenylethanol amino-N-methyltransferase (Margolis *et al.*, 1966; Parker and Noble, 1967).

The first evidence for the role of fetal endocrine function in the biochemical differentiation of fetal liver was obtained by Jost and coworkers (Jost and Hately, 1949; Jost and Jacquot, 1955). They showed that hypophysectomy of fetal rabbits by decapitation prevents the accumulation of liver glycogen and that the administration of glucocorticoids restores this capacity. Later, it was shown that enzymes necessary for glycogen formation fail to accumulate in fetal rat livers in the absence of glucocorticoid (see Table I). Thus, the correlation between the enzyme levels and the glycogen deposition must be a causal one: normally, the appearance of these enzymes precedes somewhat the accumulation of glycogen (Jacquot and Kretchmer, 1964), and in the fetus deprived of glucocorticoid the formation of both the enzymes and the glycogen is inhibited (see Fig. 2).

In rats, fetal decapitation as well as maternal adrenalectomy is necessary to prevent fetal glycogen formation (Jacquot, 1959). If, in rats, maternal glucocorticoids are transmitted to the fetus, why does the glycogen formation start only after the eighteenth day of gestation? A possible answer is that a different stimulus triggers glycogen formation and the presence of the glucocorticoid is only one of the conditions necessary for the effectiveness of this triggering stimulus. If this is so, if an as yet unknown stimulus acting on the eighteenth day is implicated, then the glucocorticoid could not cause glycogen to accumulate before this time. If, however, the glucocorticoid is the normal trigger, then its earlier administration would cause the premature formation of glycogen. Current studies tend to favor the latter possibility. Figure 3 shows that the administration of hydrocortisone results in significant concentrations of glycogen before the eighteenth day, and that on the nineteenth day the

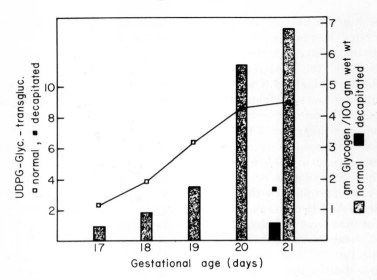

Fɪɢ. 2. The effect of fetal decapitation on liver glycogen synthesis. The values for glycogen (in normal) and for UDPG-glycogen glucosyltransferase (in normal and decapitated) rat fetuses are redrawn from Jacquot and Kretchmer (1964); the glycogen concentration after decapitation is from Jacquot (1959). Decapitations were performed on the eighteenth day of gestation.

concentration is as high as exhibited by control rats on the twenty-first day. The liver is competent to produce glycogen if exposed to glucocorticoid even on the seventeenth day of gestation. Thus, under normal conditions, fetal adrenocortical secretion may be the natural trigger for the formation of enzymes required for glycogen synthesis. The amount of glucocorticoid supplied by the maternal circulation is apparently not enough by itself to trigger glycogen formation.

Fetal decapitation inhibits the accumulation of glucose-6-phosphatase as well as that of enzymes involved in glycogen formation (Jacquot and Kretchmer, 1964). But the underlying cause must be different because the formation of glucose-6-phosphatase in fetal liver is not enhanced by hydrocortisone; in fact, it is partially inhibited (Greengard and Dewey, 1967). Although no attempt has been made to restore the glucose-6-phosphatase activity in decapitated fetuses by thyroxine administration, this hormone may be responsible for the prenatal formation of glucose-6-phosphatase since its administration to fetal rats causes premature increases in activity (Greengard and Dewey, 1968) (see Fig. 4). The response of glucose-6-phosphatase to glucagon, also shown in Fig. 4, will be discussed in the next section, in connection with the second, the early postnatal phase of development of this enzyme (see Table II).

Figure 5 depicts the enhancement of the developmental formation of NADPH dehydrogenase and of one of the urea cycle enzymes, arginase, by an injection of thyroxine to fetal rats. After birth the ability to eliminate nitrogen in the form of urea is essential and it is possible that thyroxine has an important role in preparing the fetus for this function. It is well known that thyroxine promotes the synthesis of urea cycle enzymes in metamorphosing tadpoles (Bennett and Frieden, 1962) in preparation for their terrestrial existence.

The concentration of riboflavin is as high in fetal liver, at least during the last 6 days of gestation, as in newborn or adult liver (Rivlin, 1969). The low concentrations of flavin mononucleotide (FMN) and flavin-adenine dinucleotide (FAD) in fetal liver and their sudden rise around the time of birth can be explained by the developmental formation of

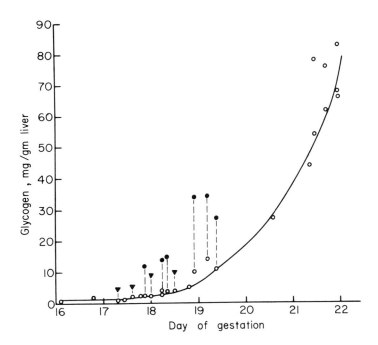

Fig. 3. The premature deposition of glycogen in fetal liver. The solid line illustrates the concentration of glycogen in untreated fetuses. Within 9 additional pregnant rats, fetuses along the uterine horns were injected intraperitoneally alternately with 0.05 ml saline and 60 μg hydrocortisone-acetate in saline 24 (▲) and 48 (●) hours before assay. The dotted lines connect the liver glycogen concentration of experimental fetuses with those of their control littermates (○). Each point is a result of duplciate assays of a pool of 4 to 6 livers. The fetal age is read off a curve of body weight against day of gestation established by Gonzales (1932), which closely agrees with that for our rats.

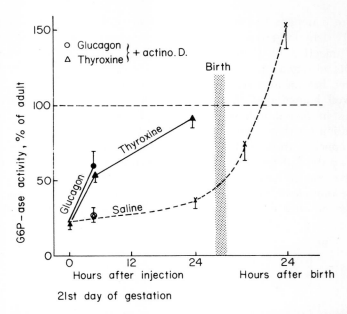

Fig. 4. The enhancement of the developmental formation of glucose-6-phosphatase by thyroxine or glucagon. The broken line indicates the glucose-6-phosphatase levels in normal, or saline-injected developing rats. Within some pregnant rats 2 days before term half of the fetuses were injected with 0.05 mg glucagon, and in other pregnant rats with 3 μg thyroxine in 0.1 ml saline. Glucose-6-phosphatase was assayed in the liver homogenates 5 hours after the injection of glucagon (●) and 5 or 24 hours after the injection of thyroxine (▲). The open symbols refer to the injection of 10 μg actinomycin D simultaneously with the hormones 5 hours before assay. Each point is a mean (±SD) of results with 12 to 30 individual fetal and 5 to 8 individual postnatal livers.

enzymes involved in the synthesis of these nucleotides: flavokinase and FAD pyrophosphorylase reach maximal levels at birth (see Table I). The formation of these enzymes in fetal liver may be initiated by the development of the secretory function of the fetal thyroid gland since hypothyroidism in adult rats is associated with low levels of flavokinase and FAD (Rivlin *et al.*, 1968).

In summary, thyroxine and glucocorticoids have been recognized to be important agents of enzymic differentiation in the late fetal rat livers. This is probably only a beginning and much more information is required about the direct and indirect action of these hormones, and of additional hormones, on the regulation of the level of individual enzymes during this period. Experimental alteration of the rate of formation of the

TABLE II

ENZYME FORMATIONS IN RAT LIVER—NEONATAL PERIOD*

Enzyme	E.C. number (IUB, 1965)	Maximum Reached — Days after birth	Maximum Reached — Relative to Adult (A)	Increase inhibited by:	Premature increase caused by:	Treatment without effect	Remarks
Tyrosine aminotransferase	2.6.1.5	0.5[i,1,2]	>A	Actinomycin[3] Puromycin, ethionine, p-fluorophenylalanine[4] Adrenalectomy,[1] glucose[i]	Premature delivery[4] Glucagon[i] Epinephrine, cAMP[k]	Prenatal hydrocortisone[i,1] Thyroxine[i]	In rabbits premature delivery evokes and postmature birth delays[5]
Serine dehydratase	4.2.1.13	2[i]	<A	Glucose[i]	Glucagon[i]	—	—
Phosphoenolpyruvate carboxylase	4.1.1.32	2[a,b,o]	>A	Glucose, puromycin, actinomycin, p-fluorophenylalanine, ethionine[6]	Premature delivery, glucagon, epinephrine, norepinephrine,[6] Cyclic AMP[k]	—	Rapid decrease to adult level in third week[k]
Glucose-6-phosphatase (see also Table I)	3.1.3.9	4[f,g,7]	—	Ethionine, puromycin, insulin, glucose[8]	Glucagon,[i] thyroxine[i] Cyclic AMP[k]	Adrenalectomy at birth[8]	Increased in rabbits by premature delivery and delayed by postmature birth[9]
Fructose-1,6-diphosphatase	3.1.3.11	5–10[a,h,m]	>A	—	—	—	—
Aspartate aminotransferase (soluble)	2.6.1.1	10[10]	>A	—	—	Cyclic AMP[k]	Decreases to adult level in third week[10]
Formamidase	3.5.1.9	1[2]	>A	—	—	—	—
Fructokinase	2.7.1.4	10[11]	>A	—	—	—	—
Glycolic acid oxidase	1.1.3.1	10[c,v]	=A	—	—	—	—
N-Dimethylase (meperidine), microsomal Pentobarbital hydroxylase, microsomal	} 12			—	Phenobarbital treatment of pregnant dam[12]	—	Shown to be absent at birth but time course of rise not determined

* The text refers to these enzymes as cluster b; they all appear and rise rapidly immediately after birth. Signs >A and <A indicate that after reaching the maximum on the indicated day, the levels will decrease and increase, respectively, toward the adult value; further information under "Remarks"; =A indicates that the further change, if any, is insignificant or very slow in comparison to the dramatic rise during early development.

Superscripts a through z, see Table I; 1 through 12 refer to the following publications: [1] Sereni et al. (1959); [2] Franz and Knox (1967); [3] Greengard et al. (1963); [4] Holt and Oliver (1968); [5] Litwack and Nemeth (1965); [6] Yeung and Oliver (1968a); [7] Kretchmer (1959); [8] Dawkins (1963); [9] Dawkins (1961); [10] Yeung and Oliver (1967); [11] D. G. Walker (1963); [12] Pantuck et al. (1968).

Olga Greengard

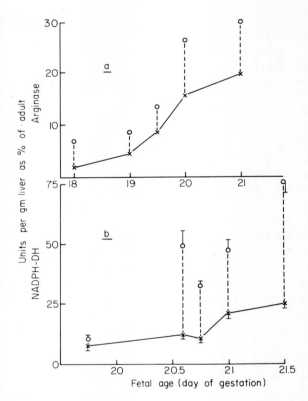

Fig. 5. The effect of thyroxine on the accumulation of arginase (a) and NADPH-dehydrogenase (b) in fetal liver. Within each pregnant rat fetuses were injected alternately with 1 μg thyroxine (○) and vehicle (×). Arginase was assayed 48 hours later in pools of 4 to 6 livers. In a different set of experiments, NADPH-dehydrogenase was assayed in 3 to 6 individual fetal livers (the values are means ±SD) 24 hours after injection. The broken lines connect the enzyme activities of the controls with those of their thyroxine-injected littermates.

majority of enzymes in cluster *a* has not even been attempted nor do we have a complete list of enzymes that belong to this cluster.

IV. NEONATAL PERIOD

Several enzymes that first appear during late fetal life (listed in Table I) continue to undergo a gradual increase in amount after birth. These will not be mentioned in this section because the major stimulus for their formation acted before birth and the reasons for their continued, relatively slow postnatal accumulation have not been sufficiently scrutinized. This section will discuss enzymes (cluster *b*) that exhibit a steep increase in amount on the first postnatal day (Table II).

Before birth most of these enzymes were absent but some were present in low amount. Of course, complete absence of enzyme cannot be proven but such will now be assumed if the activity is in the range of the blank (substratefree) value of the assay and if it does not show any increase during fetal life up to the moment of birth. By these criteria, tyrosine aminotransferase, serine dehydratase, and PEP carboxylase are absent before birth. The first phase of the accumulation of glucose-6-phosphatase occurred prenatally (see Table I and Section III) but, because of its second, neonatal phase of developmental formation, it was necessary to include it also with cluster *b* (Table II). Glucose-6-phosphatase is of historic significance in that it was the first one shown to rise precipitously during the early postnatal hours. This discovery was made by Nemeth (1954) working with guinea pigs. In rabbits, glucose-6-phosphatase rises equally fast upon premature delivery (2 days before term) as upon normal delivery at term (Dawkins, 1961). Furthermore, if pregnancy is prolonged by 3 days with chorionic gonadotrophin, the glucose-6-phosphatase remains low and rises only after the actual postmature delivery. Similarly, tyrosine aminotransferase (Holt and Oliver, 1968) and PEP carboxylase (Yeung and Oliver, 1968a) are evoked by premature delivery. On the other hand, the level of argininosuccinate synthetase, listed in Table I only, was not increased by premature delivery, indicating that its continued rise in rats born at term is *not* due to a stimulus associated by the event of birth.

What stimuli associated with the event of birth promote the formation of a group of enzymes? A clue is provided by experiments showing the inhibitory effect of postnatally administered glucose on the formation of glucose-6-phosphatase (Dawkins, 1963), tyrosine aminotransferase and serine dehydratase (Greengard and Dewey, 1967), and PEP carboxylase (Yeung and Oliver, 1968a). Severe neonatal hypoglycemia is a well-known phenomenon in all species (Dawkins, 1963; Shelley, 1966). The secretion of glucogen is known to be stimulated by hypoglycemia (Unger *et al.*, 1962). We postulated that glucagon, secreted during the neonatal hypoglycemia, may be the stimulus for the synthesis of these enzymes. To prove this, glucagon was administered to fetal rats; 5 hours later their livers exhibited considerable tyrosine aminotransferase (see Fig. 6) and serine dehydratase activity whereas in their littermates (injected with saline only) these activities remained insignificant. Thus, it becomes possible to cause premature enzyme formation in liver by hormone administration by a procedure operationally similar to enzyme induction in adult animals. The difference is, of course, that in adult animals we

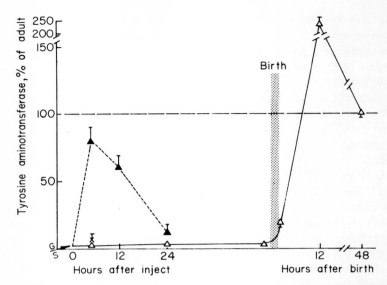

FIG. 6. The premature appearance of tyrosine aminotransferase in fetal rats injected with glucagon. Fetuses in pregnant rats during the last 2 days of gestation were injected alternately with 0.05 mg glucagon in 0.1 ml saline (- -▲- -) and with 0.1 ml saline (—△—), 5, 12, and 24 hours before assay. In additional experiments, some of the fetuses received 10 μg actinomycin simultaneously with glucagon (×). Each value is a mean (brackets = 1 SD) of results obtained with 12 to 18 individual livers; up to the time of birth, livers of untreated or saline-injected rats (—△—) contain no significant tyrosine aminotransferase activity.

are usually causing quantitative changes, rises to above normal values, whereas in these fetal animals the effect, in addition to being quantitatively significant, is qualitative: the appearance of an enzyme and its rise to almost adult levels before the time at which it would normally occur.

As discussed, the effectiveness of administered glucagon in fetal rats was predicted from the fact that normally the appearance of tyrosine aminotransferase coincides with the postnatal hypoglycemia and presumably the natural secretion of glucagon. One may ask: would this effect of glucagon also have been predictable from the facts known about the behavior of tyrosine aminotransferase in adult animals? Glucagon has substantially no effect on the tyrosine aminotransferase of normal adult animals, whereas hydrocortisone, which induces the enzyme (Lin and Knox, 1957), could not prematurely evoke it in fetal rats (Sereni *et al.*, 1959). But we found some years ago that the induction of tyrosine aminotransferase (unlike that of tryptophan oxygenase) by hydrocortisone in adrenalectomized adult rats is greater after starvation or if glucagon is administered together with hydrocortisone (Greengard and Baker, 1966; Csányi *et al.*, 1967). Thus, the answer to the posed question is a qualified yes: sufficient knowledge about the subtleties of regulation of an enzyme in the adult in different physiological states can give us valuable hints about the stimulus that promote the developmental formation of that enzyme. Conversely, experimental interference with a developing animal may show that a stimulus, in this case glucocorticoid, highly effective in the adult may also have some role during development: adrenalectomy partially inhibits (and glucocorticoid replacement restores) the neonatal accumulation of tyrosine aminotransferase (Sereni *et al.*, 1959). Thus, although glucocorticoid does not trigger the appearance of tyrosine aminotransferase, its presence may be one of the conditions necessary for the operation of the normal postnatal trigger.

The administration of glucagon to fetal rats also evoked the appearance of serine dehydratase (Greengard and Dewey, 1967) and enhanced the accumulation of glucose-6-phosphatase (Fig. 4). Glucose-6-phosphatase, like tyrosine aminotransferase, responded to epinephrine as well. During the early postnatal hours, liver glycogen is the only source of glucose that ensures the survival of the newborn and glucose-6-phosphatase is necessary for the release of free glucose. The stored glycogen is depleted within about 12 hours and thereafter gluconeogenesis *de novo* becomes important. This process also requires glucose-6-phosphatase. However, the rate-limiting factor is probably PEP carboxylase, another enzyme that can be prematurely evoked by the administration of glucagon or epinephrine to fetal rats (Yeung and Oliver, 1968a).

One may, therefore, postulate that in normal neonatal animals hypoglycemia and the consequent secretion of glucagon and epinephrine is the common stimulus for the rapid formation of a group of enzymes of great importance to the metabolism of the neonatal animal. For each of these enzymes in cluster *b* the action of glucagon and epinephrine may be mediated through cyclic AMP since this compound can be used instead of the hormones to evoke the premature formation of tyrosine aminotransferase, glucose-6-phosphatase, and PEP carboxylase in fetal rats. It is noteworthy that the actions of cyclic AMP first discovered were *activations* of preformed enzymes, such as phosphorylase, and were therefore demonstrable in cell-free systems. The effects discussed herein occur only *in vivo* and consist of changes in amounts of enzymes whose activity is not influenced by cyclic AMP or $N^6,O^{2'}$-dibutyryl adenosine $3',5'$-cyclic phosphate (dibutyryl cyclic AMP). The mechanism by which cyclic AMP, directly or indirectly, influences specific protein synthesis is of course unknown. Dibutyryl cyclic AMP is unlikely to act by a cofactor-type mechanism (Greengard, 1967) since its action is inhibited by actinomycin and since the three enzymes whose accumulation it is known to promote have entirely different molecular properties, catalytic actions and cofactor requirements.

Glucagon failed to evoke the appearance of tyrosine aminotransferase in fetuses below a certain age. Search for an earlier step in the sequence of the differentiation that renders the liver able to synthesize tyrosine aminotransferase revealed that cyclic AMP, or, more effectively, its dibutyryl derivative (Greengard, 1969a) can evoke the tyrosine amino-transferase in fetuses too young to respond to glucagon or epinephrine (Fig. 7). We thus have a unique experimental situation in which cyclic AMP is effective whereas the hormones that will later act through cyclic AMP are not yet effective. The explanation must be that the capacity to synthesize or concentrate cyclic AMP in response to glucagon or epinephrine develops relatively late during fetal life. The sequence of events that leads to the normal postnatal appearance of enzymes such as tyrosine aminotransferase will be discussed (Section VII) and illustrated later (Fig. 9).

Cofactors or substrates rather than hormones may be the direct stimuli

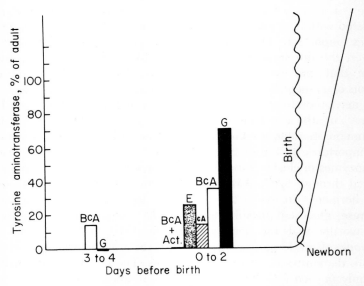

FIG. 7. Agents effective in evoking the appearance of liver tyrosine amino-transferase at two fetal ages. The height of the bars represents the increases in enzyme activity that occur in 5 hours after an injection of 0.05 mg glucagon (G), 0.01 mg epinephrine (E), 0.5 mg cyclic AMP (cA), 0.125 mg dibutyryl cyclic AMP (BcA) without and with 10 μg actinomycin D (BcA + Act). The solid line represents the level of tyrosine aminotransferase in untreated animals; see Fig. 6.

in the postnatal formation of several enzymes although the concentration of these substances may be subject to endocrine regulation. The postnatal accumulation of glycolic acid oxidase may be due to the rapidly progressing rise in the concentration of its cofactor, FMN (Rivlin, 1969). As already discussed in connection with Table I, the enzyme required for the synthesis of FMN develops just before birth, possibly under the influence of the fetal thyroid gland.

Livers of a number of mammalian species at birth are devoid of a variety of microsomal enzyme systems necessary for the metabolism of drugs. Meperidine N-dimethylase and pentobarbital hydroxylase exemplify these. Although the rate of developmental formation of these enzymes, like that of other drug metabolizing enzymes, have not been adequately studied, they are included in Table II because they have been prematurely evoked: treatment of pregnant rats with phenobarbital resulted in newborns with a significant capacity to metabolize pentobarbital and meperidien (Pantuck *et al.*, 1968). Again, it is not known whether phenobarbital affects the formation of these enzyme systems directly or with the aid of endocrine factors.

V. LATE SUCKLING PERIOD

Table III lists enzymes (cluster *c*) whose level rises rapidly around the third week of life. A multiplicity of reasons renders it very difficult to elucidate the stimuli that cause these enzymic changes. First, no new endocrine glands appear at this age but already existing ones probably have become integrated into complex regulatory circuits. Hence it is very difficult to pinpoint a causal relationship between an endocrine and an enzymic event. Second, the enzyme formations must be looked at against a background of changing diets, which in turn influence both the release of hormones (such as insulin, glucagon, and possibly the anti-insulin hormone of the anterior pituitary) and the effect of the released hormones on the enzyme levels.

Unfortunately, not much is known about the changes in the regulation of the secretion of glucagon, insulin, or thyroxine during the weaning period. However, there is a definite change in the functioning of the pituitary–adrenal axis. At the late fetal stage the pituitary can exert corticotrophic stimulation, but after birth this function is dormant and is reestablished approximately 2 weeks later (Levine and Mullins, 1966). There are many examples in the adult rat showing that dietary changes cause enzyme inductions indirectly by stimulating adrenocortical

Olga Greengard

TABLE III

ENZYME FORMATIONS IN RAT LIVER—LATE SUCKLING PERIOD*

Enzyme	E.C. Number (IUB, 1965)	Beginning of Rise: Days after birth	Maximum Reached: Days after birth	Maximum Reached: Relative to Adult (A)	Increase inhibited by:	Premature rise caused by:	Treatment without effect	Remarks
Ornithine aminotransferase	2.6.1.13	13[13,14]	23	=A	Adrenalectomy, estrogen treatment[15]	Triamcinolone[13] Hydrocortisone[15]	—	No increase in adult with triamcinolone[13]
Alanine aminotransferase	2.6.1.2	17[10,16,17]	30	>A	—	Cortisol in first week[16,17]	Cortisol in fetus[17]	—
Tryptophan oxygenase	1.13.1.12	14[a,2]	21	=A	Puromycin[18]	Hydrocortisone but only when enzyme already present[2]	Adrenalectomy, actinomycin[3]	—
Histidine-ammonia-lyase	4.3.1.3	21[b,19]	30	<A	—	—	—	Further rise during puberty particularly in female[19]
Glutamine synthetase	6.3.1.2	12[20]	20	=A	—	—	—	—
Xanthine oxidase	1.2.3.2	12[21]	after 20		—	—	—	Slow rise from 0 to 12 days[21]
Glucokinase	2.7.1.2	15[22]	27	=A	Ethionine, p-fluorophenylalanine, starvation, alloxan diabetes[22]	Repeated doses of hydrocortisone[23]	Insulin, glucose[22]	—
Malate dehydrogenase (NADP)	1.1.1.40	20[b]	30	$\geqq$A[b,x]	Weaning to high protein in solid diet[24]	Weaning, more increase with high glucose diet[24]	—	—
ATP-Citrate lyase	4.1.3.8	20[b,x]	30	=A	—	Weaning, more increase with high glucose diet[24]	—	—
Pyruvate kinase	2.7.1.40	20[b]	30	=A	Weaning to high protein or fat diet[24]	Weaning, more increase with high glucose diet[24]	—	High in fetal but decreases to minimum by 20 days[b]

* The text refers to these enzymes as cluster c. Signs >A and <A indicate that after reaching the maximum on the indicated day, the levels will decrease and increase, respectively, towards the adult value; further information under "Remarks"; =A indicates that the further change, if any, is insignificant or very slow in comparison to the dramatic rise during early development. Superscripts a through z, see Table I; 1 through 24, see Table II; 13 through 24 refer to the following publications: [13] Räihä and Kekomäki (1968); [14] Herzfeld and Knox (1968); [15] Herzfeld and Greengard, 1969; [16] Goetze and Muller (1967); [17] Harding et al. (1961); [18] Nemeth and de la Haba (1962); [19] Feigelson (1968); [20] Wu (1964); [21] Burch et al. (1958); [22] D. G. Walker and Holland (1965); [23] J. B. Walker (1963); [24] Vernon and Walker (1968b)..

secretion or insulin secretion. It is thus possible that many of the enzyme changes we see in the normal weaning rat are composite results of the dietary change and the increased secretion of adrenocortical hormones or insulin in response to the dietary change. The established pituitary–adrenocortical axis may be relevant not only to glucocorticoid secretion but also to the elaboration of catecholamines, which in turn may influence enzyme levels. In the fetal rat, as mentioned earlier, the pituitary controls the formation of epinephrine in the adrenal medulla, as it does in adult rats. But whether this system is also partially dormant during the first two postnatal weeks has apparently not been studied.

Studies on ornithine aminotransferase provide the best evidence for the role of glucocorticoids in promoting enzymic differentiation during the late suckling period. The normal rise in the level of ornithine aminotransferase coincides with the increase in the function of the pituitary–adrenocortical system. The administration of glucocorticoids, which is without effect on the ornithine aminotransferase in adult livers, causes the enzyme to accumulate prematurely, in 1 to 12-day-old rats (Räihä and Kekomäki, 1968). Furthermore, adrenalectomy prevents the normal developmental formation of ornithine aminotransferase (see Table III). The question arises as to why ornithine aminotransferase is not normally formed around the time of birth when the adrenal cortex is functioning and has not yet entered the dormant postnatal period. The explanation may be that estrogen, derived from the mother, is inhibitory: recent experiments show that administered estrogen prevents the normal, postnatal accumulation of ornithine aminotransferase as well as the premature accumulation of the enzyme induced by administered glucocorticoid (Herzfeld and Greengard, 1969).

Hydrocortisone is an inducer of alanine aminotransferase in adult rat liver (Harding *et al.*, 1961). This hormone also caused the enzyme to rise prematurely, before the third week of postnatal life (see Table III). However, tests with rats adrenalectomized during the early suckling period are needed to establish whether glucocorticoids are the natural stimuli that initiate the developmental formation of the enzyme. Another enzyme that appears in the third postnatal week, tryptophan oxygenase, is also inducible by hydrocortisone in the adult rat (Knox and Auerbach, 1955). Its developmental formation was not inhibited by adrenalectomy (Greengard *et al.*, 1963); an injection of hydrocortisone enhanced its rate of accumulation in the third week but did not cause it to appear prematurely (Franz and Knox, 1967). Our notable lack of success to evoke the premature appearance of this well-studied enzyme must be mentioned; neither its substrate nor any hormone tested was effective. In any case, the operation of a hormone-type mechanism was unlikely since actinomycin did not interfere with the developmental formation of the enzyme (Greengard *et al.*, 1963). In adult rat livers, the substrate-induced elevation of the total amount of tryptophan oxygenase is preceded by an increase in the holo- to apotryptophan oxygenase ratio (Greengard and Feigelson, 1961). During its developmental accumulation, too, most of the tryptophan oxygenase is conjugated with its heme prosthetic group (Greengard and Feigelson, 1963), and our inability to evoke it prematurely may be due to insufficient amounts of available heme in the hepatocytes of newborn rats. The level of at least one liver enzyme involved in heme synthesis was shown to be low in 1 to 2-week-old rats (Schröter and Oole, 1966).

Pyruvate kinase and ATP citrate lyase (see Fig. 8) have high activity in fetal rat liver but they are listed only with cluster *c* (Table III) because they rapidly diminish after birth and then start a precipitous rise on about the twentieth postnatal day. There is a correlation between the levels of these enzymes and the capacity for lipid synthesis. This capacity is high in fetal liver, low while the rat is on milk (high fat) but necessary again when weaned to the normal (high carbohydrate) solid diet (Ballard and Hanson, 1967a; Vernon and Walker, 1968a). NADPH malate dehydrogenase, also involved in lipid synthesis, appears for the first time at the age of 20 days. Premature weaning to a solid diet of high glucose content enhances the formation of all three of these enzymes (e.g., Fig. 8), but weaning to a high fat diet has very little or no positive effect. It has been suggested (Vernon and Walker, 1968b) that glucokinase, ap-

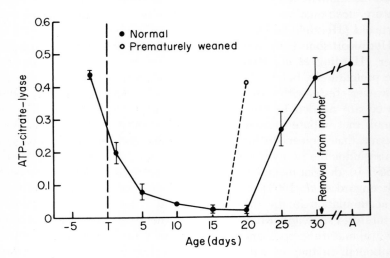

Fig. 8. The developmental formation of ATP-citrate lyase, redrawn from data by Vernon and Walker (1968a,b).

pearing on the sixteenth day, is a prerequisite for the rise of the three enzymes. This suggestion implies that glucokinase catalyzes the formation of lipogenic precursors which then stimulate the synthesis of enzymes, such as NADP malate dehydrogenase and ATP-citrate lyase.

The explanations offered for the rapid rise of several enzymes in Table III are essentially in terms of diet, a changeover from the high-protein, high-fat nature of the milk to the high carbohydrate nature of the solid diet. But in the normal rat the enzyme changes occur *before* the cessation of suckling. For example, rats were removed from the mother on the thirty-first postnatal day but the ATP-citrate lyase began its rise on the twenty-first day (see also Fig. 8). Since the effect cannot precede the cause, any "dietary theory" must be based on the reasonable assumption that the suckling rat, at some time during the second postnatal week, begins to nibble the food destined for the mother. The fact that this variable is not being controlled handicaps greatly our understanding of the stimuli that trigger the accumulation of any of the enzymes in Table III. One might postulate that these enzymes would fall into two groups, those whose rise would be delayed by preventing the premature intake of solid food and those that would rise at the normal time even if the rats were entirely restricted to suckling. The stimulus for the latter group may be an endocrine factor; this possibility has been considered for glucokinase. Insulin is a likely candidate since starvation or alloxan diabetes delay the developmental formation of this enzyme, but it has not been possible to cause glucokinase to appear prematurely by the administration of insulin or glucose (D. G. Walker and Holland, 1965), whereas treatment with large doses of hydrocortisone was somewhat effective (J. B. Walker, 1963a). Conceivably, both insulin and glucocorticoids contribute to the normal developmental formation of glucokinase.

VI. THE PROBLEMS OF THE MECHANISMS OF DEVELOPMENTAL ENZYME FORMATION

The expression of a gene in terms of measurable amounts of a specific, active enzyme depends on a number of conditions that insure, for example, the manufacture and stability of the necessary messenger RNA, its transfer to the cytoplasm, the adequacy of the ribosome, the availability of cofactors, and the stability of the subunits or of the assembled protein molecule, etc. When an enzyme has not yet appeared in the developing organ at least one of these necessary conditions has not been fulfilled. By definition this last step is accomplished by the stimulus, such as a hormone, that finally evokes the enzyme. Precise knowledge of the action of the hormone would reveal the potentiality that was missing; conversely, knowing which reaction was inoperative before the appearance of the enzyme could reveal the mode of action of the hormone. The difficulties that beset current efforts in this direction must be briefly summarized.

Knowledge of the existence of the two mechanisms of enzyme inductions in animal tissues (Greengard, 1967), the hormone type that requires RNA synthesis and the cofactor type that does not, provides only rough guidance to the underlying mechanisms. Experience accumulated so far shows that actinomycin D, which inhibits the hormonal induction of enzymes in the adult animal, also inhibits the hormone-induced premature changes in fetal liver (Greengard, 1969a) (see Figs. 4 and 6). However, it has not yet been possible to detect specific differences in the way the several hormones seem to stimulate RNA synthesis. Thus, there is no explanation for their specificity with respect to the groups of enzymes that they induce. In any case, inhibition by actinomycin merely indicates that there is an RNA-dependent step somewhere in the chain of events. It does not prove that the hormone directly influenced the RNA species specifically related to the induced enzyme. This RNA species may already be available, but the final assembly of our enzyme may await, for example, the generation of a prosthetic group. If the formation of the prosthetic group is hormone-dependent, then actinomycin will still inhibit the synthesis of the enzyme that we actually measure, even though the RNA-requiring step is, in fact, related to the synthesis of another enzyme, one involved in the manufacture of the prosthetic group.

A simple model of one specific interaction between a hormone and the genetic material that results in more enzyme synthesis is clearly unsatisfactory. Any one of the many reactions interposed between the gene and its finished product may be rate limiting. Even for the same enzyme, the limiting step varies with the physiological and developmental states of the animal (Knox *et al.*, 1956; Greengard, 1969a). Thus, the hormone important for the developmental formation of an enzyme may be effective only during a limited period; prior to this period the tissue may not yet be competent to respond to this hormone, and after this period the enzyme may no longer be inducible by the same mechanism.

The competence of a tissue to synthesize an enzyme when exposed to the appropriate regulator develops in a sequential manner. By preventing the appearance of an enzyme through endocrine ablations or dietary deprivations (and with the necessary restitution experiments), one may identify the several factors that contribute to this aspect of differentiation. It is much more complicated to ascertain the temporal hierarchy between these stimuli, i.e., the order in which they contributed to the sequential development of competence. There is even difficulty in identifying the last stimulus of the sequence, the immediate trigger. The hormone whose experimental elimination prevents the appearance of an enzyme is not necessarily the one that normally triggers its formation: we may have merely reduced the availability of a normally nonlimiting factor. On the other hand, the hormone whose administration to the *intact* organism (prior to its normal appearance) evokes the enzyme prematurely may indeed qualify as the natural trigger, i.e., the ultimate stimulus in the sequence. If an earlier stage of development at which this hormone is not yet effective can be determined, this pinpoints the time at which a previous step in the sequence must occur. This approach could lead to the identification of the nature of the penultimate step, of the preceding one, and so on.

A little has been achieved in this respect and one can at least begin to visualize the type of information needed to analyze the sequential development of competence. The scheme in Fig. 9 is based on studies of tyrosine aminotransferase. Except for the part relating to adult animals, it is probably also applicable to a group of enzymes, such as serine dehydratase, glucose-6-phosphatase, or PEP carboxylase that all rise precipitously on the day after birth (see Section IV).

The arrows in Fig. 9 do not imply mechanism but rather a competence to respond to the stimulus (at the origin of the arrow) with an increase in the amount of a substance (pointed at by the arrow). For the purposes of this scheme, dibutyryl cyclic AMP will be considered to be equivalent to cyclic AMP. Four days before birth the enzyme can be evoked only by an injection of dibutyryl cyclic AMP; 2 days before birth it can be

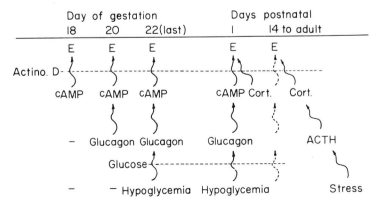

FIG. 9. The sequential development of competence for regulating the level of an enzyme. E = enzyme; cAMP = cyclic AMP; Actin. = actinomycin D; cort. = glucocorticoids.

evoked by either dibutyryl cyclic AMP or glucagon (or epinephrine); and on the last day of gestation it can be evoked by premature delivery, which, like normal birth, results in a period of hypoglycemia. Thus, the capacity to synthesize tyrosine aminotransferase (when exposed to cyclic AMP) is present 4 days before birth, the capacity to raise adequately the concentration of cyclic AMP (when exposed to glucagon or epinephrine) develops during the ensuing 2 days and the ability of the organism to secrete glucagon or epinephrine (when hypoglycemic) is present 1 day before birth. Consequently, the newborn begins to synthesize tyrosine aminotransferase because hypoglycemia can stimulate the secretion of glucagon (or epinephrine), which can cause an increase in the concentration of cyclic AMP, a compound that in turn can initiate the synthesis of the enzyme. This scheme depicting the sequential development of these steps also illustrates that glucose inhibits the normal chain of events if administered *at birth*, whereas actinomycin inhibits equally well the prematurely induced (with glucagon or dibutyryl cyclic AMP) and the normal postnatal accumulation of tyrosine aminotransferase.

The development of the competence for the regulation of tyrosine aminotransferase does not stop at birth. Soon after this event, while the enzyme is still responsive to glucagon, it becomes inducible also by hydrocortisone. Throughout postnatal life the administration of cortisone (or hydrocortisone) can induce four- to tenfeld increases in the amount of liver tyrosine aminotransferase within a few hours. After the age of approximately 2 weeks, when the function of the pituitary–adrenocortical axis is established, tyrosine aminotransferase is also inducible by "stress" (Knox and Auerbach, 1955; Schapiro *et al.*, 1966). By this time, the glucagon pathway has become vestigial (see broken arrows) in normal rats but is still detectable in adrenalectomized rats (see Section IV). As indicated in Fig. 9 by the arrow labeled "cort.," the mechanism by which glucocorticoids act is independent from the one involving cyclic AMP.

Each arrow in Fig. 9 reflects a series of unknown reactions where neither the nature nor the site of action of the immediate stimuli are known. The purpose of the scheme is to illustrate a way in which one can resolve into sequential steps during both prenatal and postnatal differentiation the development of competence of the liver to synthesize an enzyme and to permit its level to be regulated in accordance with physiological requirements.

In adult tissues the levels of individual enzymes rise and fall depending on physiological, endocrine, and nutritional states. If, during development similar mechanisms regulate gene expression, why does differentiation appear to be an essentially irreversible process? The answer formulated by Knox (1961) is that a "long series of individually reversible adaptive changes, each of which alters the adaptability of the system, can also result in essentially irreversible differentiation . . . because of the unlikelihood that all of the steps would be reversed in the appropriate order." The reversibility can however be demonstrated with individual enzymes evoked prematurely: tyrosine aminotransferase, evoked in fetal liver by an injection of glucagon, reaches almost adult levels in 5 hours, disappears by 24 hours (Fig. 5) to emerge again after birth due to the natural neonatal secretion of glucagon. But after this time the effect of the stimulus is no longer completely reversible: additional regulators came into play (e.g., cortisone, Fig. 9) that reenforce the original stimuli, maintain a finite level of the enzyme throughout the postnatal life of the animal, and permit quantitative fluctuations in enzyme amount to fit the physiological requirements.

As mentioned in Section II, the slow change in cell population of developing liver is not significant in relation to the rapid and several-fold rise of enzyme levels reviewed herein. One may ask whether an increase with age in the capacity to form enzyme after induction could be related to an increased proportion of hepatocytes. For example, tyrosine aminotransferase, absent at all fetal ages, is raised by glucagon in 5 hours to 10 and 30 units per gram liver on the twentieth and twenty-second days of gestation, respectively; dibutyryl cyclic AMP, effective already on the eighteenth day of gestation, evokes twice as much tyrosine aminotransferase on the twentieth day (see Fig. 7). These increases cannot be accounted for by the percent of liver volume occupied by hepatocytes, which increases only from about 50 to 70 during this time interval, at the expense of hemotopoietic elements (Oliver *et al.*, 1963). It would appear that the capacity to synthesize tyrosine aminotransferase increased per hepatocyte as well as per gram liver. Thus, quantitative changes in enzyme response to the same stimulus occur with age in addition to the sequential development of the competence to respond to qualitatively different stimuli.

VII. BIOCHEMICAL DIFFERENTIATION OF LIVER IN SPECIES OTHER THAN RAT

Although the information available about enzymic differentiation in livers of mammalian species other than the rat is limited, some comparisons can be made. It appears that the order in which different metabolic functions develop is similar. The capacity for glycogen and urea synthesis, which develops during late fetal life, usually precedes the formation of several enzymes required for gluconeogenesis and amino-acid catabolism that occur in early or late postnatal life. The development of the endocrine glands that influence these aspects of enzymic differentiation presumably also occurs at similar, relative stages of gestation in the different species. However, in considering individual enzymes, the length of gestation and the maturity of the species at birth may greatly influence the time of their formation. In guinea pigs, for example, cytochrome oxidase and succinoxidase accumulate in the liver during the second half of gestation, whereas in the rat, which is less mature at birth, the rapid phase of increase in the level of these enzymes occurs after birth (Flexner *et al.*, 1953; Hamburgh and Flexner, 1957; Potter *et al.*, 1945). Another well-known species difference of this sort is exemplified by tryptophan oxygenase. This enzyme appears in the guinea pig or rabbit immediately after birth but in the rat only in the third week after birth (Nemeth, 1959).

It is important to emphasize those events in enzymic differentiation whose timing is unrelated to the length of the gestation period or the maturity of the organism at birth. These events would be expected to include those that are indispensable for the early adaptation to the extra-uterine environment, a problem that affects each species uniformly. Enzymes required for glycogen synthesis appear in both rats and guinea pigs about 4 days before birth (Jacquot and Kretchmer, 1964; Kornfeld and Brown, 1963). In each mammalian species tested, the amount of glycogen in the liver reaches its peak at term and rapid depletion occurs during the first postnatal hours. Significantly, the developmental formation of glucose-6-phosphatase in the livers of six different mammalian species shows striking similarities (Dawkins, 1966). At the moment of birth the livers of each species contain *some* glucose-6-phosphatase (10 to 30% of the adult level) which rises steeply again during the early postnatal period of glycogen depletion. Consequently, the release of free glucose can start at birth and can then proceed at an increasing rate. Tyrosine aminotransferase is uniformly absent from fetal livers of all species tested and appears within hours after birth in guinea pigs, and rabbits, as well as in rats (Litwack and Nemeth, 1965). One would expect that the stimuli for these analogous steps in enzymic differentiation at birth may also be analogous in the different species. Thus, glucagon (or epinephrine), released by the postnatal hypoglycemia and acting through cyclic AMP, may be responsible in all mammalian species for the accumulation of tyrosine aminotransferase, serine dehydratase, and gluconeogenic enzymes. In fact, the uniform behavior of tyrosine aminotransferase and glucose-6-phosphatase at the time of birth in different species provided one of the clues to the nature of the stimulus: it had to be one related to the cessation of the supply of glucose upon birth, the factor common to each species, species that differ so much in other aspects of maturity. In contrast, the clue to the stimulus that evokes the formation of tryptophan oxygenase, for example, is that species differ strikingly with respect to the time at which the enzyme appears: there must be a "maturity-related" stimulus that exerts its effect at birth in some species and much later in others.

Some events of biochemical differentiation that occur around the time of birth in mammals also occur during the metamorphosis of amphibia. In mammals liver glycogen reaches a peak at birth and in amphibia at the time of the metamorphic climax (Bilewitcz, 1938). Glycogen must serve a similar purpose in the two classes: it is the only source of energy for the newborn mammal and for the tadpole, which refrains from food intake during the last phases of metamorphosis. One reason for testing thyroxine for an effect on glucose-6-phosphatase in fetal rat liver was that the activity of this enzyme increases in tadpole livers during metamorphosis (Bennett and Frieden, 1962). Our results indicate that thyroid hormone initiates the *fetal* synthesis of glucose-6-phosphatase whereas the second, *postnatal* rise of this enzyme is due to hormones whose secretion is stimulated by the hypoglycemia during the early postnatal hours of starvation. Interestingly, in tadpoles, too, glucose-6-phosphatase is subject to dual control: either thyroxine treatment or starvation can raise its level (Bennett and Frieden, 1962); thus, as in mammals, the developmental formation of this enzyme may be initiated by thyroxine and further increased during the period of starvation known to be associated with the last phases of metamorphosis.

The ability to form urea is essential both for mammals after birth and for amphibia when embarking on terrestrial existence. In tadpoles thyroxine evokes the formation of urea cycle enzymes, and we now find that the same hormone prematurely enhances the accumulation of arginase in fetal rat liver. There must be a number of additional, analogous biochemical events that prepare organisms of both classes for the aerobic, nonaquatic environment. Thyroxine may be the common trigger of the early events, those occurring during late fetal life and in the initial stages of metamorphosis; the ensuing enzymic differentiations of the neonatal period and of the late stages of metamorphosis may be promoted by additional, analogous endocrine processes.

VIII. GENERAL OBSERVATIONS

At present our only test as to whether a given gene is functioning or not is the detection of the end product, the specific protein. It is highly questionable to what extent measurements of the synthesis of RNA fractions which are usually isolated, provide biologically significant information about gene expression. For example, we have no way of isolating, recognizing, and quantifying messenger RNA molecules corresponding to a specific protein. Nor do we know how soon will the existence of a messenger RNA species result in the appearance of a protein, since both the half-life of the RNA and the rate of the complex process of protein synthesis vary unpredictably. Thus, when observing increased RNA synthesis we cannot tell which, if any, proteins structures are being transcribed, and whether these proteins are to appear within the next hour, day, or week of development. On the other hand, observations of developmental changes in enzyme patterns and the quantitation of individual enzymes reflect firm biological realities. Further advances with this approach are far from being limited by our inability to analyze the individual chemical steps involved in enzyme synthesis. A limitation probably operates in the reverse direction—more physiological information is required; matching of the enzymes with the physiological stimuli that promote their formation during development will provide the missing information for defining a system in which the molecular mechanism of gene expression can be studied in a biologically meaningful manner. The enzyme studies reviewed here point to a large number of technically feasible investigations *in vivo* that could be profitably pursued.

It is essential to obtain complete, accurate time curves for a larger number of enzymes during development. Natural or induced rises in enzyme activity during development can hardly be evaluated unless they are expressed in relation to the activity of the same enzyme in the adult organ. For many enzymes that have been shown to be absent at some fetal stage and present in adult liver, additional measurements must be taken to ascertain the exact time of their appearance. Such knowledge significantly reduces the number of stimuli that one might suspect are responsible for the appearance of the enzyme. It should be obvious from Sections II and III that birth, for example, is a critical dividing line for the operation of various regulatory factors; in assigning a role to any one of these it is essential to know whether the synthesis of the enzyme is initiated just before or just after birth. The framework used in this review, three clusters of enzyme changes corresponding to three periods in development, was designed to introduce order in the chaotic mass of available information. Because this classification is based on simple facts rather than assumptions about underlying mechanisms, it is open to additions of more enzymes and new clusters, and to further refinement with increasing knowledge about the stimuli that promote enzymic differentiation.

Descending curves of enzymatic activity are as important to the developmental changes in a metabolic state as the ascending ones. Decreases in the levels of several enzymes are associated with each of the three, relatively late stages considered in Sections III to V. The main reason for omitting them from the present review is that none of the stimuli or lack of stimuli responsible for the decrease of any enzyme in the developing liver has so far been identified. Enzymes essential for growth per se would be expected to decrease at even earlier stages of development.

Some of the data reviewed here are relevant to the way in which we can apply knowledge of enzyme regulation in the adult to developmental problems. The quantitative pattern of enzymes as well as the regulatory system evolve in the course of development. Thus, the stimuli that promote the developmental formation of an enzyme may not be important in regulating the level of the same enzyme in the adult animal. There may be traces, however, in the adult animal of the former effectiveness of these hormones apparent in certain modified physiological states. Thus, each fact about the regulation of an enzyme in the adult tissues under altered physiological conditions is of potential value for understanding the stimuli for the normal developmental formation of the same enzyme. Conversely, the elucidation of stimuli that promote enzyme formation in the normal developing organ should suggest novel ideas for approaching the regulation of enzyme levels in adult tissues in abnormal physiological states and in neoplasms with dedifferentiated enzymic patterns.

An important pointer for future studies is the limited, but definite, success achieved by the "premature induction" experiments. A long series of morphological and metabolic events precedes the appearance of every new enzyme in a developing organ. If these events occur in extremely rapid succession it may not be possible to evoke the formation of an enzyme even a few hours before the normal time because the tissue is not ready to respond to the experimental stimulus even if this stimulus is identical to the subsequently acting physiological one. This thought, together with early unsuccessful attempts to evoke the formation of an enzyme prematurely discouraged extensive experimentation in this direction. But it appears that the process of enzymic differentiation is not an unresolvable succession of predestined events—it is possible to alter it in a specific, positive, and physiologically meaningful direction by a single injection of an appropriate hormone. There are periods, as long as several days, when *an* enzyme can be formed "out of step": the proper stimulus can evoke its accumulation to levels normally associated with larger organ size, higher protein content, and a different overall enzymic profile. Going backwards in time, it may be possible to elucidate more and more steps in the sequence of events that are necessary for the eventual expression of the gene. The appearance of an enzyme cannot be explained in terms of a single, magic substance and one crucial moment in the life of the embryo but is the result of a series of events. An approach to studying the sequential development of the competence to regulate the amount of an enzyme was discussed in Section VI.

The possibility of manipulating the course of enzymic differentiation may eventually be of medical, therapeutic significance. That treatment during gestation can produce newborn rabbits and rats with a capacity to metabolize drugs (Pantuck *et al.,* 1968) has already been mentioned in Section IV. Furthermore, we found that fetal rats injected with thyroxine 1 day before term were born with increased levels of glucose-6-phosphatase and NADPH dehydrogenase (Greengard, 1969a). The latter enzyme is believed to be an essential component of the microsomal system that catalyzes the metabolism of drugs and steroids, and it is conceivable that a high level of this enzyme may permit the newborn to detoxify harmful substances. The metabolic consequences of a precociously mature enzyme profile and the possible benefit to prematurely born animals remains to be evaluated.

The developmental formation of only a very few enzymes has so far been experimentally altered; here is a vast area of unexploited possibilities. Many more endocrine and metabolic factors should be tested for their ability to enhance the developmental formation of different series of enzymes involved in various catabolic and anabolic pathways and localized in different subcellular compartments. With this type of information, it may be possible to discern whether a hormone acts on one specific enzyme-forming system or simultaneously on many, whether there is sequential triggering of enzyme formation by metabolites and whether the morphological differentiation of subcellular fractions can be understood in terms of their developing enzyme patterns.

IX. BRIEF SUMMARY

The enzymic pattern characteristic of adult liver evolves in a stepwise fashion. New enzymes emerge in clusters during the late fetal, the neonatal, and the late suckling periods. Each of these stages is associated with endocrine changes that may be causally related to the formation of these three clusters of enzymes. Experiments demonstrating such causal relationships between single enzymes and individual hormones have been reviewed. These consist of the premature evocation of appropriate enzymes by an injection of hormones such as thyroxine, glucagon, and hydrocortisone, or the elimination of the expected emergence of enzymes by endocrine ablations. In addition to the stepwise emergence of different enzymes under a succession of hormonal and nutritional influences, the competence of the liver to regulate the level of any one enzyme develops sequentially. The early part of this sequence culminates in the first appearance of the enzyme; subsequent changes in the course of development may eliminate the responsiveness to certain stimuli and enable the enzyme to respond to new regulators.

ACKNOWLEDGMENTS

The author would like to thank Dr. W. E. Knox for criticism of the manuscript and valuable suggestions. Thanks are due to Mrs. M. A. Lunetta and Mrs. N. S. Taylor for preparation of the manuscript. Experimental work by the author presented in this article was supported by United States Public Health Service Grant CA 08676 from the National Cancer Institute of the National Institutes of Health, and by United States Atomic Energy Commission Contract AT(30-1)-3779 with the New England Deaconess Hospital.

REFERENCES

Auerbach, V. H., and Waisman, H. A. (1959). *J. Biol. Chem.* **234**, 304.
Ballard, F. J., and Hanson, R. W. (1967a). *Biochem. J.* **102**, 952.
Ballard, F. J., and Hanson, R. W. (1967b). *Biochem. J.* **104**, 866.
Ballard, F. J., and Oliver, I. T. (1962). *Nature* **195**, 498.
Ballard, F. J., and Oliver, I. T. (1963). *Biochim. Biophys. Acta* **71**, 578.
Bennett, T. P., and Frieden, E. (1962). *Comp. Biochem.* **4**, 483–556.
Bilewitcz, S. (1938). *Biochem. Z.* **297**, 379.
Burch, H. B. (1965–1966). *Biol. Neonatorum* [N.S.] **9**, 176.
Burch, H. B., Lowry, O. H., de Gubareff, T., and Lowry, S. R. (1958). *J. Cellular Comp. Physiol.* **52**, 503.
Burch, H. B., Lowry, O. H., Kuhlman, A. M., Skerjance, J., Diamant, E. J., Lowry, S. R., and von Dippe, P. (1963). *J. Biol. Chem.* **238**, 2267.
Charbonneau, R., Roberge, A., and Berlinguet, L. (1967). *Can. J. Biochem.* **45**, 1427.
Coquoin-Carnot, M., and Roux, J. M. (1962). *Compt. Rend. Soc. Biol.* **156**, 442.
Csányi, V., Greengard, O., and Knox, W. E. (1967). *J. Biol. Chem.* **242**, 2688.
Dallner, G., Siekevitz, P., and Palade, G. E. (1965). *Biochem. Biophys. Res. Commun.* **20**, 135.
Dawkins, M. J. R. (1959). *Proc. Roy. Soc.* **B150**, 284.
Dawkins, M. J. R. (1961). *Nature* **191**, 72.
Dawkins, M. J. R. (1963). *Ann. N. Y. Acad. Sci.* **111**, 203.
Dawkins, M. J. R. (1966). *Brit. Med. Bull.* **22**, 27.
Feigelson, M. (1968). *J. Biol. Chem.* **243**, 5088.

Feldman, J. D., Vazquez, J. J., and Kurtz, S. M. (1961). *J. Biophys. Biochem. Cytol.* **11**, 365.

Flexner, L. B., Belknap, E. L., and Flexner, J. B. (1953). *J. Cellular Comp. Physiol.* **42**, 151.

Franz, J. M., and Knox, W. E. (1967). *Biochemistry* **6**, 3464.

Goetze, T., and Müller, K. P. (1967). *Acta Biol. Med. Ger.* **18**, 351.

Gonzales, A. W. A. (1932). *Anat. Record* **52**, 117.

Gorbman, A., and Evans, H. M. (1943). *Endocrinology* **32**, 113.

Greengard, O. (1967). *Enzymol. Biol. Clin.* **8**, 81.

Greengard, O. (1969a). *Science* **163**, 891.

Greengard, O. (1969b). *Advan. Enzyme Regulation* **7**, 283.

Greengard, O. (1969c). *Biochem. J.* **115**, 19.

Greengard, O., and Baker, G. T. (1966). *Science* **154**, 1461.

Greengard, O., and Dewey, H. K. (1967). *J. Biol. Chem.* **242**, 2986.

Greengard, O., and Dewey, H. K. (1968). *J. Biol. Chem.* **243**, 2745.

Greengard, O., and Feigelson, P. (1961). *J. Biol. Chem.* **236**, 158.

Greengard, O., and Feigelson, P. (1963). *Ann. N. Y. Acad. Sci.* **111**, 227.

Greengard, O., Smith, M. A., and Acs, G. (1963). *J. Biol. Chem.* **238**, 1548.

Hamburgh, M., and Flexner, L. B., (1957). *J. Neurochem.* **1**, 279.

Harding, H. R., Rosen, F., and Nichol, C. A. (1961). *Am. J. Physiol.* **201**, 271.

Herrmann, H., and Tootle, M. L. (1964). *Physiol. Rev.* **44**, 289.

Herzfeld, A., and Greengard, O. (1969). *J. Biol. Chem.* **244**, 4894.

Herzfeld, A., and Knox, W. E. (1968). *J. Biol. Chem.* **243**, 3327.

Holt, P. G., and Oliver, I. T. (1968). *Biochem. J.* **108**, 333.

Isselbacher, K. J. (1957). *Science* **126**, 652.

Jacquot, R. (1959). *J. Physiol. (Paris)* **51**, 655.

Jacquot, R., and Kretchmer, N. (1964). *J. Biol. Chem.* **239**, 1301.

Jost, A. (1953). *Recent Progr. Hormone Res.* **8**, 379.

Jost, A. (1954). *Cold Spring Harbor Symp. Quant. Biol.* **19**, 167.

Jost, A., and Hatley, J. (1949). *Compt. Rend. Soc. Biol.* **143**, 146.

Jost, A., and Jacquot, R. (1955). *Ann. Endocrinol. (Paris)* **16**, 849.

Kennan, A. L., and Cohen, P. P. (1959). *Develop. Biol.* **1**, 511.

Kitchell, R. L., and Wells, L. Y. (1952). *Endocrinology* **50**, 83.

Knox, W. E. (1961). *In* "Synthesis of Molecular and Cellular Structure" (Society for the Study of Development and Growth, Symp. No. 19, Brandeis Univ., 1960) (D. Rudnick, ed.), pp. 13–33. Ronald Press, New York.

Knox, W. E., and Auerbach, V. H. (1955). *J. Biol. Chem.* **214**, 307.

Knox, W. E., Auerbach, V. H., and Lin, E. C. C. (1956). *Physiol. Rev.* **36**, 164.

Kornfeld, R., and Brown, D. H. (1963). *J. Biol. Chem.* **238**, 1604.

Kretchmer, N. (1959). *Pediatrics* **23**, 606.

Lang, C. A. (1965). *Biochem. J.* **95**, 365.

Levine, S., and Mullins, R. F. (1966). *Science* **152**, 1585.

Lin, E. C. C., and Knox, W. E. (1957). *Biochim. Biophys. Acta* **26**, 85.

Litwack, G., and Nemeth, A. M. (1965). *Arch. Biochem. Biophys.* **109**, 316.

Makoff, R., and Baldridge, R. C. (1964). *Biochim. Biophys. Acta* **90**, 282.

Margolis, F. L., Roffi, J., and Jost, A. (1966). *Science* **154**, 275.

Moog, F. (1965). *In* "The Biochemistry of Animal Development" (R. Weber, ed.), Vol. 1, pp. 307–365. Academic Press, New York.

Nemeth, A. M. (1954). *J. Biol. Chem.* **208**, 773.

Nemeth, A. M. (1959). *J. Biol. Chem.* **234**, 2921.

Nemeth, A. M., and de la Haba, G. (1962). *J. Biol. Chem.* **237**, 1190.

Oliver, I. T., Blumer, W. F. C., and Witham, I. J. (1963). *Comp. Biochem. Physiol.* **10**, 33.

Pantuck, E., Conney, A. H., and Kuntzman, R. (1968). *Biochem. Pharmacol.* **17**, 1441.

Parker, L. N., and Noble, E. P. (1967). *Proc. Soc. Exptl. Biol. Med.* **216**, 734.

Potter, V. R., Schneider, W. C., and Liebl, G. J. (1945). *Cancer Res.* **5**, 21.

Räihä, N. C. R., and Kekomäki, M. P. (1968). *Biochem. J.* **108**, 521.

Räihä, N. C. R., and Suihkonen, J. (1968). *Biochem. J.* **107**, 793.

Rivlin, R. S. (1969). *Am. J. Physiol.* **216**, 979.

Rivlin, R. S., Mendendez, C., and Langdon, R. G. (1968). *Endocrinology* **83**, 461.

Roos, T. B. (1967). *Endocrinology* **81**, 716.

Schapiro, S., Yuwiller, A., and Geller, E. (1966). *Science* **152**, 1642.

Schröter, W., and Oole, A. (1966). *Nature* **211**, 1406.

Sereni, F., Kenney, F. T., and Kretchmer, N. (1959). *J. Biol. Chem.* **234**, 609.

Shelley, H. J. (1966). *Brit. Med. Bull.* **22**, 34.

Unger, R. H., Eisentraut, A. M., McCall, M. S., and Madison, L. I. (1962). *J. Clin. Invest.* **41**, 682.

Vernon, R. G., and Walker, D. G. (1968a). *Biochem. J.* **106**, 321.

Vernon, R. G., and Walker, D. G. (1968b). *Biochem. J.* **106**, 331.

Walker, D. G. (1963). *Biochem. J.* **87**, 576.

Walker, D. G., and Holland, G. (1965). *Biochem. J.* **97**, 845.

Walker, J. B. (1963). *Advan. Enzyme Regulation* **1**, 151.

Willier, B. H. (1955). *In* "Analysis of Development" (B. H. Willier, P. A. Weiss, and V. Hamburger, eds.), pp. 574–619. Saunders, Philadelphia, Pennsylvania.

Wu, C. (1964). *Arch. Biochem. Biophys.* **106**, 394.

Yeung, D., and Oliver, I. T. (1967). *Biochem. J.* **103**, 744.

Yeung, D., and Oliver, I. T. (1968a). *Biochem. J.* **108**, 325.

Yeung, D., and Oliver, I. T. (1968b). *Biochemistry* **7**, 3231.

Yeung, D., Stanley, R. S., and Oliver, I. T. (1967). *Biochem. J.* **105**, 1219.

CHAPTER 3

Regulation of Protein Synthesis by Growth and Developmental Hormones

J. R. Tata

I. INTRODUCTION

It can be said that since the publication of *Molecular Actions of Hormones* (Litwack and Kritchevsky, 1964) there have been no major conceptual advances in our understanding of hormonal control of protein synthesis. What has happened during the last 5 years is the consolidation of the tenous or reappraisal of the overoptimistic conclusions drawn from the work done in the early sixties. There are many chapters in *Molecular Actions of Hormones* in which the control of messenger RNA synthesis has been suggested as an important mechanism of hormone action. The reason for a reappraisal of some concepts is necessitated by the evolution of changes in our thinking of the question of regulation of protein synthesis in higher organisms in general.

There is good agreement among molecular biologists that the rapid modulation of messenger RNA synthesis as established in microbial enzyme synthesis is unlikely to be a key or sole mechanism for regulating protein synthesis in animal cells. It is now accepted that more than one type of mechanism must be involved at both the transcriptional and translational sites, many of which are unique to nucleated cells (see Tomkins and Ames, 1967). It is in the light of these possible mechanisms of higher organisms that have been recently postulated, and summarized here, that I wish to discuss the question of how hormones influence protein synthesis and the importance of these mechanisms. Because of the necessity of conserving a link between biochemical and physiological actions only growth and developmental hormones will be considered. Much of the experimental work described has been performed in our laboratory although it is largely used to emphasize phenomena also observed by other workers that are common features of responses evoked by most growth and developmental hormones in their target cells.

II. REGULATORY MECHANISMS OF PROTEIN SYNTHESIS IN ANIMAL CELLS

Numerous sites of control of protein synthesis in animal cells have been proposed in the last 5 years and this number is bound to increase as more unforeseen phenomena crop up. Some of the currently popular ones are summarized in Table I. The evidence that any of these mechanisms may be rate-limiting in protein synthesis *in vivo* is often circumstantial. However, we shall consider the following mechanisms in particular because of their relevance to hormone action.

A. NUCLEAR RESTRICTION OF RNA

A large amount of the RNA synthesized in animal cells is ribosomal RNA with the result that much of the rapidly labeled RNA is ribosomal

TABLE I

SOME MECHANISMS PROPOSED FOR THE REGULATION OF NEW OR PREFERENTIAL
ENZYME SYNTHESIS IN ANIMAL CELLS

1. DNA synthesis
    a. New cell population
    b. Gene "amplification"
2. Gene activation
    a. New genes unmasked
    b. Increased rate of transcription
3. Messenger RNA utilization
    a. Selective transfer from nucleus to cytoplasm
    b. Cytoplasmic stability and activation
4. Regulation of translation
    a. Polypeptide chain assembly and release
    b. Polysome deployment and cell structure, attachment to membranes
5. Regulation of degradation of proteins

precursor RNA but not mRNA. It has also been established that a substantial amount of RNA synthesized in the nucleus is rapidly turning
over, has an extremely high molecular weight (60–120 S), and is heterodisperse. It is not a precursor of messenger or any other cytoplasmic RNA
(Harris, 1964; Attardi *et al.*, 1964; Scherrer and Marcaud, 1969). The
function of this giant, labile nuclear RNA is not known, but some preliminary reports suggest that it may be of some importance during the
process of growth or enzyme induction in cells of higher organisms (see
Scherrer and Marcaud, 1969; Kijima and Wilt, 1969). However before
this could be ascertained it is important to know if the heterodisperse
RNA, which is also known to hybridize very rapidly with DNA, is made
on unique DNA sequences (as much of messenger RNA would be expected to be) or on repeating sequences that are now known to exist in
most animal cells (Britten and Kohne, 1968). Recent DNA–RNA hybridization studies have shown that only a fraction of the species of RNA
present in the nucleus is present in the cytoplasm, but the mechanism
of this selective restriction of RNA to the nucleus remains unknown
(Georgiev, 1966; Shearer and McCarthy, 1967).

B. NUCLEAR–CYTOPLASMIC RNA TRANSFER

The transfer of RNA from the nucleus to the cytoplasm is a process
that requires the formation and maturation of ribonucleoprotein particles.
From experiments with inhibitors of RNA and protein synthesis it has
been concluded that continued synthesis of both RNA (Tamaoki and
Mueller, 1965) and protein (Higashi *et al.*, 1968) is essential for the

processing and transfer of RNA from the nucleus to the cytoplasm. Two transfer mechanisms have been suggested. One is that mRNA enters into the cytoplasm as a complex with subribosomal particles or in combination with protein only, both of which may then be directly assembled into polysomes (McConkey and Hopkins, 1965; Henshaw *et al.*, 1965). The other possibility is that free messenger does not complex with ribosomal precursors but that it is released into the cytoplasm as ribonucleoprotein particles, also called "informosomes" (see Spirin, 1969), and which are then somehow incorporated into polysomes. The role of the protein associated with mRNA would be to modulate the activity of the template. Such particles have been detected both in the nucleus and in the cytoplasm (Samarina *et al.*, 1968; Perry and Kelly, 1968; Henshaw, 1968). The relevance of the process of nuclear–cytoplasmic transfer of RNA to the question of hormone action is that the speed of response to growth and developmental hormones would be determined by the rate at which such ribonucleoprotein particles could be generated. It is known that RNP particles, whether ribosomal or "informosomal" have to mature within the nucleus but very little is known about the conditions governing the synthesis and interaction of proteins necessary for the continuous generation of the particles.

C. Structural Requirement for Protein Synthesis

It is well known that free polyribosomes with endogenous or synthetic messenger will effect the incorporation of amino acids into protein. However, in intact cells it seems that some form of structural requirement is involved in the synthesis of proteins, mainly involving binding of polysomes to membranes of the endoplasmic reticulum (Campbell, 1965; Hendler, 1968). It is of some interest that the latter are themselves being continuously formed and broken down according to the demands for protein synthesis (Siekevitz *et al.*, 1967; Tata, 1968a). Unfortunately, so far, much of the work done on the proliferation of the endoplasmic reticulum has been carried out on predominantly protein-secreting tissues such as the liver and pancreas. The well-known participation of both the rough and smooth endoplasmic reticulum (see Palade, 1966) in the process of transport of secretory proteins has therefore tended to mask possible other roles for the attachment of ribosomes to endoplasmic membranes, especially during growth. However, it is important to note that in bacteria and nonsecretory animal cells the attached ribosomes appear to be functionally very active in intact cells (Hendler, 1968; Andrews and Tata, 1968). One possible significance of the nonsecretory aspect of ribosome-membrane attachment will be discussed later (see page 120).

III. HORMONES AND PROTEIN SYNTHESIS

Most tissues in higher animals are to some degree dependent on hormones for their normal growth and development. Until recently the most prevalent explanation of hormone action was in terms of a direct hormone–enzyme interaction resulting in the modification of enzymic activity (see Tepperman and Tepperman, 1960). The classical work from Knox's laboratory on the rapid induction of adaptive enzymes upon the administration of steroid hormones (see Knox *et al.,* 1956) however, later led to the acceptance of the idea that a selective regulation of synthesis of enzymes or proteins could explain both the growth-promoting and metabolic actions of hormones (Tata, 1964). Although there is good evidence that many metabolic effects of hormones are independent of inductive processes (Hechter and Halkerston, 1964) there is no doubt that processes of growth and development have an absolute requirement for a *de novo* synthesis of specific proteins. For this reason, I shall mainly restrict this discussion of hormonal control of protein synthesis to hormones with pronounced growth-promoting and developmental properties. Because many of the phenomena to be described require a long lag period to be manifested after hormone administration I shall not be dealing with the problem of initial site of action, which may be remote from those directly concerned with protein synthesis.

Before dealing with the question of protein synthesis, however, it is well worth considering the following features of hormone action.

(a) Most hormones exhibit multiple actions, some hormones regulating both growth or development and a variety of metabolic functions in adult tissues. This multiplicity raises the question, as yet unanswered, of whether the hormone has a single site of action leading to all the different actions or multiple sites of actions for each of the major effects.

(b) There is a high degree of tissue or cell specificity of response to hormones. This specificity may arise from the presence of the right receptor molecules in those cells that have become dependent on hormones for their growth or function. Therefore whether or not a response is evoked and the type of response depend as much on the target tissue as on the hormone provoking it.

(c) The same tissue may be dependent on or responsive to more than one growth-promoting hormone. Conversely, different tissues of an organism may respond differently to the same hormone (see Barrington, 1964; Bern and Nicoll, 1968). The diversity of enzymes synthesized in different tissues of anuran larvae during thyroid-hormone-induced metamorphosis is a good example of this feature.

(d) Most growth and developmental hormones are active at extremely low concentrations; at high doses they may be toxic or provoke other effects. Each hormone also has a very characteristic lag period before provoking growth, and therefore the biochemical response studied should fit into this lag period if it is to bear any causal significance.

A. HORMONES AND RNA SYNTHESIS

It is now quite well established that growth and developmental hormones, when administered precociously or to animals experimentally deprived of them, markedly affect the protein synthesizing activity of their target cells (see Korner, 1965a; Mueller, 1965; Williams-Ashman *et al.,* 1964; Tata, 1964, 1967a). It is also known that the large majority of growth-promoting hormones, when administered *in vivo,* markedly affect protein synthesis *in vivo* or *in vitro* at the level of the ribosome but fail to influence amino acid incorporation when added *in vitro* to ribosomes from their target cells (see Korner, 1965a; Tata, 1967a). This finding prompted investigations of RNA metabolism and soon led to observations that RNA synthesis in target cells is very sensitive to growth and developmental hormones, and experiments with inhibitors of RNA synthesis revealed that part of the RNA synthesized under hormonal influences is essential for the biological expression of hormonal activity (Tata, 1966a). Even before these observations were made, it had been suggested that hormones may control protein synthesis by acting as gene derepressors, much in the same way as microbial protein synthesis is regulated via messenger RNA (mRNA) synthesis (see Karlson, 1963; Sekeris, 1967). However, in recent years it has become quite clear that protein synthesis in nucleated animal cells may be regulated by many processes not directly associated with mRNA transcription (see N. Cohen, 1966; Tomkins and Ames, 1967; Tomkins and Geleherter, Vol. 2).

The effect of hormones on RNA synthesis has been studied in two ways: (1) by following the incorporation of radioactive precursors into nuclear RNA *in vivo* following hormonal stimulation *in vivo;* and (2) by examining the effect of hormones administered *in vivo* or added *in vitro* on isolated nuclei or chromatin.

1. Nuclear RNA Synthesis in Vivo

A rapid stimulation of nuclear RNA synthesis in the target cells is now a well-known feature of the administration of growth and developmental hormones to immature animals or in animals in which the endogenous hormone was experimentally eliminated. The relatively rapid effect on RNA synthesis, anticipating that on protein synthesis has been observed in a variety of hormone-induced growth systems (see Tata, 1966a, 1967a; Sekeris, 1967; Hamilton, 1968). This feature is illustrated in Fig. 1 for the fast-acting estrogen, as well as for the slower effects of thyroid hormone. A stimulation of synthesis of rapidly labeled nuclear RNA of the uterus can be observed within minutes after the administration of estrogen and the relatively delayed stimulation by thyroid hormone is still one of its earliest actions (Means and Hamilton, 1966; Hamilton *et al.,* 1968; Tata and Widnell, 1966). When studying RNA synthesis *in vivo* it is important to distinguish between the possible rapid changes in the uptake of the labeled precursor or in the size of the precursor pool and a true net synthesis of RNA in the initial phase of hormone action. Almost every hormone, growth promoting or not, is known to have some rapid influence on permeability barriers for nucleotides, sugars, and amino acids (see Hechter and Halkerston, 1964). Means and Hamilton (1966), while detecting a very rapid increase in the incorporation of ^{3}H-uridine into the rapidly labeled nuclear RNA of uterus of ovariectomized rats, found that the action was also accompanied by an enhanced rate of entry of the labeled precursor into the tissue. Recently we performed some experiments to look for a possible early effect of thyroid hormone on uptake of labeled precursors for RNA that might possibly lead to only an apparent increase in specific activity of RNA. As can be seen in Fig. 1b it was indeed found that a part or all of the very early stimulation of RNA synthesis *in vivo* could be accounted for by an enhanced uptake of ^{14}C-labeled orotic acid caused by tri-iodothyronine administration. When corrections based on changes in acid-soluble radioactivity were made in the specific activity of nuclear RNA, the time-course of stimulation of nuclear RNA synthesis *in vivo* approached that for RNA polymerase activity. The latter activity assayed *in vitro* of course is independent of any hormonal effects on changes in permeability toward the precursors of RNA or their availability. Similar results have been obtained by Yu and Feigelson (1969) in studying the stimulation of nuclear RNA synthesis caused by hydrocortisone. Taking this effect into consideration, the stimulation of nuclear RNA synthesis by hormones is still a real one and it precedes by several hours sustained elevation of the protein synthesizing capacity of cytoplasmic ribosomes.

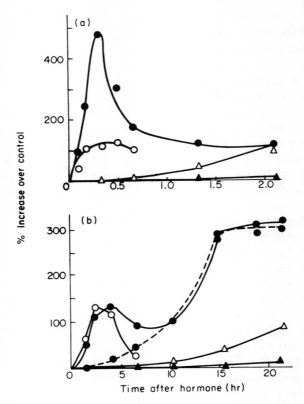

F IG. 1. Time course of stimulations of specific activity of nuclear RNA labeled
in vivo and RNA synthesis by isolated nuclei in (a) the uterus of ovariectomized
rats after a single injection of estradiol-17β and (b) the liver of the thyroidectomized rat following a single injection of 3,3′,5-triiodothyronine. Labeling *in vivo*
was achieved by 2–10-minute pulses of (a) ³H-uridine and (b) ¹⁴C-orotic acid. ●,
rapidly labeled nuclear RNA (dashed line represents values obtained after correcting
for the increase in acid-soluble fraction); △, RNA polymerase assayed at low ionic
strength (product mainly ribosomal RNA); ▲, RNA polymerase assayed at high
ionic strength (product mainly DNA-like RNA). Note the differences in the time
scales for the two hormones. Curves derived from data of Hamilton *et al.* (1968)
and Tata and Widnell (1966). (○) radioactivity in acid-soluble fraction

2. RNA Synthesis in Vitro

Evidence for the regulation of RNA synthesis independent of hormonal
effects on precursor pools can be demonstrated by a stimulated RNA
polymerase activity in isolated nuclear preparations or when chromatin
template efficiency is measured (Tata and Widnell, 1966; Widnell and

Tata, 1966a; Hamilton *et al.*, 1968; Barker and Warren, 1966; Dahmus and Bonner, 1965; Liao *et al.*, 1966a; Kim and Cohen, 1966). Table II shows that hormonal stimulation of the capacity of isolated nuclei or chromatin to synthesize, or prime the synthesis of RNA *in vitro* is manifested after an increase in nuclear RNA *in vivo* has taken place. Another interesting feature shown in Table II for a variety of hormones is that the response of RNA polymerase assayed at low ionic strength was, in every instance, more rapid and more pronounced than when the polymerase was assayed at high ionic strength or when the isolated chromatin was transcribed by a bacterial polymerase. The significance of this finding lies in the fact that the product of the first reaction is rich in ribosomal RNA and that of the other two in DNA-like or messenger RNA (Widnell and Tata, 1966b; Marushige and Bonner, 1966). It means that the transcription of rRNA cistrons is more sensitive to hormonal stimulus for growth than that of other cistrons.

There have been reports on the ability of hormones to stimulate RNA synthesis directly when added to nuclei or chromatin *in vitro* (Sekeris, 1965, 1967; Beato *et al.*, 1968; Ohtsuka and Koide, 1969). This is particularly reported with steroid hormones such as cortisol, testosterone, estrogen, and ecdysone. To some extent, attempts to demonstrate a direct action of steroid hormones have been encouraged by the observation that these hormones are often found to be localized in high concentrations in nuclei following their administration *in vivo* (Wilson and Loeb, 1965; Karlson *et al.*, 1964; King *et al.*, 1965; Mangan *et al.*, 1968; Stumpf, 1969). However, most workers who have tried have failed to observe a direct effect of hormones on RNA synthesis by isolated nuclei. In those instances where an effect has been demonstrated the conditions (nucleoside or nucleotide requirements, preparation of nuclei, magnitude of the effect, concentration of hormone) necessary to produce it are so special as to make its relevance to the hormonal stimulation of RNA synthesis *in vivo* very restricted. Suggestions have been made about the possible sites in the nuclear complex, such as interaction with DNA, histones, RNA polymerase, but by and large we still do not know the mechanism by which hormones influence nucleic acid synthesis *in vitro* or *in vivo*.

3. *Nature of RNA Synthesized under Hormonal Influence*

Much work has been done over the last 5 or 6 years on the nature of RNA, whose synthesis is preferentially influenced by hormones (see Tata, 1966a; Korner, 1965a; Hamilton, 1968). All the classical techniques for extraction and characterization of RNA have been used, especially sucrose gradient analysis, base analysis, differential extractibility, template

TABLE II

LAG PERIOD AND MAXIMUM STIMULATION OF NUCLEAR RNA SYNTHETIC CAPACITY[a]

Hormone[b]	Target	RNA labeled in vivo[d]	Lag period (time) and maximal stimulation (%)[c]		
			RNA polymerase, low ionic strength	RNA polymerase, high ionic strength	Chromatin activation
Estrogen	Rat uterus	2–10 min., 500%	1 hr, 150%	24 hr, 50%	2 hr, 70%
	Chick oviduct	—	24 hr, 1600%	24 hr, 1100%	—
Progesterone	Chick oviduct	—	—	12 hr, 500%	—
Growth hormone	Rat liver	1 hr, 50–100%	2 hr, 80%	No effect	—
	Rat muscle	—	18 hr, 50%	18 hr, 50%	Inhibition
Hydrocortisone	Rat liver	1 hr, 300%	2–4 hr, 75%	No effect	4 hr, 30%
Testosterone	Rat prostate	90 min., 300–500%	2 hr, 120%	20%	No effect
	Seminal vesicles	1 hr, 450–600%	2–3 hr, 180%	10%	—
Thyroid hormone	Rat liver	3 hr, 350%	12 hr, 200%	24 hr, 50%	4 days, 50%
	Tadpole liver	8 hr, 600%	—	—	—
Insulin	Rat liver	30 min., 200%	2 hr, 150%	90%	—

[a] Measured in different ways after hormone administration in vivo.

[b] Hormones administered to immature animals or animals made hormone-deficient.

[c] Lag period is the time elapsed between hormone administration and a 10% stimulation of RNA synthesis. Stimulation is expressed as percent increase above control levels.

[d] For estrogen, hydrocortisone, and triiodothyronine, data are available on the extent to which the incorporation of the labeled precursor represents a net synthesis of RNA or may be due to specific activity changes in the acid-soluble components.

activity, electrophoresis, and hybridization to DNA. Every technique has its own particular disadvantage and it is best to assess the nature of RNA synthesized from the results of several different methods. For example DNA-like RNA in the nucleus is not likely to be mRNA or that 45 S RNA and the heterodisperse DNA-like RNA may be superimposed on density gradients.

Briefly, the synthesis of all classes of RNA is affected by hormone administration or withdrawal (Tata, 1966a, 1967a; Greenman *et al.*, 1966; Hamilton, 1968). The earlier claims or hopes of a selective modulation by hormones of specific messenger RNA (Karlson, 1963; Sekeris, 1965) have not been held up. At some stage of hormonal control of specific protein synthesis, as in hormone-induced differentiation (Lockwood *et. al.*, 1967; O'Malley and McGuire, 1968) or metamorphosis (Tata, 1967b; Nakagawa and Cohen, 1967; see Frieden and Just, this volume; Wyatt, Vol. 2) mRNA must play a key role. The stimulation of template activity in chromatin isolated from hormone-primed animals has been suggested to be a reflection of mRNA control by hormones (Dahmus and Bonner, 1965; Kim and Cohen, 1966; Barker and Warren, 1966). But the real problem still remains: to identify the small amounts of messenger RNA formed in the midst of vast quantities of other types of RNA in the intact nucleus.

With most growth and developmental hormones, at the time of a peak shift in the rate of RNA synthesis, the major effect is on the synthesis of ribosomal RNA (see Tata, 1966a, 1967a; Liao *et al.*, 1966a,b; Hamilton, 1968; Drews, 1969). It is interesting to note, in retrospect, that in most of the observations on the abolition by actinomycin D of the growth-promoting or even metabolic actions of hormones that the antibiotic is very effective at doses that are too low to block all RNA synthesis (see Tata, 1966a). Synthesis of ribosomal RNA is inhibited to a greater extent than that of DNA-like RNA by low doses of the antibiotic. However, at early time intervals after hormonal administration, when the overall rate of RNA synthesis is unaffected, it is likely that there may be a subtle qualitative change in the nature of RNA synthesized without much effect on ribosomal RNA synthesis. This seems to be so in the estrogen-primed synthesis of avidin synthesis in the chick oviduct (O'Malley and McGuire, 1968; Hahn *et al.*, 1968) as well as with cortisol (Drews and Brawerman, 1967) and thyroid hormones (see Fig. 2) in mammalian tissues.

Many of the aforementioned changes in nature of RNA synthesized at early time-intervals after hormone administration have been demonstrated by the technique of RNA–DNA hybridization. Recent work from our laboratory has shown that the hybridization efficiency of newly syn-

TABLE III

Effect of Hormone Administration on the Hybridization with Homologous DNA of Nuclear and Cytoplasmic RNA Labeled for Different Periods of Time[a]

Species	Source of RNA	Hormonal treatment	Length of pulse (min)	Sp. activity (cpm./μg RNA)	Hybridization efficiency (%)
Rat	Rapidly labeled nuclear RNA	Hx,[b] control	10	1850	6.9
Rat	Rapidly labeled nuclear RNA	Hx, 2.0 hr. after HGH[c]	10	1490	6.8
Rat	Rapidly labeled nuclear RNA	Hx, control	35	2004	6.5
Rat	Rapidly labeled nuclear RNA	Hx, 2 days after HGH + T_3[d]	35	3630	4.3
Rat	Rapidly labeled nuclear RNA	Tx,[e] control	10	1480	6.3
Rat	Rapidly labeled nuclear RNA	Tx, 3.2 hr. after T_3	10	1756	8.0
Rat	Rapidly labeled nuclear RNA	Tx, 30 hr. after T_3	10	3130	4.4
Rat	Long-term labeled microsomal RNA	Tx, control	200	220	0.6
Rat	Long-term labeled microsomal RNA	Tx, 3 days after T_3	200	395	0.7
Bullfrog	Rapidly labeled nuclear RNA	Premetamorphosis,	45	30	6.9
Bullfrog	Rapidly labeled nuclear RNA	metamorphosis induced	45	155	3.2
Xenopus	Total body long-term labeled RNA	Premetamorphosis,	650	87	4.8
Xenopus	Total body long-term labeled RNA	metamorphosis induced	650	629	2.5

[a] [3H]-labeled RNA ([3H] orotic acid for rats, [3H]-uridine for tadpoles) was used on cellulose nitrate membranes on which denatured homologous DNA was trapped. The hybridization plateau level was determined by hybridizing a constant amount of RNA with different amounts of DNA bound to membranes. Hybridization efficiency is the percent of radioactive RNA input recovered as the hybrid at saturation levels of DNA/RNA. Data adapted from Wyatt and Tata (1968) and Tata (unpublished).

[b] Hx = hypophysectomized.

[c] HGH = human growth hormone.

[d] T_3 = triiodothyronine.

[e] Tx = thyroidectomized.

thesized RNA can vary in both directions according to the time that has elapsed after hormone administration. Wyatt and Tata (1968) found that at peak stimulation of RNA synthetic rate the hybridization efficiency was depressed in a number of systems (Table III). This was interpreted to mean that small increases in the synthesis of rapidly hybridizable RNA were swamped by a massive stimulation of ribosomal RNA, which has low (0.3–0.4%) hybridization efficiency. The same studies, when performed at early time intervals, showed that triiodothyronine, but not growth hormone, caused a slight but significant increase in hybridizable RNA. This biphasic effect is illustrated schematically in Fig. 2. Thus the direction of change in the labeling of RNA varies according to the time at which the isotope is administered after the hormone. As for growth hormone, it is interesting that at no time after its administration did it increase the hybridization efficiency of nuclear or total cellular RNA, a finding also reported by Drews and Brawerman (1967) and Gupta and Talwar (1968). Competition studies from other laboratories have also

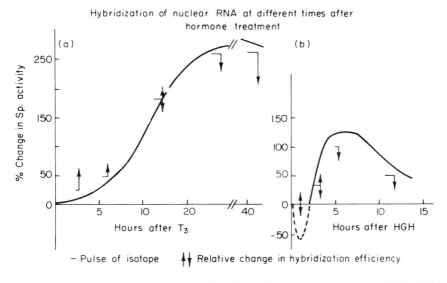

Fig. 2. Schematic representation of the effect of hormone treatment on DNA–RNA hybridization experiments with rapidly labeled nuclear RNA. The curves represent the change in specific activity of hepatic nuclear RNA obtained at different times after the administration of (a) 3,3′,5-triiodothyronine (T_3) to thyroidectomized rats and (b) human growth hormone to hypophysectomized rats. The length of the upward or downward pointing arrows denotes the increase or decrease in the fraction of rapidly hybridizable RNA. The length of horizontal bars adjoining the arrows indicates the relative duration of the pulse of ³H-labeled orotic acid, which varied from 10–35 mins. Other conditions as in Table III.

shown that hormones do increase the content of highly hybridizable RNA in the nucleus (Drews and Brawerman, 1967; O'Malley and McGuire, 1968; O'Malley *et al.*, 1968; Hahn *et al.*, 1968). It is important to realize that the nature of highly hybridizable RNA from the nucleus is still in doubt. Much of it may not be mRNA but represent the product of highly repetitive sequences of genes whose function is as yet unknown (Britten and Kohne, 1968). Britten and Davidson (1969) have recently suggested that this type of RNA may be of considerable importance in differentiation and postdifferentiation adaptation processes.

If the nature of the RNA made at early time intervals is not clear, it is certain that when overall rates of RNA synthesis are drastically affected it is the synthesis of ribosomal RNA that is elevated (as in growth) or depressed (as in tissue involution). It is interesting, as already mentioned, that hormonal stimulation of RNA polymerase *in vitro* is most marked under conditions in which the product is ribosomal RNA (see Tata, 1967a, 1968b; Hamilton, 1968; Liao *et al.*, 1966a,b). Studies in which nucleoli or nucleolar RNA were isolated have emphasized the preferential effect of growth and developmental hormones on ribosomal RNA synthesis. Such a high sensitivity of ribosomal cistrons is unlikely to be a specific property of hormones but seems to be a common response of cells that have to grow rapidly, as during regeneration (Tsukada *et al.*, 1968) or in chemical carcinogenesis (Steele and Busch, 1966). An exaggerated acceleration of the rate of rRNA synthesis may perhaps facilitate the transfer of ribosomes and messenger RNA from the nucleus to the cytoplasm.

4. Transfer of RNA from the Nucleus to the Cytoplasm

Very little is known yet about the possible effects of hormones on the selective transfer of RNA from the nucleus to the cytoplasm. It may be that the hormone triggers off a qualitative or quantitative change in the synthesis of RNA but that it does not control the eventual selection and transfer of the different species of RNA made. In any case, Table III gives an idea of the importance of the process of selection. It can be seen that there was very little effect of hormone treatment on cytoplasmic RNA when compared with that on nuclear RNA. Recently Dingman *et al.* (1969) have also found that in the chick oviduct, estrogen, which has a marked effect on the pattern of RNA synthesized in the nucleus (O'Malley and McGuire, 1968; O'Malley *et al.*, 1968), provoked only minor changes in cytoplasmic RNA when it was analyzed by acrylamide gel electrophoresis.

It is interesting that in two studies, growth hormone and cortisol were found to accelerate the rate of appearance of 40–50 S particles in rat liver (Sells and Takahashi, 1967; Finkel *et al.*, 1966). These particles are thought to be precursors to polysomes and contain mRNA attached to the small ribosomal subunits (McConkey and Hopkins, 1965; Henshaw *et al.*, 1965). However, it is possible that they also contained "informosomes" or messenger ribonucleoprotein particles, which have been identified in rat liver (Henshaw, 1968). Further work is needed to discover if hormones do indeed play a direct role in the transfer of RNA from the nucleus to the cytoplasm.

5. Cytoplasmic RNA and Ribosomes

Soon after the stimulation of nuclear RNA synthesis by many growth-promoting hormones, there occurs a gradual buildup of cytoplasmic RNA and ribosomes. In immature tissues or in tissues of animals deprived of the hormone the increase is very rapid and often most impressive. Growth-hormone treatment can almost double the population of hepatic polyribosomes in hypophysectomized rats and androgen and estrogen can cause a four- to eightfold increase in cytoplasmic RNA of their target accessory sexual tissues in castrated rats. To a large extent the accumulation of cytoplasmic RNA is a consequence of enhanced RNA synthesis in the nucleus but there may also be a concommitant stabilization or reduction in turnover of RNA. Recently Brewer *et al.* (1969) have looked at the problem of RNA degradation. They find that ribonuclease activity of the postmitochondrial fraction of hypophysectomized rat liver is double that in normal animals and that treatment of the hypophysectomized animals with growth hormone reduced it to normal levels. In thyroid hormone-induced metamorphosis of bullfrog tadpoles the degradation of cytoplasmic ribosomes was found to be selective in that the population accumulating after hormone treatment was more stable but at the same time the breakdown of the "older" ribosomes was accelerated (Tata, 1967b).

Accompanying the appearance of newly formed RNA into the cytoplasm following hormonal induction is a gradual change in the polyribosomal profile. In virtually every instance of a growth and developmental system it has been shown that lack or withdrawal of the hormone causes a shift to smaller aggregates and an increase in the monomeric ribosomal peak, whereas hormone administration causes a shift in the opposite direction (see Korner, 1965a,b; Tata, 1966a, 1967b; Staehelin, 1965; Earl and Korner, 1966; Tata and Widnell, 1966; Garren *et al.*, 1967; Teng and Hamilton, 1967). From the earlier studies on amino acid incorporation, in which the response to exogenous synthetic messenger was assayed, it was concluded that the hormone was correcting a deficiency of messenger content in the cytoplasm (Liao and Williams-Ashman, 1962; Korner, 1965b). However, later studies have shown that this does not constitute the principal mode of regulation of cytoplasmic protein synthesis. There is good evidence now to show that hormone deficiency leads to an inherent defect in the capacity of the ribosome itself and that hormone replacement corrects the defect, either directly or through the generation of new, more active population of ribosomes (Tata and Widnell, 1966; Earl and Korner, 1966; Tata and Williams-Ashman,

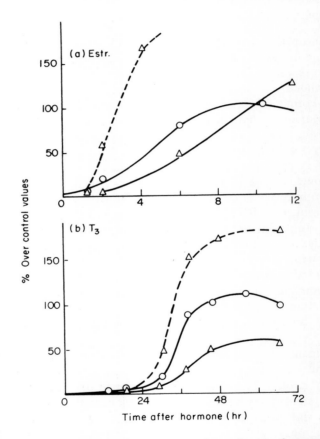

Fig. 3. Increase in protein synthetic capacity of cytoplasmic ribosomes coinciding with the appearance of additional polysomes formed as a result of hormone administration. (a) Effect of a single injection of estradiol on ovariectomized rat uterus; (b) effect of a single injection of triiodothyronine on thyroidectomized rat liver. △, increase in amount of cytoplasmic ribosomal population (dashed line indicates the increase in radioactivity of the newly labeled polysomes; ○, amino acid incorporation *in vitro* expressed per unit ribosomal RNA. Curves derived from data of Hamilton *et al.* (1968), Teng and Hamilton (1967), and Tata and Widnell (1966).

1967; Garren *et al.*, 1967; Wool, 1965; Wool *et al.*, 1968). The question of a direct translational control will be discussed briefly in Section III,B.

The relevance of the accumulation or alteration of cytoplasmic RNA to the question of hormonal regulation of protein synthesis becomes most obvious when the timing of changes in protein synthetic activity is taken into account. For many hormones, including androgens, estrogens, thyroid hormones and growth hormone, the rate of protein synthesis increases rather abruptly following a relatively long lag period after hormone replacement (Tata, 1966a, 1967a, 1968a). The onset of increased protein synthetic activity coincides with the accumulation in the cytoplasm of the hormone-induced newly formed ribosomes. This feature is illustrated in Fig. 3 for the stimulation of growth of the uterus by estrogen and that of liver by triiodothyronine. Similar results were observed with triiodothyronine-induced metamorphosis of bullfrog tadpoles (Tata, 1967b). It appears therefore that a large part of the hormonal effect on protein synthesis is incorporated into the new ribosomes formed after hormone treatment but it is not certain whether these ribosomes play a passive role as mere transporters of messenger RNA or whether their intrinsic amino acid incorporation activity is also under hormonal influence. In any case, it seems unlikely that hormones control protein synthesis merely by increasing the number of ribosomes, although this would certainly be important for a sustained growth action. Recent work from our laboratory has also underlined the importance of distribution of ribosomes in the cytoplasm, which will be discussed in Section IV.

B. DIRECT TRANSLATIONAL CONTROL OF PROTEIN SYNTHESIS

The early observations on the inability of hormones to affect ribosomal amino acid incorporation when added *in vitro* have been confirmed in most hormone-dependent growth systems. It was concluded that hormones do not act directly at the level of polypeptide chain assembly. However the concept of translational control has been recently invoked to account for a few situations in which a hormone brings about a rapid anabolic change or induces specific enzyme synthesis.

Much of the evidence in favor of a direct translational control is indirect and often based on the differential effect of inhibitors of RNA and protein synthesis. Garren *et al.* (1965) observed that actinomycin D failed to prevent the ACTH-induced steroid production by adrenal quarters, and Gorski and Padnos (1965) made similar observations on the incubation of ovaries with FSH. Notides and Gorski (1966) had also noticed that actinomycin D failed to completely suppress the formation of a rapidly labeled soluble protein in the uterus 30 minutes after the administration of estrogen. Similarly, the early part of growth hormone effect on amino acid incorporation into protein is insensitive to the antibiotic and therefore independent of RNA synthesis (Korner, 1969). Such findings have often been interpreted to mean that the hormone directly controls the synthesis of a single or few specific proteins that have a very short half-life (usually a few minutes) but synthesized on relatively stable templates. As a consequence of such a preferential synthesis the tissue may further respond with a massive RNA synthesis. However, it is important to establish the identity of such proteins because the hormonal effect would not be detectable on the basis of an overall incorporation of amino acids into protein. Garren (1968) has suggested that an important short-lived steroidogenic enzyme is itself one of these proteins and that ACTH may act initially via a mechanism involving cyclic AMP. The increase in adrenal RNA synthesis associated with an anabolic effect of ACTH would then be a secondary effect.

Tomkins has also made a good case for translational control in the induction by cortisol of tyrosine transaminase in cultured human hepatoma cells (Tomkins and Thompson, 1967; Tomkins, 1968; Tomkins and Geleherter, Vol. 2). He has proposed an ingenious model, which obviates the need for a Jacob-Monod type of enzyme induction process but which involves the interaction of the hormone with a cytoplasmic translation repressor. Such models have to be seriously considered because there is no doubt that the bacterial model of modulation of messenger RNA levels is too simple to account for the complexities of highly structured animal and plant cells. However, Kenney *et al.* (1968) have argued that the Tomkins model has been too much based on differential effects of actinomycin D at low and high doses in cultured hepatoma cells and that the situation may be quite different in the induction by cortisol of tyrosine transaminase in intact rat liver. In the latter system it is known that the full induction of the transaminase is sensitive to low doses of actinomycin D.

Perhaps the most convincing case for a direct translational control by hormones is that provided by Wool for the anabolic action of insulin in diaphragm muscle (Wool and Cavicchi, 1967; Martin and Wool, 1968; Wool *et al.*, 1968). Insulin stimulates the incorporation of amino acid into protein by muscle ribosomes within 5 minutes after the exposure of diaphragm to the hormone. Martin and Wool (1968) succeeded in reassociating the large and small ribosomal subunits into functional particles capable of responding to poly U. They then showed that the defect of alloxan diabetes was associated with the large (60 S) subunit and that insulin corrected this deficient amino acid incorporation capacity within

5 minutes. In similar reassociation studies with monomeric ribosomes from normal and hypophysectomized rat liver, Foster and Sells (1969) found that all possible combinations of 40 S and 60 S subunits produced monosomes that were equally responsive to poly U. It is also not known whether the effect of insulin is a direct one since it fails to correct the defect when added *in vitro* to ribosomes or subunits from diabetic animals.

A direct effect of hormone *in vitro* on amino acid incorporation by cell-free preparations has been consistently reported by Sokoloff and his colleagues (see Sokoloff, 1968). They have shown that thyroxine can stimulate the incorporation of amino acid by rat liver microsomes or ribosomes in the presence of mitochondria. In the absence of mitochondria in the incubation medium, thyroxine fails to affect the ribosomal activity, as has also been observed by other workers (Tata *et al.*, 1963). It seems that thyroxine releases some factor from mitochondria which is beneficial for ribosomal incorporation. It is of course well known that thyroxine and its analogs are potent mitochondrial swelling agents and would be expected to release a wide variety of mitochondrial components (see Lehninger, 1962). The beneficial effect may then only be an artificial one since conditions (pH, ionic strength, nucleotides, salts, etc.) that are optimal for maintenance of mitochondria and microsomes *in vitro* are not the same. An additional complication is that direct addition of thyroxine or tri-iodothyronine can itself enhance the incorporation of amino acids by mitochondria. Furthermore it is difficult to correlate these *in vitro* effects with the phenomena observed *in vivo*. Thyroid hormones have a long lag period for protein synthesis *in vivo* (Tata, 1964), affecting mitochondrial protein synthesis simultaneously with, and independently of, ribosomal response (Roodyn *et al.*, 1965) and small doses of actinomycin D abolish not only the anabolic but also the calorigenic function of the hormones (Tata, 1963). Recently, Sokoloff *et al.* (1968) have suggested that there may be two actions of thyroid hormones administered *in vivo*—an early mitochondrial dependent effect on microsomal amino acid incorporation followed by a second mitochondria independent action that would be based on microsomal RNA synthesis.

The question of an early and a late stimulation of protein synthesis raises the very likely possibility that the two may arise from different actions of the hormone. It may also be that one does not necessarily lead to the other. Both these possibilities deserve attention in interpreting sequential phenomena. Some recent work on the control of protein synthesis by growth hormone is most compatible with a dual temporal action. Growth hormone has a very rapid effect on the transport of amino acids, especially into muscle (Kostyo, 1968; Åhrén and Hjalmarson,

1968). An increased availability of amino acids has been shown to increase the activity of ribosomes (Munro, 1968), and Korner (1969) has recently shown that growth hormone administration very rapidly increases the ratio of active to inactive ribosomes. It is also interesting that a growth hormone effect, unrelated to its own protein synthetic action (that of depressing the cortisol-induced hepatic enzymes activity), was abolished by amino acid administration (Labrie and Korner, 1968). Kostyo (1968) has suggested that the early action which may involve the synthesis of a few specific proteins is not directly related to the slow, overall enhancement of protein anabolism by growth hormone. On the other hand it is possible that increased transport of amino acids may have a "permissive" action in a sustained increase in the rate of protein synthesis (see Snipes, 1968).

IV. THE ROLE OF CELL STRUCTURE

It has been estimated that protein synthesis in cell-free systems has an efficiency less than 1% of that *in vivo*. Thus, the disintegration of the structure of the cell must cause the loss of some vital factor(s) for protein synthesis. The importance of cellular architecture in the control of protein synthesis is now being realized (see Hendler, 1968) but it has not yet drawn much attention in problems concerning hormonal regulation of protein synthesis.

A. Cytoplasmic Distribution of Ribosomes

My attention to the importance of structural considerations in evaluating the action of growth and developmental hormones was first drawn in the studies on the timing of hormone-induced acceleration of protein synthesis and the accumulation of newly formed RNA in the cytoplasm.

At the same time as finding additional ribosomes accompanying the stimulation of protein synthesis, we observed in mammalian and amphibian tissues that the polysomes were more firmly bound to microsomal membranes in hormonally stimulated tissues as judged by the ease with which the particles were released from membrane complexes with detergents. Both these effects are illustrated in Table IV with hepatic ribosomes from bullfrog tadpoles in which metamorphosis was precociously induced with triiodothyronine (Tata, 1967b).

A firmer attachment of this type also caused a shift in the distribution

TABLE IV

Effect of Inducing Metamorphosis on the Relative Distribution of Newly Synthesized RNA[a]

Tadpoles	Concentration of Na deoxycholate (%)	Specific activity (cpm/E_{260}) and distribution (%) of RNA in fractions[b]			
		Membrane-bound ribosomes	Polysomes	Dimers + Monomers[c]	50 S
Control	0.08	295 (4.7)	227 (21.5)	107 (56.6)	58 (12.0)
	0.16	418 (2.0)	254 (22.8)	92 (53.0)	41 (8.8)
	0.30	— (0)	238 (18.7)	122 (62.5)	73 (14.5)
6 d. after 0.7 μg T$_3$	0.08	875 (20.5)	430 (33.5)	492 (26.0)	196 (10.5)
	0.16	990 (12.8)	518 (35.1)	631 (32.9)	281 (15.1)
	0.30	1185 (1.5)	550 (25.8)	675 (29.0)	255 (11.9)

[a] In membrane-bound and free ribosomal fractions from liver mitochondria-free supernatants treated with different amounts of Na deoxycholate. Microsomal RNA was labeled by injecting 11.5 μCi of ^{3}H-uridine per tadpole 22.5 hours before killing them. Equal amounts of mitochondria-free supernatants were treated with different quantities of Na deoxycholate, indicated by their final concentration before the sucrose density gradient centrifugation was carried out. 1-ml fractions were then pooled, after determination of E_{260}, into the four fractions. The "membrane-bound" ribosomal fraction is that which did not sediment through the 2.0 M sucrose interface (from Tata, 1967b).

[b] Figures in parenthesis indicate the percent of total radioactivity delivered on the gradient that was recovered in each of the fractions.

[c] Also includes ribosomal precursor particles smaller than 78 S monomers.

of ribosomes from the free polysome fraction to those attached to rough endoplasmic reticulum membranes as the predominant type. Qualitatively similar, but less pronounced, changes were also observed in tissues of young, thyroidectomized or hypophysectomized rats whose rate of growth was stimulated by growth hormone and thyroid hormone (Tata and Widnell, 1966; Tata and Williams-Ashman, 1967). Although free ribosomes detached with detergents from membranes can incorporate amino acids into protein *in vitro,* it is believed that much of protein synthesis *in vivo* may take place on those ribosomes that are attached to membranes of the endoplasmic reticulum or even other structures (Henshaw *et al.,* 1963; Campbell *et al.,* 1967; Hendler, 1968).

In the next series of experiments it was decided to compare the activities *in vitro* of bound and free ribosomes from tissues of animals deprived of or treated with hormones. That it is not necessary to have membrane-attached ribosomes *in vitro* to reflect a hormonal stimulation *in vivo* is quite well established in numerous studies on ribosomes prepared with detergent treatment (see Korner, 1965b; Tata, 1967a; Hamilton, 1968). However if hormonal stimulation caused ribosomes to be redistributed in the intact cell between free and membrane-bound fractions, it became imperative to prepare submicrosomal fractions *without the use of detergents* and under very mild conditions to cause minimal damage to bound ribosomes. A method, based on differential centrifugation, was devised that permitted the separation of microsomes into at least four major fractions: smooth membranes, light rough membranes, heavy rough membranes, and free polysomes (Tata, 1969a). The difference between the light and heavy rough microsomes, as revealed by chemical analysis and electron microscopy, is that the ratio of bound ribosomes per unit of membrane in higher in the latter fraction. Table V summarizes the results of some experiments on the effect of hypophysectomy and combined treatment with growth hormone and triiodothyronine on the capacity of submicrosomal fractions to incorporate amino acids into protein, both with endogenous and synthetic mRNA (Tata and Williams-Ashman, 1967). When the ability to incorporate ^{14}C-phenylalanine and ^{14}C-isoleucine were measured, in the presence and absence of synthetic messengers (polyuridylic acid and copolymer of uridylic and adenylic acids), it was found that hormone treatment corrected the lowered incorporation capacity caused by hypophysectomy in all three types of submicrosomal fractions. The effect of hormone deprivation or replacement was of greater magnitude in the heavy rough membranes than in the light rough membranes. To a large extent, the response to synthetic messengers of both the membrane-bound and free ribosomes paralleled that to endogenous messenger, whether growth had

TABLE V

INCORPORATION OF ¹⁴C-PHENYLALANINE AND ¹⁴C-ISOLEUCINE INTO PROTEIN[a]

Rats	Polysomes	mg RNA/gm	¹⁴C-Phe incorporated (cpm/10 min/mg RNA)		¹⁴C-Ile incorporated (cpm/10 min/mg RNA)	
			−Poly U	+Poly U	−Poly UA	+Poly UA
Normal	Free	0.57	13,590	38,090	5,320	6,383
	Light membranes	0.51	18,620	41,840	3,590	5,748
	Heavy membranes	1.62	58,800	128,400	23,800	29,980
Hx	Free	0.44	6,700	30,520	3,120	6,150
	Light membranes	0.46	14,550	44,250	3,560	5,036
	Heavy membranes	0.59	40,100	102,900	18,550	21,190
Hx + HGH + T₃	Free	0.66	26,700	86,300	10,900	20,720
	Light membranes	0.47	22,630	101,130	6,980	11,590
	Heavy membranes	1.40	66,000	144,000	32,100	45,700

[a] Incorporation of amino acids into protein by "free" polysomes and polysomes in light and heavy rough membrane fractions of liver microsomes from normal and hypophysectomized rats with or without hormonal treatment: Response to poly U and poly UA. Hormonal treatment consisted of three injections of 75 μg of human growth hormone (HGH) at 21, 47, and 74 hours before killing and two injections of triiodothyronine (T₃) at 47 and 74 hours. Light and heavy rough membrane fractions consist of ribosomes attached to membranes of the endoplasmic reticulum and differ from one another by the density of ribosome packing. Abbreviations as in Table II and further details are given in Tata and Williams-Ashman (1967).

been retarded or accelerated. Under the conditions of the rather prolonged hormonal treatment used in these experiments, the population of hepatic ribosomes would be 50–60% higher than in the control hypophysectomized rats. Thus there is a distinct possibility that the newly formed ribosomes upon hormone administration were inherently more efficient in handling synthetic or natural messengers. At the same time, the relative stimulation by synthetic polynucleotides was slightly higher in the less active preparations, which indicated that a small part of hormonal effect could be due to an increase in the polysomal mRNA content. This type of result raises the possibility that the relatively slow anabolic and developmental actions of hormones may be restricted to a small population of newly generated ribosomes rather than modify the activity of all the ribosomes in the cytoplasm.

B. Coordination between the Proliferation of Microsomal Membranes and Ribosomes and Accelerated Protein Synthesis in Vivo

The foregoing findings on the distribution of ribosomes and their amino acid incorporating activity *in vitro* posed two important questions. (a) Are the new ribosomes formed upon hormonal stimulation merely redistributed upon existing membranes or are there simultaneous alterations in the rate or type of membranes formed? (b) Does the activity of bound and free ribosomes *in vitro* truly reflect the protein synthetic capacity of the different populations of ribosomes in the intact cell? Both these questions have been attacked together in a series of experiments in our laboratory over the past 5 years (Tata, 1967b,c, 1968a, 1970; Kerkof and Tata, 1967, 1969; Andrews and Tata, 1968).

The proliferation of membranes of the endoplasmic reticulum was followed by measuring the incorporation of ^{32}P-phosphate and ^{14}C-labeled choline and glycerol into membrane phospholipids. In order to correlate the effect of hormones on this process with those on biosynthetic activity of the tissue we studied the rate of incorporation of radioactive amino acids into nascent proteins of the different submicrosomal fractions simultaneously with the accumulation of newly synthesized microsomal RNA in the following hormonal systems: (a) growth of liver induced by a single injection of growth hormone, triiodothyronine, and testosterone in hypophysectomized, thyroidectomized, and castrated rats, respectively; (b) growth and maturation of the seminal vesicle of the castrated rat when stimulated by testosterone; (c) precocious initiation of enzyme and protein synthesis in bullfrog tadpole liver during thyroid hormone-induced metamorphosis; (d) accelerated synthesis of thyroglobulin or iodoprotein by thyroid tissue under the influence of thyrotrophic hormone (TSH).

Initial studies revealed that administration of these hormones accelerated the synthesis of phospholipids, after different lag periods and to different extents, in the microsomal as well as the mitochondrial and nuclear fractions (Tata, 1967c). It was, however, in the microsomes that the effect of the hormone was most prominent, at least as far as the proliferation of membrane components is concerned.

Figure 4 compares the rates of formation of liver microsomal phospholipids with those of microsomal RNA and of nascent protein on microsomes following the combined administration of growth hormone and tri-iodothyronine to hypophysectomized rats. Since the two hormones have very different lag periods it was quite simple to detect a temporally coordinated enhancement by the hormones of microsomal phospholipid formation with that of the rates of microsomal RNA and protein synthesis. Thus, growth hormone (Fig. 4a) stimulated the protein synthetic capacity of hepatic ribosomes several hours earlier than did tri-iodothyronine (Fig. 4b), and the same pattern was followed for the accelerated formation of polysomes (much of the additional microsomal RNA appeared as polysomes). In another type of experiment (Tata, 1970) hypophysectomized rats were killed at a fixed time corresponding to the peak stimulation for each hormone (i.e., the hormones were not administered together as in Fig. 4). This led to additive stimulations in all three newly made constituents of the rough endoplasmic reticulum. It should be emphasized that in all these studies of combined treatment the maximal dose of each hormone was used. It is interesting to note that similar additive or sequential stimulations were observed a few hours earlier with nuclear RNA polymerase activity when different combinations of growth hormone, thyroid hormone, and testosterone were administered to study the growth of liver (Widnell and Tata, 1966a) or muscle (Breuer and Florini, 1966).

Such coordination of proliferation of cellular structures and biosynthetic activity is not a unique property of growth hormone and thyroid hormones. A good coordination in the onset of accelerated synthesis of phospholipid, RNA, and protein was also observed in microsomes isolated from the seminal vesicles of castrated rats following growth stimulation with testosterone, as shown in Fig. 5. Attempts to obtain mutually uncontaminated sub-microsomal fractions from seminal vesicles were unsuccessful. In earlier studies in which both the liver and seminal vesicles were studied the effect of testosterone was shown to be highly tissue specific (Tata, 1967c). Ultrastructural studies on seminal vesicles are also compatible with the foregoing biochemical findings (Szirmai and Van der Linde, 1964). In another system, although ribosomes and membranes were not actually isolated, a coordinated synthesis of phospholipid and RNA in their respective target tissues may underlie the same process

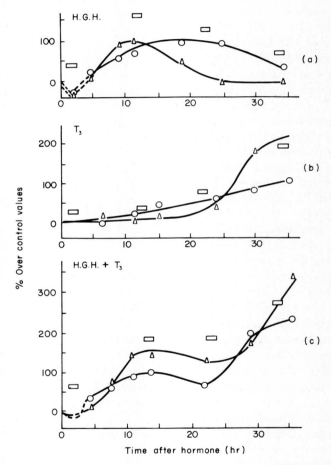

FIG. 4. Coordination of the appearance of additional newly formed hepatic microsomal phospholipids (○) and RNA (△) and the recovery of nascent microsomal protein formed *in vivo* (□) following the administration to hypophysectomized rats of (a) growth hormone alone, (b) triiodothyronine alone, or (c) the two together. The rate of formation of microsomal RNA and phospholipids was determined from the incorporation of ^{32}P after about a 10-hour exposure to the isotope whereas the rate of protein synthesis *in vivo* was derived from the incorporation of ^{14}C-labeled amino acids within 10 minutes after their administration. The results are expressed as percent increase in specific radioactivities in hormone-treated animals over the values obtained in untreated controls (Tata, 1968a).

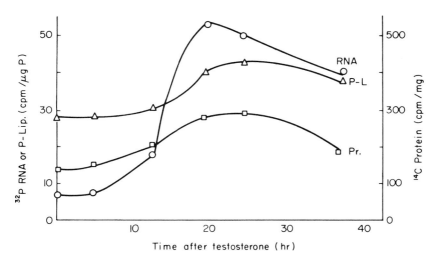

FIG. 5. Coordinated acceleration of formation of microsomal phospholipid (△), RNA (○) and protein (□) following the single administration of 250 μg of testosterone propionate to castrated rats. Phospholipid and RNA were both labeled with 95 μCi of ^{32}P-orthophosphate administered 1.5 and 3.5 hours before death, whereas newly synthesized protein was labeled with 15 μCi of ^{14}C-labeled amino acids given 15 minutes before death. Corrections were made for isotope uptake in each determination. Six castrated rats (160–180 gm) were used for each time interval. Seminal vesicles weighed 14 ± 4 mg in control rats (time 0) and 32 ± 6 mg at 35.5 hours after hormone injection (from Tata, 1970).

in the case of estrogen (Aizawa and Mueller, 1961; Nishigori and Aizawa, 1968). This coordination is in fact a common feature of cells undergoing rapid development in general, irrespective of whether the stimulus is hormonal or not. During this period new biochemical functions tend to be concentrated in cytoplasmic structures of increasing complexities (see Siekevitz *et al.*, 1967; Dallner *et al.*, 1966; Pollak and Ward, 1967).

Where then does the specificity of individual hormones lie in terms of such seemingly nonspecific phenomena? There are two indirect approaches that provide a partial answer to this important question. First, the experiment in which growth hormone and tri-iodothyronine were administered to hypophysectomized rats simultaneously and in maximal growth-promoting amounts (Fig. 4c) produced two stepwise bursts of additional microsomal RNA and phospholipids, each burst corresponding in its time course and magnitude to the effects of the individual hormones shown in Fig. 4a and b. The rate of protein synthesis *in vivo* was elevated in a manner corresponding to the two bursts of microsomal proliferation and it is therefore of some interest that the two hormones have additive effects on the growth of the tissue. The nature of proteins synthesized under the influence of the two hormones is also different. It is hence possible that some degree of hormonal specificity may be incorporated into the additional ribosome-membrane units formed in response to the individual hormones.

Other evidence for hormonal specificity in microsomal structures is provided by systems in which the hormone induces the synthesis *de novo* of specific enzymes or proteins. Two such systems have been studied in our laboratory: (a) The induction of urea cycle enzymes and serum albumin during tri-iodothyronine induced metamorphosis in bullfrog tadpoles, which is largely based on the classical work from the laboratories of Cohen and Frieden (see P. P. Cohen, 1966; Frieden, 1967; and in this issue). (b) The enhancement of thyroglobulin formation by thyroid cells under the influence of thyrotrophic hormone (see Freinkel, 1964).

In the latter system, TSH causes an almost simultaneous increase in the rate of whole thyroid phospholipid and RNA synthesis *in vivo* (see Fig. 6). What is particularly interesting is that the onset of this change coincides with increasing amounts of a thyroglobulinlike protein being

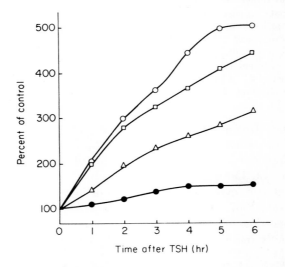

Time after TSH (hr)

Fig. 6. Simultaneous stimulation *in vivo* by TSH of the incorporation of ^{32}P into RNA and phospholipid and of ^{125}I into protein of guinea pig thyroid. A 0.5 unit dose of TSH was given to each animal 1–6 hours before killing. ^{32}P (50 μCi) and ^{125}I (3.75 μCi) were injected 1 hour before killing. RNA, phospholipid and iodoprotein were extracted and analyzed as described in the original paper. Each point represents the average of at least 3 determinations (9 animals) and the values are expressed as the percent of those of control animals (time 0). ○, specific activity of RNA; △, specific activity of phospholipid; □, total protein-bound ^{125}I; ●, total uptake of ^{32}P. (From Kerkof and Tata, 1967.)

formed (Kerkof and Tata, 1967). Since one of the multiple actions of TSH is to stimulate the secretion of thyroglobulin, it could be argued that additional membrane synthesis would be necessary to perform the vectorial discharge of extra iodoprotein (Ekholm and Strandberg, 1968). Later studies have confirmed this effect *in vitro* using pig thyroid slices in which it was shown that much of the additional phospholipid, RNA, and iodoprotein formed in response to TSH accumulated in the smooth and rough microsomal fraction (Kerkof and Tata, 1969). The effect of TSH on phospholipid synthesis is particularly striking and has been studied in detail for some time (Freinkel, 1964), but what was not known

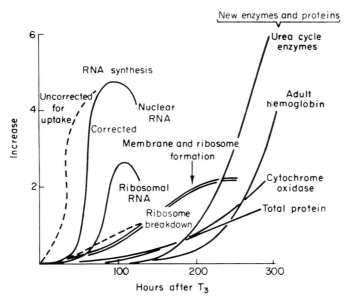

FIG. 7. Schematic representation of sequential stimulation of rates of RNA and phospholipid synthesis in relation to the increases in enzymes or protein synthesized upon the precocious induction of metamorphosis in *Rana catesbeiana* tadpoles with triiodothyronine. Curves show the rate of rapidly labeled nuclear RNA synthesis; specific activity of RNA in cytoplasmic ribosomes; breakdown of ribosomes labeled before induction; rate of microsomal phospholipid synthesis; urea cycle enzymes (carbamyl phosphate synthetase); cytochrome oxidase per mg mitochondrial protein; appearance of adult hemoglobin in the blood; total liver protein per mg wet weight. The values are expressed as percentage increases over those in the noninduced control tadpoles. The decreasing values in curves of RNA synthesis reflect the dilution of specific radioactivity in precursor molecules due to the onset of regression of tissues such as the tail and intestine. (Data from Tata, 1967b).

until our studies was that this effect was part of the general effect of growth and developmental hormones in enhancing membrane proliferation.

The system of artificial induction of metamorphosis in amphibia has received much attention in our laboratory over the last 6 years (Tata, 1967c). In Fig. 7 are summarized some of our findings on major biosynthetic events that occur during the lag period preceding the appearance of newly formed proteins as a result of administration of triiodo-

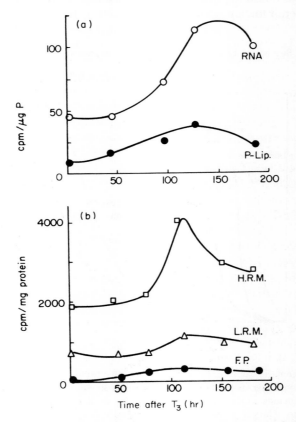

FIG. 8. Coordinated proliferation of endoplasmic reticulum and the increase in protein synthesis *in vivo* in the heavy rough membranes (densely packed ribosomes attached to membranes) during triiodothyronine-induced metamorphosis of young bullfrog tadpoles. (a) The appearance of newly synthesized (^{32}P-labeled) heavy rough membrane phospholipids (●) and RNA (○); (b) the recovery of labeled nascent proteins formed *in vivo* after a short pulse of radioactive amino acids in heavy rough membranes (□), light rough membranes (△), and free polysomes (●). For details see Tata (1967b).

thyronine to immature *Rana catesbeiana* tadpoles. It can be seen that there occurred, well within the latent period (5–6 days) for new proteins to be detected, an acceleration of the rate of nuclear and cytoplasmic RNA synthesis. Of interest are the events that occur between the initial burst of RNA synthesis following triiodothyronine administration and the appearance of newly synthesized proteins. Unlike the mammalian systems that we noted earlier, there occurs during this period a more complex process of breakdown of "old" RNA, alterations in polysome profiles, and a redistribution of ribosomes attached to membranes of the endoplasmic reticulum. The latter process is accompanied by a simultaneous increase in the synthesis of ribosomes and membranes of the endoplasmic reticulum as judged by membrane phospholipid synthesis (Fig. 8a). It is interesting to note that this simultaneous increase in the formation of the two rough endoplasmic reticulum components is accompanied by an enhanced rate of protein synthesis (Fig. 8b). These biochemical changes are so marked that it is easy to observe structural changes by electron microscopy. Figure 9 shows schematically that during metamorphosis there is a shift in the distribution of ribosomes from around the simple vesicular membrane structures of the immature larvae to the more complex double lamellar structures more commonly seen in mature tissues. It is interesting that this shift in structural organization of the endoplasmic reticulum coincided temporally with the changes in the formation of microsomal RNA and phospholipids and the synthesis of proteins by polyribosomes. Similar changes have been observed in the ecdysone-induced maturation of insect wing epidermal cells (Ebstein *et al.*, personal communication) in the androgen-dependent growth of male accessory sexual tissues (prostate. seminal vesicles) in rodents (Szirmai and Van der Linde, 1964) and in the induction of phosvitin by estrogen (Nicholls *et al.*, 1968).

As regards membrane proliferation, these studies describe only the rate of formation but not turnover of membrane constituents. It is quite possible that the hormonal stimulus leads to both accelerated formation and retarded degradation of membranes for which the demand is most acute, as for example the rough endoplasmic reticulum. The question of membrane stability is an important one and ought to be studied along the lines recently laid down by the groups of Palade, Dallner, and Schimke in studying drug-induced proliferation of the endoplasmic reticulum (Omura *et al.*, 1967; Orrenius and Ericsson, 1966; Dallner *et al.*, 1966; Arias *et al.*, 1969). How the phospholipid and protein components of membranes are assembled in an orderly fashion to yield precise structures is not known. It may be that the initial response to a growth stimulus may be to accelerate the assembly or "crystallization"

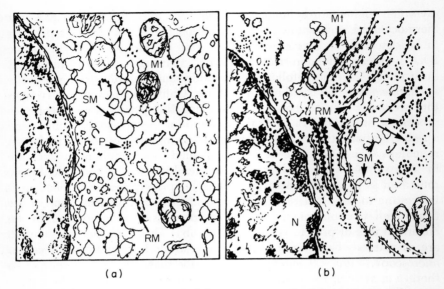

(a)   (b)

FIG. 9. Schematic representation of electron micrographs showing the reorganization of the cytoplasmic membranes and ribosomes during hormone-induced metamorphosis in bullfrog tadpole liver cells. (a) Hepatocyte in a premetamorphic tadpole showing small groups of ribosomes around simple vesicular structures. (b) Similar cells in tadpoles 6 days after induction of metamorphosis with triiodothyronine, showing dense ribosomal accumulation often attached to a more differentiated double-lamellar type of reticulum. N, nucleus, Mt, mitochondrion; SM, smooth membranes; RM, rough membranes; P, typical polysomal chains, rosettes and spirals. See Tata (1967a,b) for details.

of rigid structures from existing components whose depletion in turn would trigger off the synthesis of additional membrane phospholipids and proteins.

The preferential accumulation of rough endoplasmic reticulum which, as this work has shown, also contains the ribosomal fraction most active in amino acid incorporation *in vivo,* underlines the importance in protein synthesis of the attachment of ribosomes to membranes (see also Henshaw *et al.,* 1963; Campbell, 1965; Campbell *et al.,* 1967; Hendler, 1968). The effect of hormonal stimulation on protein synthesis *in vivo* on membrane-bound relative to free ribosomes was considerably greater than when amino acid incorporation was measured with isolated preparations (compare Table V and Fig. 8b). Until now the major emphasis on ribosome-membrane attachment in animal cells has been focused on the export of proteins in predominantly secretory cells (Palade, 1966; Siekevitz *et al.* (1967). However, recent studies from our laboratory on nonsecretory tissues, such as brain and muscle, have shown that the membrane-attached ribosomes play an important role in synthesizing proteins for intracellular destinations (Andrews and Tata, 1968; Unpublished data). A preferential increase in the proliferation of rough endoplasmic reticulum of the predominantly nonsecretory cells of the kidney has been observed both in neonatal (Priestly and Malt, 1969) and androgen-induced growth (Failoni and Scarpelli, 1965). One has to consider the possibility that some factor determining the efficiency of protein synthesis may be dependent on the interaction between the ribosome and membrane (see Hendler, 1968; Mainwaring, 1969).

From the work described, it can be concluded that there exists some mechanism in the cell that tightly couples the formation of rough endoplasmic reticulum in response to an increased demand for protein synthesis following stimulation with a variety of growth and developmental hormones. Perhaps a common fundamental mechanism may also underlie the numerous observations of a marked acceleration of phospholipid synthesis or membrane proliferation anticipating or accompanying the initial burst of protein synthesis in apparently a variety of situations of growth and development that are independent of hormones (Dallner *et al.*, 1966; Pollak and Ward, 1967; Leduc *et al.*, 1968; Fisher and Mueller, 1968; Ursprung and Schabtach, 1968; Priestly and Malt, 1969; Tata, 1970). These systems vary from the regenerating liver in the rat, immune response in spleen cells, and lymphocytes, to imaginal discs in developing *Drosophila* larvae. What could be the meaning of an enhanced coupled formation of membranes and ribosomes during growth and development? It has already been suggested elsewhere (Tata, 1968a,b) that, besides satisfying a need for secretion of proteins, such a coupling may reflect a topographical segregation of different populations of ribosomes, presumably differently precoded according to the developmental or environmental stimulus. The advantage of such a segregation in cells that have to adapt rapidly to such external stimuli as those regulating growth, development, detoxication, etc., would be to preferentially synthesize proteins involved in the adaptation response with the minimum of perturbation of synthesis of those proteins that are not involved in the response to the stimulus. The additive effect of different stimuli on the proliferation of membrane-bound ribosomes can be interpreted as a reflection of such a process in which different types of proteins are preferentially made in response to different agents. Of course, such results do not constitute direct evidence for this idea of segregation. However it can be tested as a first step by determining histochemically whether or not new enzymes formed during development are initially localized in the region of newly formed rough endoplasmic reticulum.

V. PHENOMENOLOGY AND MECHANISM OF ACTION

For those studying the biochemical actions of hormones it is often tempting to interpret a relatively early phenomenon provoked by the hormone as the basis for its mechanism of action. However, it is essential to distinguish between the two for an eventual understanding of the chemical basis of hormonal action. It is nonetheless important to study "phenomenology" because a chemical or molecular interpretation must be compatible with the cellular phenomena provoked by the hormone. Following is a summary and an attempt to integrate the principle cellular responses relevant to hormonal regulation of protein synthesis that have been described in this chapter.

A. SUMMARY AND INTEGRATION OF PHENOMENA

It is clear from what we have seen in Sections III and IV that growth and developmental hormones affect biosynthetic functions of their target cells at multiple steps of genetic transcription and translation. Figure 10 presents a schematic, and obviously simplified, summary of the main

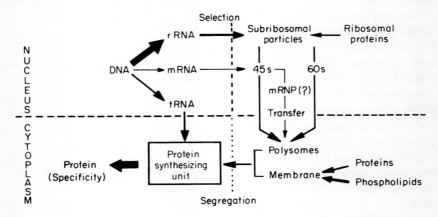

FIG. 10. Scheme attempting to integrate some of the processes regulating protein synthesis in nucleated cells and which respond to the growth-promoting stimulus of hormones. It is proposed that the type of growth or development would be determined genetically via mRNA coding for specific proteins but that its expression requires the generation of ribosomes and mRNA protein particles and that their topographical segregation may be achieved by a firm attachment to membranes. The width of the arrows is roughly related to the magnitude of response of the target cell to growth and developmental hormones with respect to the process studied.

phenomena and how they may be interrelated. It is assumed that to a large extent growth and development eventually depend on the induction or preferential synthesis of a predetermined protein pattern. This may even apply to control of metabolic activity in adult tissues as seems to be the case with aldosterone (see Edelman and Fimognari, 1968; Edelman and Fanestil, Chapter 8, Vol. 1) and thyroid hormones (see Tata, 1964, 1969b). Among the earliest events occurring in target cells following the administration of growth and developmental hormones is a marked alteration in the rate and nature of nuclear RNA synthesis. [Uterine nuclei may respond as early as 2 minutes after the administration of estrogen to ovariectomized rats (Hamilton, 1968).] A direct and selective control of messenger RNA synthesis, as predicted by Karlson (1963), still remains one of the simplest explanations of hormone specificity. However, it has not yet been possible to provide any convincing experimental evidence for direct interaction between hormones and genes or repressors, and many now hold the view that hormonal activation of genetic transcription can be only indirect. Recently some attempt has been made to search for events that would directly lead to the stimulation of nuclear RNA synthesis. Among these are the effects on the acetylation or phosphorylation of histones and other basic proteins of the nucleus (see Allfrey, 1968) and the interesting findings of a firm correlation between polyamine metabolism and RNA synthesis following hormonal stimulus (see Williams-Ashman and Reddi, Vol. 2). However, an important technical problem has yet to be resolved, namely, detecting very small changes in what must be a minute fraction of nuclear RNA, especially when a massive increase in the synthesis of ribosomal RNA and nonmessenger, DNA-like RNA are provoked. Perhaps, as Fig. 2 suggests, the search for such subtle changes ought to be extended to a period when no substantial increases in the overall rate of RNA synthesis have occurred following hormone administration.

The extreme sensitivity of ribosomal cistrons may not be a specific property of hormones but it has been observed in a variety of growth and maturational processes. An exaggerated increase in ribosomal RNA synthesis and ribonucleoprotein particles (including "informosomes") may be a common feature of nucleated cells in order to facilitate the transport of messenger RNA from the nucleus to the cytoplasm. But before the process of transport must come that of selection of the right species of RNA for utilization in the cytoplasm. Little is known as yet about the role of the extensive synthesis of rapidly turning over RNA that is restricted to the nucleus (see Shearer and McCarthy, 1967; Britten and Davidson, 1969). Until this is achieved it will be impossible to say how, if at all, hormones may affect the process of discrimination between those species of RNA that do not leave the nucleus and those that do. But, as a practical measure, the high degree of nuclear restriction makes it imperative to characterize more carefully both the nuclear *and* cytoplasmic RNA formed under the influence of the hormone.

Regardless of the mechanism of selection of RNA, hormonal stimulation gradually leads to an accumulation of polysomes that are precoded with hormone-specific messengers. Figure 10 indicates that when newly formed RNA accumulates in the cytoplasm there occurs a simultaneous increase in the rate of formation of membranes, especially those to which the ribosomes are attached. There seems to be some mechanism in the cell that coordinates the formation or assembly of membranes of the endoplasmic reticulum according to the demands for protein synthesis, especially during growth and development. Thus the terminal stages leading to a rather abrupt increase in protein synthesis are complex and include

(a) an increase in overall content of cytoplasmic RNA

(b) a shift toward heavier polysomal aggregates suggesting a relative increase in messenger content

(c) An elevation of the intrinsic capacity of the ribosome to incorporate amino acids

(d) a shift of polysomal distribution from free to membrane-bound

(e) a coordinated proliferation of membranes to which the ribosomes are bound.

So far, virtually all the attention on ribosome-membrane attachment has been directed toward the function of export of proteins in secondary cells. However, the marked proliferation of the rough endoplasmic reticulum that one observes during rapid growth (when relatively more protein would be made for intracellular use) in both secretory and nonsecretory cells suggests that the attachment may serve some other function. One such role that I have suggested (see Tata, 1968a) is that the ribosome-membrane association could conceivably restrict the exchange between all the populations of ribosomes and messengers so as to achieve a topographical segregation of polysomes. The main advantage of such a segregation would be eventually to isolate responses (based on selective synthesis of proteins) to hormonal or nonhormonal stimuli from the orderly synthesis of proteins that are not involved initially in the growth or developmental response.

There is still little evidence that sustained growth and development can be explained by a direct translational control by the hormone at the level of the ribosome. In some instances, such as enzyme induction by cortisol and ACTH, or the early phase of action of insulin and growth hormone, it is possible that the hormone may modulate the synthesis of proteins on relatively stable templates (see Tomkins, Vol. 2; Wool *et al.*, 1968; Korner, 1969; Garren, 1968). However, even with insulin, whose action has been localized to the large ribosomal subunit, the nature of the hormonal interaction in controlling translation is not known. One of the salient features of hormonal regulation of protein synthesis is that it is not possible to mimic the action of the hormone *in vivo*, however rapid this may be, by its addition to a cell-free system of protein synthesis.

It has not been possible to cover all the recent developments in the field of hormonal regulation of protein synthesis, some of which present promising approaches. Among these are the role of a limited DNA synthesis prior to induction of specific protein synthesis, which is discussed by Topper (Vol. 2). The examples of prolactin-induced formation of milk proteins (Lockwood *et al.*, 1967) and erythroprotein-induced hemoglobin synthesis (Paul and Hunter, 1969) may serve as useful models for other hormone-dependent systems of differentiation in which a round of cell division or restricted DNA synthesis is a prerequisite for competence for full developmental expression. This certainly seems to be important in insect metamorphosis as suggested in two recent studies (Crouse, 1968; Kafatos and Feder, 1968). In this connection, it would also be useful to investigate the possible effects of developmental hormones on mitochondrial nucleic acid and protein synthesis since recent work points to the importance of cytoplasmic DNA in early development (see Gurdon and Woodland, 1968).

An aspect of hormonal regulation of protein synthesis that does not often attract attention deserves to be mentioned. It has to do with the problem of regression or cell death, which is often an important part of the process of development of the whole organism. There appear to be two main pathways. The first one involves inhibition of RNA and protein synthesis, often by the same hormone that promotes growth and protein synthesis in other tissues. The involution of thymic cells by cortisol is a classical example of this feature, in which the hormone suppresses RNA and protein synthesis (Makman *et al.*, 1967; Drews, 1969). Another example is the inhibition by thyroxine of protein synthesis by pituitary cells, which Tonoue and Yamamoto (1967) have explained is the basis for the negative feedback system operating via TSH production. Similar suppressive actions should also be observed in the action of other hormones on the hypothalamus–pituitary axis. In the second pathway, cell death or tissue regression is brought about by additional protein synthesis. At the onset of regression of the tadpole tail by thyroid hormone there occurs a substantial activation of RNA synthesis, some of the additional RNA being essential for regression to occur since the process is very sensitive to actinomycin D (Tata, 1966b; Weber, 1965). This suggests that during development the growth and multiplication of one type of cells and the death of another, initiated by the same stimulus, may only be a question of the nature of proteins synthesized.

B. SITES OF ACTION

The importance of searching for the earliest event in sequential biochemical actions is to get closer to the initial site of interaction of the hormone. The identification of the latter is essential to building a molecular model explaining the physiological actions of hormones. At the moment we do not know of any cellular constituent(s) whose interaction with a growth and developmental hormone will lead to the chain of events that characterize the multiple hormonal actions *in vivo*. But before a rational appraisal is possible it is essential to decide from the indirect evidence available whether or not there need only be a unique site of action or whether the multiplicity of actions could be due to some extent to more than one site of action.

Currently the concept of a unique site of action is much in favor, whether it is the gene or the cell membrane (see Hechter and Halkerston, 1964). Certainly a single fundamental interaction explaining the diversity of hormonal actions would be more attractive than having to consider each action separately. On the other hand there is no theoretical or experimental argument against multiple sites of action, acting separately or in concert. Indeed the evolutionary considerations of hormonal function and the multiplicity of actions could be better explained on the basis of more than a single site of action (see Section II). Figure 11 schematically summarizes three of the many possible models, the first two based on a single site of action of hormones and the third depicting the situation with multiple sites.

Adenyl cyclase, the ubiquitous constituent of plasma membrane, is perhaps the closest one has got to the site of action of hormones. A large and ever-growing list of hormones can now be drawn up in which a very rapid activation or inhibition of adenyl cyclase is either a major response to hormone administration or that many biochemical and physiological actions of the hormone, specifically in its target cell, are mimicked by cyclic AMP (see Butcher *et al.*, 1968; and Vol. 2). Perhaps even the steroid hormones, which do not fit into this list, may eventually be included if the right experimental conditions are worked out. Certainly the cyclogenic action is the best explanation of the physiological proper ties of the rapid metabolic regulation by hormones such as adrenaline,

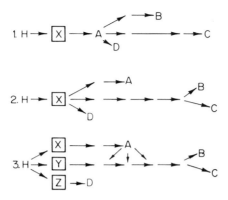

Fig. 11. Three hypothetical models suggesting how multiple biological effects (A, B,C,D) of a hormone (H) may be derived from either a single primary site of interaction (X), as in models 1 and 2, or multiple sites (X,Y,Z) as in model 3. In the latter model, the result of interaction with one of the sites (X) facilitates the expression of slower events via another site (Y). The number and length of arrows have been varied to suggest that the lag period and degree of remoteness of the various actions from the initial site of interaction are different. From Tata (1968a).

glucagon, and several pituitary trophic hormones. Cyclic AMP has also been convincingly invoked in the induction of enzymes for ACTH-induced adrenal steroidogenic enzymes (Garren, 1968). Indeed, Garren (1968) has proposed that cyclic AMP may be the agent responsible for the translational control of protein synthesis exerted by ACTH on adrenal tissue.

Even if cyclic AMP were the active agent, it is difficult to account for the chain of events that would lead from a rapid interaction of cyclic AMP with some cellular constituent(s) to the extremely slow responses of growth and developmental hormones. However, there is a good possibility that some of the early hormonal events associated with RNA and protein synthesis may arise from an activation of the adenyl cyclase or through some permeability control mechanism, for example, the early action of growth hormone on amino acid uptake and incorporation or the effect of tri-iodothyronine and estrogen on nucleotide uptake and metabolism (see Fig. 1). But an important question that is seldom asked is whether all the rapid effects bear a causal or only permissive relationship to the later events or whether the two are unrelated *in vivo*. This is indeed a difficult question to answer directly and is illustrated by the formation of products A and D in models 1 and 2 of Figure 11. A partial practical solution will be made possible by the discovery of a highly specific inhibitor of adenyl cyclase. Until this or some other solution is found, the mere observation of rapid and slow events in itself does not constitute the basis for a cause-and-effect relationship. Recently, in a study of the mimicry by dibutyryl cyclic AMP of many of the actions of TSH on thyroid cells it was found that the mimicry by the cyclic nucleotide was convincing for the rapid actions of the hormone but was only an apparent one for the slower growth-promoting actions—those of increased phospholipid (see Pastan and Macchia, 1967) and RNA synthesis (Kerkof and Tata, 1969). Whereas TSH caused a slow but net increase in phospholipid and RNA, of thyroid slices *in vitro,* dibutyryl cyclic AMP increased the specific activity of these constituents almost immediately upon its addition. This effect was later found to be due to an enhancement of the uptake of the radioactive precursor but not a true mimicry of the hormone action. A correction for isotope uptake completely abolished the mimicry of the biosynthetic actions of TSH but not as regards the rapid effects on iodine incorporation and discharge.

The almost universal occurrence of adenyl cyclase in cell membranes (from bacteria to mammals) and the mimicry by cyclic AMP of almost every type of biochemical and physiological function suggests that "cyclogenicity" maybe a primitive, rapid "reflex" of every type of living organism to almost any form of rapid or slow adjustment to environmental change. Such a reflex may or may not have a causal relationship with later events.

Sutherland has introduced the concept that cyclic AMP is the "second messenger" so that the specificity of eventual actions depends on the nature of the cell according to its pattern of differentiation (Sutherland *et al.,* 1967). This still leaves unanswered the important question of whether or not the hormone or any other cyclogenic agent interacts with adenyl cyclase itself. At the moment we have no suitable technique to distinguish between the site of action, often now termed receptors, and site of localization of a biologically active substance in that the latter may represent a site of storage, a "buffering capacity" or a site of metabolism. Wurtman (1968) has argued that the currently available isotopic or immunological methods of localization of hormones in intact cells (Stumpf, 1969; Greenspan and Hargadine, 1965; Pastan *et al.,* 1966; Gorski *et al.,* 1968; Shyamala and Gorski, 1969) or their interaction with extracts (Talwar *et al.,* 1964; Jensen *et al.,* 1968; Wilson and Loeb, 1965) does not allow the possibility of making the distinction. Since, on only theoretical considerations it would be expected that the "active" sites (high binding, affinity, low capacity) may be extremely few and the others (relatively low affinity, high capacity) numerous the problem is one of detecting a needle in a haystack. It is not unreasonable to predict that more powerful techniques will be developed to make such a distinction. It will be a major step in bringing closer the multiple biochemical phenomena of a hormone with its mechanism of action.

REFERENCES

Ahrén, K., and Hjalmarson, A. (1968). *In* "Growth Hormone" (A. Pecile and E. Müller, eds.), p. 143. Excerpta Med. Found., Amsterdam.

Aizawa, Y., and Mueller, G. C. (1961). *J. Biol. Chem.* **236**, 381.

Allfrey, V. G. (1968). *In* "Regulatory Mechanisms for Protein Synthesis in Mammalian Cells" (A. San Pietro, M. R. Lamborg, and F. T. Kenney, eds.), p. 65. Academic Press, New York.

Andrews, T. M., and Tata, J. R. (1968). *Biochem. Biophys. Res. Commun.* **32**, 1050.

Arias, I. M., Doyle, D., and Schimke, R. T. (1969). *J. Biol. Chem.* **244**, 3303.

Attardi, G., Parnas, H., Hwang, M., and Attardi, B. (1964). *J. Mol. Biol.* **20**, 145.

Barker, K. L., and Warren, J. C. (1966). *Proc. Natl. Acad. Sci. U. S.* **56**, 1298.

Barrington, E. J. W. (1964). "Hormones and Evolution." English Univ. Press, London.

Beato, M., Homoki, J., Lukacs, I., and Sekeris, C. E. (1968). *Z. Physiol. Chem.* **349**, 1099.

Bern, H. A., and Nicoll, C. S. (1968). *Recent Progr. Hormone Res.* **24**, 681.

Breuer, C. B., and Florini, J. R. (1966). *Biochemistry* **5**, 3857.

Brewer, E. N., Foster, L. B., and Sells, B. H. (1969). *J. Biol. Chem.* **244**, 1389.

Britten, R. J., and Davidson, E. H. (1969). *Science* **165**, 349.

Britten, R. J., and Kohne, D. E. (1968). *Science* **161**, 529.

Butcher, R. W., Robison, G. A., Hardman, J. G., and Sutherland, E. W. (1968). *Advan. Enzyme Regulation* **6**, 357.

Campbell, P. N. (1965). *Progr. Biophys. Mol. Biol.* **15**, 3.

Campbell, P. N., Lowe, E., and Serck-Hanssen, G. (1967). *Biochem. J.* **103**, 280.

Cohen, N. (1966). *Biol. Rev.* **41**, 503.

Cohen, P. P. (1966). *Harvey Lectures* **60**, 119.

Crouse, H. V. (1968). *Proc. Natl. Acad. Sci. U. S.* **61**, 971.

Dahmus, M. E., and Bonner, J. (1965). *Proc. Natl. Acad. Sci. U. S.* **54**, 1370.

Dallner, G., Siekevitz, P., and Palade, G. E. (1966). *J. Cell Biol.* **30**, 73.

Dingman, C. W., Aronow, A., Bunting, S. L., Peacock, A. C., and O'Malley, B. W. (1969). *Biochemistry* **8**, 489.

Drews, J. (1969). *European J. Biochem.* **7**, 200.

Drews, J., and Brawerman, G. (1967). *Science* **156**, 1385.

Earl, D. C. N., and Korner, A. (1966). *Arch. Biochem. Biophys.* **115**, 445.

Ebstein, M., Greenstein, M., and Wyatt, G. R. Personal communication.

Edelman, I., and Fimognari, G. M. (1968). *Recent Progr. Hormone Res.* **24**, 1.

Ekholm, R., and Strandberg, U. (1968). *J. Ultrastruct. Res.* **22**, 252.

Failoni, D., and Scarpelli, D. G. (1965). *Federation Proc.* **24**, 428.

Finkel, R. M., Henshaw, E. C., and Hiatt, H. H. (1966). *Mol. Pharmacol.* **2**, 221.

Fisher, D. B., and Mueller, G. C. (1968). *Proc. Natl. Acad. Sci. U. S.* **60**, 1396.

Foster, L. B., and Sells, B. H. (1969). *Arch. Biochem. Biophys.* **132**, 561.

Freinkel, N. (1964). *In* "The Thyroid Gland" (R. Pitt-Rivers and W. R. Trotter, eds.), Vol. I, p. 131. Butterworth, London and Washington, D. C.

Frieden, E. (1967). *Recent Progr. Hormone Res.* **23**, 139.

Garren, L. D. (1968). *Hormones Vitamins* **26**, 119.

Garren, L. D., Ney, R. L., and Davis, W. W. (1965). *Proc. Natl. Acad. Sci. U. S.* **53**, 1443.

Garren, L. D., Richardson, A. P., Jr., and Crocco, R. M. (1967). *J. Biol. Chem.* **242**, 650.

Georgiev, G. P. (1966). *Progr. Nucleic Acid Res. Mol. Biol.* **6**, 259.

Gorski, J., and Padnos, D. (1965). *Federation Proc.* **241**, 600.

Gorski, J., Toft, D., Shyamala, G., Smith, D., and Notides, A. (1968). *Recent Progr. Hormone Res.* **24**, 45

Greenman, D. L., Wicks, W. D., and Kenney, F. T. (1966). *J. Biol. Chem.* **240**, 4420.

Greenspan, F. S., and Hargadine, J. R. (1965). *J. Cell Biol.* **26**, 177.

Gupta, S. L., and Talwar, G. P. (1968). *Biochem. J.* **110**, 401.

Gurdon, J. B., and Woodland, H. R. (1968). *Biol. Rev.* **13**, 233.

Hahn, W. E., Church, R. B., Gorbman, A., and Wilmot, L. (1968). *Gen. Comp. Endocrinol.* **10**, 438.

Hamilton, T. H. (1968). *Science* **161**, 649.

Hamilton, T. H., Widnell, C. C., and Tata, J. R. (1968). *J. Biol. Chem.* **243**, 408.

Harris, H. (1964). *Nature* **202**, 249.

Hechter, O., and Halkerston, I. D. K. (1964). *Hormones* **5**, 697.

Hendler, R. W. (1968). "Protein Biosynthesis and Membrane Biochemistry." Wiley, New York.

Henshaw, E. C. (1968). *J. Mol. Biol.* **36**, 401.

Henshaw, E. C., Bojarski, T. B., and Hiatt, H. H. (1963). *J. Mol. Biol.* **7**, 122.

Henshaw, E. C., Revel, M., and Hiatt, H. H. (1965). *J. Mol. Biol.* **14**, 241.

Higashi, K., Matsuhisa, T., Kitao, A., and Sakamoto, Y. (1968). *Biochim. Biophys. Acta* **166**, 388.

Jensen, E. V., Suzuki, T., Kawashima, T., Stumpf, W. E., Jungblut, P. W., and De Sombre, E. R. (1968). *Proc. Natl. Acad. Sci. U. S.* **59**, 632.

Kafatos, E. F., and Feder, N. (1968). *Science* **161**, 470.

Karlson, P. (1963). *Angew. Chem.* **2**, 175.

Karlson, P., Sekeris, C. E., and Maurer, R. (1964). *Z. Physiol. Chem.* **336**, 100.

Kenney, F. T., Reel, J. R., Hager, B. C., and Wittliff, J. L. (1968). *In* "Regulatory Mechanisms for Protein Synthesis in Mammalian Cells" (A. San Pietro, M. R. Lamborg, and F. T. Kenney, eds.), p. 269. Academic Press, New York.

Kerkof, P. R., and Tata, J. R. (1967). *Biochem. Biophys. Res. Commun.* **28**, 111.

Kerkof, P. R., and Tata, J. R. (1969). *Biochem. J.* **112**, 729.

Kijima, S., and Wilt, F. H. (1969). *J. Mol. Biol.* **40**, 235.

Kim, K.-H., and Cohen, P. P. (1966). *Proc. Natl. Acad. Sci. U. S.* **55**, 1251.

King, R. J. B., Gordon, J., and Inman, D. R. (1965). *J. Endocrinol.* **32**, 9.

Knox, W. E., Auerbach, V. H., and Lin, E. C. C. (1956). *Physiol. Rev.* **36**, 164.

Korner, A. (1965a). *Recent. Progr. Hormone Res.* **21**, 205.

Korner, A. (1965b). *Biochem. J.* **92**, 449.

Korner, A. (1969). *Biochim. Biophys. Acta* **174**, 351.

Kostyo, J. L. (1968). *Ann. N. Y. Acad. Sci.* **148**, 389.

Labrie, F., and Korner, A. (1968). *J. Biol. Chem.* **243**, 1120.

Langan, T. A. (1968). *In* "Regulatory Mechanisms for Protein Synthesis in Mammalian Cells" (A. San Pietro, M. R. Lamborg, and F. T. Kenney, eds.), p. 101. Academic Press, New York.

Leduc, E. H., Avrameas, S., and Bouteille, M. (1968). *J. Exptl. Med.* **127**, 109.

Lehninger, A. L. (1962). *Physiol. Rev.* **42**, 467.

Liao, S., and Williams-Ashman, H. G. (1962). *Proc. Natl. Acad. Sci. U. S.* **48**, 1956.

Liao, S., Barton, R. W., and Lin, A. H. (1966a). *Proc. Natl. Acad. Sci. U. S.* **55**, 1593.

Liao, S., Lin, A. H., and Barton, R. W. (1966b). *J. Biol. Chem.* **241**, 3869.

Litwack, G., and Kritchevsky, D. (eds.) (1964). "Molecular Actions of Hormones," Wiley, New York.

Lockwood, D. H., Stockdale, F. E., and Topper, Y. J. (1967). *Science* **156**, 945.

McConkey, E. H., and Hopkins, J. W. (1965). *J. Mol. Biol.* **14**, 257.

Makman, M. H., Nakagawa, S., and White, A. (1967). *Recent Progr. Hormone Res.* **23**, 195.

Mainwaring, W. I. P. (1969). *Biochem. J.* **113**, 869.

Mangan, F. R., Neal, G. E., and Williams, D. C. (1968). *Arch. Biochem. Biophys.* **124**, 27.

Martin, T. E., and Wool, I. G. (1968). *Proc. Natl. Acad. Sci. U. S.* **60**, 569.

Marushige, K., and Bonner, J. (1966). *J. Mol. Biol.* **15**, 160.

Means, A. R., and Hamilton, T. H. (1966). *Proc. Natl. Acad. Sci. U. S.* **56**, 1594.

Mueller, G. C. (1965). *In* "Mechanisms of Hormone Action" (P. Karlson, ed.), p. 228. Thieme, Stuttgart.

Munro, H. N. (1968). *In* "Regulatory Mechanisms for Protein Synthesis in Mammalian Cells" (A. Sam Pietro, M. R. Lamborg, and F. T. Kenney, eds.), p. 183. Academic Press, New York.

Nakagawa, H., and Cohen, P. P. (1967). *J. Biol. Chem.* **242**, 642.

Nicholls, T. J., Follett, B. K., and Evennett, P. J. (1968). *Z. Zellforsch. Mikrokop. Anat.* **90**, 19.

Nishigori, H., and Aizawa, Y. (1968). *Endocrinol. Japon.* **15**, 209.

Notides, A., and Gorski, J. (1966). *Proc. Natl. Acad. Sci. U. S.* **56**, 230.

Ohtsuka, E., and Koide, S. S. (1969). *Biochem. Biophys. Res. Commun.* **35**, 648.

O'Malley, B. W., and McGuire, W. L. (1968). *Proc. Natl. Acad. Sci. U. S.* **60**, 1527.

O'Malley, B. W., McGuire, W. L., and Middleton, P. A. (1968). *Nature* **218**, 1249.

Omura, T., Siekevitz, P., and Palade, G. E. (1967). *J. Biol. Chem.* **242**, 2389.

Orrenius, S., and Ericsson, J. L. E. (1966). *J. Cell Biol.* **28**, 181.

Palade, G. E. (1966). *J. Am. Med. Assoc.* **198**, 815.

Pastan, I., and Macchia, V. (1967). *J. Biol. Chem.* **252**, 5757.

Pastan, I., Roth, J., and Macchia, V. (1966). *Proc. Natl. Acad. Sci. U. S.* **56**, 1802.

Paul, J., and Hunter, J. A. (1969). *J. Mol. Biol.* **42**, 31.

Perry, R. P., and Kelly, D. E. (1968). *J. Mol. Biol.* **35**, 37.

Pollak, J. K., and Ward, D. B. (1967). *Biochem. J.* **103**, 730.

Priestly, G. C., and Malt, R. A. (1969). *J. Cell Biol.* **41**, 886.

Roodyn, D. B., Freeman, K., and Tata, J. R. (1965). *Biochem. J.* **94**, 628.

Samarina, O. P., Lukanidin, E. M., Molnar, J., and Georgiev, G. P. (1968). *J. Mol. Biol.* **33**, 251.

Scherrer, K., and Marcaud, L. (1969). *J. Cell. Physiol. Suppl.* **1**, 181.

Sekeris, C. E. (1965). *In* "Mechanisms of Hormone Action" (P. Karlson, ed.), p. 149. Thieme, Stuttgart.

Sekeris, C. E. (1967). *Colloq. Ges. Physiol. Chem.* **18**, 126–151.

Sells, B. H., and Takahashi, T. (1967). *Biochim. Biophys. Acta* **134**, 69.

Shearer, R. W., and McCarthy, B. J. (1967). *Biochemistry* **6**, 283.

Shyamala, G., and Gorski, J. (1969). *J. Biol. Chem.* **244**, 1097.

Siekevitz, P., Palade, G. E., Dallner, G., Ohad, I., and Omura, T. (1967). *In* "Organizational Biosynthesis" (H. J. Vogel, J. O. Lampen, and V. Bryson, eds.), p. 331.

Snipes, C. A. (1968). *Quart. Rev. Biol.* **43**, 127.

Sokoloff, L. (1968). *In* "Regulatory Mechanisms for Protein Synthesis in Mammalian Cells" (A. San Pietro, M. R. Lamborg, and F. T. Kenney, eds.), p. 345. Academic Press, New York.

Sokoloff, L., Roberts, P. A., Januska, M. M., and Kline, J. E. (1968). *Proc. Natl. Acad. Sci. U. S.* **60**, 652.

Spirin, A. S. (1969). *European J. Biochem.* **10**, 20.

Staehelin, M. (1965). *Biochem. Z.* **342**, 459.

Steele, W. J., and Busch, H. (1966). *Biochem. Biophys. Acta* **119**, 501.

Stumpf, W. E. (1969). *Endocrinology* **85**, 31.

Sutherland, E. W., Butcher, R. W., Robison, G. A., and Hardman, J. G. (1967). *In* "Wirkungsmechanismon der Hormone" (P. Karlson, ed.), p. 1. Springer, Berlin.

Szirmai, J. A., and Van der Linde, P. C. (1964). *J. Ultrastruct. Res.* **12**, 380.

Talwar, G. P., Segal, S. J., Evans, A., and Davidson, O. W. (1964). *Proc. Natl. Acad. Sci. U. S.* **52**, 1059.

Tamaoki, T., and Mueller, G. C. (1965). *Biochim. Biophys. Acta* **108**, 73.

Tata, J. R. (1963). *Nature* **197**, 1167.

Tata, J. R. (1964). *In* "Actions of Hormones on Molecular Processes" (G. Litwack and D. Kritchevsky, eds.), p. 58. Wiley, New York.

Tata, J. R. (1966a). *Progr. Nucleic Acid Res. Mol. Biol.* **5**, 191.

Tata, J. R. (1966b). *Develop. Biol.* **13**, 77.

Tata, J. R. (1967a). *Biochem. J.* **104**, 1.

Tata, J. R. (1967b). *Biochem. J.* **105**, 783.

Tata, J. R. (1967c). *Nature* **213**, 516.

Tata, J. R. (1968a). *BBA Library* **11**, 222.

Tata, J. R. (1968b). *Nature* **219**, 331.

Tata, J. R. (1969a). *In* "Subcellular Components" (G. D. Birnie and S. Fox, eds.), p. 83. Butterworth, London and Washington, D. C.

Tata, J. R. (1969b). *Gen. Comp. Endocrinol. Suppl.* **2**, 385.

Tata, J. R. (1970). *Biochem. J.* (in press).

Tata, J. R., and Widnell, C. C. (1966). *Biochem. J.* **98**, 604.

Tata, J. R., and Williams-Ashman, H. G. (1967). *European J. Biochem.* **2**, 366.

Tata, J. R., Ernster, L., Lindberg, O., Arrhenius, E., Pedersen, S., and Hedman, R. (1963). *Biochem. J.* **86**, 408.

Teng, C. S., and Hamilton, T. H. (1967). *Biochem. J.* **105**, 1091.

Tepperman, J., and Tepperman, H. M. (1960). *Pharmacol. Rev.* **12**, 301.

Tomkins, G. M. (1968). *In* "Regulatory Mechanisms for Protein Synthesis in Mammalian Cells" (A. San Pietro, M. R. Lamborg, and F. T. Kenney, eds.), p. 269. Academic Press, New York.

Tomkins, G. M., and Ames, B. N. (1967). *Nat. Cancer Inst. Monograph* **27**, 221.

Tomkins, G. M., and Thompson, E. B. (1967). *Colloq. Ges. Physiol. Chem.* **18**, 107.

Tonoue, T., and Yamamoto, K. (1967). *Endocrinology* **81**, 1029.

Tsukada, K., Takako, M., Doi, O., and Lieberman, I. (1968). *J. Biol. Chem.* **243,** 1160.

Ursprung, H., and Schabtach, E. (1968). *Entwicklungsmech. Organ. Arch.* **160,** 243.

Weber, R. (1965). *Experientia* **21,** 665.

Widnell, C. C., and Tata, J. R. (1966a). *Biochem. J.* **98,** 621.

Widnell, C. C., and Tata, J. R. (1966b). *Biochim. Biophys. Acta.* **123,** 478.

Williams-Ashman, H. G., Liao, S., Hancock, R. L., Jurkovitz, L., and Silverman, D. A. (1964). *Recent Progr. Hormone Res.* **20,** 247.

Wilson, J., and Loeb, P. (1965). *19th Ann. Symp. Fundamental Cancer Res. Houston, Texas,* p. 375. Williams & Wilkins, Baltimore, Maryland.

Wool, I. G. (1965). *Federation Proc.* **24,** 1060.

Wool, I. G., and Cavicchi, P. (1967). *Biochemistry* **6,** 1230.

Wool, I. G., Stirewalt, W. S., Kurihara, K., Low, R. B., Bailey, P., and Oyer, D. (1968). *Recent Progr. Hormone Res.* **24,** 139.

Wurtman, R. J. (1968). *Science* **159,** 1261.

Wyatt, G. R., and Tata, J. R. (1968). *Biochem. J.* **109,** 253.

Yu, F. L., and Feigelson, P. (1969). *Arch. Biochem. Biophys.* **129,** 152.

CHAPTER 4

The Regulation of Some Biochemical Circadian Rhythms

Ira B. Black and Julius Axelrod

I. INTRODUCTION

Biological periodicity has been demonstrated in virtually all plant and animal species ranging from unicellular organisms to the most complex vertebrates. Biorhythms serve to synchronize the activities and capabilities of a species with a periodically varying environment. In addition, biological cycles synchronize the individuals within a species with one another, and synchronize multiple processes occurring within a single organism. In this context, such rhythms are of obvious survival value. For example, the probability of procreation will vary directly with the number of males and females simultaneously sexually active. Furthermore, in an oscillating environment, those individuals conceiving and delivering at the most propitious times (with respect to predation, food availability, ambient temperature, etc.) would be expected to produce viable progeny in largest numbers. Within the reproductive individual, clearly, synchronization of the physiological capability for reproduction with relevant sexual behavior is obligatory for the preservation of its genetic complement.

The form and timing of biorhythms in a species will not only alter its probability of survival, but will help to determine its evolutionary progression. Thus, with the evolutionary conversion of an organism from a diurnal to nocturnal creature, a new constellation of environmental pressures will affect the species' characteristics.

Biological rhythms may be endogenous to the organism or may be driven by environmental cues. Although the driving oscillation of a rhythm may reside within the organism, synchronization in time may depend upon external entraining agents. Such environmental factors, capable of entraining a rhythm, have been termed Zeitgeber by Aschoff (1951). To establish a periodicity as endogenous, it is necessary to exclude all environmental factors capable of functioning either as Zeitgeber or driving oscillations. With an organism placed in a constant environment, continuation of the periodicity [free-running period (Pittendrigh, 1958)] constitutes evidence for its endogenous character. Classically, light and temperature have been considered the critical variables. However, recent work has demonstrated that other geophysical factors such as weak magnetic fields (Brown, 1962a) (as in the case of *dugesia*), weak electrostatic fields (Brown, 1962b) (*dugesia*), and weak gamma fields (Brown, 1963) (*dugesia*) are capable of altering biological rhythms.

Biorhythms vary in period from minutes, as in the case of cyclic ribosomal aggregation (Kaempfer *et al.*, 1968), to decades (as in the cases of sexual maturation and climacteric). The most commonly studied cycles are circadian, with a period varying about a mean of approximately 24 hours. Confusion has arisen in use of the term "circadian." In this chapter, circadian is used to denote any rhythm with a period approximating 24 hours, whether endogenous or exogenous. Regardless of this period, these rhythms may be either unimodal or multimodal depending not only upon the nature of interaction of driving oscillation and measured parameter, but also upon the interaction of the measured parameter with other variables in the organism. The existence of endogenous rhythms with periods approximating environmental oscillations, implies, in a Darwinian sense, the natural selection of such cycles.

Functioning at the interface of organism and environment, the nervous system plays a role in transducing environmental information to biochemical cycles. This has been extensively documented in the activity rhythms of both primitive and complex forms. In the case of endogenous rhythms, the role of the nervous system may have changed from that of transducer to that of generator. In 1938, Kalmus reported a brain hormone that controlled the daily pigmentation rhythm in *carausius*. Similarly, Harker (1956) demonstrated that the activity rhythm in the cockroach, *periplaneta*, was lost upon decapitation and restored by transplantation of the subesophageal ganglion from a normally rhythmic animal. In vertebrates, the arguments are more complex but appear to support the role of central nervous system in driving rhythms throughout the organism. The well-recognized circadian variation in urinary (Pincus, 1943) (and plasma) adrenal corticoids persists during most diseases, and conditions that alter the normal sleep–wakefulness cycle (Migeon *et al.*, 1956), such as night work and total bed rest, but is disrupted by central nervous system disorders involving the temporal lobe, pretectal (Krieger, 1961) or hypothalamic (Hökfelt and Luft, 1959) areas. The central nervous system, through the mediation of ACTH, regulates the daily corticoid rhythm (Harris, 1960).

Additional lines of evidence support the contention that the central nervous system contains the driving oscillations of rhythms throughout the organism. The daily rat hepatic glycogen rhythm persists during fasting (Agren *et al.*, 1931). Recent work has demonstrated that hypothalamic and peripheral neural stimulation markedly alter the activities of glycogen synthetase, phosphorylase and glucose-6-phosphatase in rat liver (Shimazu and Fukuda, 1965; Shimazu, 1967), suggesting a neural role in the glycogen cycle. The driving oscillation of biorhythms may be obscured by numerous mediators. Thus the circadian rhythm in the activity of certain hepatic, microsomal enzymes that oxidatively metabolize drugs is dependent on the daily corticoid rhythm (Radzialowski and Bousquet, 1968), which is driven by cyclic pituitary ACTH secretion, which, in turn, is generated by hypothalamic factors.

Subsequent sections of this chapter will examine biochemical rhythms within the pineal gland and the rhythm in hepatic tyrosine transaminase activity in detail in an effort to elucidate the neural and molecular basis of such cycles.

II. CIRCADIAN RHYTHMS IN THE PINEAL GLAND

Mammalian pineal gland has high concentrations of the biogenic amines serotonin and norepinephrine, as well as the enzymes involved in their synthesis and metabolism. In the pineal gland biogenic amines undergo changes in content every 24 hours. The mammalian pineal gland is richly innervated by sympathetic nerves that contain both serotonin and norepinephrine. The activity of these nerves markedly influences biochemical reactions involving these biogenic amines.

A. SEROTONIN

The concentration of serotonin in most mammalian pineal glands is several times higher than that of any other organ (Giarman *et al.*, 1960). Its distribution within the pineal gland is unusual; it is present both in parenchymal cells and sympathetic nerves (Owman, 1964). In the sympathetic nerves, it is stored in dense core granules that also contain norepinephrine (Wolfe *et al.*, 1962). The biosynthesis of serotonin in the pineal gland proceeds through the following pathway: tryptophan → 5-hydroxytryptophan → 5-hydroxytryptamine (serotonin). The initial step is catalyzed by tryptophan hydroxylase, probably the rate-limiting enzyme. A fraction of the serotonin, which is synthesized in parenchymal cells, enters the sympathetic nerve and is taken up and stored in the intraneural granule (Owman, 1964). The remainder is metabolized via two pathways; the major metabolic pathway involves (1) deamination by monoamine oxidase to form 5-hydroxyindole acetic acid, and (2) transformation to *N*-acetyl serotonin by an acetylase. *N*-Acetyl serotonin is then methylated by hydroxyindole-*O*-methyltransferase (HIOMT) (Axelrod and Weissbach, 1961).

The concentration of serotonin in the rat pineal gland rises and falls over a 24-hour period (Quay, 1963). The maximum concentration (70 ng) occurs about 1 P.M., and the lowest (20 ng) about 11 P.M. (Fig. 1). This circadian rhythm appears to be endogenous since it persists in blinded rats and in rats exposed to constant darkness (Snyder *et al.*, 1965) (Fig. 1). However, it can be abolished when rats are kept in continuous light. With lighting schedule reversal (lights on during the night and darkness during the day) the phase of the rhythm was shifted about 180° over a period of 6 days, indicating that environmental lighting served as a Zeitgeber. Interrupting the sympathetic nerve to the pineal by ganglionectomy suppresses the serotonin rhythm (Fig. 1).

The serotonin rhythm may be generated by daily changes in the synthesis, metabolism, or release of this amine. To establish whether there are daily changes in the synthesis of serotonin, the precursors tryptophan and 5-hydroxytryptophan were administered at several times during the 24-hour day (Snyder *et al.*, 1967). Administration of these amino acids caused a marked increase in pineal serotonin. However, the magnitude of rise did not vary with the time of administration. These results indicated that changes in the rates of hydroxylation of tryptophan or

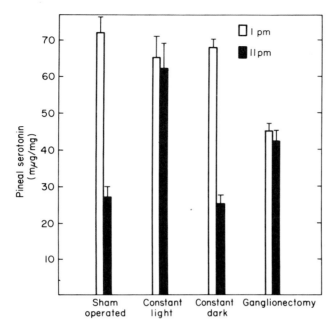

Fɪɢ. 1. Neural control of the circadian rhythm in pineal serotonin. Sham-operated and (superior cervical) ganglionectomized rats were exposed to light from 5 ᴀ.ᴍ. to 7 ᴘ.ᴍ. for 1 week after surgery. Normal rats were exposed to constant light or constant darkness. Vertical bars indicate standard errors of the mean.

decarboxylation of 5-hydroxytryptophan does not account for the daily changes in the serotonin content of the pineal gland. To determine whether there were changes in the rate of metabolism of serotonin, mono-amine oxidase activity was examined around the clock. No difference was observed. Experiments using monoamine oxidase inhibitors showed that more serotonin was released at night than during the day (Snyder *et al.*, 1967).

B. Norepinephrine

The content of norepinephrine in the rat pineal is high (3 to 12 $\mu g/gm$) (Wurtman *et al.*, 1967). This amine is confined mainly to the sympathetic nerves; denervation results in almost complete disappearance of the catecholamine (Zieher and Pellegrino de Iraldi, 1966). Norepinephrine is formed from tyrosine by the following sequence of reactions: tyrosine → dopa → dopamine → norepinephrine. In contrast to serotonin, all of the norepinephrine is stored in dense core vesicles of sympathetic nerves. Norepinephrine content of the rat pineal gland varied with time of day (Wurtman *et al.*, 1967). In rats exposed to alternating 12-hour periods of light and darkness, pineal norepinephrine levels peaked at the end of the dark period and fell continuously during the light period (Fig. 2). The rhythm in pineal norepinephrine was abolished by blinding (Fig. 2) continuous light, or continuous darkness. These results suggested that, in contrast to the pineal serotonin rhythm, the rhythm of norepinephrine is exogenous; it is generated by environmental lighting. To examine whether the norepinephrine rhythm was mediated by the flow of impulses from the central nervous system, pineal sympathetic nerves were interrupted by cutting the preganglionic fibers to the superior cervical ganglia. The norepinephrine rhythm was abolished. To determine the neural pathway through which environmental lighting generates the norepinephrine rhythm, the main optic tract and the inferior accessory optic tract were transected. The rhythm disappeared in rats in which the inferior accessory optic tract was cut, while it persisted after transection of the main optic tract, indicating that light-generated impulses reach the pineal via the inferior accessory optic tract.

Norepinephrine and serotonin appear to be stored in the same vesicle

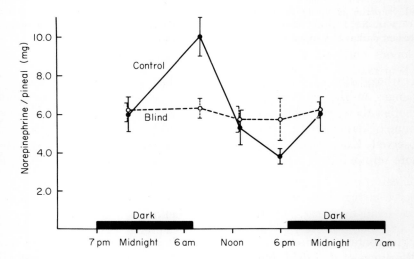

FIG. 2. Twenty-four-hour variation in pineal norepinephrine levels and the effect of blinding. Rats were blinded and maintained with sham-operated controls under diurnal lighting for 5 days. (Results are shown as mean ± SE.) (Wurtman *et al.*, 1967.)

in sympathetic nerves of the pineal gland and both undergo a 24-hour rhythm in concentration. This suggested that the content of these biogenic amines might be interrelated. The effect of changing the levels of norepinephrine on the content of pineal serotonin (Zweig and Axelrod, 1969) was examined. Norepinephrine content was selectively decreased by inhibition of its synthesis by α-methyl-*p*-tyrosine. Under these conditions, the serotonin content was elevated. The administration of norepinephrine blocked the increase of pineal serotonin by α-methyl tyrosine. These observations indicated a reciprocal relationship between norepinephrine and serotonin in the pineal gland.

C. REGULATION OF HYDROXYINDOLE-*O*-METHYLTRANSFERASE
ACTIVITY IN THE PINEAL GLAND BY
ENVIRONMENTAL LIGHTING

In the mammal, hydroxyindole-*O*-methyltransferase (HIOMT) is uniquely localized to the pineal gland (Axelrod *et al.*, 1961). This enzyme transfers the methyl group of S-adenosylmethionine to the hydroxyl group of *N*-acetylserotonin to form melatonin (5-methoxy-*N*-acetylserotonin). Melatonin is involved in the inhibition of the estrous cycle in rats (Wurtman *et al.*, 1963), and in blanching the skin of amphibians (Lerner *et al.*, 1958). Hydroxyindole-*O*-methyltransferase activity was increased more than twofold when rats were kept in continuous darkness as compared with those in continuous light (Fig. 3) (Wurtman *et al.*, 1963). The effects of environmental lighting on the melatonin-forming enzyme were abolished when the rats were blinded (Fig. 3). Removal of the sympathetic ganglia that innervate the pineal gland (Axelrod *et al.*, 1965) suppressed these differences in HIOMT between rats exposed to constant darkness and those exposed to constant light (Fig. 3). These results indicated that the environmental lighting message is transmitted by the retina via noradrenergic nerves to the pineal gland. To determine the specific pathways through which the nerve impulses reach the pineal, the inferior accessory optic tract and/or the main optic tract were cut and the effect of light and darkness on hydroxyindole-*O*-methyltransferase was examined (Moore *et al.*, 1967). Transection of the main optic tract caused an elevation of hydroxyindole-*O*-methyltransferase in darkness. When the inferior accessory optic tract was cut, darkness or light no longer altered hydroxyindole-*O*-methyltransferase activity. From these experiments, it can be concluded that information about lighting reaches the pineal gland as follows: retina →

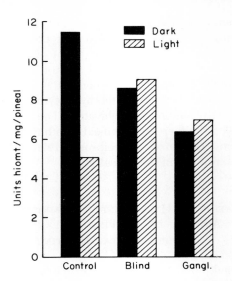

Fɪɢ. 3. Neural control of pineal HIOMT activity. Sham-operated (bilateral orbital), enucleated and ganglionectomized rats were exposed to normal diurnal lighting for 7 days. One unit of HIOMT equals 1 μmole of melatonin formed per hour after incubation with ^{14}C-methyl-S-adenosylmethionine and N-acetylserotonin.

inferior accessory optic tract → superior cervical ganglia → postganglionic sympathetic nerves → parenchymal cells of the pineal gland.

The sympathetic nerves to the pineal liberate norepinephrine as the neurotransmitter (von Euler, 1954). It thus seems possible that the liberated norepinephrine might influence the changes in hydroxyindole-O-methyltransferase. To approach this problem, pineal glands in organ culture were used. Rat pineal glands maintained in organ culture converted ^{14}C-tryptophan to ^{14}C-melatonin (Wurtman *et al.*, 1968a). Addition of norepinephrine to the culture medium caused a two- to threefold stimulation (Axelrod *et al.*, 1969) of the conversion of ^{14}C-tryptophan to ^{14}C-melatonin. The formation of ^{14}C proteins from ^{14}C-tryptophan was also increased by the addition of norepinephrine or related catecholamines (Wurtman *et al.*, 1969) by enhancing the cellular uptake of this amino acid.

Inhibition of protein synthesis *in vivo* prevented the stimulatory effect of darkness on the melatonin-forming enzyme (Axelrod *et al.*, 1965). It thus appears that the sympathetic nerve, by releasing norepinephrine, stimulates the activity of the hydroxyindole-O-methyltransferase, possibly by increasing enzyme synthesis.

III. CIRCADIAN RHYTHM OF HEPATIC TYROSINE TRANSAMINASE ACTIVITY

Tyrosine-α-ketoglutarate transaminase is the first in a sequence of enzymes that metabolize the amino acid tyrosine (Schepartz, 1951). Hepatic tyrosine transaminase, a soluble, pyridoxal-requiring enzyme, has been of particular interest in the sphere of regulatory biochemistry. As the initial (Canellakis and Cohen, 1956), and probably rate-limiting enzyme in tyrosine metabolism, tyrosine transaminase determines the degradative flux of an amino acid that is converted to Kreb's cycle intermediates (Edwards and Knox, 1956), as well as the neurotransmitter norepinephrine, the hormone epinephrine (Udenfriend and Wyngaarden, 1956), and the pigment melanin (Mason, 1948). The enzyme turns over with a half-life of approximately 1.5 hours (Kenney, 1967a), allowing fine control of its activity and experimental use as a convenient model in regulatory, biochemistry.

In 1957, Lin and Knox demonstrated that rat hepatic tyrosine transaminase activity increases several-fold 4 hours after the administration of hydrocortisone or tyrosine. Only the steroid, however, was associated with increased activity in the adrenalectomized rat. Steroids increase tyrosine transaminase activity through an actinomycin-sensitive process (Greengard *et al.*, 1963), due to increased synthesis of tyrosine transaminase protein (Granner *et al.*, 1968). Although several amino acids are capable of elevating enzyme activity in the intact rat, only tryptophan (Rosen and Milholland, 1963) is effective in the adrenalectomized animal. Several other compounds elevate enzyme activity in the adrenalectomized rat. Thus, glucagon (Greengard and Baker, 1966) and insulin (Holten and Kenney, 1967), for example, cause an actinomycin-sensitive increase in enzyme activity, secondary to an increase in enzyme synthesis. Evidence has recently been presented suggesting that growth hormone (Kenney, 1967b) suppresses enzyme activity through inhibition of tyrosine transaminase synthesis.

In 1966, Potter *et al.* demonstrated that rat hepatic tyrosine transaminase undergoes a 24-hour rhythm in activity, varying over a three- to fourfold range daily. Subsequent investigations have indicated that the rhythm persists in the absence of the pituitary or adrenal glands (Civen *et al.*, 1967; Shambaugh *et al.*, 1967; Wurtman and Axelrod, 1967). Enzyme activity reaches a peak between 8 and 11 P.M., rapidly falls to nadir values by 8 A.M., and remains at basal levels until the early evening rise (Fig. 4).

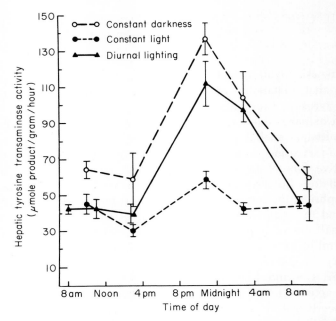

FIG. 4. Effect of environmental lighting on the hepatic tyrosine transaminase rhythm. Controls were subjected to the normal diurnal light cycle with lights on from 5 A.M. to 7 P.M. Experimental groups were exposed to either constant light or constant darkness for 1 week. Each group at each time consisted of six animals. Vertical bars indicate standard errors of the mean. In all groups the 11 P.M. value differs from the 3 P.M. value at $p < 0.001$. (Black and Axelrod, 1968a).

A. CHARACTERISTICS OF THE TYROSINE TRANSAMINASE RHYTHM

1. Environmental Lighting

Investigations were undertaken to elucidate the relationship of the hepatic enzyme rhythm to the environment (Black and Axelrod, 1968a). Intact rats were exposed to the normal diurnal lighting schedule (cool white fluorescent lights on at 50 to 75 ft-c illumination from 5 A.M. to 7 P.M.) while other groups were exposed to constant light or constant darkness for 1 week (seven cycles). In constant darkness, the rhythm persisted essentially unchanged. Seven days of constant light resulted in unaltered period or phase, but reduced the rhythm's amplitude (Fig. 4). Persistence of the rhythm during constant lighting conditions indicates that the enzyme cycle is not generated by external light cues and thus is endogenous. Amplitude reduction in constant light suggests that either the amplitude (and/or basal level) of the driving oscillation, or the sensitivity of the measured parameter (enzyme activity) to that oscillation, decreases in constant light.

To determine whether a combination of light and dark stimuli during the 24-hour day serves to synchronize the rhythm in time, groups of rats were exposed to either the normal or a reversed lighting schedule. Those rats exposed to schedule reversal exhibited a nearly 180° shift of rhythm phase (Black and Axelrod, 1968a), indicating that environmental lighting is capable of entraining the enzyme rhythm (Fig. 5), and that both a light signal and a dark signal, at critical times of the 24-hour day, are necessary for synchronization. Thus, the enzyme rhythm is endogenous to the rat and is entrained by environmental lighting.

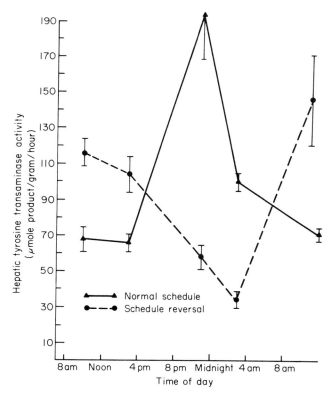

Fig. 5. Synchronization of the hepatic tyrosine transaminase rhythm by environmental lighting. Control rats were exposed to the normal diurnal light–dark cycle (see Fig. 4). The experimental group was subjected to a reversed lighting cycle with lights on from 7 P.M. to 5 A.M. Vertical bars indicate standard errors of the mean. Both rhythms are statistically significant at $p < 0.001$. (Black and Axelrod, 1968a.)

2. Feeding

Because amino acids induce tyrosine transaminase, and because the rat almost doubles its food intake between 4 and 10 P.M., cyclic feeding might generate the enzyme rhythm (Wurtman *et al.*, 1968b). If the peak in tyrosine transaminase activity is dependent upon the peak in food ingestion, the enzyme rhythm should extinguish when rats are deprived of food for 6 or more hours (i.e., from before 2 P.M. or earlier). Groups of rats were fasted for 6, 8, 10, and 12 hours before death and were killed at 8 A.M. and 8 P.M., times corresponding to nadir and peak enzyme activities.

Controls were offered food ad libitum. Both normal and adrenal-ectomized animals were studied to eliminate the possibility that stress due to fasting (e.g., hypoglycemia) might cause increased adrenal steroid secretion with elevation of enzyme activity. The enzyme rhythm persisted in rats fasted up to and including 10 hours (Black and Axelrod, 1968a) (Table I). After 12 hours, a significant rhythm was observed in approximately one-half of the experiments, but a statistically significant rhythm was not discernible after a 24-hour fast. Similar results were obtained with intact rats. Thus, the increased food ingestion after 4 P.M. does not appear responsible for the 8 P.M. peak in tyrosine transaminase activity, since rats fasted up to at least 10 hours before the normal peak time

TABLE I

THE EFFECT OF FASTING ON THE TYROSINE TRANSAMINASE
RHYTHM IN ADRENALECTOMIZED RATS[a]

Hours fasted	Tyrosine transaminase activity	
	8 A.M.	8 P.M.
0	32.3 ± 5.8	75.8 ±8.8[b]
8	20.8 ± 2.5	48.7 ± 3.9[b]
9	32.2 ± 4.9	60.4 ± 5.7[b]
10	34.9 ± 3.7	69.3 ± 11.2[b]
12	43.6 ± 4.1	87.6 ± 8.6[b]
12	57.1 ± 3.4	84.5 ± 18.3[c]
24	62.4 ± 5.3	80.2 ± 18.4[c]

[a] Rats were fasted for varying periods of time prior to death, e.g., those fasted for 10 hours were deprived of food from 10 P.M. to 8 A.M., and from 10 A.M. to 8 P.M. Controls were provided with food ad libitum. Each group consisted of 6 to 8 rats. Results are expressed as μmole product/gm/hour ± standard error of the mean. (Black and Axelrod, 1968a)

[b] Differs from 8 A.M. group at $p < 0.02$.

[c] No significant difference.

(i.e., from 10 A.M. to 8 P.M.) demonstrate a clear rhythm. The enzyme cycle is occasionally obscured by the modestly elevated basal activities observed in those groups fasted 12 hours. This may reflect an imposed hypoglycemia with secondary secretion of glucagon (Greengard and Baker, 1966). In addition, in an enzyme with a half-life of approximately 1.5 hours, a 12-hour fast may result in a relative lack of amino acid precursors for the synthesis of tyrosine transaminase or its degrading system, rather than in an alteration of the driving oscillation of the rhythm. Other investigators have demonstrated that there is a peak in enzyme activity during fasting equal in amplitude to that observed in the fed animal (Potter *et al.*, 1968). Although the ingestion of food per se does not appear to constitute the driving oscillation of the enzyme activity rhythm, cyclic feeding may serve to synchronize the diurnal enzyme variation in time. Fuller and Snoddy (1968) have demonstrated that the phase of the rhythm may be shifted by an imposed change in the availability of food, suggesting that feeding may function as a Zeitgeber (analogous to the observations with lighting). It is possible that some correlate of the complex act of feeding, other than the ingestion of food itself, may be the true Zeitgeber.

3. Adrenal and Pituitary Glands

The enzyme rhythm persists for 2 weeks after adrenalectomy or hypophysectomy (Civen *et al.*, 1967; Shambaugh *et al.*, 1967; Wurtman and Axelrod, 1967). Since the effects of steroids could conceivably persist for a longer period of time, adrenalectomized rats were examined 1, 2, and 8 weeks after surgery. No consistent change in the enzyme rhythm was discernible (Black and Axelrod, 1968a).

B. The Role of Norepinephrine

The tyrosine transaminase activity rhythm is endogenous to the rat, and can be entrained by the lighting and/or feeding schedules. The enzyme cycle may be driven by phenomena intrinsic to the hepatic cell, or may be controlled by humoral or neural mechanisms. The last alternative was examined through the use of pharmacological tools that allow manipulation of specific neurotransmitters. Since glucocorticoids and amino acids increase tyrosine transaminase activity, only adrenalectomized rats were used, and were fasted during the time of study.

Reserpine, a depletor of biogenic amines, was administered to rats in a dose of 2 mg/kg. Whole brain norepinephrine was employed as an index of depletion of tissue norepinephrine. Tyrosine transaminase activity exhibited a threefold increase in activity within 8 hours, while brain norepinephrine showed greater than a 90% depletion (Black and Axelrod, 1968b). Doses of less than 1 mg/kg caused erratic depletion of brain norepinephrine, and inconsistent increases of tyrosine transaminase activity. In experiments dealing with biological rhythms, dosage and time of drug administration are of critical importance. Variable increases in tyrosine transaminase activity were obtained when norepinephrine depletion was less than 90%. Some property of the reserpine molecule other than its ability to cause amine depletion could theoretically be responsible for the elevation of tyrosine transaminase activity. To exclude this possibility, reserpine was administered after pretreatment with catron, a monoamine oxidase inhibitor. This regimen prevents norepinephrine depletion. Reserpine administered alone was associated with the expected threefold elevation in enzyme activity, whereas the catron-pretreated rats showed no depletion of brain norepinephrine and no significant rise in tyrosine transaminase activity (Black and Axelrod, 1968c).

To determine whether the increased enzyme activity was attributable to the synthesis of new enzyme protein, puromycin, an inhibitor of protein synthesis was administered to rats previously treated with reserpine. Reserpine caused the expected rise in tyrosine transaminase activity, whereas puromycin reduced activity to control levels in rats pretreated with reserpine (Black and Axelrod, 1968b) (Fig. 6).

Because reserpine depletes serotonin as well as norepinephrine, the effect of depletion of norepinephrine alone was studied. α-Methyl-p-tyrosine (α-m-t) inhibits tyrosine hydroxylase (Spector *et al.*, 1965), the rate-limiting enzyme in norepinephrine biosynthesis (Levitt *et al.*, 1965), which catalyzes the conversion of L-tyrosine to L-DOPA. Norepinephrine is selectively depleted whereas the levels of serotonin are not affected. Norepinephrine stores may be repleted by giving precursors distal to the block in norepinephrine synthesis. L-DOPA was employed for this purpose. The effect of α-m-t was to increase tyrosine transaminase activity nearly fivefold and reduce brain norepinephrine by approximately 90% (Table II). L-DOPA significantly elevated brain norepinephrine in rats treated with the tyrosine hydroxylase inhibitor and reversed the effect of α-m-t in raising tyrosine transaminase activity (Black and Axelrod, 1968b).

Thus, depletion of tissue norepinephrine was associated with a three- to fivefold rise in tyrosine transaminase activity. This rise was abolished by puromycin. These observations are consistent with a mechanism in which norepinephrine, either directly or indirectly, suppresses the synthesis of tyrosine transaminase activity. Alternatively, norepinephrine may suppress the synthesis of a tyrosine transaminase activating protein. In

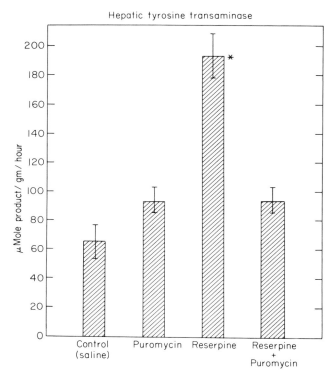

FIG. 6. Elevation of hepatic tyrosine transaminase activity by reserpine. One group received reserpine 2 mg/kg at 12 midnight. Those treated with puromycin alone received 50 mg/kg at 8 A.M. and 10 A.M. Rats given the combination were treated with reserpine 2 mg/kg at 12 midnight, and puromycin 50 mg/kg at 8 A.M. and 10 A.M. Controls were treated with saline at appropriate times. All injections were intraperitoneal. All rats were killed at 12 noon. Vertical bars indicate standard errors of the mean. The point indicated by the asterisk (*) differs from control at $p <$ 0.001, differs from reserpine + puromycin at $p < 0.001$. (Black and Axelrod, 1968b.)

the absence of the adrenal glands, norepinephrine is restricted to, and must be operating via, the central and/or peripheral nervous system(s), and may exert its effect through neural or blood-borne mediation.

Theoretically, elevation of tissue norepinephrine should abolish the daily rhythm by suppressing the synthesis of tyrosine transaminase. Norepinephrine was elevated by blocking intraneural degradation by monoamine oxidase. In groups killed 24 hours after the administration of β-phenylisopropylhydrazine (Catron), the enzyme rhythm was abolished between basal and peak levels, whereas brain norepinephrine exhibited a significant (60%) increase in concentration (Axelrod and Black, 1968).

TABLE II

The Effect of Depletion and Repletion of Brain Norepinephrine
on Hepatic Tyrosine Transaminase Activity[a]

Group	Hepatic tyrosine transaminase (μmole product/ gm/hour)	Brain Norepinephrine (NE) (μg NE/gm brain)
Control	43.4 ± 12.3	0.458 ± 0.023
α-Methyl-p-tyrosine	190.1 ± 18.4^b	0.056 ± 0.016^c
L-DOPA	34.6 ± 4.1	0.431 ± 0.037
α-Methyl-p-tyrosine + L-DOPA	51.1 ± 5.9	0.206 ± 0.034

[a] Rats receiving α-methyl-p-tyrosine were injected with 200 mg/kg at 12 midnight, and 50 mg/kg at 8 A.M. Those treated with L-DOPA alone received 100 mg/kg at 8 A.M. The group treated with the combination was injected with α-methyl-p-tyrosine 200 mg/ kg at 12 midnight, and 50 mg/kg at 8 A.M., and L-DOPA 100 mg/kg at 8 A.M. Controls were treated with 1 ml of saline at appropriate times. All rats were killed at 12 noon. All injections were intraperitoneal. Results expressed as mean $\pm$ standard error. (Black and Axelrod, 1968b)

[b] Differs from control at $p < 0.001$, differs from α-methyl-p-tyrosine + L-DOPA at $p < 0.001$.

[c] Differs from control at $p < 0.001$, differs from α-methyl-p-tyrosine + L-DOPA at $p < 0.05$.

Because monoamine oxidase inhibitors elevate endogenous serotonin as well as norepinephrine, the tissue catecholamine content was selectively increased by the administration of large doses of L-DOPA. This precursor of norepinephrine caused a 15% increase in brain norepinephrine and suppressed the tyrosine transaminase activity rhythm by abolition of the normal evening peak (Axelrod and Black, 1968). Enzyme activity was equal to or below baseline values at all times (Fig. 7).

Thus, two structurally dissimilar compounds, Catron and L-DOPA, which raise tissue norepinephrine by different mechanisms, suppress the characteristic 10 P.M. peak in hepatic tyrosine transaminase activity. The evening elevation may result from decreased neuronal norepinephrine release, secondary either to a reduction in neural activity, or to a decrease in the effective neural concentration of norepinephrine: Norepinephrine, directly or indirectly, may repress the synthesis of tyrosine transaminase, whereas daily variations in the neural catecholamine release may generate the rhythm in tyrosine transaminase activity. Such an hypothesis is consistent with the observations that the norepinephrine concentration of various areas of the rat brain varies daily (Friedman and Walker, 1968; Reis *et al.*, 1968). If this formulation is correct, circadian variation in the concentration of norepinephrine may constitute the driving oscillation of the tyrosine transaminase activity rhythm. In turn, the oscillation in neuronal norepinephrine concentration may be determined by daily variations in the activity of the rate-limiting enzymes in norepinephrine synthesis and/or inactivation. Such a rhythm has already been documented in the case of pineal tyrosine hydroxylase (Mc-Geer and McGeer, 1966), the rate-limiting enzyme in norepinephrine biosynthesis. Since norepinephrine is restricted to the sympathetic nerves impinging on the pinealocytes (Zieher and Pellegrino de Iraldi, 1966), these data are consistent with the present formulation.

Subsequent studies have demonstrated that norepinephrine, by competing with apotyrosine transaminase for the binding of the pyridoxal-5′-phosphate cofactor, inhibits enzyme activity *in vitro*. Investigations indicate that the neuromediator may regulate tyrosine transaminase

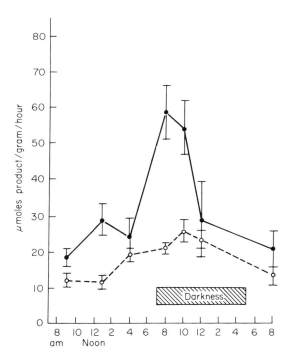

FIG. 7. Effect of L-DOPA on the hepatic tyrosine transaminase activity rhythm. Each group of rats was treated with a suspension of L-DOPA, 100 mg/kg intraperitoneally in a volume of 1 ml 4 hours before death. Controls were injected with saline at appropriate times. Vertical bars indicate standard errors of the mean. ●——● = saline, ○——○ = L-DOPA. (Axelrod and Black, 1968.)

turnover *in vivo* by binding cofactor (Black and Axelrod, 1969b). The rhythm in enzyme activity may therefore be dependent on daily fluctuations in the norepinephrine/pyridoxal-5'-phosphate ratio.

IV. CONCLUSIONS: POSSIBLE DRIVING OSCILLATIONS OF BIOCHEMICAL RHYTHMS

If the central nervous system contains the driving oscillation(s) of endogenous biological rhythms, central neural rhythmic correlates should be identifiable. In fact, a number of biogenic amines that may function as neuromediators exhibit rhythmicity in discrete brain areas. Norepinephrine, serotonin (Friedman and Walker, 1968; Reis *et al.*, 1968), and histamine (Friedman and Walker, 1968) undergo dissynchronous circadian variation in regions of the rat midbrain and brain stem, and a seasonal rhythm in toad brain epinephrine, norepinephrine, and serotonin has been identified (Segura *et al.*, 1967). Temporal variation in the concentration of agents that presumably function as central neurotransmitters allows for obvious mechanisms of transmission of information concerning rhythmic functions. Of greater interest, perhaps, is the fact that neuromediator rhythms may constitute part of the driving oscillator mechanism itself.

Recent work has shown a daily rhythm in the rate of depletion of brain norepinephrine by reserpine (Black and Axelrod, 1969). Because this cycle is restricted to the brain, an inherent characteristic of the central nervous system, rather than a generalized oscillation in the organism affecting reserpine metabolism is indicated. Circadian variation in the sensitivity of the noradrenergic storage vesicle to norepinephrine release by reserpine may reflect a rhythm residing within the vesicle or an oscillation of factors affecting vesicles, such as nerve impulse frequency.

If the central nervous system generates endogenous biological rhythmicity, one might expect that (1) single neurons, or at least groups of neurons, should function rhythmically in the absence of exogenous stimuli, and (2) the "clock" function should have already been incorporated into the evolutionarily primitive nervous system. The studies of Strumwasser (1965) document these points. Nerve Cell 3 of the parietovisceral ganglion of the sea hare, *Aplysia californica*, exhibits an endogenous, circadian rhythm in spontaneous spike frequency for days after removal from its host. The phase-timing of this rhythm can be changed by the intracellular injection of actinomycin D, implicating a messenger

RNA role. In addition, this isolated neuron contains an endogenous lunar rhythm in spike frequency; a parabolic rhythm describes the successive intervals between action potentials over a course of minutes.

Little is known concerning the subcellular localization of driving mechanisms in animal forms. Work with the unicellular green alga *acetabulariae* (Schweiger and Schweiger, 1965) has indicated that the nucleus is capable of controlling a cytoplasmic rhythm. In these experiments, transplanted nuclei generated their own rhythms in foreign cytoplasm.

Periodicity in the concentration of neuromediators in the brain clearly implies the existence of rhythms in the metabolism of these amines. Whether such temporal variation is an immutable characteristic of a particular series of biochemical reactions or whether it is secondary to factors that affect enzyme activity (e.g., nerve impulse frequency, inhibitor concentration) has yet to be resolved.

REFERENCES

Agren, G., Wilander, O., and Jorpes, E. (1931). *Biochem. J.* **25**, 777.
Aschoff, J. (1951). *Naturwissenchaften* **38**, 506.
Axelrod, J., and Black, I. B. (1968). *Nature* **220**, 161.
Axelrod, J., and Weissbach, H. (1961). *J. Biol. Chem.* **236**, 211.
Axelrod, J., MacLean, P. D., Albers, R. W., and Weissbach, H. (1961). In "Regional Neurochemistry" (S. S. Kety and J. Elkes, eds.), pp. 307–311. Pergamon Press, Oxford.
Axelrod, J., Wurtman, R. J., and Snyder, S. H. (1965). *J. Biol. Chem.* **240**, 949.
Axelrod, J., Shein, H. M., and Wurtman, R. J. (1969). *Proc. Natl. Acad. Sci. U. S.* **62**, 544.
Black, I. B., and Axelrod, J. (1968a). *Proc. Natl. Acad. Sci. U. S.* **61**, 1287.
Black, I. B., and Axelrod, J. (1968b). *Proc. Natl. Acad. Sci. U. S.* **59**, 1231.
Black, I. B., and Axelrod, J. (1968c). Unpublished observations.
Black, I. B., Parker, L., and Axelrod, J. (1969a). *Biochem. Pharmacol.* **18**, 2688.
Black, I. B., and Axelrod, J. (1969b). *J. Biol. Chem.* **244**, 6124.
Brown, F. A., Jr. (1962a). *Biol. Bull.* **123**, 264.
Brown, F. A., Jr. (1962b). *Biol. Bull.* **123**, 282.
Brown, F. A., Jr. (1963). *Biol. Bull.* **125**, 206.
Canellakis, Z. N., and Cohen, P. P. (1956). *J. Biol. Chem.* **222**, 53.
Civen, M., Ulrich, R., Trimmer, B. M., and Brown, C. B. (1967). *Science* **157**, 1563.
Edwards, S. W., and Knox, W. E. (1956). *J. Biol. Chem.* **220**, 79.
Friedman, A. H., and Walker, C. A., (1968). *J. Physiol. (London)* **197**, 77.
Fuller, R. W., and Snoddy, H. D. (1968). *Science* **159**, 738.
Giarman, N. J., Freedman, D. X., and Picard-Ami, L. (1960). *Nature* **186**, 480.
Granner, D. K., Hayashi, S., Thompson, E. B., and Tomkins, G. (1968). *J. Mol. Biol.* **35**, 291.

Greengard, O., and Baker, G. T. (1966). *Science* **154**, 1461.

Greengard, O., Smith, M. A., and Acs, G. (1963). *J. Biol. Chem.* **238**, 1548.

Harker, J. E. (1956). *J. Exp. Biol.* **33**, 224.

Harris, G. W. (1960). *In* "Handbook of Physiology" (Am. Physiol. Soc., J. Field, ed.), Sect. 1, Vol. II, pp. 1007–1038. Williams & Wilkins, Baltimore, Maryland.

Hökfelt, B., and Luft, R. (1959). *Acta Endocrinol.* **32**, 177.

Holten, D., and Kenney, F. T. (1967). *J. Biol. Chem.* **242**, 4372.

Kaempfer, R. O. R., Meselson, M., and Raskas, H. J. (1968). *J. Mol. Biol.* **31**, 277.

Kalmus, H. (1938). *Z. Vergleich. Physiol.* **25**, 494.

Kenney, F. T., (1967a). *Science* **156**, 525.

Kenney, F. T. (1967b). *J. Biol. Chem.* **242**, 4367.

Krieger, D. T. (1961). *J. Clin. Endocrinol. Metab.* **21**, 695.

Lerner, A. B., Case, J. D., Takahashi, Y., Lee, T. H., and Mori, W. (1958). *J. Am. Chem. Soc.* **80**, 2587.

Levitt, M., Spector, S., Sjoerdsma, A., and Udenfriend, S. (1965). *J. Pharmacol. Exptl. Therap.* **148**, 1.

Lin, E. C. C., and Knox, W. E. (1957). *Biochim. Biophys. Acta* **26**, 85.

McGeer, E. G., and McGeer, P. L. (1966). *Science* **153**, 73.

Mason, H. S. (1948). *J. Biol. Chem.* **172**, 83.

Migeon, C. J., Tyler, F. H., Mahoney, J. P., Florentin, A. A., Castle, H., Bliss, E. L., and Samuels, L. T. (1956). *J. Clin. Endocrinol. Metab.* **16**, 622.

Moore, R. Y., Heller, A., Wurtman, R. J., and Axelrod, J. (1967). *Science* **155**, 220.

Owman, C. (1964). *Intern. J. Neuropharmacol.* **3**, 105.

Pincus, G. (1943). *J. Clin. Endocrinol.* **3**, 195.

Pittendrigh, C. S. (1958). *In* "Symposium on Perspectives in Marine Biology" (A. A. Buzzati-Traversa, ed.), pp. 239–268. Univ. of California Press, Berkeley, California.

Potter, V. R., Gebert, R. A., Pitot, H. C., Peraino, C., Lamar, C., Jr., Lesher, S., and Morris, H. P. (1966). *Cancer Res.* **26**, 1547.

Potter, V. R., Baril, E. F., Watanabe, M., and Whittle, E. D. (1968). *Federation Proc.* **27**, 1238.

Quay, W. B. (1963). *Gen. Comp. Endocrinol.* **3**, 474.

Radzialowski, F. M., and Bousquet, W. F. (1968). *J. Pharmacol. Exptl. Therap.* **163**, 229.

Reis, D. J., Weinbren, M., and Corvelli, A. (1968). *J. Pharmacol. Exptl. Therap.* **164**, 135.

Rosen, F., and Milholland, R. J. (1963). *J. Biol. Chem.* **238**, 3730.

Schepartz, B. (1951). *J. Biol. Chem.* **193**, 293.

Schweiger, H. G., and Schweiger, E. (1965). *In* "Circadian Clocks" (J. Aschoff, ed.), pp. 195–197. North Holland Publ., Amsterdam.

Segura, E. T., Biscardi, A. M., and Apelbaum, J. (1967). *Comp. Biochem. Physiol.* **22**, 843.

Shambaugh, G. E., III, Warner, D. A., and Beisel, W. R. (1967). *Endocrinology* **81**, 811.

Shimazu, T. (1967). *Science* **156**, 1256.

Shimazu, T., and Fukuda, A. (1965). *Science* **150**, 1607.

Snyder, S. H., Zweig, M., Axelrod, J., and Fischer, J. E. (1965). *Proc. Natl. Acad. Sci. U. S.* **53**, 301.

Snyder, S. H., Zweig, M., and Axelrod, J. (1967). *J. Pharmacol. Exptl. Therap.* **158**, 206.

Spector, S., Sjoerdsma, A., and Udenfriend, S. (1965). *J. Pharmacol. Exptl. Therap.* **147**, 86.

Strumwasser, F. (1965). *In* "Circadian Clocks" (J. Aschoff, ed.), pp. 442–462. North-Holland Publ., Amsterdam.

Udenfriend, S., and Wyngaarden, J. B. (1956). *Biochim. Biophys. Acta* **20**, 48.

von Euler, U. S. (1954). *Pharmacol. Rev.* **6**, 15.

Wolfe, D. E., Potter, L. T., Richardson, K. C., and Axelrod, J. (1962). *Science* **138**, 440.

Wurtman, R. J., and Axelrod, J. (1967). *Proc. Natl. Acad. Sci. U. S.* **57**, 1594.

Wurtman, R. J., Axelrod, J., and Chu, E. W. (1963). *Science* **141**, 277.

Wurtman, R. J., Axelrod, J., Sedvall, G., and Moore, R. Y. (1967). *J. Pharmacol. Exptl. Therap.* **157**, 487.

Wurtman, R. J., Larin, F., Axelrod, J., Shein, H. M., and Rosasco, K. (1968a). *Nature* **217**, 953.

Wurtman, R. J., Shoemaker, W. J., and Larin, F. (1968b). *Proc. Natl. Acad. Sci. U. S.* **59**, 800.

Wurtman, R. J., Shein, H. M., Axelrod, J., and Larin, F. (1969). *Proc. Natl. Acad. Sci. U. S.* **62**, 749.

Zieher, L. M., and Pellegrino de Iraldi, A. (1966). *Life Sci.* **5**, 155.

Zweig, M., and Axelrod, J. (1969). *J. Neurobiol.* **1**, 87.

CHAPTER 5

Hormones
and Transport
across Cell Membranes

Thomas R. Riggs

I. INTRODUCTION

The cell membrane was early suggested as a possible site of hormone action. The proposal was premature at the time that it was made, however, because biologists then lacked the tools to test the hypothesis adequately. Subsequently, enzymology and biochemical genetics have in turn appeared as productive and, consequently, popular approaches to biochemical problems; and so, not unexpectedly, both have been proposed as holding the key to the way hormones act. Each of these successive theories was conceived as putting the explanation one step closer to the primary action of the hormone. First, effects of hormones on transports, as well as on other metabolism, were imagined as in reality resulting from modifications of enzyme activities that are either directly or indirectly involved in the transport processes. The gene hypothesis, on the other hand, proposes that enzyme activities are controlled by modification of genetic production of enzymes. These enzymes would then include those that affect transport processes.

Present evidence does not rule out the possibility that hormonal actions on transport are produced in any one of these ways. Very little is yet known about the biochemical steps of any transport process, so we can do no more than speculate on how any agent might affect these steps. Nevertheless, it does not seem likely that a hormone acts directly on a transport process. The probabilities for direct action are very limited: for example, the hormone molecule would have to be a part of the transport carrier system itself; or, it would have to act directly with a molecular species of the carrier system. Neither of these possibilities would be expected for several reasons. First, in many cases, transport of a given substrate can be altered by two or more hormones of quite different chemical structures. In addition, a single hormone often alters transport of more than one type of chemical substance at the same time—i.e., inorganic anions and cations, sugars, amino acids—even though there may be little or no evidence that the transports of these substances are linked directly. In fact, only rarely is the action of a hormone limited to the transport of only one type of substance.

The importance of hormonal action on transmembrane transport should not be minimized, even if the effect does not prove to be produced directly. In several instances, of course, the effects of hormones on transports are clearly of major physiological importance. In many cases, however, the effects in themselves cannot explain very much of what the hormone does. Yet a rather large number of these more modest effects are known, a fact that in itself suggests that modification of transport is a necessary part of the total hormonal action. A cell or tissue will respond as an integrated unit to a given hormone, each biochemical change being an important part of the total physiological response. Whenever altered transport of one or more nutrients is among the changes, the response is not complete unless this change in transport has taken place. Part of the hormonal regulation of metabolism may depend upon control of access of substrates or cofactors to enzymes, an access determined by transport across the various membranes of the three-dimensional cell structure. For this reason, the action on transport needs to be examined if the total effect of the hormone is to be understood, even though the change in transport may be small. Recognition of this fact by investigators has undoubtedly contributed to the increase in transport literature within recent years; more and more work is appearing in which transport studies have been made as part of investigations into many other areas of metabolism.

The major purpose of the present chapter is to review the more recent literature as a means of assessing current knowledge on effects of a number of the hormones on transport systems. The various theories of hormone action will be discussed only incidentally. Rather, attention will be directed toward the evidence upon which any theory must finally be based. The discussion also does not include the major transport effects related to several hormones and actions that are considered elsewhere in this volume: primarily, parathyroid hormone, thyrocalcitonin, and aldosterone; the actions of insulin on adipose tissue or on protein synthesis, and its reaction with cell membranes; or, the role of 3′,5′-cyclic adenylic acid in transport. Nor has an attempt been made to cover the remaining literature exhaustively for any one of the other hormones or topics. Instead, a brief, broad description has been attempted in most cases, because such a presentation has seemed most appropriate for covering the wide variety of subjects within a reasonable space.

II. SOME HORMONAL EFFECTS ON TRANSPORTS

A. NEUROHYPOPHYSEAL HORMONES

1. Action on Water Movement

These compounds are unique among the hormones that alter transport in that they apparently increase the movement of molecules across membranes by removing barriers to passive transfer, rather than by modifying transport carrier systems. Koefoed-Johnsen and Ussing (1953) first proposed that vasopressin increases net water movement by enlarging the radii of pores in the membrane, through which the water molecules move by bulk flow. They conceived that many small pores may be converted into fewer larger ones, the total surface area of the pores being enlarged very little. The larger pores would permit water to move more rapidly, since they could accommodate the larger, more highly aggregated clusters of water molecules that normally are present (see the more extended discussion by Leaf, 1967). On the bases of this scheme, Leaf (1961) has calculated a mean pore radius for water movement across toad bladder of 8 Å in the absence of vasopressin, and 40 Å in its presence; while Whittembury *et al.* (1960) calculated values of 5.6 and 6.5 Å, respectively, in necturus kidney.

The extensive studies of Leaf and associates (see, for example, Leaf, 1964, 1965, 1967, for reviews) has helped describe the nature of the water movement across the isolated toad bladder and its modification by vasopressin. In this tissue, no net water movement is found even in the presence of a water gradient across the bladder if vasopressin is not added. If the serosal fluid is made hypertonic to that bathing the mucosal side, water will move from the mucosal to the serosal side, but only if vasopressin is present. A barrier at the mucosal surface is decreased by the hormone, and water then can move in proportion to the osmotic gradient (Hays and Leaf, 1962). Net water movement can be shown in the absence of Na^+, however, showing that the former is not dependent directly on the active transport of Na^+. In the situation *in vivo*, the osmotic gradient would be produced by the active Na^+ transport, but the water could not follow the Na^+ unless hormone was present. Stein (1967) has pointed out that the mucosal surface of the bladder, in the absence of hormone, has a much lower water permeability than found in other epithelial cells, and addition of vasopressin makes it more typical.

The view that the mucosal surface is the barrier to water movement is supported by the histological finding that mucosal cells of the toad bladder do not swell in hypotonic solution unless vasopressin is present (Peachey and Rasmussen, 1961; Jard *et al.*, 1966). The serosal surface swells even in the absence of hormone. MacRobbie and Ussing (1961) have shown similar results in the frog skin, i.e., the skin will swell in response to hypotonicity only when vasopressin is present.

2. *Action on Movement of Sodium Ion*

Most of the evidence suggests that vasopressin also increases Na^+ movement across membranes, such as toad bladder and frog skin, by removing a barrier to passive transfer across the mucosal surface (Leaf *et al.*, 1958; Curran *et al.*, 1963; Herrera and Curran, 1963; Civan *et al.*, 1966; Snart *et al.*, 1968). Leaf and Dempsey (1960) showed that the increase in Na^+ movement produced by vasopressin is from the mucosal to the serosal side of the toad bladder. Active Na^+ transport, which has been localized at the serosal surface, results in pumping of Na^+ out of the cells into the medium. As a result, the intracellular $[Na^+]$ is kept low, and Na^+ is therefore believed to enter the cells by passive diffusion across the mucosal surface even at low external levels. Civan *et al.* (1966) found that vaso-pressin had no effect on Na^+ transport if the driving force for the pas-sive Na^+ movement was removed. They concluded that the hormone acts on the permeability barrier on the mucosal side to permit more Na^+ to enter the cell. More Na^+ is therefore available to be pumped out on the serosal side.

Snart *et al.* (1968) showed that both vasopressin and amphotericin B added to toad bladder, and oxytocin added to frog skin, altered the tem-perature dependence of the short circuit current in a way that suggests a lowering of the permeability barrier. Since the short circuit current can be taken as a measure of Na^+ movement, they concluded that the hor-mones, as well as the amphotericin, act on Na^+ transfer by altering its passive movement.

Morel and associates, in contrast, interpret some of their results with frog skin as suggesting that neurohypophyseal hormones can directly alter active Na^+ transport. Morel and Bastide (1965) found that with very low Na^+ levels in the mucosal bathing medium, a net outward flux of Na^+ occurs, and that oxytocin can reverse this net flux to an inward direction. They argue (Bastide *et al.*, 1968) that a likely explanation of this result would be that the electrochemical gradient for Na^+ at the mucosal border of the frog skin is reversed by the hormone; and that a stimulation of a step in active transport could well be involved, presumably at the mucosal surface.

The relation between energy metabolism and the actions of the hor-mone is, nevertheless, not clear. Metabolic energy is required for vaso-pressin to stimulate Na^+ transport, as shown by the facts that the stimu-lation is accompanied by elevated oxygen consumption and utilization of substrates (Leaf, 1960; Leaf and Dempsey, 1960; Leaf and Renshaw, 1957a); and that it is reduced by anaerobiosis or the presence of metabolic inhibitors (Handler *et al.*, 1966; Leaf and Renshaw, 1957b). Hong *et al.* (1968) have recently shown a seasonal variation in sensitivity of Na^+ transport in the frog skin to the hormone, and their results suggest that supply of substrate may be a controlling factor. Skins taken from sum-mer frogs are normally insensitive to vasopressin, but they can be made responsive if either pyruvate or β-hydroxybutyrate is added to the buffer medium. Skins from winter frogs are normally responsive to the hormone, and they show no further effect in the presence of the substrates. The glycogen content of the skins was much greater in the winter than in the summer, a fact that suggested that substrate availability was important for the hormone action. The energy requirement may reflect the elevated active Na^+ transport produced in response to the elevated cell Na^+ levels (see discussion in Section II,A,5, however).

3. Independence of Hormone Actions on Water and Sodium Movements

Although most of the evidence suggests that vasopressin and related compounds alter movements of both water and Na$^+$ by removing barriers to their free movement, it is quite clear that the actions on the two substances are independent of one another. As cited, Hays and Leaf (1962) showed that the hormone can increase net water movement across toad bladder membrane in the absence of Na$^+$. Several other pieces of evidence also support this conclusion. Lichtenstein and Leaf (1965, 1966) found that amphotericin B added to the serosal surface would stimulate Na$^+$ transfer across the toad bladder, but that it had no effect on water movement. Vasopressin had no further effect on Na$^+$ movement beyond that given by the amphotericin B. The authors construct a model for neurohypophyseal hormone action based partly on these results. The fact that amphotericin B had different effects on the transfers of water and Na$^+$ again suggests that a single action did not produce both results.

Results with a wide range of octapeptide analogs also lead to the conclusion that their actions on water and Na$^+$ movements are independent of each other. For example, vasopressin and oxytocin affect permeability to water in the toad skin to the same extent, but show quite different actions on Na$^+$ transports (Elliott, 1967). In the dog and rat, oxytocin is more active than vasopressin in increasing Na$^+$ excretion (Kramar *et al.*, 1966). Bourguet and Morel (1967) studied a series of analogs of vasopressin and found different orders of their potencies for stimulating Na$^+$ transport and water movement. The results from a number of other investigations also support the general conclusion (e.g., Bentley, 1960; Bourguet and Maetz, 1961, among others). One purpose of many of these studies has been to determine the chemical functional groups that are responsible for the different physiological actions of the hormones.

4. Specificity of Hormone Action on Transport

Vasopressin alters movements of several other substances in addition to water and Na$^+$. Nevertheless, the effect shows a high degree of specificity—a fact that has led investigators to doubt that movement is produced by simple bulk flow of water plus solutes through pores. Na$^+$ is apparently the only inorganic cation affected in toad bladder. Urea transfer in bladder is increased by the hormone, but that of thiourea is not. Of 40 compounds tested by Leaf and Hays (1962) only 12 besides water had their transfers increased by vasopressin. These were all low molecular weight alcohols and amides. Vasopressin is also reported to increase renal Ca^{++} excretion in man, however (Thorn, 1961).

5. Possible Biochemical Mechanism of Action of the Hormones

Very little is known about the biochemical mechanism by which the neurohypophyseal hormones act on bladder, skin, or kidney. Some 200 analogs of the hormone have been prepared and tested for various types of biological activity. Walter *et al.* (1967) discuss the effects of structural variations on activities (cf. Pickering, 1968; Rudinger *et al.*, 1968; Morel *et al.*, 1968; Berde, 1968). Perhaps most significant has been the question of the role of the disulfide bridge present in all natural forms of the hormones. Most of the early evidence pointed to the necessity of a disulfide interchange with sulfur groups of the membrane. For example, physiological activity of various compounds gave a high correlation with the binding of hormone to rat kidney and toad bladder through an S-S linkage (Fong *et al.*, 1960; Schwartz *et al.*, 1960, 1964a; Rasmussen *et al.*, 1960, 1963; Rasmussen and Schwartz, 1964; Schwartz, 1965). However, recently, Schwartz *et al.* (1964b; cf. Schwartz, 1965), and Pliska *et al.* (1968) have prepared several active compounds that do not contain sulfur. The activities of the derivatives were relatively low compared with the disulfide-containing parent compounds, suggesting that the S—S linkage may be important in determining the affinity of hormone with receptor. The S-free analogs may well be held in the proper site only loosely as, for example, by hydrophobic bonds. The cyclic structure of the compound appears to be an essential requirement for activity, on the other hand, since no active acylic structure has yet been found (Walter *et al.*, 1967). Attempts to identify the nature of a stabilizing S—S linkage between octapeptide and membrane have not been successful because of the large number of sulfur-binding sites on cells, most of which are undoubtedly not related to the biological function of the hormone. It is interesting to note that low levels of NEM can substitute for vasopressin in increasing water movement (Rasmussen, 1965).

A great amount of work has been directed toward discovering the possible role of 3′,5′-cyclic adenylic acid as the mediator of vasopressin action on water and Na^+ movements. The importance of this compound in actions of hormones is discussed by Butcher *et al.* in a separate chapter in Volume 2, so it will not be considered extensively here. It may be pointed out, however, that cyclic-AMP can substitute for vasopressin in toad bladder (Orloff and Handler, 1962), frog skin (Bastide and Jard, 1968) and mammalian kidney tubules (Grantham and Burg, 1966). Handler *et al.* (1965) have shown that neurohypophyseal hormones will increase the cyclic AMP levels of toad bladders, and also (Handler and Orloff, 1963) that either neurohypophyseal hormones or cyclic AMP will increase phosphorylase activity. Whether or not cyclic AMP is the direct mediator of changes in water movements, the intervention of one or more steps involving small molecules seems likely in view of the fact that in the toad bladder vasopressin must be added to the serosal bathing fluid in order to alter permeability at the mucosal surface. As Leaf (1967) has suggested, small molecules such as cyclic AMP would more likely have access to the interior of the bladder cell than would an octapeptide. He proposes that the mucosal membrane may be affected at its inner surface by some such small molecule that is formed at the serosal surface either directly or indirectly in response to vasopressin.

Vasopressin also produces several other biochemical changes in the toad bladder, but these may or may not be related to the action of the hormone to alter transports. In several cases, however, the change in transport, rather than the actual presence of the hormones, may account for the changes in metabolism. For example, the oxygen consumption of the membrane is increased in the presence of the hormone, and this increase is found only if Na^+ is present in the incubation medium (Leaf and Dempsey, 1960). This result suggests that the increased intracellular Na^+ level produced by vasopressin is responsible for an elevated respiration. It seems less likely that the increased respiration is needed to produce the elevated Na^+ transfer, since the hormone is generally believed not to alter active Na^+ transport. Vasopressin is also reported to increase the activities of phosphofructokinase and pyruvate kinase, as well as phosphorylase, in toad bladder (Handler *et al.*, 1968). Handler *et al.* (1968) suggest that these activities might be changed as a result of the altered cellular Na^+ levels produced by the hormone, although other factors undoubtedly are also involved. They suggest, further, that vasopressin may control glycogenolysis in this tissue through regulation of Na^+ transport. The energy metabolism of the toad bladder parallels the Na^+ transport, i.e., the rates of glycogenolysis and O_2 consumption are decreased by Na^+ removal. They are also increased by vasopressin, but only when Na^+ is present (Leaf *et al.*, 1959; Leaf and Dempsey, 1960). Phosphofructokinase and phosphorylase were activated very little when Na^+ transport was prevented in intact tissues; but their activities were not affected by the absence of Na^+ when homogenates of the tissue were used (Handler *et al.*, 1968). The membrane may, therefore, be a site of control of the Na^+ activation of the enzymes, and the various neurohypophyseal hormones could control enzyme activities in intact tissues by controlling Na^+ transport. The hormones could also regulate glycogenolysis in this way, since rate of glycogenolysis was found to depend upon phosphofructokinase activity(Handler *et al.*, 1968). Control of ion movement may be a means by which metabolism is regulated more generally. The rate of glycolysis in several tissues, for example, is related to the rate of cation movement (see Handler *et al.*, 1968, for discussion and references).

Rasmussen (1968) has suggested a °possible relation of neurohypophyseal hormone action to Ca^{++} binding or permeability at the plasma membrane. Schwartz and Walter (1968) have reported an interesting oscillation of Ca^{++} binding by bladder homogenates treated with vasopressin. Zadunaisky *et al.* (1968), using the electron microscope, have found that vasopressin causes movement of Na^+ from the nucleus to the cytoplasm of the frog skin cell, and that Ca^{++} uptake by the mitochondria is increased. They propose that the hormone elevates Na^+ transport by increasing the Na^+ level in the cytoplasm in two ways: by increased Na^+ movement across the external membrane into the cell, made possible because Ca^{++} moves from the membrane to the mitochondria; and by increased release of Na^+ from the nucleus. The increased cytoplasmic Na^+ levels would then increase the active transport of Na^+ out of the cell, as suggested by Leaf (1960).

Apparently no study has been made of the possible dependence of Na^+ transport in the toad bladder or frog skin on a Na^+–K^+-sensitive ATPase. The presence of this type of enzyme in toad bladder has been established (Bonting and Canady, 1964). One would not except vasopressin to alter its activity if the hormone does not affect active Na^+ transport. A test of this possibility would, therefore, be of interest.

6. Miscellaneous Related Studies

The effect of vasopressin on amino acid uptake is of interest because of the dependence of some amino acid transports on Na^+ levels. Lowenstein *et al.* (1968) tested the effects of vasopressin and aldosterone on transport of α-aminoisobutyric acid (AIB) and 1-aminocyclopentanecarboxylic acid in the rat renal papilla. No effect of either hormone was found at any of several Na^+ levels. Uptakes of both of these model amino acids were shown to vary markedly with the Na^+ levels used. Unfortunately no measurement was made to determine if Na^+ transport was indeed altered by the hormones in their experiments. Thier (1968) also found a Na^+ dependence for transport of AIB into the toad bladder. The transport occurred only at the serosal surface and was independent of the absence of Na^+ from the medium bathing the mucosal surface. These facts suggest that transepithelial Na^+ transport may not be needed for amino acid transport. The effect of vasopressin on the latter transport was not tested, but such experiments might also shed light on the relations between the transports of Na^+ and amino acids.

B. Natriuretic Hormone

A substance has been detected in plasma of a number of species (man, dog, cat, cow) that will increase Na⁺ excretion in various animals, and also inhibit Na⁺ transport in the frog skin (Cort, 1966; Lichardus and Pearce, 1966). The effect on excretion is apparently due to a direct action on the proximal tubule of the kidney to inhibit Na⁺ reabsorption (Dirks *et al.*, 1965). The compound has been separated from the plasma of cats and found to be a polypeptide with a molecular weight below 20,000, and to contain at least one basic amino acid and a free terminal N group (Cort *et al.*, 1968a,b). It is believed to be released from the posterior hypothalamus (Cort, 1966) in response to a number of hemodynamic stimuli (e.g., carotid occlusion), and it may be identical with material isolated from either the mitochondrial fraction or an acetone powder of the posterior hypothalamus that has similar activity.

The hormone is quite distinct from vasopressin, oxytocin and other known, physiologically active polypeptides, although it may be similar chemically to the neurohypophyseal hormones (Cort *et al.*, 1968a). This last suggestion is based on a number of similarities between the natriuretic hormone and the active neurohypophyseal octapeptides: e.g., both vasopressin and oxytocin produce a transitory natriuresis; and a number of synthetic oxytocin antagonists can counteract the natriuretic response to carotid occlusion (Cort *et al.*, 1966). In addition, as pointed out by Cort *et al.* (1968a), a prolonged natriuretic response, compared to vasopressin, is given by synthetic vasopressin derivatives containing extended chains with additional amino acid residues attached to the first cysteine (Cort, 1964).

C. Insulin

1. Effects on Sugar Transport

Levine *et al.* (1949) were the first to propose that insulin may exert its control over glucose metabolism by regulating the glucose transport across cell membranes. In the intervening years it has become clear that transport is only one of the sites of control by the hormone over carbohydrate metabolism (see Levine, 1965). Nonetheless, glucose utilization is limited by transport in both muscle (Morgan *et al.*, 1961a) and adipose tissue (Crofford and Renold, 1965a), and insulin makes possible increased glucose utilization by elevating its transport. Consideration here will be limited to a brief summary of results obtained primarily on muscle tissues.

Glucose entry into muscle, as well as into erythrocytes, has the general characteristics of a carrier-mediated transport. It shows saturation kinetics, is stereospecific, and shows competition from other sugars, as well as counterflow (Morgan *et al.*, 1964; Regen and Morgan, 1964; Wilbrandt and Rosenberg, 1961). This last fact supports the idea that a movable carrier is necessary (Bowyer, 1957; Wilbrandt and Rosenberg, 1961). In muscle, insulin accelerates the entry of both glucose and a variety of other sugars (Park *et al.*, 1959; Randle and Smith, 1958a). The hormone has been found to increase the V_{max} of sugar transport by rat heart (Post *et al.*, 1961) and frog sartorius muscle (Narahara and Ozand, 1963). The effect on apparent K_m, however, seems to depend on the tissue studied. Fisher and Zachariah (1961), and Morgan *et al.* (1964) find that insulin decreases apparent glucose transport affinity in rat heart, whereas Narahara and Ozand (1963) find no effect in frog sartorius; and Guidotti *et al.* (1966) find that insulin produces a decreased K_m in 10-day chick embryo heart. A decrease in apparent K_m is also reported for insulin action on glucose uptake by adipose tissue (Baker and Rutter, 1964; Crofford and Renold, 1965b).

Puromycin or actinomycin D does not block the uptake of D-galactose, D-xylose, or D-glucose by rat diaphragm (Wool and Moyer, 1964; Burrow and Bondy, 1964; Carlin and Hechter, 1964; Eboue-Bonis *et al.*, 1963). These results show that synthesis of new RNA and protein is not necessary for the insulin-induced increase in transport. Narahara and Ozand (1963), however, interpret their results with 3-O-methyl glucose to suggest that insulin increases the number of sugar transport sites in the cells of frog sartorius muscle. If insulin induces similar biochemical changes when it alters sugar transport in rat diaphragm and frog sartorius, we may conclude that the sugar sites are not protein that is synthesized *de novo* in response to the hormone. (See further discussion on this point in Section II,C,4.)

A potentially useful system for studying insulin action on sugar uptake has been introduced by Foa *et al.* (1965). These investigators found that chick embryo heart is freely permeable to glucose until the seventh day of its development. At that time a saturable transport process appears that limits the rate of glucose utilization by the tissue. At the same time the uptake also becomes sensitive to stimulation by insulin. Foa *et al.* (1965) show that changes in lipid metabolism produced by insulin cannot be explained entirely by the hormone's ability to elevate glucose transport. The tissue might prove to be especially useful for studying biochemical changes leading to formation of the glucose transport system and its modification by insulin.

Ungar and Psychoyos (1963) report that insulin decreases the diffusion across rat diaphragm of those sugars whose uptakes are known to be accelerated by the hormone. Diffusion of glucose was also slowed by anoxia and electrical stimulation, and it was accelerated by adrenaline and 2,4-dinitrophenol.

Insulin has also been reported to be necessary for glucose uptake by the isolated toad bladder (Nusynowitz, 1967). The effect was antagonized by epinephrine.

Few effects of insulin on intestinal absorption have been reported. Dubois and Roy (1968) report, however, that the intestinal transport of 3-*O*-methyl glucose was increased in both experimental and clinical diabetes mellitus. The change was insensitive to insulin. When rats were made diabetic with guinea pig anti-insulin serum, however, insulin increased the rate of absorption in the perfused intestine. The effect could not be shown with alloxanized rats.

Insulin *in vivo* could not be shown to alter the intestinal absorption of D-glucosamine, N-acetyl-D-glucosamine, or D-glucose (Capps *et al.*, 1966). Metabolism of the compounds was increased, however, a fact that led to the suggestion that insulin may alter the transport of the amino sugars into some tissues. Wick *et al.* (1955) have shown that insulin can stimulate glucosamine entry into muscle cells of eviscerated rats.

Glucose metabolism in diaphragm, heart, and epididymal fat tissue is decreased after rats are made diabetic (Gregor *et al.*, 1963; Dixit *et al.*, 1963; Jefferson *et al.*, 1968). Jefferson *et al.* (1968) suggest that in perfused heart the effect may be due to elevated free fatty acid levels, which reduce the sensitivity of glucose transport to insulin.

Katzen (1967) has proposed the interesting theory that hexokinase may serve as the transport carrier for glucose. From a study of a wide range of tissues, he has found that one of the electrophoretically distinct forms of hexokinase, hexokinase I, occurs in high activity in tissues in which glucose transport is not responsive to insulin. Hexokinase I also has a much lower K_m for glucose than do the other forms of the enzyme. Hexokinase II, in contrast, is the predominant form in insulin-sensitive tissues. Katzen proposes that when type I is present in large amounts, transport is already maximal without insulin. When type II is the major form, and type I is deficient, insulin would react with type II to increase its activity as a carrier. The idea is supported by the demonstration that the activity of the type II form is decreased in adipose tissue during conditions that produce low blood insulin levels [e.g., starvation, diabetes (Moore *et al.*, 1964; McLean *et al.*, 1966; Katzen, 1966)]. Walters and McLean (1967, 1968) have shown, furthermore, that the sensitivity of the rat mammary gland to insulin *in vitro* is related to the ratio of hexokinase II to hexokinase I. This gland shows a variation in response to insulin with the stages of the lactation cycle, the response being high during lactation, and low during pregnancy and during involution of the gland following lactation. The ratio of hexokinase II/I rose from 1 during pregnancy to 3 at midlactation, and returned to 1 at involution. Diabetes produced by either alloxan or anti-insulin serum decreased the amount of hexokinase in the particulate fraction of the gland and significantly decreased the ratio of type II to type I in the soluble fraction.

The hypothesis of Katzen is unique in that it conceives of an efficient transfer of glucose from outside the cell to its phosphorylated form on the same molecule. In addition, the scheme can account for the insulin stimulation of glucose transport without synthesis of new protein.

2. Insulinlike Effects on Sugar Transport

Over a decade ago, Randle and Smith (1958a,b) found that a number of cell poisons that interfere with energy production would stimulate monosaccharide transport into muscle. They proposed that high-energy compounds are a hindrance to transport, and that insulin stimulated the uptake of sugar by diverting energy-rich substances from the transport site. The possibility of a common method of action of the two agents is also supported by the finding of Morgan *et al.* (1961b) that anoxia will accelerate transport in alloxan-diabetic hearts. Recently, Morgan *et al.* (1965) have tested this hypothesis with new experiments. They found that neither insulin treatment nor anaerobiosis interfered with counterflow or stereospecificity of sugar transport in perfused rat heart. Likewise, V_{max} of transport was increased, but K_m was essentially unchanged under either condition. Stimulation produced by both conditions could be blocked by brief treatment of tissue with N-ethylmaleimide. All of these similarities are consistent with a common action of the two conditions. The data lead the authors to conclude that both insulin and anoxia stimulate the specific sugar carrier transport system. The stimulation of transport by anoxia was also found in the goose erythrocyte, however, a cell that does not respond to insulin. This last fact suggests some difference between the actions of anoxia and insulin on glucose transport. The proposal of Randle and Smith also cannot explain the effect of insulin on amino acid transport, since this process requires energy. Glucose and amino acid transports are both altered at the same time by insulin.

Increased sugar transports have also been found in the presence of such other agents as lipolytic and proteolytic enzymes (Blecher, 1967; Kuo *et al.*, 1967; Kuo, 1968), phospholipase (Rodbell, 1966) and as low a Li^+ level as 5 mM in the extracellular fluid (Clausen, 1968b). The pattern of changes in glycogen deposition and lactate production in the latter case differed both quantitatively and qualitatively from those produced by insulin, however. 3',5'-Cyclic AMP has also been reported to increase glucose uptake by striated muscle, a fact that has led to the suggestion that this compound may be the mediator of insulin action on transport (Edelman *et al.*, 1966).

Bihler (1968) has reported that ouabain and other cardiac glycosides and aglycones will stimulate the transport of 3-O-methyl glucose into diaphragm muscle. The effect could be enhanced by submaximal levels of insulin but not when maximal stimulation was given by the hormone. The author suggests that the various steroids may be affecting the insulin-sensitive sugar transport process.

3. *Effects of Insulin on Transport of Amino Acids*

The action of the hormone has been tested on the transport of nearly every natural amino acid, and on a large number of model amino acids as well. Excised rat diaphragm, perfused rat heart (see Section III), and the rat levator ani muscle (Adolfsson *et al.*, 1967) have been used for studies *in vitro*. The nonmetabolizable model amino acids, AIB and 1-aminocyclopentanecarboxylic acid, have also been studied *in vivo* with results on muscle tissues similar to those found *in vitro*. An effect of insulin on transport into the liver was also apparent both *in vivo* (Sanders and Riggs, 1967a) and in the perfused liver (Chambers *et al.*, 1965). Debons and Pittman (1966) report that insulin increases AIB uptake by thyroid tissue.

Wool and associates have found that the insulin stimulation of transport of the metabolizable amino acids may be obscured by their incorporation into protein. When puromycin was used to inhibit protein synthesis, significant increases in transport became apparent for a number of amino acids (Castles and Wool, 1964; Wool *et al.*, 1965; Scharff and Wool, 1965; cf. Wool, 1965). Their results, as well as those of others, are summarized in Table I and are discussed in more detail in Section III.

Manchester (1968) has questioned the results showing that the presence of puromycin can uncover an action of insulin to increase amino acid transport. He calculates that much more free radioactivity appears in the cell in the presence of this compound than can be accounted for by the reduction of incorporation of ^{14}C-amino acid into protein. He suggests that the puromycin may be slowing the decay of the amino acid carrier of the membrane. A similar idea has been suggested by Dawson and Beck (1968) for the action of actinomycin D on growth hormone stimulation of amino acid uptake. This latter antibiotic prolongs the period over which growth hormone is active *in vitro* (see Section II,D,2).

Oddly, amino acid transport has been found to be increased, rather than decreased, by diabetes produced by either alloxan, partial pancreatectomy, or anti-insulin serum (Castles *et al.*, 1965; Scharff and Wool, 1966;

Manchester and Young, 1960b). This increase occurs whether the diabetes decreases or elevates protein synthesis. Somewhat different patterns of cell amino acids are found for the three types of diabetes. In contrast, the transport of glucose was below normal in hearts removed from rats treated with anti-insulin serum and perfused *in vitro* (Jefferson *et al.*, 1968).

Manchester discusses the general question of insulin and protein synthesis in Chapter 7 in this volume. It seems necessary here, however, to consider the evidence bearing on the question of whether or not insulin alters amino acid transport by increasing the synthesis of protein involved in the transport process. Numerous investigators have shown that protein synthesis in muscle tissue can be inhibited by puromycin without a change in insulin stimulation of amino acid transport (Fritz and Knobil, 1963; Wool and Moyer, 1964; Burrow and Bondy, 1964; Carlin and Hechter, 1964; Castles and Wool, 1964; Wool *et al.*, 1965; Scharff and Wool, 1965). In these cases, however, puromycin was present during incubation periods of generally less than 3 hours. The fact that insulin still stimulated the uptake showed not only that new protein did not need to be synthesized, but it also provided evidence that any protein component of the amino acid transport system did not break down during that time. Several reports have appeared, however, that show that preincubation of tissues for 2 to 3 hours or more with puromycin or cycloheximide results in a substantial decrease in the subsequent baseline uptake of several amino acids, including AIB, glycine, proline, leucine and 1-aminocyclopentane-carboxylic acid (Adamson *et al.*, 1966; Elsas *et al.*, 1967; Elsas and Rosenberg, 1967; Manchester 1967). Elsas *et al.* (1968) found that puromycin did not alter a variety of other cellular functions (O_2 consumption, tissue Na^+, K^+, and water content, nonsaturable entry, or binding of amino acid, among others); they therefore concluded that the most likely cause of the altered transport was inhibition of protein synthesis. Their results also suggested that the long preincubation with puromycin affected the influx of AIB and not its efflux (Elsas and Rosenberg, 1967). Later they reported that the V_{max} of AIB uptake was reduced by the preincubation with puromycin to about one-half the normal value (Elsas *et al.*, 1968), a fact that suggests that AIB carrier had been lost through catabolism. The half-life of the protein was estimated to be about 3.5 hours (Elsas *et al.*, 1967).

The insulin stimulation of AIB uptake could be inhibited by a 3-hour preincubation with actinomycin D and the aminonucleoside of puromycin, as well as by puromycin and cycloheximide (Elsas *et al.*, 1968). The degree of inhibition paralleled the inhibition of incorporation of L-lysine into protein. Insulin alone lowered the K_m of AIB entry to half the normal value, but it did not affect the V_{max}. Puromycin, on the other hand, not only decreased the V_{max} in the presence of insulin (as it did in the absence of insulin), but it also raised the K_m somewhat, from 3.0 mM to 4.0 mM. This latter change may not be significant, however, in view of the error inherent in its estimation (see Dowd and Riggs, 1965). The nonsaturable entry of AIB was not altered by either puromycin or insulin. The results provide good evidence that protein synthesis is necessary for the action of insulin on amino acid transport, and seem to contradict the earlier findings obtained with shorter incubation periods.

There are, theoretically, several possible reconciliations, however. The presence of puromycin reduced the uptake whether or not insulin was used. This fact suggests that the insulin did not exert its effect through altering protein synthesis, but rather by acting on a protein present after a 1- or 2-hour treatment with puromycin, but absent after longer times with the antibiotic. Protein synthesis was needed for insulin stimulation only because specific protein had decayed and had to be replaced before the hormone could act. The subsequent steps could involve, for example, an action of insulin to convert an inactive, precarrier molecule into its active carrier form. The long-term incubation with puromycin or other agents would prevent the normal formation of precarrier protein, and insulin would be unable to exert its effect on amino acid transport. A similar reaction may also occur in the insulin stimulation of sugar transport (see Section II,C,1). It is interesting to note in this connection that such proteolytic enzymes as trypsin and chymotrypsin will accelerate the accumulation of L-proline and sugars by rat diaphragm (Rieser and Rieser, 1964); and that insulin can catalyze proteolysis (Rieser, 1966). A part of the action of insulin could conceivably be produced by splitting peptide bonds. Some of these bonds might be in precarrier molecules of sugar and amino acid transport. The carriers themselves would then also be protein in nature, and would not be formed in the presence of puromycin (shown at least in the case of amino acid transport); whereas the action of insulin would be limited to a late step in the formation of the active carriers, a step beyond those involving *de novo* protein synthesis.

The results of Elsas *et al.* (1968) confirm qualitatively the earlier report of Akedo and Christensen (1962) that insulin decreases the K_m of AIB uptake by isolated diaphragm without altering V_{max} appreciably. These calculations were based on results obtained after incubations of 1 hour; values given at this time were shown to be essentially proportional to initial rate uptakes. Manchester (1968a), on the other hand, used data and calculations based on steady state conditions, and concluded that insulin increased the V_{max} of AIB uptake by rat diaphragm, the K_m remaining unchanged. His original calculation (Manchester, 1968a) was based on the assumption that efflux from diaphragm at the steady state is equal to nonsaturable influx—a condition that is probably not met [see the evidence of Christensen and Handlogten (1968) that amino acid exodus from cells may be mediated]. Nevertheless, when this factor is taken into account, the data still show that insulin alters maximum AIB transport capacity rather than K_m (Manchester, 1968b). There is, therefore, lack of complete agreement at present as to what kinetic parameter is altered when insulin increases the transport of either sugars (see Section II,C,1) or amino acids.

4. Insulin Modification of Ion Transports and Its Relation to Sugar and Amino Acid Transports

The hormone has been shown to alter transport of both Na^+ and K^+ in several tissues. On the other hand, the transports of both sugars (Bihler and Crane, 1962; Kleinzeller and Kotyk, 1961; Ricklis and Quastel, 1958; Clausen, 1965; Letarte and Renold, 1967; Clausen *et al.*, 1968), and some amino acids (see Wheeler and Christensen, 1967, for references) into a number of tissues have been shown to depend upon the presence of extracellular Na^+. It has often been suggested that the energy for active transport of sugars and amino acids may derive from the high Na^+ and K^+ transports. Such a scheme would be relevant, of course, only if the hormone produced changes in transports of Na^+ and K^+ as well as of the organic substances.

Several reports have appeared with results that bear on this subject. Kostyo (1964), and Kipnis and Parrish (1965) have shown that Na^+ is needed for the hormone to alter transport of glycine and AIB, respectively. An examination of the other data suggests that the amino acids whose uptakes require Na^+ are those whose transports are most readily stimulated by insulin. This subject is discussed in greater detail in Section III. It seems likely, therefore, that insulin does act on a Na^+-sensitive amino acid transport system. This does not mean, however, that insulin acts only on the Na^+ transport system and not on one of the systems used by amino acids. The results of Elsas and Rosenberg (1967) show that Na^+ and K^+ gradients are maintained in rat diaphragm after a 3-hour incubation with puromycin. Such an incubation resulted in decreased AIB transport. The authors conclude that the half-life of the alkali metal pump (or pumps), if protein, is considerably longer than the 3.5 hours assigned to the amino acid carrier protein. The results show that AIB uptake depends upon more than the proper Na^+ and K^+ levels. It will be important to know whether insulin affects Na^+ and K^+ transports after prolonged incubations with puromycin, since it does not affect AIB uptake under these conditions. Crabbe (1968) has found that neither actinomycin D nor puromycin will inhibit the insulin stimulation of Na^+ transport in toad skin in 2 hours. Effects on both Na^+ and amino acid need to be tested at the same time in a single tissue, and for longer incubation periods than 2 hours.

Studies of insulin actions on Na^+ and sugar transports have given varying results depending upon the tissue used. Letarte and Renold (1967; cf. Clausen *et al.*, 1968) found that Na^+ was necessary for the insulin stimulation of glucose uptake by isolated adipose tissue; whereas Kipnis and Parrish (1965) could not find a Na^+ dependence of sugar uptake in the rat diaphragm, although the tissue is insulin-sensitive. Clausen (1966) has concluded that effects of insulin on Na^+ and glucose transports in diaphragm are not directly related to one another. His results (Clausen, 1968a) show that glucose uptake by this tissue is not completely dependent on Na^+. Ouabain gave only a small depression of glucose uptake in the presence of insulin (Clausen, 1966). The situation may be different in the fat pad, because in this tissue ouabain, like insulin, stimulates uptake of glucose (Ho and Jeanrenaud, 1967). Kestens *et al.* (1963) have found, however, that K^+ uptake is increased when insulin is added to the isolated perfused liver of the dog, although glucose uptake is not affected. Glucose is likewise not needed to obtain the insulin effect on cation transport (Zierler, 1959; Hechter and Lester, 1960).

An interesting related phenomenon is the finding of Milner and Hales (1967; cf. 1968) that a number of stimuli of insulin secretion (glucose, L-leucine, glucagon, tolbutamide) all cause Na^+ entry into the β cells of the pancreas. Preventing or enhancing Na^+ entry produced less and more insulin release, respectively. They suggest that the secretion is controlled by the extent of Na^+ entry.

D. GROWTH HORMONE

1. Effect on Sugar Transport

Pituitary growth hormone also produces increased uptakes of amino acids, sugars, and some inorganic ions. However, most of its ability to increase glucose uptake by tissues *in vivo* has generally been attributed to insulin that is secreted in response to growth hormone administration (see review by de Bodo and Altszuler, 1957). Nonetheless, direct actions of the hormone on sugar transport have been shown in studies *in vitro*. The hormone will increase uptake of glucose and other sugars by diaphragm and adipose tissue if it is given *in vivo* within 1 hour before tissues are removed from hypophysectomized rats, or if it is added *in vitro* (Park *et al.*, 1952; Mezey *et al.*, 1961; Goodman, 1963, 1966, 1968). At times longer than 1 hour *in vivo*, however, the stimulatory action is not apparent; in fact, uptake *in vitro* may be decreased, especially after repeated injections of the hormone (Goodman, 1966, 1967b; Riddick *et. al.*, 1962; Henderson *et al.*, 1961). The results are not due to an increased lipolytic activity (Goodman, 1967b). Goodman (1967b), and Hjalmarson and Ahren (1965, 1967a) found that diaphragms from growth hormone-treated, hypophysectomized rats did not show increased uptake of glucose, xylose, or AIB in response to addition of the hormone *in vitro*. A large response was found in the absence of prior hormone injection, however. Even a 2-hour preincubation of the diaphragm with growth hormone *in vitro* eliminated the response to hormone added along with either xylose or AIB (Hjalmarson and Ahren, 1967a). In the light of these results it is not surprising that growth hormone does not stimulate uptake in tissues from rats still with their hypophyses (Henderson *et al.*, 1961; Riddick *et al.*, 1962; Goodman, 1965a).

The ability of growth hormone to inhibit glucose uptake by tissues can be prevented by treatment of the rats with actinomycin. The effect is seen in either adipose tissue or diaphragm (Goodman, 1965b, 1967b, 1968). The antibiotic given *in vivo* did not alter the stimulation of glucose uptake by growth hormone added *in vitro*, however, nor did it remove the refractoriness of the tissue to *in vitro* stimulation in diaphragms from rats given growth hormone *in vivo* for 3 hours. Actinomycin and growth hormone added together *in vitro*, on the other hand, produced stimulation of arabinose uptake by adipose tissue under conditions in which neither agent was effective by itself. Goodman (1968) concludes that in adipose tissue an increased entry of sugars leads to the other early changes in metabolism produced by the hormone. One might conclude that protein synthesis is not required for the response, since it is not altered until after sugar transport is changed. However, the results do not rule out the possibility that one or a few proteins need to be formed as Kostyo (1968) has observed for growth hormone stimulation of amino acid transport (see next section).

Goodman (1967a) presents data suggesting that the action of growth hormone on sugar uptake into adipose tissue is not mediated by insulin.

2. *Effect on Amino Acid Transport*

Growth hormone alters movement of several amino acids into muscle tissue, but it does not affect others. For a fuller discussion of which amino acids are affected, see Section III of this chapter. An increased transport is always found in association with the increased protein synthesis that is a part of cell growth. Increased capture of extracellular amino acids is necessary if the cell is to have the raw materials from which the new protein can be made.

Results suggest, however, that both amino acid transport and protein synthesis can be increased by growth hormone independently. For example, under suitable incubation conditions puromycin will inhibit protein synthesis nearly completely without preventing the action of growth hormone to stimulate AIB uptake by rat diaphragm (Knobil, 1966). In addition, growth hormone can increase incorporation into protein of amino acids whose transports are not stimulated significantly (e.g., leucine, valine, phenylalanine) (Knobil, 1966), or under conditions in which transport is severely inhibited and not altered by the hormone (Kostyo, 1964; Dawson *et al.*, 1966). Kostyo (1964) used a Na^+-free medium to eliminate growth hormone action on transport and still obtained elevated incorporation. At normal Na^+ levels, the hormone acted within 10–20 minutes *in vitro* on both transport and synthesis in diaphragm (Kostyo, 1968).

The foregoing results do not rule out the possibility, however, that a specific protein is affected quite soon by the hormone, even though the bulk of the proteins may be altered only later. Recent work by Kostyo (1968) supports this possibility. He found that preincubation of rat diaphragm for 1 hour with puromycin did not alter the baseline uptake of AIB, but it abolished stimulation by growth hormone. Similar results were obtained when cycloheximide was used to inhibit protein synthesis, although the hormone did produce a small amount of stimulation. Cycloheximide did not inhibit protein synthesis as much as did puromycin, however. Kostyo (1968) showed, further, that growth hormone added *in vitro* or injected for 1 hour *in vivo* stimulated synthesis of protein first in the "heavy" fraction of the diaphragm cell (sedimented at $700\,g$). The increase was in the actomyosin portion of the fraction, but it could be shown not to be actomyosin. Proteins from the mitochondria, microsomes, and cell sap were not labeled until later.

Growth hormone added *in vitro* increased AIB uptake by the rat diaphragm during a 2-hour incubation, but the effect was no longer apparent after 3 hours (Hjalmarson and Ahren, 1967a,b; Dawson and Beck, 1968). Stimulation of incorporation was evident over the entire 3 hours. When actinomycin D was added to the incubation flask, the hormone stimulated the AIB transport in 3 hours as well as at 1 hour, but incorporation was altered only at 1 hour, but not at 3 hours. Protein synthesis was inhibited 98% by the actinomycin even at 1 hour. Dawson and Beck (1968) suggest that different mechanisms act to stimulate protein synthesis at short and long times, and that uptake is controlled by a regulatory mechanism that depends upon both RNA and protein synthesis. The results also suggest that the hormone induces formation of a protein transport carrier even in the presence of actinomycin-inhibited RNA and protein synthesis. Furthermore, this carrier protein has a shorter half-life in the presence of continued RNA and/or protein syntheses than in their absence.

Kostyo and Schmidt (1962) and Manchester and Young (1959) have presented evidence that insulin is not needed for growth hormone to stimulate amino acid uptake. The former workers have shown that the hormone added *in vitro* will stimulate AIB uptake in the diaphragm from alloxan-diabetic, hypophysectomized rats. These results provide additional evidence that the actions of the two hormones are at least partly independent of one another. The growth hormone stimulation can be prevented by a 1-hour pretreatment of diaphragm with puromycin or cycloheximide, whereas a 2 to 3-hour preincubation is necessary to show effects on the stimulation by insulin (see Section II,C). The 3-hour preincubation with antibiotic decreased baseline AIB uptake, whereas the 1-hour preincubation did not. These facts suggest that the longer preincubation period led to destruction of the carrier already present in nontreated diaphragm, and that the additional uptake produced by insulin in nontreated tissue did not require protein synthesis. In contrast, the increased transport produced by growth hormone did probably require some protein synthesis.

The time courses for action of insulin and growth hormone on AIB uptake also support the conclusion that insulin acts more directly on the transport system than does the pituitary hormone. Insulin increases AIB uptake by diaphragm *in vitro* within 5 minutes, while growth hormone must be present for more than 10 minutes (Kostyo, 1968).

Recently, evidence has been presented that the decreased amino acid transport found in vitamin B_6-deficient rats may be more directly related to a deficiency of growth hormone than to a direct lack of the vitamin (Heindel and Riggs, 1968). Huber and Gershoff (1965) had found earlier that a nutritional deficiency of vitamin B_6 resulted in decreased levels of growth hormone in the pituitaries of rats. The earlier postulate (Christensen *et al.*, 1954), that some form of vitamin B_6 may be an important part of the amino acid transport system of cells, has not been supported by the subsequent evidence. It would now appear that the effects of the vitamin deficiency on amino acid transport may, in part, be explained as due to alteration in growth hormone supply (Heindel and Riggs, 1969).

E. Glucocorticoids

Changes in amino acid transport appear to be essential parts of the actions of the glucocorticoids to increase amino acid and protein catabolism and to elevate gluconeogenesis. The steroids both increase amino acid transport into the liver (Noall *et al.*, 1957; Chambers *et al.*, 1965) and decrease it in muscle (Wool, 1960; Kostyo and Schmidt, 1963), in spleen and thymus (Kaplan and Nagareda, 1961), and in tissue culture of HeLa, JTC-4 and L-929 cells (Mohri, 1967). They also decrease the rate of incorporation of amino acids into proteins of various extrahepatic tissues independently of an action on transport (Manchester *et al.*, 1959; Wool and Weinshelbaum, 1959; Pena *et al.*, 1966; Mankin and Conger, 1966). It has been found, furthermore, that in at least one tissue, the thymus, there is an increased release of endogenous amino acids from cells into the surrounding medium in response to cortisol (Sutherland and Haynes, 1967). Presumably the amino acids would come from the protein of the cells. The evidence supports the idea that glucocorticoids cause a loss of amino acids from the extrahepatic tissues followed by their increased capture by the liver. Amino acid N is then converted into urea in the liver, and the carbon skeletons are available for formation into glucose. The glucogenic steroids such as cortisol have been shown to produce increases in the activities of a number of enzymes that catalyze these conversions.

O. K. Smith and Long (1967) have recently presented results that support the view that glucocorticoids act independently on liver and extrahepatic tissues to produce the above chain of events. The high plasma amino-N levels found in diabetic rats were markedly reduced by adrenalectomy, and cortisol restored them. Even in the eviscerated rat, the hormone could increase protein catabolism, showing that the liver was not needed for this effect. The investigators conclude, furthermore, that the cortisol-induced increases in urinary-N and body glucose are so large that they could be derived only from extrahepatic tissues.

Kostyo and Redmond (1966) have examined the action of corticosteroids on isolated rat diaphragm in an attempt to determine how they might act biochemically to alter amino acid transport. They found that corticosterone would inhibit subsequent AIB uptake roughly in proportion to the length of a preincubation time with the steroid prior to addition of amino acid; i.e., very little effect was found after a 1-hour preincubation, with progressively more inhibition occurring as the preincubation period was extended up to 4 hours. The action of the steroid paralleled that of puromycin and, as shown subsequently, other inhibitors of protein synthesis. When preincubation was carried out in the presence of both puromycin and corticosterone, inhibition of AIB uptake was the same as given by either agent alone. The investigators suggest that glucocorticoids may be inhibiting amino acid uptake by preventing the synthesis of a specific protein of the transport system. Glucocorticoids have been shown to inhibit protein synthesis in muscle tissue. As discussed in Section II,C,3, the half-life of a protein of the AIB-transport system in rat diaphragm is estimated to be about 3.5 hours *in vitro* (Elsas *et al.*,

1967). The decay of existing molecules would continue without replacement, of course, if protein synthesis were blocked.

Munck and associates have used the thymus cell to study the action of glucocorticoids on glucose metabolism, including transport, and have attempted to relate the binding of the steroid with the cell to its physiological effects. Glucocorticoids added to suspensions of thymus cells can produce general effects similar to those given *in vivo* (Bartlett *et al.*, 1962; Morita and Munck, 1964; Kattwinkel and Munck, 1966; Munck, 1968; Munck and Brinck-Johnsen, 1968). The observed decrease in glucose utilization is due to a block in either transport or phosphorylation within 15 to 20 minutes. Interestingly, cortisone is inactive for the thymus cell *in vitro*, presumably because of the inability of this tissue to convert it to cortisol (Dougherty *et al.*, 1964; Burton, 1965). When such considerations were taken into account, these investigators found generally good correlation between the ability of a steroid at physiological levels to inhibit glucose uptake *in vitro* and its glucocorticoid activity *in vivo*. At higher levels *in vitro*, however, nonspecific effects are found (Munck, 1965; Kattwinkel and Munck, 1966). The steroids have been found to bind with thymus cells in two ways that can be related to their specific and nonspecific effects. One fraction binds weakly and nonspecifically, and dissociates rapidly. A smaller fraction appears to include binding that leads to specific glucocorticoid activity as measured by glucose uptake. Binding in this fraction is strong and it dissociates slowly; binding is, furthermore, believed to be rapid enough to account for any known glucocorticoid activity. The specific binding also depends upon cellular ATP levels, which would explain the fact that glucocorticoid effects are abolished by anaerobiosis. Competition for binding of cortisol seems to be in proportion to glucocorticoid activity, although some compounds, such as cortexolone, showed binding but also inhibited glucose uptake. It will be of interest to learn if the binding is also related to other metabolic effects of the glucocorticoids, including actions on the transports of amino acids and ions.

The glucocorticoids also possess some activity for altering cation transport, although, of course, they are much less effective than aldosterone. Robb *et al.* (1968) report, however, that the renal tubule of the rabbit is especially sensitive to the Na^+-retaining activity of cortisone. As a result, large quantities of salt and water are retained, and vascular congestion occurs following large doses of the steroid. DOCA has much less effect. The adrenal glands were not necessary for this action of cortisone, nor could the effect be attributed to changes in renal hemodynamic function. It is not clear whether the cortisone acts directly on the tubule, or is responsible for the release of another factor that makes the tubules unusually responsive. Some evidence has been given suggesting the presence of an extra-adrenal Na^+-retaining hormone (Davis *et al.*, 1966). Gaunt *et al.* (1967) also present indirect evidence for a Na^+-retaining agent that acts following adrenal enucleation of rats but which is apparently not identical with aldosterone.

Manitius *et al.* (1968) have attempted to relate the Na^+-retaining action of the glucocorticoids to the Na^+-K^+-sensitive ATPase of kidney membranes. Methylprednisolone increased the specific activity of the enzyme in whole homogenates but not in a fraction that should have contained plasma membranes. They conclude that the glucocorticoids increase the Na^+-K^+-sensitive ATPase activity in this tissue by increasing the quantity of plasma membrane per cell rather than by increasing the activity per weight of membranes. Jorgensen (1968) concludes from his studies, however, that the kidney Na^+-K^+-ATPase is not directly under the control of the adrenal glands. The decrease in activity of the enzyme following adrenalectomy corresponded to the change in plasma Na^+ and K^+ levels and could be partially prevented by a high-Na^+ diet. This latter fact suggests that the Na^+ level is at least partly responsible for the activity of the enzyme in the kidney.

Martonosi (1968) has reported that a number of steroids with glucocorticoid activity can inhibit Ca^{++} transport into microsomes of rabbit skeletal muscle. The effective compounds also increased the microsomal total ATPase activity and promoted hemolysis of human red blood cells.

Llaurado and Brito (1967) could find no effect of adrenalectomy, or addition of aldosterone, cortisol, epinephrine, or norepinephrine, on K^+ influx into rat erythrocytes.

Weissmann and co-workers (1966; Bangham *et al.*, 1965) have found that cortisone and cortisol decrease the leakage of Na^+, K^+, anions, glucose, and glycine from artificial phospholipid membranes. They suggest that the action of these steroids on natural membranes results from their interaction with lipid, independent of polysaccharide and protein. This view seems an oversimplification for explaining action on transports, especially since the transports of amino acids and Na^+ are uphill, and changes in them cannot be explained in terms of simple modification of nonmediated movements.

F. Estrogens

These steroids modify transports generally into tissues that show the more dramatic responses to the hormone, suggesting that the changes in transport are important parts of the physiological effects. The uterus has usually been chosen for study because it is easily removed for study, and because of its high sensitivity to estrogens.

Estradiol-17-β can stimulate the transport of both sugars and amino acids into uteri if it is injected into rats before tissues are removed for study *in vitro*, but the effect is produced only with difficulty if the hormone is added *in vitro*. The stimulation can apparently be prevented by injecting inhibitors of protein or RNA synthesis (puromycin, cycloheximide, actinomycin D), which have been reported to block all of the classical responses of the uteri to estrogen (Gorski and Axman, 1964; Mueller *et al.*, 1961).

Estradiol accelerates metabolism of glucose in the uterus within 1 hour after its administration *in vivo* (Nicolette and Gorski, 1964; Barker and Warren, 1966; Barker *et al.*, 1966; D. E. Smith, 1967). Generally, the evidence has favored the conclusion that a major change had occurred in the transport step. Spaziani and Gutman (1965) showed effects on transport of nonmetabolizable sugars within 1-2 hours. Uptakes into psoas muscle and ileum were unaltered. They concluded that estradiol altered rate of entry of the sugars into uteri, but not the steady state of their distribution.

D. E. Smith and Gorski (1968) have used 2-deoxyglucose to study the first two steps of sugar metabolism in the uterus. This compound is transported and very rapidly converted to the 6-phosphate in uteri, but it is not metabolized further. The two steps are not easily separated, however, so that it is not possible to determine if the estradiol influences the transport step or the phosphorylation. Nonetheless, the combined steps were increased by a half-hour treatment of rats *in vivo* with 5 μg estradiol. The V_{max} associated with the two steps was increased, but the apparent K_m was not.

Different sugars may respond in different ways, however. Roskoski and Steiner (1967a), and Levin and Gorski (unpublished observations mentioned in D. E. Smith and Gorski, 1968) did not find an effect of estradiol on uptake of 3-O-methyl glucose 1 hour after estrogen treatment. The hormone did produce a large increase after 2 hours (Roskoski and Steiner, 1967a). D. E. Smith and Gorski (1968) present evidence, however, that 2-deoxyglucose and 3-O-methylglucose may use different transport systems in the uterus, the former but not the latter going by the same system as glucose. Discrepancies concerning the minimum time needed for estradiol stimulation of sugar transports may be due to the presence of more than one transport system.

Cycloheximide, puromycin, and actinomycin D block the estrogen-stimulated sugar metabolism, and presumably sugar transport, if they are given *in vivo* at the same time as the estradiol (as short a time as

30-90 minutes before removing uteri) (Nicolette and Gorski, 1964; Gorski and Morgan, 1967; Roskoski and Steiner, 1967a; D. E. Smith and Gorski, 1968; Spaziani and Suddick, 1967). Actinomycin D also inhibits the estrogen-stimulated uterine weight increase in mice (Bialy and Pincus, 1966) and adrenalectomized rats (Nicolette and Mueller, 1966). In the latter case, the inhibition of RNA synthesis prevented the early response of the tissue to estrogen, but not all of the response was sensitive. The inhibitors had no effect on baseline uptake of 3-O-methyl glucose when they were given 3 hours *in vivo* before uteri were removed for study *in vitro* (Roskoski and Steiner, 1967a). Cortisol did not block the estrogen stimulation, showing that the effect of the cycloheximide or actinomycin in these cases was not due to increased secretion of adrenocortical hormone, which may occur in response to actinomycins (Planelles *et al.*, 1962). Cortisol can prevent other responses of the uterus to estrogen, including uptakes of water, electrolytes and glucose (Szego and Roberts, 1953; Spaziani and Szego, 1959; Bitman and Cecil, 1967; Nicolette and Gorski, 1964). The data of Spaziani and Suddick (1967) suggest that actinomycin D but not puromycin may exert its action on sugar and water uptake by inducing glucocorticoid secretion. Adrenalectomy prevented the depression in uterine 3-O-methyl glucose uptake given by actinomycin, but it did not alter the action of puromycin. However, other adverse actions of the latter compound (decreased sucrose space and blood flow, increased hematocrit) raised questions as to interpretation of results.

The data of Roskoski and Steiner (1967b) support the view that a carrier-mediated transport process is present in the uterus for 3-O-methyl glucose. This conclusion is based on the demonstration of saturation kinetics and countertransport for 3-O-methyl glucose uptake, and inhibition of its uptake by several sugars, including D-mannose, D-glucose, 2-deoxy-D-glucose, and D-xylose. D-Galactose, L-arabinose, and D-xylose were ineffective. The transport of 3-O-methyl glucose was not altered by various metabolic inhibitors (2,4-dinitrophenol, N-ethylmaleimide, iodoacetate, p-chloromercuribenzoate, diiosopropyl phosphofluoridate, cyanide). Treatment of rats with estradiol 4 hours before removing uteri resulted in nearly a doubling of the V_{max} of uptake of the sugar *in vitro*, while the K_m was unchanged. This fact, along with the results obtained after actinomycin treatment, suggests that the hormone is increasing the amount of a protein necessary for the carrier transport of the sugar. The results support the idea that the hormone acts on either RNA or protein synthesis, or both, before an effect on transport occurs.

Very similar results to these have been reported for the action of estradiol on amino acid uptake by the uterus. The uptake as measured by AIB is saturable and shows competition by other amino acids (Roskoski and Steiner, 1967c; Riggs *et al.*, 1968). In contrast to results on sugar uptake, the transport of AIB is inhibited by cyanide, DNP, *N*-ethylmaleimide and iodoacetate (Riggs *et al.*, 1968; Feng *et al.*, 1967). The latter two agents at low levels (0.05 mM) only stimulate uptakes of L-valine and L-phenylalanine; the difference in the action on these latter amino acids may be related to the fact that AIB uses predominantly a different amino acid transport route than do valine and phenylalanine. The presence of more than one amino acid transport system in the uterus is suggested by the pattern of competitive inhibition of AIB uptake, and by the fact that uptake of only some amino acids is Na$^+$-sensitive (Riggs *et al.*, 1968; Feng *et al.*, 1967). A possible relationship between transport system and estradiol stimulation of amino acid transport is discussed in Section III.

Estradiol given *in vivo* will stimulate subsequent uptake of several amino acids by the uterus *in vitro* when it is given for as short a time as 30 to 60 minutes before animals are killed (Noall and Allen, 1961; Roskoski and Steiner, 1967c; Riggs *et al.*, 1968; see, however, Coulson and Gorski, 1967). A maximum response is given within 3 hours when 1 μg of hormone is injected into immature rats. Some amino acids do not show the effect even after a 3-hour priming with the hormone, however, unless the incubation period is prolonged (up to 4 hours). If a 6-hour incubation period is used, a 10^{-6} M level of estradiol added *in vitro* produces as great a stimulation of AIB uptake as does an injection of 1 μg of the steroid 1 hour before uteri are removed for study *in vitro* (Riggs *et al.*, 1968). A 3-hour incubation does not show the stimulation. Estradiol stimulates only those amino acids that require Na$^+$ for their uptake, and Na$^+$ is needed for the stimulation (Feng *et al.*, 1967).

Injection of rats with cycloheximide or actinomycin D 1 hour before the estradiol can prevent the hormone stimulation of AIB uptake by uteri *in vitro* (Roskoski and Steiner, 1967a). As in the case of sugar uptake, cortisol injection cannot produce this same inhibition. Estradiol given *in vivo* for 3 hours can double the V_{max} of AIB uptake without altering the K_m (Riggs *et al.*, 1968). No effect was found on the non-saturable entry. Again, the results suggest that the hormone acts within a very short time to produce synthesis of large molecules (RNA and/or protein), and the action of the hormone on amino acid transport is secondary to this effect. A secondary action of the hormone on transport is also suggested by the results cited that a long incubation period is needed if the steroid is to stimulate AIB uptake when it is added *in vitro*. This fact shows, furthermore, that the hormone can act directly on the tissue to change transport. Any change needed in the molecule itself, before it can affect transport, is not produced exclusively by the liver, since partial or complete hepatectomy does not abolish the response of the uterus to estradiol when AIB uptake is measured *in vitro* (Daniels and Kalman, 1963).

Considerable evidence has been obtained regarding the biochemical action of estrogens with the uterine cell that presumably precedes the observed biochemical and physiological changes that they produce. Jensen reviews this subject in his chapter in Volume 2, so it will not be discussed at length here. It should be evident, however, that any reaction that alters transport of amino acids or sugars must occur *in vivo* within 1 hour after hormone administration, and the evidence suggests the reaction must lead to an increase in synthesis of specific RNA or protein molecules involved in their carrier systems. In this regard, it is of special interest to note that Notides and Gorski (1966) have given evidence for the presence of a uterine protein whose synthesis is increased in response to estrogen before any increase in net protein synthesis can be measured. This protein (or proteins) is believed to be necessary for the uterine response to the hormone in times of 1 hour or less. These workers have separated one protein that was stimulated 30 minutes after estrogen treatment, and its formation could be reduced by actinomycin D injection. Whether or not this protein is related to either the electrolyte, sugar, or amino acid carrier system is, of course, not known. It is not likely that an increase in a single protein would change the transport of all three types of substances, although the estrogen-induced changes in water, Na^+, Cl^-, K^+, and glucose uptakes are also altered in the same way by cortisol (Bitman and Cecil, 1967).

The foregoing results show that estradiol alters transports probably secondarily to a direct action on other cell metabolism. The effect, furthermore, is on mediated transport, and not on a nonsaturable, or difficultly saturable, entry. The work of Weissmann and associates (Bangham *et al.*, 1965; Weissmann *et al.*, 1966; Weissmann and Sessa, 1967; Sessa and Weissmann, 1968) has shown nevertheless, that steroids, including estradiol, progesterone, deoxycorticosterone, cortisone, and cortisol, as well as diethylstilbestrol, can alter the permeability of artificial lipid spherules to anions, cations, glucose, or glycine. The ability of the estrogen to render the membrane less permeable to anions does not have any apparent relation to the physiological action of the hormone, however.

Estradiol benzoate has also been reported to stimulate iodide uptake by thyroid tissue taken from hypophysectomized rats (Yamada *et al.*, 1966). It also increased the uptake of thyroxine by rat erythrocytes and diaphragm. Again, the relation of these effects to the physiological function of estradiol is not immediately apparent.

G. Androgens

Several androgenic steroids have been shown to increase the uptake by various muscle tissues of inorganic phosphate (Fleischmann and Fleischmann, 1952–1953), the model amino acids, AIB and cycloleucine (Metcalf and Gross, 1960; Riggs and Walker, 1963; Riggs *et al.*, 1963; Riggs and Wegrzyn, 1966; Mills and Spaziani, 1968), and the model sugar, 2-deoxyglucose (Mills and Spaziani, 1968). Most of the measurements have been made *in vivo* after repeated injections of hormone, or after treatment for several days. Mills and Spaziani (1968) have shown, however, that testosterone can increase the transport of both AIB and 2-deoxyglucose by prostate, seminal vesicle, and levator ani muscle of castrate rats within 6 to 18 hours *in vivo*. Most significant is the finding that a 12-hour treatment *in vivo* produces an increased ability of these tissues to take up both substances during a 1-hour incubation *in vitro* (the exception being 2-deoxyglucose uptake by levator ani muscle). The increased AIB uptake due to testosterone required energy, and could be inhibited by the absence of buffer Na⁺, the presence of ouabain, or by high levels of a competitor amino acid, alanine. Accumulation of 2-deoxyglucose was depressed by glucose or phlorizin. These results show that the steroid hormone alters active transport in the tissues studied, presumably by affecting a membrane transport carrier. Because the transports can be altered within a few hours after androgen injection, they may be important among the early metabolic changes produced by the hormone. Increased synthesis of RNA and protein in some of these tissues occurs within 1 to 6 hours after treatment with androgens (Wicks *et al.*, 1965; Greenman *et al.*, 1965; Butenandt *et al.*, 1960).

Although the exact relationships between changes in transport and cell metabolism are not known, Farnsworth (1968) has suggested that testosterone may regulate growth and function of the prostate gland by controlling the Na⁺ pump of the plasma membrane. He has found that a 15-minute pretreatment of prostate microsomes with 10^{-8} to $10^{-6}\ M$ testosterone can stimulate the Na⁺–K⁺-dependent, ouabain sensitive, ATPase. On the basis of these results, one would expect testosterone would also control Na⁺ transport in the prostate. It does greatly stimulate K⁺ uptake (Farnsworth, 1968). If Na⁺ transport is also regulated, the possibility must be considered that testosterone may regulate amino acid transport through its control of Na⁺ transport. If such a sequence is correct, then one can predict that androgens will alter transports of only those amino acids that require Na⁺ for maximal uptake in the affected tissue.

Klienman *et al.* (1966) report that the rate of PAH movement into renal cortical slices and intact kidneys is 50% higher in male rats than in females. Gonadectomy abolished the differences, and administration of testosterone to gonadectomized rats increased the PAH transport.

H. Thyroid Hormones

Thyroid hormones have been found to stimulate uptake of some amino acids, inhibit uptake of others, and exert no significant effect on still others. The effect also varies with the tissue. Hence, any attempt to relate an effect of these hormones on amino acid transport to their action on protein synthesis would have limited meaning unless both studies were made at the same time on the same amino acids and on a single tissue.

Adamson and Ingbar (1967b,c) have studied the properties of amino acid uptake by embryonic chick bone and its modification by several iodinated tyrosines and thyronines. Triiodothyronine was the most effective compound of those used. In some cases, levels as low as $10^{-7} M$ were effective, and within times as short as 2 minutes. They obtained evidence for the presence of at least two transport sites for neutral amino acids in this tissue (Adamson and Ingbar, 1967a), which seem closely analogous to the A and L sites described by Oxender and Christensen (1963) for Ehrlich ascites tumor cells. With minor exceptions, those amino acids that were transported well by the L site were stimulated by triiodothyronine, whereas those with high specificity for the A site were unaffected (see Table I, and further discussion in Section III). Uptakes of glycine, valine, and isoleucine were inhibited by the hormone, however. Increased incorporation of amino acids into protein did not occur under conditions in which methionine transport was increased. Neither actinomycin D nor puromycin affected cycloleucine uptake nor its stimulation by thyroid hormones within 1 hour. After 1 hour, however, these agents inhibited further amino acid accumulation (Adamson and Ingbar, 1967a; Adamson *et al.*, 1966); and the stimulation by triiodothyronine and thyroxine was inhibited by actinomycin D after 4 hours (Adamson and Ingbar, 1967c). The lack of immediate inhibition by either actinomycin D or puromycin suggests that the stimulation of transport does not require prior synthesis of new protein or RNA. The effect at longer times is doubtless due to the decay of normal transport molecules that cannot be formed again in the presence of the inhibitors.

Thyroid hormone also stimulates the uptake of methionine by costal and xiphoid cartilage of mature thyroidectomized rats (Adamson and Ingbar, 1967c). Potchen and Watts (1967) report that thyroxine suppresses uptake of selenomethionine by thyroid tissue, while uptake by the parathyroid gland is not affected. AIB uptake by rat pituitary gland is also inhibited by thyroxine and stimulated by thyroidectomy (Tonoue and Yamamoto, 1967). Interestingly, the hypophysis was found to take up AIB to a level about five times that found in diaphragm. The hormone did not affect uptake by this latter tissue. Tonoue and Yamamoto (1967) suggest that the thyroid hormone may exert its effect on the pituitary gland by way of control of amino acid uptake.

Studies on the effect of thyroid hormones on intestinal transport of sugars have given conflicting results. The early work of Althausen and Stockholm (1938) suggested that the intestinal absorption of glucose and xylose was increased by thyroxine administration and decreased by thyroidectomy. However, Broitman *et al.* (1961), and Bronk and Parsons (1966a) could not find any consistent effect of a deficiency or excess of the hormone on absorption of xylose or galactose; while Halliday *et al.* (1962), Levin and Smyth (1963), and London and Segal (1967) report that hyperthyroidism decreases and hypothyroidism increases the serosal to mucosal concentration ratios of glucose across the everted rat gut sac *in vitro*. Several reports present results showing this latter effect on intestinal amino acid transport, i.e., a decrease in the presence of an excess of the hormone, and an increase in its deficiency (Matty and Seshardi, 1965; Bronk and Parsons, 1966b; London and Segal, 1967). In some cases the nonmetabolizable models AIB, cycloleucine, and α-methyl-D-glucose were used and gave the same results as obtained with natural compounds. This last fact suggests that the hormone acts on the transport step itself. London and Segal (1967), for example, found that intestinal segments from hypothyroid rats would take up greater than normal levels of cycloleucine, histidine, valine, or α-methyl glucose during incubation *in vitro*. Differences could be shown after uptakes of 5 minutes. The effects were diminished by treatment of the donor animals for 4 to 5 days with triiodothyronine, but thyroxine added *in vitro* was ineffective. Flux measurements showed that the rate of loss of valine from the tissue was unchanged when the uptake was increased, whereas kinetic studies showed that the maximum velocity of transport had been elevated by the absence of the hormone.

Bauman and Earls (1967) report that triiodothyronine retards the excretion of water loads and increases urine osmolarity in hypophysectomized rats. Sodium ion retention was also increased during the first few hours after water or saline loading. Aldosterone failed to produce the same pattern of effects. The authors propose that triiodothyronine affects the renal tissue in some way that is independent of aldosterone and the adrenal cortex.

TABLE I

SUMMARY OF REPORTED EFFECTS OF INSULIN, GROWTH HORMONE,
ESTRADIOL, AND TRIIODOTHYRONINE ON TRANSPORTS OF NEUTRAL AMINO ACIDS[a]

Amino acid	Insulin: diaphragm[b]	Insulin + puromycin: diaphragm[c]	Insulin + puromycin: heart[d]	Growth hormone: diaphragm[e]	Estradiol: uterus[f]	Triiodo-thyronine: embryonic bone[g]	Major transport system used[a]
L-Proline	+	—	+61[h]	+	+47[h]	0	A
L-Serine	+	—	+54[h]	+	+23[h]	0	A
L-Threonine	+	—	+50	+	—	0	A
L-Alanine	0	+36[h]	+46[h]	+	+30[h]	0	A
Glycine	+	—	+28[h]	+	+21[h]	—	A
L-Glutamine	—	—	—	+	—	—	A
L-Asparagine	—	—	—	+	—	—	A
Sarcosine	+++	—	—	—	—	—	A
AIB	++	—	—	+[i]	+100[h]	0	A
L-Hydroxyproline	+	—	—	—	—	—	A
1-Aminocyclopentane-carboxylic acid	+	—	—	—	+57[h]	+	A, L
L-Methionine	+	—	+32[h]	0	—	+	A, L

L-Histidine	0	+35[h]	+17	+	—	+	A, L
DL-Norleucine	0	—	—	—	-9[i]	—	A, L
L-Valine	0	+21[h]	+25	0[i]	-7[i]	+	L
L-Leucine	0	+18[h]	+22[h]	0	-46[i]	—	L
L-Isoleucine	0	+18[h]	+10	—	—	+	L
L-Tryptophan	0	—	+8	+	—	++	L
L-Phenylalanine	0	+18[h]	-6	0	-2	++	L
L-Tyrosine	0	+18[h]	-9	0	—	+	L

[a] Classification of amino acids according to major transport system used; based primarily on the division found in Ehrlich ascites cells.
[b] Data of Kipnis and Noall (1958); Manchester and Young (1960a); Akedo and Christensen (1962); Wool (1964); Rieser and Rieser (1964); Snipes (1967).
[c] Data of Castles and Wool (1964); Wool et al. (1965).
[d] Data of Scharff and Wool (1965).
[e] Data of Snipes and Kostyo (1962); Knobil (1966).
[f] Data of Riggs et al. (1968).
[g] Data of Adamson and Ingbar (1967b).
[h] Change shown to be significant by statistical test.
[i] Same qualitative result found in presence of puromycin.
[j] Significant increase found after a 4-hour incubation.

I. Thyroid-Stimulating Hormone

This protein controls iodide transport, which is the first step in I⁻ metabolism in the thyroid gland (although not the first response to TSH), and it also influences the transport of amino acids and sugars into this tissue. The action on iodide transport has also been shown in single cells cultured in suspension (Dickson, 1966). The effect on I⁻ is by far the most pronounced of the effects on transport; thyroid:serum ratios can be raised from near unity to around 400 by treatment of hypophysectomized rats with the hormone. The increase is apparently due to both a decreased efflux and an increased influx (Surks, 1967; Wollman and Reed, 1959). Attempts have been made to identify the chemical changes associated with the membrane that might account for this large effect. The work particularly of Wolff (Wolff and Maurey, 1961; Wolff and Halmi, 1963), and Turkington (1962) had suggested that TSH may stimulate I⁻ uptake indirectly by increasing Na⁺ and/or K⁺ transport. In glands from guinea pigs, the hormone produced parallel increases in thyroidal Na⁺-K⁺-sensitive ATPase activity, iodide transport, and sensitivity to inhibition of both activities by cardiac glycosides. More recently, however, Brunberg and Halmi (1966) have concluded that the TSH-induced increase in ouabain-sensitive ATPase activity in the thyroid gland of the rat is not directly related to stimulation of I⁻ transport by the gland. Although a close relation between the two activities could be shown in some conditions that increased TSH output (e.g., on low iodide intake), poor correlations were found after hypophysectomy of the rats, or after treatment with either propylthiouracil or triiodothyronine. The independence of the two factors was especially pronounced when hypophysectomized rats were given TSH plus propylthiouracil. Wolff and Rall (1965) had reported earlier that they were unable to detect changes in ouabain-sensitive ATPase activity in thyroids of rats under some conditions in which the thyroid:serum ratios had been raised by cystamine or cysteamine; and when both did change, no close correlation between the responses was found. The relation between the two activities in the rat thyroid is, therefore, not at all clear. Comparable experiments need to be done in thyroid tissue from rat and thyroid tissue from guinea pig to determine if the two are different. Scranton and Halmi (1965) obtained results suggesting that in the rat thyroid, ouabain interferes with the ability of the gland to retain iodide, and does not affect its entry.

Conflicting reports have also appeared regarding the effect of actinomycin D on the TSH stimulation of I⁻ uptake by the thyroid gland. A. B. Schneider and Goldberg (1965), and Niccolini and Mack (1965) have reported in abstract that the compound inhibits I⁻ uptake *in vitro* in glands from hypophysectomized rats; Dumont *et al.* (1964) found an increase in the 3-hour I⁻ uptake (as percent of dose) by the thyroids of mice pretreated with actinomycin D. Halmi *et al.* (1966, 1967) failed to find a consistent increase in thyroidal I⁻ uptake *in vivo* within 4 hours after giving the antibiotic; they thus disagree with Dumont *et al.* They also could not confirm the results of Schneider and Goldberg or Niccolini and Mack with studies *in vitro*. However, Halmi and co-workers did show a large stimulation of I⁻ uptake 16 hours after actinomycin D treatment *in vivo*. This result could not at first be shown to be independent of the presence of TSH; but later work showed that the effect was as great in hypophysectomized as in normal rats. Actinomycin D also produced an early depression in thyroid:serum ratios of iodide (Halmi *et al.*, 1967), an effect that is also given by TSH (Halmi *et al.*, 1960). These facts suggested to the investigators that TSH acts on organic binding of I⁻ before transport is altered (see also Isaacs and Rosenberg, 1967). The results do not show consistently, however, that nucleic acid synthesis, and presumably also protein synthesis, is necessary for TSH stimulation of I⁻ transport. Dumont *et al.* (1964) and Halmi *et al.* (1966, 1967) suggest, on the other hand, that the stimulation by actinomycin may be due to repression of the formation of an inhibitor of the iodide pump of the thyroid gland. Such an inhibitor had been postulated earlier by Halmi and Spirtos (1955).

Although their experiments had another purpose, the results of Taurog and Thio (1966) are consistent with the conclusion that protein synthesis is not needed for I⁻ transport. These workers found that infusion of puromycin into the thyroid gland by way of the carotid artery did not alter the release of ^{131}I-thyroxine in rabbits. Because the labeled thyroxine was formed from injected radioiodide, we may conclude that inhibition of protein synthesis by the puromycin did not decrease any of the intermediate steps involved in thyroxine formation, including the transport of iodide into the cells.

Macchia and Pastan (1967) have presented evidence that TSH action on thyroid cells depends upon a membrane phospholipid, and they suggest that the hormone becomes bound to the cell membrane. Dog thyroid slices preincubated with TSH and then washed thoroughly show the same increase in oxidation of glucose-1-^{14}C to ^{14}CO$_2$ as found if TSH is present along with the glucose (Pastan *et al.*, 1966). This effect could be abolished, however, by exposing the tissue to either anti-TSH antibody or trypsin before incubating it with glucose. The action of TSH could also be prevented by adding an enzyme, identified as phospholipase C, obtained from the culture medium of *Clostridium perfringens* (Macchia and Pastan, 1967). The enzyme-treated cells had normal basal glucose oxidation and showed normal stimulation of glucose oxidation by acetylcholine. The results therefore suggest that the phospholipid is not important for all actions at the membrane, but that it is necessary for the effect of TSH.

A possible role of phospholipid in transport carrier processes in the thyroid has also been suggested by Vilkki (1962), and by P. Schneider and Wolff, (1964). Kogl and van Deenen (1961) have shown, furthermore, that phospholipid synthesis in thyroid tissue is sensitive to TSH. Phospholipase C has been reported to decrease the baseline iodide transport in thyroid slices (Larsen and Wolff, 1967), and so presumably it would modify the TSH stimulation of this transport. The enzyme also affects the activities of various membrane-bound enzymes, however, including a muscle ATPase (see Macchia and Pastan, 1967), so the action is not solely on transport. Nevertheless it will be of importance to learn if phospholipase C produces its effects by modifying transport sites normally affected by TSH.

Cyclic 3',5'-AMP has also been suggested as the mediator of TSH actions on metabolism of I⁻ and glucose in thyroid cells. Gilman and Rall (1968a) have shown that TSH increases the content of this compound in bovine thyroid slices *in vitro*, with a maximum value being found after 3 to 6 minutes and at a level of 10 munits/ml. The response is rapid enough to account for the TSH effects. High concentrations of ACTH, LH, FSH, growth hormone, human chorionic gonadotropin, and prolactin produced effects that could be accounted for on the basis of their contamination with TSH. The effect of TSH was potentiated by theophylline, a competitive inhibitor of the phosphodiesterase that catalyzes the hydrolysis of cyclic AMP. Bastomsky and McKenzie (1967) have found that cyclic AMP as well as theophylline alters I⁻ metabolism in rat and mouse thyroid tissue in a manner similar to that shown by TSH; while Gilman and Rall (1968b) report evidence suggesting that cyclic AMP mediates the TSH-induced changes in glucose metabolism in bovine thyroid slices. In the latter case, however, the authors conclude that the altered glucose oxidation was not dependent upon glucose uptake from the medium, since dibutyryl cyclic AMP did not affect uptake. It should be noted that TSH causes a decrease in conversion of glucose-1-^{14}C to $^{14}CO_2$ in bovine thyroid tissue, in contrast to the increase produced by the hormone in tissues from calves (Field *et al.*, 1960) as well as other species. Pastan (1966; cf. Pastan and Macchai, 1967) has shown, in addition, that in dog thyroid slices, dibutyryl cyclic AMP can substitute for TSH in stimulating glucose oxidation. Furthermore, TSH has been reported to stimulate glucose uptake by sheep and calf thyroid slices (Freinkel, 1960; Field *et al.*, 1960); and both TSH and cyclic AMP enhance pentose transport in thyroid slices from calves (Tarui *et al.*, 1963). Bovine thyroid tissue is apparently unique in its response to TSH, so that TSH and cyclic AMP may have different actions on transport as well as on other metabolism in glands from this species. Such a possibility suggests the need to test the effect of TSH on cyclic AMP levels in thyroid glands from other animals.

TSH stimulates the uptake of some amino acids by dog and bovine thyroid gland cells (Debons and Pittman, 1962; Segal *et al.*, 1966; Tong, 1964, 1967), although no effect was found in sheep thyroid tissue (Raghupathy *et al.*, 1964). Elevated amino acid uptake alone apparently cannot account entirely for the TSH-induced protein synthesis, however. A similar conclusion has been reached with regard to actions of other hormones on protein synthesis. Tong (1967) has suggested that the augmentation by TSH of both amino acid accumulation and protein synthesis may be secondary to an effect of the hormone to stimulate energy metabolism and respiration.

Both bovine and dog thyroid slices have been used by Segal *et al.* (1966) to study the kinetics of amino acid uptake. TSH produced a significant increase in uptake of AIB but not of the other amino acids tested (glycine, L-histidine, L-tyrosine, L-valine, 1-aminocyclopentanecarboxylic acid). The action on AIB became greater with time of incubation up to 90 minutes. Uptake of AIB from a 0.067 mM solution was biphasic, and did not reach a steady state within 210 minutes; while the steady state was given by the other amino acids within 30 to 90 minutes. These facts led Segal *et al.*, to the conclusion that, in thyroid tissue, AIB does not serve as a good model for the natural amino acids tested. The response in amino acid uptake and metabolism to TSH appears to be quite complex, however. The hormone stimulates protein synthesis in the thyroid gland (e.g., Tong, 1967); and it also has been reported to increase the α-amino-N in the tissue (Poffenbarger *et al.*, 1963), presumably as a consequence of its ability to stimulate hydrolysis of thyroglobulin. It seems relevant to refer again, therefore, to the finding of Scharff and Wool (1965) that the effect of insulin on amino acid transport can be obscured by the action of the insulin to increase protein synthesis. One recalls in this connection the difficulty in demonstrating an action of insulin on transport of amino acids other than AIB and glycine (see Manchester and Young, 1961). Clearly, the action of TSH on amino acid transport needs to be tested under conditions in which both synthesis and hydrolysis of protein are brought to a minimum before effects can be evaluated. It also seems likely that not all amino acids will show significant stimulation of their transports by TSH (see discussion in Section III).

J. Other Tropic Hormones of the Pituitary Gland

Luteinizing hormone, follicle-stimulating hormone, and human chorionic gonadotropin have all been found to stimulate glucose uptake by isolated ovaries from prepubertal or hypophysectomized rats (Ahren and Kostyo, 1963; Armstrong *et al.*, 1963; Hamberger and Ahren, 1967). The effects have been shown when the hormone was given *in vivo* or added *in vitro*. Intravenously injected FSH also stimulated AIB uptake by ovaries *in vitro*, but LH had no effect (Ahren and Kostyo, 1963).

A possible action on substrate or cofactor movement across the membrane of adrenal mitochondria has been suggested as one way in which ACTH may modify adrenal steroidogenesis (Koritz, 1968a,b). This hormone (probably through mediation of cyclic AMP) stimulates the conversion of cholesterol to pregnenolone in reactions that take place within adrenal mitochondria (Halkerston *et al.*, 1961). The conversion can also be stimulated by a number of unrelated agents and conditions that cause mitochondrial swelling (e.g., Ca^{++}, proteolytic enzymes, fatty acids, detergents, freezing the tissue) (Hirshfield and Koritz, 1964). Inhibiting the swelling by ATP prevents the stimulation of pregnenolone synthesis. Because swelling of mitochondria changes the permeability of their membranes, it is possible that a change in entry or exit of substrates or cofactors could control steroid synthesis.

De Nicola *et al.* (1968) have proposed that the well-known ability of ACTH to cause depletion of adrenal ascorbic acid levels may result from inhibition of transport of ascorbate. Uptake of the vitamin into the gland *in vitro* was shown to have some of the properties of active transport, and it could be inhibited not only by ACTH but also by estradiol, progesterone, aldosterone, and corticosterone. The inhibition by ACTH was correlated with increased steroidogenesis. ACTH was also inhibitory when transport was measured in isolated zona fasciculata-reticularis. The inhibition by ACTH required protein synthesis, since it was abolished by addition of puromycin. The antibiotic did not alter baseline transport of ascorbate, however. The inhibition could also be produced by a factor isolated from the incubation medium in which adrenal glands were exposed to ACTH. This factor was not believed to be corticosteroid in nature.

K. Epinephrine and Norepinephrine

Epinephrine has long been known to lower blood levels of amino acids and increase their uptake by tissues. Sanders and Riggs (1967b) have recently studied this effect in somewhat more detail in rats, using the model nonmetabolizable amino acids, 1-aminocyclopentanecarboxylic acid and AIB. Their results suggest that the hormone acts directly on muscle tissues and liver to increase amino acid uptake. The epinephrine inhibitor, dihydroergotaminemethanesulfonate, blocked the epinephrine stimulation of uptake especially in heart muscle and liver; and removal of adrenal or pituitary glands did not greatly alter effects of injected epinephrine on amino acid distribution. The large increase in uptake of 1-aminocyclopentanecarboxylic acid produced by insulin injection could be attributed to a hypoglycemia-induced secretion of epinephrine in these rats rather than to a large direct action of insulin itself (Sanders and Riggs, 1967a).

Because epinephrine elevates blood glucose levels, one might expect it to have an inhibitory effect, if any action at all, on sugar uptake by tissues (see, for example, Walaas and Walaas, 1950). Several reports show, however, that the hormone increases uptake by adipose tissue (Leboeuf *et al.*, 1959; Vaughan, 1961), perfused rat heart (Williamson, 1964), and isolated frog sartorius muscle (Saha *et al.*, 1968). In the latter case, the nonutilizable 3-O-methyl-D-glucose was used, so that the effect was isolated on the transport process. The effects of insulin and epinephrine on the transport were compared and believed to be similar, suggesting that the two hormones may act in the same way on this process. Glucose was found to compete with 3-O-methyl glucose for transport and also to induce countertransport of the latter sugar. Cyclic AMP did not alter uptake of the methyl glucose over a 3.5 hour incubation with the frog sartorius muscle, however, in contrast to the effect of the cyclic compound on glucose uptake by rat diaphragm *in vitro* (Edelman *et al.*, 1966). The evidence therefore does not support the possibility that cyclic AMP may mediate the action of epinephrine on sugar transport as it does on glycogenolysis.

Epinephrine and/or norepinephrine have been shown to alter the movement of Na^+ and/or K^+ out of a variety of tissues, including the sinus venosus and atrium of the frog heart (Haas and Trautwein, 1963), and intestinal smooth muscle depolarized by high K^+ levels (Jenkinson and Morton, 1967). Gonzales *et al.* (1967) have also presented evidence that norepinephrine is responsible for the changes in potential difference and short-circuit current across isolated toad skin when innervating nerve fibers are stimulated. The norepinephrine is liberated from sympathetic fibers following electrical stimulation. The changes in potential difference and short-circuit current are ordinarily taken to indicate a movement of Na^+ across the skin.

Bastide and Jard (1968), and Jard *et al.* (1968) have compared the effects of oxytocin and norepinephrine on the transport of Na^+ and water across the frog skin. The results suggest that cyclic AMP mediates the actions of both hormones to increase movements of the two substances. Because a number of differences were found, however, the authors conclude that oxytocin and norepinephrine have different mechanisms for binding to their specific receptor sites on the membrane.

L. Minor Actions of Parathormone and Thyrocalcitonin

The effects of these hormones on calcium metabolism are dealt with in detail in Chapter 9 in this volume. Several studies have been reported, however, on the effects of one or both of these substances on amino acid and sugar transport in bone as a part of the effort to determine what general effects the hormones may have on metabolism. Rosenbusch and Nichols (1967) found, for example, that AIB uptake by bone cells from metaphyses of 40-day-old rats is stimulated 8 to 12 hours after treatment of animals with parathyroid hormone. Inhibition was produced after 48 to 72 hours of treatment, however. Similar effects were shown on bone from hypophysectomized and parathyroidectomized animals, a fact that suggests that the action was produced directly by parathormone. The changes also mirror the alterations in biosynthesis of collagen produced by the hormone. The same workers (Dos Reis *et al.*, 1968) could not find an effect of either parathyroid extract or thyrocalcitonin on uptake of 3-*O*-methyl-D-glucose by these bone cells.

An interesting observation has been reported by Fujita *et al.* (1966), who found that valine or tryptophan would elevate the plasma Ca^{++} level in parathyroidectomized rats. Methionine decreased the Ca^{++} level, whereas thirteen other amino acids were without effect. The authors conclude that the phenomena are not directly related to the mechanism of action of the parathyroid hormone. Whether or not it is related to transport effects is also of interest.

III. EVIDENCE THAT HORMONES AFFECT ONLY ONE OF THE TRANSPORT SYSTEMS FOR NEUTRAL AMINO ACIDS

As discussed, a number of hormones alter transport of some of the neutral amino acids into specific tissues. In cases in which a variety of amino acids have been tested, however, results have shown that not all of them are affected by any one of the hormones. One possible explanation for this observation rests in the fact that probably every cell contains more than one transport system for neutral amino acids, not all of which may be altered by a given hormone. Oxender and Christensen (1963; see also Christensen, 1966, 1967) have described in considerable detail the evidence for multiple neutral amino acid transport systems in the Ehrlich ascites carcinoma cell. The two major systems have been designated A and L, the former serving most efficiently for short-chain, more polar compounds such as glycine, L-alanine and L-serine; while the latter is more effective for transporting the branched-chain, less polar substances, such as L-leucine, L-valine and L-phenylalanine. Members of the first group are also distinguished in that their uptakes require the presence of extracellular Na^+ and are quite sensitive to metabolic inhibitors. The transport systems are not discrete, however. All of the natural neutral amino acids have been found to be transported by both the A and L systems, and the foregoing division has been made on the basis of the system that is used predominantly by a given amino acid. Compounds such as L-methionine, L-histidine and 1-aminocyclopentanecarboxylic acid appear to be transported quite well by both the A and the L systems, at least in the Ehrlich cell.

The amino acid transport systems have not been described in great detail for any of the hormone-sensitive tissues. Nevertheless, systems quite similar to the A and L of Ehrlich cells have been reported for a variety of tissues, including several that respond to hormones, e.g., bone (Finerman and Rosenberg, 1966; Adamson and Ingbar, 1967a), uterus (Riggs *et al.*, 1968), and diaphragm (see Kipnis and Parrish, 1965).

Table I summarizes the reported effects of insulin and growth hormone on neutral amino acid uptake by diaphragm and heart muscle; the action of estradiol on their uptake by the uterus; and the effect of triiodothyronine on their uptake by embryonic chick bone. Quantitative values are given in some instances, in terms of per cent increase in uptake produced by the hormone. In column 8 of the table is listed the major transport system used by each of the amino acids, based primarily, although not entirely, on the evidence obtained from Ehrlich cells. The designation is in each case consistent with that found in the hormone-sensitive tissue in question, in those instances in which it has been tested.

A study of the results in Table I shows that insulin, growth hormone, and estradiol produce the greatest stimulation of uptake of those amino acids that are transported very well by the A system; while triiodothyronine affects only those that use predominantly the L system. These facts suggest that the first three hormones may affect only the A system, and triiodothyronine acts on only the L. Upon closer examination, several apparent exceptions to this generalization can be seen not to be inconsistent. For example, the relatively small but significant response of leucine uptake to insulin (columns 3 and 4) is to be expected even though insulin may act only on the A system. The increased uptake would result because leucine probably enters the tissues to some extent by way of the A system, even though less well than by the L system.

The available data on actions of hormones other than these four are not extensive enough to permit classification in the manner shown in Table I. Nonetheless, the glucocorticoids, testosterone, TSH, FSH, and parathormone all have been reported to affect uptake of AIB; and, at least in the case of testosterone, this action requires Na^+. The results suggest that these latter five hormones, also, may well affect a transport system similar to the A, since this system is used best by AIB.

It is clear that any interpretation of hormonal effects on amino acid transport must take into account the probable presence of more than one transport system in a tissue.

IV. CONCLUDING REMARKS

The foregoing survey shows the continued abundance of descriptive information being reported concerning the hormones that affect transport systems in different tissues. This description is important as a first step in identifying areas for further investigation, and also to emphasize the integral part that transport processes play in the total action of a hormone. Research must move beyond this purely descriptive stage, however, and toward a dissection of the molecular steps of transport processes that are affected by hormones. Some progress has already been made in this direction, as the present review has made clear, but more intensive effort can be expected in the future. It seems appropriate, in conclusion, to call attention to a few of the approaches that seem necessary, or appear to hold special promise, at this stage of our knowledge.

First, it is clearly not possible to understand what chemical changes a hormone produces in a transport process until the molecular steps of the process are known. One attack on this problem is that of learning the three-dimensional, physical-chemical nature of membranes. A closely related aspect is that of how a given hormone reacts with the membrane to affect a transport, whether this reaction is a direct one, or whether it is mediated through some molecule such as 3′,5′-cyclic adenylic acid.

Current effort should continue, of course, toward identifying the primary reaction of the hormone with the cell, whether it be at the membrane or elsewhere, and toward describing the subsequent sequence of events that leads to the altered transport.

On the other hand, work should also continue to attack directly the problem of how transport processes work. Changes induced by hormones may prove especially helpful here. For example, a hormone may produce an increase in the amount of a specific protein that can thereby be associated with a carrier transport system. Experiments along this line may be modeled after those carried out with bacteria. Several groups of investigators (e.g., Pardee, 1966, 1967; Piperno and Oxender, 1966; Penrose *et al.*, 1968; Anraku, 1968a,b,c) have isolated bacterial proteins, generally believed to have been associated with cell membranes, that have characteristics of transport carriers for specific substances. In these studies, transportless mutants, and induction of transport, have both been important in providing evidence that the transport was associated with the specific protein—it was absent in the transportless strain and present in proportion to induced transport under the conditions of induction. In mammalian tissues, hormone stimulation might be used to increase the amount of a transport constituent present in a membrane, or, alternatively, to increase the affinity of binding of substrate to carrier. As described earlier (Section II,D,2), Kostyo (1968) has already used this approach in his attempt to separate a specific protein from rat diaphragm, which may presumably be formed in parallel to the increased amino acid transport produced by growth hormone. Other hormone-sensitive tissues could be examined in the same way. Kostyo's results should serve to emphasize the need to work increasingly in purified systems if results are to be interpreted with meaning. Gross changes in protein or nucleic acid synthesis probably have little significance in this connection, since a change in only one or a few specific compounds may be all that is necessary for a hormone to bring about a change in transport.

As a final comment, the twofold nature of investigations regarding hormones and transport should be stressed again. Any study in this area can, potentially, advance present knowledge concerning both the way hormones act and the way ions and molecules are transported across membranes. The current literature suggests that investigators of the subject are at the present time more interested in the former aspect than in the latter. In some cases (although by no means all), an apparent unfamiliarity with, or inattention to, fundamental transport theory has resulted in more poorly planned experiments, or more imprecise or superficial interpretation than is necessary. Greater attention to transport itself appears to be a general need in future investigations of effects of hormones on transport.

REFERENCES

Adamson, L. F., and Ingbar, S. H. (1967a). *J. Biol. Chem.* **242**, 2646.
Adamson, L. F., and Ingbar, S. H. (1967b). *Endocrinology* **81**, 1362.
Adamson, L. F., and Ingbar, S. H. (1967c). *Endocrinology* **81**, 1372.
Adamson, L. F., Langeluttig, S. G., and Anast, C. S. (1966). *Biochim. Biophys. Acta* **115**, 355.
Adolfsson, S., Arvill, A., and Ahren, K. (1967). *Biochim. Biophys. Acta* **135**, 176.
Ahrén, K., and Kostyo, J. L. (1963). *Endocrinology* **73**, 81.
Akedo, H., and Christensen, H. N. (1962). *J. Biol. Chem.* **237**, 118.
Althausen, T. L., and Stockholm, M. (1938). *Am. J. Physiol.* **123**, 577.
Anraku, Y. (1968a). *J. Biol. Chem.* **243**, 3116.
Anraku, Y. (1968b). *J. Biol. Chem.* **243**, 3123.
Anraku, Y. (1968c). *J. Biol. Chem.* **243**, 3128.
Armstrong, D. T., Kilpatrick, R., and Greep, R. O. (1963). *Endocrinology* **73**, 165.
Baker, W. K., and Rutter, W. J. (1964). *Arch. Biochem. Biophys.* **105**, 68.
Bangham, A. D., Standish, M. M., and Weissmann, G. (1965). *J. Mol. Biol.* **13**, 253.
Barker, K. L., and Warren, J. C. (1966). *Endocrinology* **78**, 1205.
Barker, K. L., Nielson, M. H., and Warren, J. C. (1966). *Endocrinology* **79**, 1069.
Bartlett, D., Morita, Y., and Munck, A. (1962). *Nature* **196**, 897.
Bastide, F., and Jard, S. (1968). *Biochim. Biophys. Acta* **150**, 113.
Bastide, F., Bourguet, J., Jard, S., and Morel, F. (1968). In "Protein and Polypeptide Hormones" (M. Margoulies, ed.), pp. 257–259. Excerpta Med. Found., Amsterdam.
Bastomsky, C. H., and McKenzie, J. M. (1967). *Am. J. Physiol.* **213**, 753.
Bauman, J. W., and Earls, C. (1967). *Endocrinology* **80**, 1185.
Bentley, P. J. (1960). *J. Endocrinol.* **21**, 161.
Berde, B. (1968). In "Protein and Polypeptide Hormones" (M. Margoulies, ed.), pp. 222–223. Excerpta Med. Found., Amsterdam.
Bialy, G., and Pincus, G. (1966). *Endocrinology* **78**, 286.
Bihler, I. (1968). *Biochim. Biophys. Acta* **163**, 401.
Bihler, I., and Crane, R. K. (1962). *Biochim. Biophys. Acta* **59**, 78.
Bitman, J., and Cecil, H. C. (1967). *Endocrinology* **80**, 423.
Blecher, M. (1967). *Biochim. Biophys. Acta* **137**, 557.
Bonting, S. L., and Canady, M. R. (1964). *Am. J. Physiol.* **207**, 1005.
Bourguet, J., and Maetz, J. (1961). *Biochim. Biophys. Acta* **52**, 552.
Bourguet, J., and Morel, F. (1967). *Biochim. Biophys. Acta* **135**, 693.
Bowyer, F. (1957). *Intern. Rev. Cytol.* **6**, 469.
Broitman, S. A., Small, M. D., Vitale, J. J., and Zamcheck, N. (1961). *Gastroenterology* **41**, 24.
Bronk, J. R., and Parsons, D. S. (1966a). *J. Physiol. (London)* **179**, 323.

Bronk, J. R., and Parsons, D. S. (1966b). *J. Physiol.* (*London*) **184**, 942.
Brunberg, J. A., and Halmi, N. S. (1966). *Endocrinology* **79**, 801.
Burrow, G. N., and Bondy, P. K. (1964). *Endocrinology* **75**, 455.
Burton, A. F. (1965). *Endocrinology* **77**, 325.
Butenandt, A., Gunther, H., and Turba, F. (1960). *Z. Physiol. Chem.* **322**, 28.
Capps, J. C., Shetlar, M. R., and Bradford, R. H. (1966). *Biochim. Biophys. Acta* **127**, 205.
Carlin, H., and Hechter, O. (1964). *Proc. Soc. Exptl. Biol. Med.* **115**, 127.
Castles, J. J., and Wool, I. G. (1964). *Biochem. J.* **91**, 11c.
Castles, J. J., Wool, I. G., and Moyer, A. N. (1965). *Biochim. Biophys. Acta* **100**, 609.
Chambers, J. W., Georg, R. H., and Bass, A. D. (1965). *Mol. Pharmacol.* **1**, 66.
Christensen, H. N. (1966). *Federation Proc.* **25**, 850.
Christensen, H. N. (1967). *Perspectives Biol. Med.* **10**, 471.
Christensen, H. N., and Handlogten, M. E. (1968). *J. Biol. Chem.* **243**, 5428.
Christensen, H. N., Riggs, T. R., and Coyne, B. A. (1954). *J. Biol. Chem.* **209**, 413.
Civan, M. M., Kedem, O., and Leaf, A. (1966). *Am. J. Physiol.* **211**, 569.
Clausen, T. (1965). *Biochim. Biophys. Acta* **109**, 164.
Clausen, T. (1966). *Biochim. Biophys. Acta* **120**, 361.
Clausen, T. (1968a). *Biochim. Biophys. Acta* **150**, 56.
Clausen, T. (1968b). *Biochim. Biophys. Acta* **150**, 66.
Clausen, T., Letarte, J., and Rodbell, M. (1968). *In* "Protein and Polypeptide Hormones" (M. Margoulies, ed.), pp. 282–284. Excerpta Med. Found., Amsterdam.
Cort, J. H. (1964). *In* "Oxytocin, Vasopressin and their Structural Analogues" (J. Rudinger, ed.), Vol. 10, pp. 72–73. Pergamon Press, Oxford.
Cort, J. H. (1966). "Electrolytes, Fluid Dynamics, and the Nervous System." Academic Press, New York.
Cort, J. H., Rudinger, J., Lichardus, B., and Hagemann, I. (1966). *Am. J. Physiol.* **210**, 162.
Cort, J. H., Lichardus, B., Pliska, V., Uhrin, V., Barth, T., and Rudinger, J. (1968a). *In* "Protein and Polypeptide Hormones" (M. Margoulies, ed.), pp. 523–525. Excerpta Med. Found., Amsterdam.
Cort, J. H., Dousa, T., Pliska, V., Lichardus, B., Safárová, J., Vranesić, M., and Rudinger, J. (1968b). *Am. J. Physiol.* **215**, 921.
Coulson, P., and Gorski, J. (1967). *Endocrinology* **80**, 357.
Crabbé, J. (1968). *In* "Protein and Polypeptide Hormones" (M. Margoulies, ed.), pp. 260–263. Excerpta Med. Found., Amsterdam.
Crofford, O. B., and Renold, A. E. (1965a). *J. Biol. Chem.* **240**, 14.
Crofford, O. B., and Renold, A. E. (1965b). *J. Biol. Chem.* **240**, 3237.
Curran, P. F., Herrera, F. C., and Flanigan, W. J. (1963). *J. Gen. Physiol.* **46**, 1011.
Daniels, J. R., and Kalman, S. M. (1963). *J. Endocrinol.* **28**, 73.
Davis, J. O., Urquhart, J., Higgins, J. T., Jr., Johnston, C. I., and Brown, T. C. (1966). *Endocrinology* **78**, 316.
Dawson, K. G., and Beck, J. C. (1968). *Proc. Soc. Exptl. Biol. Med.* **127**, 617.
Dawson, K. G., Patey, P., Rubinstein, D., and Beck, J. C. (1966). *Mol. Pharmacol.* **2**, 269.
de Bodo, R. C., and Altszuler, N. (1957). *Vitamins Hormones* **15**, 205.
Debons, A. F., and Pittman, J. A. (1962). *Endocrinology* **70**, 937.
Debons, A. F., and Pittman, J. A. (1966). *Am. J. Physiol.* **210**, 395.

de Nicola, A. F., Clayman, M., and Johnstone, R. M. (1968). *Endocrinology* **82**, 436.

Dickson, J. A. (1966). *Endocrinology* **79**, 721.

Dirks, J. H., Cirksena, W. J., and Berliner, R. W. (1965). *J. Clin. Invest.* **44**, 1160.

Dixit, P. K., Morgan, C. R., Lowe, I. P., and Lazarow, A. (1963). *Metab., Clin. Exptl.* **12**, 642.

Dos Reis, L., Rosenbusch, J., and Nichols, G., Jr. (1968). *Biochim. Biophys. Acta* **150**, 311.

Dougherty, T. F., Berliner, M. L., Schneebeli, G. L., and Berliner, D. L. (1964). *Ann. N. Y. Acad. Sci.* **113**, 825.

Dowd, J. E., and Riggs, D. S. (1965). *J. Biol. Chem.* **240**, 863.

Dubois, R. S., and Roy, C. C. (1968). *Gastroenterology* **54**, 1292.

Dumont, J. E., Rodesch, F. R., and Rocmans, P. (1964). *Biochem. Pharmacol.* **13**, 935.

Eboué-Bonis, D., Chambout, A. M., Volfin, P., and Clauser, H. (1963). *Nature* **199**, 1183.

Edelman, P. M., Edelman, J. C., and Schwartz, I. L. (1966). *Nature* **210**, 1017.

Elliott, A. B. (1967). *Experientia* **23**, 220.

Elsas, L. J., and Rosenberg, L. E. (1967). *Proc. Natl. Acad. Sci. U. S.* **57**, 371.

Elsas, L. J., Albrecht, I., Koehne, W., and Rosenberg, L. E. (1967). *Nature* **214**, 916.

Elsas, L. J., Albrecht, I., and Rosenberg, L. E. (1968). *J. Biol. Chem.* **243**, 1846.

Farnsworth, W. E. (1968). *Biochim. Biophys. Acta* **150**, 446.

Feng, H. W., Pan, M. W., and Riggs, T. R. (1967). *Federation Proc.* **26**, 535.

Field, J. B., Pastan, I., Johnson, P., and Herring, B. (1960). *J. Biol. Chem.* **235**, 1863.

Finerman, G. A. M., and Rosenberg, L. E. (1966). *J. Biol. Chem.* **241**, 1487.

Fisher, R. B., and Zachariah, P. (1961). *J. Physiol. (London)* **158**, 73.

Fleischmann, W., and Fleischmann, S. K. (1952–1953). *J. Mt. Sinai. Hosp., N. Y.* **19**, 228.

Foa, P. P., Melli, M., Berger, C. K., Billinger, D., and Guidotti, G. G. (1965). *Federation Proc.* **24**, 1046.

Fong, C. T. O., Silver, L., Christman, D. R., and Schwartz, I. L. (1960). *Proc. Natl. Acad. Sci. U. S.* **46**, 1273.

Freinkel, N. (1960). *Endocrinology* **66**, 851.

Fritz, G. R., and Knobil, E. (1963). *Nature* **200**, 682.

Fujita, T., Orimo, H., and Yoshikawa, M. (1966). *Endocrinology* **78**, 1082.

Gaunt, R., Renzi, A. A., Gisoldi, E., and Howie, N. C. (1967). *Endocrinology* **81**, 1331.

Gilman, A. G., and Rall, T. W. (1968a). *J. Biol. Chem.* **243**, 5867.

Gilman, A. G., and Rall, T. W. (1968b). *J. Biol. Chem.* **243**, 5872.

Gonzales, C., Sanchez, J., and Concha, J. (1967). *Biochim. Biophys. Acta* **135**, 167.

Goodman, H. M. (1963). *Endocrinology* **72**, 95.

Goodman, H. M. (1965a). *Endocrinology* **76**, 216.

Goodman, H. M. (1965b). *Endocrinology* **76**, 1134.

Goodman, H. M. (1966). *Endocrinology* **78**, 819.

Goodman, H. M. (1967a). *Endocrinology* **80**, 45.

Goodman, H. M. (1967b). *Endocrinology* **81**, 1099.

Goodman, H. M. (1968). *Ann. N. Y. Acad. Sci.* **148**, 419.

Gorski, J., and Axman, S. M. E. (1964). *Arch. Biochem. Biophys.* **104**, 517.

Gorski, J., and Morgan, M. S. (1967). *Biochim. Biophys. Acta* **149**, 282.
Grantham, J. J., and Burg, M. B. (1966). *Am. J. Physiol.* **211**, 255.
Greenman, D. L., Wicks, W. D., and Kenney, F. T. (1965). *J. Biol. Chem.* **240**, 4420.
Gregor, W. H., Martin, J. M., Williamson, J. R., Lacy, P. E., and Kipnis, D. M. (1963). *Diabetes* **12**, 73.
Guidotti, G. G., Loreti, L., Gaja, G., and Foa, P. P. (1966). *Am. J. Physiol.* **211**, 981.
Haas, H. G., and Trautwein, W. (1963). *Nature* **197**, 80.
Halkerston, I. D. K., Eichhorn, J., and Hechter, O. (1961). *J. Biol. Chem.* **236**, 374.
Halliday, G. J., Howard, R. B., and Munro, A. F. (1962). *J. Physiol. (London)* **164**, 28P.
Halmi, N. S., and Spirtos, B. N. (1955). *Endocrinology* **56**, 157.
Halmi, N. S., Granner, D. K., Doughman, D. J., Peters, B. H., and Muller, G. (1960). *Endocrinology* **67**, 70.
Halmi, N. S., Westra, J. P., and Polly, R. E. (1966). *Endocrinology* **79**, 424.
Halmi, N. S., Gifford, T. H., and Glesne, R. E. (1967). *Endocrinology* **81**, 893.
Hamberger, L. A., and Ahrén, K. E. B. (1967). *Endocrinology* **81**, 93.
Handler, J. S., and Orloff, J. (1963). *Am. J. Physiol.* **205**, 298.
Handler, J. S., Butcher, R. W., Sutherland, E. W., and Orloff, J. (1965). *J. Biol. Chem.* **240**, 4524.
Handler, J. S., Peterson, M., and Orloff, J. (1966). *Am. J. Physiol.* **211**, 1175.
Handler, J. S., Preston, A. S., and Rogulski, J. (1968). *J. Biol. Chem.* **243**, 1376.
Hays, R. M., and Leaf, A. (1962). *J. Gen. Physiol.* **45**, 905.
Hechter, O., and Lester, G. (1960). *Recent Progr. Hormone Res.* **16**, 139.
Heindel, J. J., and Riggs, T. R. (1968). *Federation Proc.* **27**, 553.
Heindel, J. J., and Riggs, T. R. (1969). Unpublished results.
Henderson, M. J., Morgan, H. E., and Park, C. R. (1961). *J. Biol. Chem.* **236**, 2157.
Herrera, F. C., and Curran, P. F. (1963). *J. Gen. Physiol.* **46**, 999.
Hirshfield, I. N., and Koritz, S. B. (1964). *Biochemistry* **3**, 1994.
Hjalmarson, A., and Ahren, K. (1965). *Life Sci.* **4**, 863.
Hjalmarson, A., and Ahren, K. (1967a). *Life Sci.* **6**, 809.
Hjalmarson, A., and Ahren, K. (1967b). *Acta Endocrinol.* **54**, 645.
Ho, R. J., and Jeanrenaud, B. (1967). *Biochim. Biophys. Acta* **144**, 61.
Hong, S. K., Park, C. S., Park, Y. S., and Kim, J. K. (1968). *Am. J. Physiol.* **215**, 439.
Huber, A. M., and Gershoff, S. N. (1965). *J. Nutr.* **87**, 407.
Isaacs, G. H., and Rosenberg, I. N. (1967). *Endocrinology* **81**, 981.
Jard, S., Bourguet, J., Carasso, N., and Favard, P. (1966). *J. Microscopie* **5**, 31.
Jard, S., Bastide, F., and Morel, F. (1968). *Biochim. Biophys. Acta* **150**, 124.
Jefferson, L. S., Exton, J. H., Butcher, R. W., Sutherland, E. W., and Park, C. R. (1968). *J. Biol. Chem.* **243**, 1031.
Jenkinson, D. H., and Morton, I. K. M. (1967). *J. Physiol. (London)* **188**, 373.
Jorgensen, P. L. (1968). *Biochim. Biophys. Acta* **151**, 212.
Kaplan, S. A., and Nagareda, C. S. (1961). *Am. J. Physiol.* **200**, 1035.
Kattwinkel, J., and Munck, A. (1966). *Endocrinology* **79**, 387.
Katzen, H. M. (1966). *Biochem. Biophys. Res. Commun.* **24**, 531.
Katzen, H. M. (1967). *Advan. Enzyme Regulation* **5**, 335.

Kestens, P. J., Haxhe, J. J., Lambotte, L., and Lambotte, C. (1963). *Metab., Clin. Exptl.* **12**, 941.

Kipnis, D. M., and Noall, M. W. (1958). *Biochim. Biophys. Acta* **28**, 226.

Kipnis, D. M., and Parrish, J. E. (1965). *Federation Proc.* **24**, 1051.

Kleinzeller, A., and Kotyk, A. (1961). *Biochim. Biophys. Acta* **54**, 367.

Klienman, L. I., Loewenstein, M. S., and Goldstein, L. (1966). *Endocrinology* **78**, 403.

Knobil, E. (1966). *Physiologist* **9**, 25.

Koefoed-Johnsen, V., and Ussing, H. H. (1953). *Acta Physiol. Scand.* **28**, 60.

Kogl, F., and van Deenen, L. L. M. (1961). *Acta Endocrinol.* **39**, 9.

Koritz, S. B. (1968a). In "Protein and Polypeptide Hormones" (M. Margoulies, ed.), pp. 171–175. Excerpta Med. Found., Amsterdam.

Koritz, S. B. (1968b). In "Function of the Adrenal Cortex" (K. W. McKerns, ed.), Vol. I., p. 27. Appleton, New York.

Kostyo, J. L. (1964). *Endocrinology* **75**, 113.

Kostyo, J. L. (1968). *Ann. N. Y. Acad. Sci.* **148**, 389.

Kostyo, J. L., and Redmond, A. F. (1966). *Endocrinology* **79**, 531.

Kostyo, J. L., and Schmidt, J. E. (1962). *Endocrinology* **71**, 513.

Kostyo, J. L., and Schmidt, J. E. (1963). *Am. J. Physiol.* **204**, 1031.

Kramar, J., Grinnel, E. H., and Duff, W. M. (1966). *Am. J. Med. Sci.* **252**, 53.

Kuo, J. F. (1968). *J. Biol. Chem.* **243**, 211.

Kuo, J. F., Dill, I. K., and Holmlund, C. E. (1967). *Biochim. Biophys. Acta* **144**, 252.

Larsen, P. R., and Wolff, J. (1967). *Science* **155**, 335.

Leaf, A. (1960). *J. Gen. Physiol.* **43**, Suppl., 175.

Leaf, A. (1961). In "Membrane Transport and Metabolism" (A. Kleinzeller and A. Kotyk, eds.), pp. 247–55. Academic Press, New York.

Leaf, A. (1964). In "The Biochemical Aspects of Hormone Action" (A. B. Eisenstein, ed.), pp. 95–124. Little, Brown, Boston, Massachusetts.

Leaf, A. (1965). *Ergeb. Physiol. Biol. Chem. Exptl. Pharmakol.* **56**, 216.

Leaf, A. (1967). *Am. J. Med.* **42**, 745.

Leaf, A., and Dempsey, E. (1960). *J. Biol. Chem.* **235**, 2160.

Leaf, A., and Hays, R. M. (1962). *J. Gen. Physiol.* **45**, 921.

Leaf, A., and Renshaw, A. (1957a). *Biochem. J.* **65**, 82.

Leaf, A., and Renshaw, A. (1957b). *Biochem. J.* **65**, 90.

Leaf, A., Anderson, J., and Page, L. B. (1958). *J. Gen. Physiol.* **41**, 657.

Leaf, A., Page, L. B., and Anderson, J. (1959). *J. Biol. Chem.* **234**, 1625.

Leboeuf, B., Finn, R. B., and Cahill, G. F. (1959). *Proc. Soc. Exptl. Biol. Med.* **102**, 527.

Letarte, J., and Renold, A. E. (1967). *Nature* **215**, 961.

Levin, R. J., and Smyth, D. H. (1963). *J. Physiol. (London)* **169**, 755.

Levine, R. (1965). *Federation Proc.* **24**, 1071.

Levine, R., Goldstein, M., Huddlestun, B., and Klein, S. (1949). *J. Biol. Chem.* **179**, 985.

Lichardus, B., and Pearce, J. W. (1966). *Nature* **209**, 407.

Lichtenstein, N. S., and Leaf, A. (1965). *J. Clin. Invest.* **44**, 1328.

Lichtenstein, N. S., and Leaf, A. (1966). *Ann. N. Y. Acad. Sci.* **137**, 556.

Llaurado, J. G., and Brito, A. (1967). *Endocrinology* **80**, 375.

London, D. R., and Segal, S. (1967). *Endocrinology* **80**, 623.

Lowenstein, L. M., Smith, I., and Segal, S. (1968). *Biochim. Biophys. Acta* **150**, 73.

Macchia, V., and Pastan, I. (1967). *J. Biol. Chem.* **242**, 1864.

McLean, P., Brown, J., Greenslade, K. R., and Brew, K. (1966). *Biochem. Biophys. Res. Commun.* **23**, 117.

MacRobbie, E. A. C., and Ussing, H. H. (1961). *Acta Physiol. Scand.* **53**, 348.

Manchester, K. L. (1967). *Nature* **216**, 394.

Manchester, K. L. (1968a). In "Protein and Polypeptide Hormones" (M. Margoulies, ed.), pp. 296–299. Excerpta Med. Found., Amsterdam.

Manchester, K. L. (1968b). Personal communication.

Manchester, K. L., and Young, F. G. (1959). *J. Endocrinol.* **18**, 381.

Manchester, K. L., and Young, F. G. (1960a). *Biochem. J.* **75**, 487.

Manchester, K. L., and Young, F. G. (1960b). *Biochem. J.* **77**, 386.

Manchester, K. L., and Young, F. G. (1961). *Vitamins Hormones* **19**, 95.

Manchester, K. L., Randle, P. J., and Young, F. G. (1959). *J. Endocrinol.* **18**, 395.

Manitius, A., Bensch, K., and Epstein, F. H. (1968). *Biochim. Biophys. Acta* **150**, 563.

Mankin, H. J., and Conger, K. A. (1966). *Lab. Invest.* **15**, 794.

Martonosi, A. (1968). *Arch. Biochem. Biophys.* **125**, 295.

Matty, A. J., and Seshardi, B. (1965). *Gut* **6**, 200.

Metcalf, W., and Gross, E. (1960). *Science* **132**, 41.

Mezey, A. P., Foley, H. T., and Altszuler, N. (1961). *Proc. Soc. Exptl. Biol. Med.* **107**, 689.

Mills, T. M., and Spaziani, E. (1968). *Biochim. Biophys. Acta* **150**, 435.

Milner, R. D. G., and Hales, C. N. (1967). *Biochim. Biophys. Acta* **135**, 375.

Milner, R. D. G., and Hales, C. N. (1968). *Biochim. Biophys. Acta* **150**, 165.

Mohri, T. (1967). *Endocrinology* **81**, 454.

Moore, R. O., Chandler, A. M., and Tettenhorst, N. (1964). *Biochem. Biophys. Res. Commun.* **17**, 527.

Morel, F., and Bastide, F. (1965). *Biochim. Biophys. Acta* **94**, 609.

Morel, F., Jard, S., Bourguet, J., and Bastide, F. (1968). In "Protein and Polypeptide Hormones" (M. Margoulies, ed.), pp. 219–221. Excerpta Med. Found., Amsterdam.

Morgan, H. E., Henderson, M. J., Regen, D. M., and Park, C. R. (1961a). *J. Biol. Chem.* **236**, 253.

Morgan, H. E., Cadenas, E., Regen, D. M., and Park, C. R. (1961b). *J. Biol. Chem.* **236**, 262.

Morgan, H. E., Regan, D. M., and Park, C. R. (1964). *J. Biol. Chem.* **239**, 369.

Morgan, H. E., Neely, J. R., Wood, R. E., Liebecq, C., Liebermeister, H., and Park, C. R. (1965). *Federation Proc.* **24**, 1040.

Morita, Y., and Munck, A. (1964). *Biochim. Biophys. Acta* **93**, 150.

Mueller, G. C., Gorski, J., and Aizawa, Y. (1961). *Proc. Natl. Acad. Sci. U. S.* **47**, 164.

Munck, A. (1965). *Endocrinology* **77**, 356.

Munck, A. (1968). *J. Biol. Chem.* **243**, 1039.

Munck, A., and Brinck-Johnsen, T. (1968). *J. Biol. Chem.* **243**, 5556.

Narahara, H. T., and Ozand, P. (1963). *J. Biol. Chem.* **238**, 40.

Niccolini, R., and Mack, R. E. (1965). *Clin. Res.* **13**, 407.

Nicolette, J. A., and Gorski, J. (1964). *Arch. Biochem. Biophys.* **107**, 279.

Nicolette, J. A., and Mueller, G. C. (1966). *Endocrinology* **79**, 1162.

Noall, M. W., and Allen, W. M. (1961). *J. Biol. Chem.* **236**, 2987.

Noall, M. W., Riggs, T. R., Walker, L. M., and Christensen, H. N. (1957). *Science* **126**, 1002.

Notides, A., and Gorski, J. (1966). *Proc. Natl. Acad. Sci. U. S.* **56**, 230.

Nusynowitz, M. L. (1967). *Endocrinology* **80**, 788.

Orloff, J., and Handler, J. S. (1962). *J. Clin. Invest.* **41**, 702.

Oxender, D. L., and Christensen, H. N. (1963). *J. Biol. Chem.* **238**, 3686.

Pardee, A. B. (1966). *J. Biol. Chem.* **241**, 5886.

Pardee, A. B. (1967). *Science* **156**, 1627.

Park, C. R., Brown, D. H., Cornblath, M., Daughaday, W. H., and Krahl, M. E. (1952). *J. Biol. Chem.* **197**, 151.

Park, C. R., Reinwein, D., Henderson, M. J., Cadenas, E., and Morgan, H. E. (1959). *Am. J. Med.* **26**, 684.

Pastan, I. (1966). *Biochem. Biophys. Res. Commun.* **25**, 14.

Pastan, I., and Macchia, V. (1967). *J. Biol. Chem.* **242**, 5757.

Pastan, I., Roth, J., and Macchia, V. (1966). *Proc. Natl. Acad. Sci. U. S.* **56**, 1802.

Peachey, L. D., and Rasmussen, H. (1961). *J. Biophys. Biochem. Cytol.* **10**, 529.

Pena, A., Dvorkin, B., and White, A. (1966). *J. Biol. Chem.* **241**, 2144.

Penrose, W. R., Nichoalds, G. E., Piperno, J. R., and Oxender, D. L. (1968). *J. Biol. Chem.* **243**, 5921.

Pickering, B. T. (1968). *In* "Protein and Polypeptide Hormones" (M. Margoulies, ed.), pp. 214–216. Excerpta Med. Found., Amsterdam.

Piperno, J. R., and Oxender, D. L. (1966). *J. Biol. Chem.* **241**, 5732.

Planelles, J., Ozeretskovsky, N., and Djeksenbaev, O. (1962). *Nature* **195**, 713.

Pliska, V., Rudinger, J., Dousa, T., and Cort, J. H. (1968). *Am. J. Physiol.* **215**, 916.

Poffenbarger, P. L., Powell, R. C., and Deiss, W., Jr. (1963). *J. Clin. Invest.* **42**, 239.

Post, R. L., Morgan, H. E., and Park, C. R. (1961). *J. Biol. Chem.* **236**, 269.

Potchen, E. J., and Watts, H. G. (1967). *Endocrinology* **80**, 467.

Raghupathy, E., Abraham, S., Kerkof, P. R., and Chaikoff, I. L. (1964). *Endocrinology* **74**, 468.

Randle, P. J., and Smith, G. H. (1958a). *Biochem. J.* **70**, 490.

Randle, P. J., and Smith, G. H. (1958b). *Biochem. J.* **70**, 501.

Rasmussen, H. (1965). *In* "Mechanisms of Hormone Action" (P. Karlson, ed.), p. 125. Thieme, Stuttgart.

Rasmussen, H. (1968). *In* "Protein and Polypeptide Hormones" (M. Margoulies, ed.), pp. 247–256. Excerpta Med. Found., Amsterdam.

Rasmussen, H., and Schwartz, I. L. (1964). *Proc. 2nd Intern. Pharmacol. Meeting, Prague, 1963* Vol. 10, p. 41. Pergamon Press, Oxford.

Rasmussen, H., Schwartz, I. L., Schoessler, M. A., and Hochster, G. (1960). *Proc. Natl. Acad. Sci. U. S.* **46**, 1278.

Rasmussen, H., Schwartz, I. L., Young, R., and Marc-Aurele, J. (1963). *J. Gen. Physiol.* **46**, 1171.

Regen, D. M., and Morgan, H. E. (1964). *Biochim. Biophys. Acta* **79**, 151.

Ricklis, E., and Quastel, J. H. (1958). *Can. J. Biochem.* **36**, 347.

Riddick, F. A., Jr., Reisler, D. M., and Kipnis, D. M. (1962). *Diabetes* **11**, 171.

Rieser, P. (1966). *Am. J. Med.* **40**, 759.

Rieser, P., and Rieser, C. H. (1964). *Proc. Soc. Exptl. Biol. Med.* **116**, 669.

Riggs, T. R., and Walker, L. M. (1963). *Endocrinology* **73**, 781.

Riggs, T. R., and Wegrzyn, S. W. (1966). *Endocrinology* **78**, 137.

Riggs, T. R., Sanders, R. B., and Weindling, H. K. (1963). *Endocrinology* **73**, 789.

Riggs, T. R., Pan, M. W., and Feng, H. W. (1968). *Biochim. Biophys. Acta* **150**, 92.

Robb, C. A., Davis, J. O. Johnston, C. I., and Hartroft, P. M. (1968). *Endocrinology* **82**, 1200.

Rodbell, M. (1966). *J. Biol. Chem.* **241**, 130.

Rosenbusch, J. P., and Nichols, G., Jr. (1967). *Endocrinology* **81**, 553.

Roskoski, R., Jr., and Steiner, D. F. (1967a). *Biochim. Biophys. Acta* **135**, 347.

Roskoski, R., Jr., and Steiner, D. F. (1967b). *Biochim. Biophys. Acta* **135**, 717.

Roskoski, R., Jr., and Steiner, D. F. (1967c). *Biochim. Biophys. Acta* **135**, 727.

Rudinger, J., Krejci, I., Polacek, I., and Kupkova, B. (1968). *In* "Protein and Polypeptide Hormones" (M. Margoulies, ed.), pp. 217–218. Excerpta Med. Found., Amsterdam.

Saha, J., Lopez-Mondragon, R., and Narahara, H. T. (1968). *J. Biol. Chem.* **243**, 521.

Sanders, R. B., and Riggs, T. R. (1967a). *Endocrinology* **80**, 29.

Sanders, R. B., and Riggs, T. R. (1967b). *Mol. Pharmacol.* **3**, 352.

Scharff, R., and Wool, I. G. (1965). *Biochem. J.* **97**, 272.

Scharff, R., and Wool, I. G. (1966). *Biochem. J.* **99**, 173.

Schneider, A. B., and Goldberg, I. H. (1965). *Federation Proc.* **24**, 383.

Schneider, P., and Wolff, J. (1964). *Biochim. Biophys. Acta* **94**, 114.

Schwartz, I. L. (1965). *In* "Mechanisms of Hormone Action" (P. Karlson, ed.), pp. 121–122. Thieme, Stuttgart.

Schwartz, I. L., and Walter, R. (1968). *In* "Protein and Polypeptide Hormones" (M. Margoulies, ed.), pp. 264–269. Excerpta Med. Found., Amsterdam.

Schwartz, I. L., Rasmussen, H., Schoessler, M. A., Silver, L., and Fong, C. T. O. (1960). *Proc. Natl. Acad. Sci. U. S.* **46**, 1288.

Schwartz, I. L., Rasmussen, H., Livingston, L. M., and Marc-Aurele, J. (1964a). *Proc. 2nd Intern. Pharmacol. Meeting, Prague, 1963* Vol. 10, p. 125. Pergamon Press, Oxford.

Schwartz, I. L., Rasmussen, H., and Rudinger, J. (1964b). *Proc. Natl. Acad. Sci. U. S.* **52**, 1044.

Scranton, J. R., and Halmi, N. S. (1965). *Endocrinology* **76**, 441.

Segal, S., Roth, H., Blair, A., and Bertoli, D. (1966). *Endocrinology* **79**, 675.

Sessa, G., and Weissmann, G. (1968). *Biochim. Biophys. Acta* **150**, 173.

Smith, D. E. (1967). *Proc. Soc. Exptl. Biol. Med.* **124**, 747.

Smith, D. E., and Gorski, J. (1968). *J. Biol. Chem.* **243**, 4169.

Smith, O. K., and Long, C. N. H. (1967). *Endocrinology* **80**, 561.

Snart, R. S., Sanyal, N. N., and Dalton, T. (1968). *In* "Protein and Polypeptide Hormones" (M. Margoulies, ed.), pp. 519–522. Excerpta Med. Found., Amsterdam.

Snipes, C. A. (1967). *Am. J. Physiol.* **212**, 279.

Snipes, C. A., and Kostyo, J. L. (1962). *Am. J. Physiol.* **203**, 933.

Spaziani, E., and Gutman, A. (1965). *Endocrinology* **76**, 470.

Spaziani, E., and Suddick, R. P. (1967). *Endocrinology* **81**, 205.

Spaziani, E., and Szego, C. M. (1959). *Am. J. Physiol.* **197**, 355.

Stein, W. D. (1967). "The Movement of Molecules across Cell Membranes," pp. 253–265. Academic Press, New York.

Surks, M. I. (1967). *Endocrinology* **80**, 1020.

Sutherland, E. W., III, and Haynes, R. C., Jr. (1967). *Endocrinology* **80**, 288.

Szego, C. M., and Roberts, S. (1953). *Recent Progr. Hormone Res.* **8**, 419.

Tarui, S., Nonaka, K., Ikura, Y., and Shima, K. (1963). *Biochem. Biophys. Res. Commun.* **13**, 329.

Taurog, A., and Thio, D. T. (1966). *Endocrinology* **78**, 103.
Thier, S. O. (1968). *Biochim. Biophys. Acta* **150**, 253.
Thorn, N. A. (1961). *Acta Endocrinol.* **38**, 563.
Tong, W. (1964). *Endocrinology* **75**, 527.
Tong, W. (1967). *Endocrinology* **80**, 1101.
Tonoue, T., and Yamamoto, K. (1967). *Endocrinology* **81**, 101.
Turkington, R. W. (1962). *Biochim. Biophys. Acta* **65**, 386.
Ungar, G., and Psychoyos, S. (1963). *Biochim. Biophys. Acta* **66**, 118.
Vaughan, M. (1961). *J. Biol. Chem.* **236**, 2196.
Vilkki, P. (1962). *Arch. Biochem. Biophys.* **97**, 231.
Walaas, O., and Walaas, E. (1950). *J. Biol. Chem.* **187**, 769.
Walter, R., Rudinger, J., and Schwartz, I. L. (1967). *Am. J. Med.* **42**, 653.
Walters, E., and McLean, P. (1967). *Biochem. J.* **104**, 778.
Walters, E., and McLean, P. (1968). *Biochem. J.* **109**, 737.
Weissmann, G., and Sessa, G. (1967). *J. Biol. Chem.* **242**, 616.
Weissmann, G., Sessa, G., and Weissmann, S. (1966). *Biochem. Pharmacol.* **15**, 1537.
Wheeler, K. P., and Christensen, H. N. (1967). *J. Biol. Chem.* **242**, 3782.
Whittembury, G., Sugino, N., and Solomon, A. K. (1960). *Nature* **187**, 699.
Wick, A. N., Drury, D. R., Nakada, H. I., Barnet, H. N., and Morita, T. N. (1955). *J. Biol. Chem.* **213**, 907.
Wicks, W. D., Greenman, D. L., and Kenney, F. T. (1965). *J. Biol. Chem.* **240**, 4414.
Wilbrandt, W., and Rosenberg, T. (1961). *Pharmacol. Rev.* **13**, 109.
Williamson, J. R. (1964). *J. Biol. Chem.* **239**, 2721.
Wolff, J., and Halmi, N. S. (1963). *J. Biol. Chem.* **238**, 847.
Wolff, J., and Maurey, J. R. (1961). *Biochim. Biophys. Acta* **47**, 467.
Wolff, J., and Rall, J. E. (1965). *Endocrinology* **76**, 949.
Wollman, S. H., and Reed, F. E. (1959). *Am. J. Physiol.* **196**, 113.
Wool, I. G. (1960). *Am. J. Physiol.* **199**, 715.
Wool, I. G. (1964). *Nature* **202**, 196.
Wool, I. G. (1965). *Federation Proc.* **24**, 1060.
Wool, I. G., and Moyer, A. N. (1964). *Biochim. Biophys. Acta* **91**, 248.
Wool, I. G., and Weinshelbaum, E. I. (1959). *Am. J. Physiol.* **197**, 1089.
Wool, I. G., Castles, J. J., and Moyer, A. N. (1965). *Biochim. Biophys. Acta* **107**, 333.
Yamada, T., Takemura, Y., Kobayashi, I., and Schichijo, K. (1966). *Endocrinology* **79**, 849.
Zadunaisky, J. A., Gennara, J. F., Bashirelahi, N., and Hilton, M. (1968). *J. Gen. Physiol.* **51**, 290s.
Zierler, K. L. (1959). *Am. J. Physiol.* **197**, 524.

CHAPTER 6

Binding
of Hormones
to Serum Proteins

Ulrich Westphal

I. GENERAL CHARACTERISTICS OF HORMONE–PROTEIN COMPLEXES

A few years after the isolation of the estrogenic hormones, it was discovered (Brunelli, 1934) that these steroid hormones associated spontaneously with serum proteins to form reversible complexes, predominantly with the globulin fraction. Many years passed before the binding of steroid hormones to serum proteins was studied systematically

(Bischoff and Pilhorn, 1948; Eik-Nes *et al.*, 1954; Schellman *et al.*, 1954) and recognized as a general phenomenon. Interactions of serum proteins with steroids and other hormones have been the object of intensive investigation in recent years. A number of pure proteins are known today which have the ability of associating more or less specifically with the natural hormones in the circulating blood. The influence of various factors on the plasma concentration of several hormone-binding proteins has been established, and we begin to understand some of the biological implications of the formation of the dissociable complexes.

Most of the studies in this field have been concerned with the interaction of the binding proteins with "small" molecules, i.e., with hormones of molecular weights below 1000. Such compounds dialyze through the usual dialysis membranes, and may also be separated from the macromolecules by ultrafiltration. They enter the "pores" of certain gels such as Sephadex, and therefore pass more slowly over a gel filtration column than the larger proteins. Examples for hormones of this size are the steroid hormones (e.g., progesterone, molecular weight 314) and the thyroid hormones (e.g., thyroxine, molecular weight 777). Interactions of serum proteins with these two groups of endocrines will be discussed in the present chapter.

Protein binding of hormones of larger molecular size, such as protein hormones, has not been elucidated to any great extent. Fractionation of insulin-containing serum by cold ethanol precipitation methods yielded β-globulin fractions that were associated with insulin (Beigelman *et al.*, 1956); it is not known whether this protein–protein interaction observed after the rather harsh precipitation procedures truly reflects binding occurring in the native serum. Association of insulin with β- and γ-globulins, and to some extent with albumin and α_1-globulin, has also been observed by electrophoretic techniques (Randle and Taylor, 1958). Taylor (1967) has recently reviewed the subject of insulin interaction with serum proteins. No differences have been found in the biological effects of "bound" and crystalline insulin (Antoniades and Gershoff, 1966; Gershoff *et al.*, 1966). Studies with ^{125}I-labeled insulin showed association with an α_1-globulin (Gjedde, 1967a,b).

Evidence for binding to serum proteins has been obtained for other protein hormones. Radioimmunoelectrophoresis studies (Hadden and Prout, 1964) showed that human growth hormone associates with an α_2-macroglobulin present in normal human serum; no other serum factors are involved in the interaction. Tritiated ACTH (β^{1-23} corticotropin) was found to interact with serum albumin (von Werder *et al.*, 1968a,b); the complex formation results in reduction of the steroidogenic activity (Stouffer and Hsu, 1966). Sephadex gel filtration experiments led to the conclusion (Smith and Thorn, 1965) that vasopressin forms serum protein complexes that are dissociated by calcium ions. The binding appears to be weak (Brook and Share, 1966).

A common characteristic of the hormone–protein interactions, for which the terms binding, association, attachment, complex formation, ligand-macromolecule interaction, and others have been used, is the relatively low energy of binding between the two components. Whereas the usual covalent bonds between C, H, O, or N atoms are of the order of approximately 80–110 kcal/mole, the hormones and proteins in the complexes to be discussed are held together by noncovalent bonds of 10–20 times lower energies. As a consequence, the complexes dissociate readily, especially at the temperature of the warm-blooded animal. The dissociable nature of the association products is the basis of their biological significance: since the hormonal activity is suppressed in the hormone–protein complexes as found in all cases investigated so far, the complex formation provides a mechanism to store relatively large quantities of the hormones in the circulating blood in an inactive form. Whenever active hormone is required at a target site, where the uptake by the receptors may cause a local depletion of unbound hormone, the protein complexes will dissociate spontaneously and make more of the unbound, physiologically active form available.

Another consequence of the association between protein and hormone ligand is the protection of labile hormone molecules from chemical attack by environmental factors. For example, cortisol undergoes spontaneous decomposition in aqueous solution (Kripalani and Sorby, 1967), especially when radiolabeled (Westphal et al., 1967). Addition of serum proteins to the buffer provides some protection against the chemical alterations (Hoffmann and Westphal, 1969). Conversely, sensitive proteins are protected by the interaction with steroids. This was demonstrated in studies on heat inactivation of the corticosteroid-binding globulin (Doe et al., 1964), which showed that rising amounts of cortisol stabilize this serum protein increasingly against the destructive effect of incubation at 60°. The protection of CBG[1] by association with the corticosteroid may not be essential for the glycoprotein while in the serum where it seems to be protected by interaction with other serum proteins (Westphal, 1967). It becomes important, however, for the

---

[1] Abbreviations used: AAG, α_1-acid glycoprotein or orosomucoid; CBG, corticosteroid-binding globulin or transcortin; DEAE, diethylaminoethyl; $\Delta F°$, change of free energy; $\Delta H°$, change of enthalpy; $\Delta S°$, change of entropy; HSA, human serum albumin; k, association constant; n, number of binding sites; T_3, 3,5,3'-triiodothyronine; T_4, thyroxine or 3,5,3',5'-tetraiodothyronine; TBG, thyroxine-binding globulin; TBPA, thyroxine-binding prealbumin; TSH, thyroid-stimulating hormone.

purified CBG which is a very labile protein after removal of the bound
steroid (Chader and Westphal, 1968b).

II. THYROID HORMONE-BINDING PROTEINS

The protein interactions of the thyroid hormones will be discussed
only briefly, since excellent reviews of the subject are available (Robbins
and Rall, 1957, 1960, 1967; Ingbar and Freinkel, 1960; Sterling, 1964a;
Andreoli *et al.*, 1965; Oppenheimer and Bernstein, 1965; Salvatore *et al.*,
1966) to which the present author cannot contribute from his own experience. Three distinct serum proteins have been recognized to bind
thyroxine (T_4) and other thyroid hormones in a more or less specific
manner: (1) thyroxine-binding globulin (TBG); (2) thyroxine-binding
prealbumin (TBPA); and (3) serum albumin (HSA in human blood).
Observations in several laboratories indicate the possibility that additional serum protein components are capable of associating with
thyroxine (Thorson *et al.*, 1966; Kumahara *et al.*, 1968). The nature of
these components, including the question of methodological artifacts
(Launay, 1966), remains to be elucidated.

A. THYROXINE-BINDING GLOBULIN (TBG)

1. Physicochemical Properties

Clear evidence for the presence in blood serum of a specific thyroxine-
binding protein was first obtained by Gordon *et al.* (1952), who applied
paper electrophoresis to a serum containing ^{131}I-labeled thyroxine. At
pH 8.6 in barbital buffer, T_4 migrates in a zone intermediate between
α_1- and α_2-globulin; TBG therefore also has been designated as an inter-
alpha globulin. It should be noted that the successful paper-electro-
phoretic demonstration of the T_4–TBG complex is the result of the unusually high binding affinity of this complex, which migrates in zone
electrophoresis without significant dissociation. The analogous complex
between cortisol and CBG is not stable under similar conditions of paper
electrophoresis; it dissociates almost completely during the electrophoresis (Westphal and DeVenuto, 1966), due to an association constant
that is more than 100 times smaller.

Human TBG in serum migrates slowly toward the anode in zone or
moving boundary electrophoresis at pH 4.5; the isoelectric point is close
to pH 4 (Robbins *et al.*, 1955). Determination of the sedimentation rate

TABLE I

PHYSICOCHEMICAL PROPERTIES OF THYROID HORMONE-BINDING PROTEINS[a]

Property	TBG	TBPA	HSA (1)
$s_{20,w}$	3.3 (2)	4.1 (3)	4.6
	3.6 (3)		
	3.9 (4)		
$s^0_{20,w}$	3.9 (5)	4.6 (6)	
Molecular weight $\times 10^{-3}$	40–50 (7)	70 (3)	69
	59 (3)	73 (6)	
	58 (5)		
	53 (4)		
$E^{1\%}_{1\,cm}$ at 280 nm	8.43 (3)	12.2 (3)	5.8
	8.9 (5)	13.6 (6)	
Carbohydrate content, %	32 (3)	0.9 (3)	<0.1
	13.2 (5)		

[a] Numbers in parentheses refer to the following references: (1) Schultze and Heremans, 1966; (2) Robbins *et al.*, 1955; (3) Seal and Doe, 1965a; (4) Marshall and Pensky, 1969; (5) Giorgio and Tabachnick, 1968; (6) Oppenheimer *et al.*, 1965; (7) Tata, 1961.

of TBG in whole human serum gave a value of $s_{20,w}$ of 3.3. A highly purified TBG preparation was found to have a sedimentation coefficient, $s^0_{20,w}$ of 3.9, and a molecular weight of 58,000 (Giorgio and Tabachnick, 1968); the sedimentation rate was concentration dependent (Giorgio and Tabachnick, 1968). Similar values for the sedimentation coefficient and molecular weight were obtained recently (Marshall and Pensky, 1969). These TBG preparations are homogeneous in ultracentrifugation, disc electrophoresis and immunoelectrophoresis. Tata (1961) reported a molecular weight of 40,000 to 50,000 for a purified TBG preparation. Some of the physicochemical properties of TBG are given in Table I.

TBG is an acid glycoprotein with the relatively high carbohydrate content of 32% (Seal and Doe, 1965a). It contains terminal sialic acid residues, and a comparatively large percentage of fucose. The sialic acid residues in the TBG molecule have been found (Blumberg and Warren, 1961) not to be essential for the binding activity. Table II shows the amino acid and carbohydrate composition of TBG, in comparison with those of other thyroid hormone-binding proteins to be discussed.

2. Serum Concentrations and Binding Characteristics

The concentration of TBG in normal human serum was first determined by reverse-flow zone electrophoresis and expressed as thyroxine-binding capacity (Robbins, 1956). A value of 16–25 μg/100 ml was found, cor-

TABLE II

AMINO ACID AND CARBOHYDRATE CONTENT OF
THYROID HORMONE-BINDING PROTEINS

Constituent	TBG mole/mole (1)[c]	TBG mole/mole (2)[c]	TBPA mole/mole (1)[c]	HSA mole/mole (3)[c]
Lysine	12	25	26	56
Histidine	11	10	12	15
Arginine	22	16	12	23
Aspartic acid	25	38	24	52
Threonine	18	25	31	28
Serine	19	34	22	24
Glutamic acid	34	52	36	81
Proline	27	30	24	25
Glycine	25	25	30	12
Alanine	27	31	37	62
Half cystine	5	8	2	33
Valine	12	23	36	41
Methionine	3	5	3	5
Isoleucine	8	9	15	8
Leucine	43	44	22	60
Tyrosine	7	10	15	16
Phenylalanine	14	18	15	30
Tryptophan	4	4	6[a]	1
Hexose	56	24	4	0
Hexosamine	15	15[b]	0	0
Fucose	19	<1	0	0
Sialic acid	9	5	0	0

[a] The tryptophan content of 3.15% reported by Oppenheimer *et al.* (1965) would correspond to about 12 mole/70,000 gm TBPA.

[b] Glucosamine, 12; galactosamine, 3.

[c] References used in table: (1) Seal and Doe, 1965a; (2) Giorgio and Tabachnick, 1968; (3) Schultze and Heremans, 1966.

responding to an average concentration of about $2.5 \times 10^{-7} M$ if one assumes one T_4-binding site per TBG molecule. Similar TBG levels have been observed in other laboratories, as seen in Table III. A steady decline of the TBG concentration was found in the growing human from age 5–6 to adulthood, with somewhat higher values in the female (Goldsmith *et al.*, 1967). In larger samples, the greater TBG concentration in the female sex was statistically significant (Braverman *et al.*, 1967). The TBG capacity increases in pregnancy about 2.5-fold (Robbins and Rall, 1967). Enhancement of TBG capacity can also be produced by administration of estrogens (Robbins and Rall, 1967); a converse influence is obtained with androgens (Braverman and Ingbar, 1967). TBG resembles

TABLE III

BINDING PARAMETERS FOR THYROID HORMONE–PROTEIN INTERACTIONS
IN NORMAL HUMAN SERUM

Parameter	TBG	TBPA	HSA
Concentration, mole/liter	2.5×10^{-7} (1, 2)[k] 3.2×10^{-7} (4) 2.6×10^{-7} (6) 2.7×10^{-7} (8) 4.0×10^{-7a} (8) 2.7×10^{-7b} (9) 3.1×10^{-7c} (9) 5.9×10^{-7d} (2)	2.2×10^{-6} (3) 1.9×10^{-6} (5) 3.5×10^{-6} (7)	5.1×10^{-4} to 6.5×10^{-4}
n_1[e] for T$_4$ n_2 for T$_4$	1 (10, 11) —	1 (3) —	1 (12, 13, 14) 3 or more (12) 5–6 (13, 14)
k_1[f] for T$_4$, liter/mole	$\sim 4 \times 10^{10g}$ (6) $\sim 10^{10}$ (16) 1.7×10^{10} (2)	3.6×10^{8} (15) 2.3×10^{8} (2)	1.6×10^{6h}, 26° (12) 1.6×10^{6}, 6° (13) 1.4×10^{6}, 30° (13) 2.5×10^{6}, 26° (14)
k_2 for T$_4$, liter/mole	—	—	6×10^{4}, 24° (12) 5×10^{4}, 6° (13) 8×10^{4}, 30° (13) 6×10^{4}, 26° (14)
k for T$_3$, liter/mole	2×10^{9} (6)	~ 0 (6)	2.5×10^{5i} (17) 3.8×10^{5j} (12)

[a] Normal subjects, 5–6 years old.

[b] Normal males, 20–30 years old.

[c] Normal females, 20–30 years old.

[d] Pregnant women.

[e] n_1 and n_2, number of primary and secondary binding sites, respectively.

[f] k_1 and k_2, apparent association constants for primary and secondary binding sites, respectively.

[g] pH 8.6, barbital, 26°.

[h] All k_1 and k_2 values for T$_4$-HSA in phosphate buffer, pH 7.4.

[i] nk, in phosphate buffer, pH 7.35.

[j] in phosphate buffer, pH 8.6, 26°.

[k] Numbers in parentheses refer to the following references: (1) Robbins, 1956; (2) Woeber and Ingbar, 1968; (3) Oppenheimer et al., 1965; (4) Ingbar, 1958; (5) Purdy et al., 1965; (6) Robbins and Rall, 1967; (7) Oppenheimer et al., 1966; (8) Goldsmith et al., 1967; (9) Braverman et al., 1967; (10) Seal and Doe, 1965a; (11) Giorgio and Tabachnick, 1968; (12) Steiner et al., 1966; (13) Tabachnick, 1967; (14) Tritsch, 1968; (15) Oppenheimer and Surks, 1964; (16) Sterling et al., 1967; (17) Tritsch and Tritsch, 1965.

CBG in these effects of gonadal hormones on the blood level of the glyco-protein. Increased TBG concentration was also observed in women after administration of the synthetic estrogens, diethylstilbestrol (Doe *et al.*, 1967) and ethinyl estradiol (Musa *et al.*, 1967). Another similarity to CBG may be seen in the decline of the TBG level after the adminis-tration of the modified corticosteroid hormone, prednisone (Oppenheimer and Werner, 1966). Familial decrease and increase of TBG activity have been observed and have been interpreted as X-chromosome linked ab-normalities (Nikolai and Seal, 1966, 1967; Jones and Seal, 1967).

The relatively high apparent association constant of the thyroxine–TBG complex (Table III) explains its stability during electrophoresis. Maximum binding affinity is found at neutral pH; the association becomes markedly weaker in acid, and decreases at high pH values. The number of primary T_4-binding sites has been found to be $n = 1$ (Seal and Doe, 1965a; Giorgio and Tabachnick, 1968). Structural changes in the thyrox-ine molecule result in reduced affinity to TBG; triiodothyronine (T_3) at pH 8.6 has only about one-third the strength of association of T_4. Iodo-tyrosines have been found not to be bound by TBG. The ability of a considerable number of thyroxine analogues to inhibit the binding of radiolabeled thyroxine to TBG and to TBPA has been studied (Ross and Tapley, 1966). The alanine side chain and the amino group were found to be essential components for optimal binding to TBG, but not to TBPA.

The apparent association constant of the T_4–TBG complex, $k = 1.7 \times 10^{10}$ M^{-1}, determined with TBG from normal human serum, has also been found for TBG in pregnancy serum in which the TBG concentration is elevated (Table III) and for TBG in pathological sera with reduced TBG levels (Woeber and Ingbar, 1968). It may be assumed, therefore, that the TBG molecules circulating in the blood under these different conditions are the same. Identity of the molecular species has also been concluded for CBG in the serum of normal subjects and in serum of persons with increased CBG levels due to augmented estrogenic hor-mones (Seal and Doe, 1962a).

B. Thyroxine-Binding Prealbumin (TBPA)

Binding of thyroxine to a prealbumin component of normal plasma or serum was first demonstrated by Ingbar (1958). The protein, TBPA, has been purified and characterized physicochemically (Seal and Doe, 1965a; Oppenheimer *et al.*, 1965), also in a crystalline form (Purdy *et al.*, 1965). Its molecular weight (Table I) is slightly higher than that of HSA. The relatively high extinction coefficient at 280 nm is in accordance with a high tyrosine and tryptophan (Table II) content (Oppen-heimer *et al.*, 1965). The carbohydrate content of TBPA appears minimal (Seal and Doe, 1965a) and no sialic acid has been found (Robbins and Rall, 1967).

The serum concentration of TBPA is approximately 10 times as high as that of TBG (Table III). The protein has one binding site for thyroxine, with an association constant about 100 times smaller than that of the T_4–TBG complex. No affinity has been observed for triiodothyronine (Robbins and Rall, 1967). The TBPA concentration increases in the growing human, reaches a maximal value around age 40, and declines toward older age (Braverman *et al.*, 1966); this change with age thus shows an opposite trend as TBG. Another inverse relationship between TBG and TBPA was observed when the levels of the binding proteins of males and females were compared: the TBG and TBPA values in women were respectively higher and lower than in men, as shown by paper electrophoresis in two buffer systems (Braverman *et al.*, 1967). Reduced levels of TBPA were observed in disease states of various etiology; a pregnancy serum also had a subnormal TBPA concentration (Woeber and Ingbar, 1968).

An assessment of the contribution of TBPA to the binding of T_4 in human serum has been made by immunoadsorption (Woeber and Ingbar, 1968). It was concluded that approximately 15% of endogenous thyroxine in normal human serum is bound to TBPA, whereas 75% and 10% are as-sociated with TBG and HSA, respectively. This binding distribution was obtained by immunoadsorption at pH 7.4 or pH 8.1, whereas electro-phoretic methods in agar gel or on paper show a higher percentage of T_4 bound to TBPA at pH 7.4 and particularly at pH 8.6 (Woeber and Ingbar, 1968). Recent studies on pH dependence of T_4 binding to TBPA in human serum (Lutz and Gregerman, 1969) confirmed maximal as-sociation at pH 8.6; the affinity was found to be much lower at pH 9.0 and at pH 7.8. At a physiological pH of 7.4, the binding is still weaker. Evaluation (Robbins and Rall, 1967) of the binding distribution of T_4 and T_3 among serum proteins by methods based on the concentration of unoccupied binding sites has resulted in proportional binding that shows a general similarity to these data (see Section II,D.).

C. Thyroid Hormone Interactions with Human Serum Albumin (HSA)

Of the three serum proteins involved in binding thyroxine and other thyroid hormones, albumin has by far the lowest affinity. Recent inves-tigations (Steiner *et al.*, 1966; Tabachnick, 1967) are in agreement with the assumption of one primary binding site for thyroxine, in addition to about 3–6 secondary sites of considerably smaller association constants (Table III). The effect of temperature on T_4–HSA interaction is very small (Tabachnick, 1967). The affinity constant of the T_4–HSA complex is pH-dependent (Steiner *et al.*, 1966); the highest value was observed above pH 8. Bovine serum albumin was found to bind T_4 with approximately the same affinity as determined for HSA (Steiner *et al.*, 1966); the numbers of primary and secondary binding sites were assumed to be similar to those in HSA.

HSA interacts also with 3,5,3′-triiodothyronine, but the association constant is smaller (Sterling, 1964b); only about one-fourth the k value of the T_4–HSA complex has been reported (Table III). Albumin binds T_3 much more avidly at pH 8.6 than at pH 7.4 (Sterling and Tabachnick, 1961). A systematic study of the influence on HSA interaction of structural changes in the thyroxine molecule (Sterling, 1964b) has shown that loss of the four iodine atoms reduces the binding affinity by more than 99%. Introduction of iodine substituents into thyronine at the 3,5 and 3′,5′ positions results in a gradual increase of the association constant in proportion to the number of iodine atoms. Replacement of the amino group in thyroxine by hydrogen reduces the binding affinity but little; the same alteration in T_3 strengthens the interaction (Sterling, 1964b). The affinity constant of 3,5-diiodotyrosine is only about 0.1% of that for T_4.

The primary thyroxine-binding site in HSA has been reported (Tritsch and Tritsch, 1963) to involve the region around the amino terminus of the protein. This portion of the HSA structure appears to be more sensitive to urea denaturation than the molecule as a whole (Tritsch, 1968). Chicken serum albumin has been found (Tritsch and Tritsch, 1965) to bind thyroxine at pH 7.35 with an affinity constant of $2 \times 10^7\ M^{-1}$, i.e., about 8 times that of the T_4 complex with HSA. One primary binding site is involved; five secondary sites have been observed with an apparent association constant of $1.0 \times 10^5\ M^{-1}$.

D. Distribution of Thyroid Hormones among Serum Proteins

Presence of the three binding proteins, and the relatively high affinity of TBG for thyroxine, results in almost complete ($> 99.9\%$) association of T_4 with the proteins. The thyroxine concentration in normal serum may range from approximately 5 μg/100 ml ($6.4 \times 10^{-8}\ M$) to 10 μg/100 ml ($1.3 \times 10^{-7}\ M$); the level of T_3 is much smaller (about 0.3 μg/100 ml or $4.6 \times 10^{-9}\ M$). Experimental determinations of free thyroxine in human serum at 37° gave values ranging from 3–6 $\times\ 10^{-11}\ M$ (Oppen-

TABLE IV
DISTRIBUTION OF THYROXINE (T_4) AMONG PROTEINS IN HUMAN SERUM[a]

Total T_4	Percentage binding to		
	TBG	TBPA	HSA
$5 \times 10^{-8} M$	68^b (1)[c]	25 (1)	7 (1)
$1 \times 10^{-7} M$	64^b (1)	28 (1)	8 (1)
"Normal"	43 (2)	42 (2)	15 (2)
"Normal"	57 (3)	32 (3)	11 (3)
"Normal"	75 (4)	15 (4)	10 (4)

[a] In percent of total T_4.

[b] Calculated for a TBG capacity of $2.6 \times 10^{-7} M$.

[c] Numbers in parentheses refer to the following references: (1) Robbins and Rall, 1967; (2) Ingbar and Freinkel, 1960; (3) Oppenheimer *et al.*, 1963; (4) Woeber and Ingbar, 1968.

heimer and Surks, 1964; Sterling and Brenner, 1966). Somewhat lower concentrations of free thyroxine (0.5–$2.0 \times 10^{-11} M$) have been calculated (Steiner *et al.*, 1966) for normal human plasma, and the theoretical level of free thyroxine as a function of total thyroxine concentration has been computed for total T_4 values up to 30 μg/100 ml (Robbins and Rall, 1967).

The distribution of thyroxine among the binding proteins has been assessed. Values are given in Table IV for two T_4 concentrations, and for normal serum. About 60–70% of the total thyroxine is associated with TBG and only 8–10% with HSA. In serum with higher TBG concentration, such as pregnancy serum, markedly higher portions of T_4 are bound to TBG, at the cost of the TBPA and HSA complexes (Robbins and Rall, 1967).

Whereas the free thyroxine constitutes only about 0.03–0.05% of total T_4, the fraction of free triiodothyronine is approximately 10 times greater, i.e., 0.46% of total T_3 or $2.3 \times 10^{-11} M$ (Robbins and Rall, 1967). The theoretical distribution of triiodothyronine among the binding proteins in serum is given in Table V.

Musa *et al.* (1969) have recently studied the role of TBG in the early distribution of administered T_4 and T_3. They found that elevated TBG concentration, induced by estrogens, decreases the hepatic uptake of T_4, which accounts principally for the observed retardation of its disappearance from plasma; hepatic volume of distribution and hepatic clearance are reduced. Conversely, in patients lacking TBG these two parameters and hepatic uptake were much greater than in normals. Qualitatively similar observations were made for T_3.

TABLE V

DISTRIBUTION OF TRIIODOTHYRONINE (T₃) AMONG PROTEINS IN HUMAN SERUM[a]

Total T₄	Percentage binding to		
	TBG	HSA	Free T₃
$5 \times 10^{-8} M$	74^b (1)[c]	26^b (1)	$9 \times 10^{-12} M$ (1)
$1 \times 10^{-7} M$	71^b (1)	29^b (1)	$1 \times 10^{-11} M$ (1)
"Normal"	72 (2)	15^d (2)	—

[a] In percent of total T₃.

[b] Calculated for total T₃ of $5.5 \times 10^{-9} M$.

[c] Numbers in parentheses refer to the following references: (1) Robbins and Rall, 1967; (2) Braverman and Ingbar, 1965.

[d] The remaining 13% were present in an area cathodal to TBG in this agar gel electrophoresis experiment at pH 7.4.

The physiological significance of protein binding of thyroid hormones in many ways parallels the consequences of steroid hormone interaction with serum proteins. Ample evidence is available that it is the unbound form that is responsible for the manifold hormonal effects. Metabolism and excretion also involve the free hormone. Increase in the level of binding protein, e.g., of TBG, results in an increased reservoir of biologically inactive thyroid hormone that can become immediately available to the organism in active form by dissociation. The decrease of TBPA in the diseased or the postoperative state may be an important mechanism for ready availability of the biologically active hormone. These and related problems have been discussed recently (Robbins and Rall, 1967).

III. STEROID HORMONE-BINDING PROTEINS

A. GENERAL IMPLICATIONS OF THE INTERACTIONS

1. Quantitative Relationships and Binding Distribution

The interactions of the steroid hormones with serum proteins are comparable, in a general way, with the protein binding of the thyroid hormones. In either case we have a limited number of proteins capable of associating with a given hormone in a more or less specific manner. For either type of hormone, highly specific proteins are available in very low concentration which provide binding with a very high affinity: TBG as discussed in the preceding sections, the corticosteroid-binding globulin

(CBG, transcortin), which also binds progesterone, and high-affinity binding proteins for estradiol and testosterone. Binding affinities several orders of magnitude lower are provided by TBPA for thyroxine; α_1-acid glycoprotein (AAG, orosomucoid) interacts with progesterone and other steroid hormones with similarly reduced affinities. Serum albumin plays the role of a general binding protein, for thyroid hormones as well as for steroids; the association constants of the complexes are relatively low, but this is compensated by the high concentration of this protein in the blood serum, so that the proportional binding to HSA may be substantial.

For general orientation, Table VI shows the approximate serum concentrations of the three types of steroid-binding proteins in a pregnancy serum, together with their molecular weights. Similar data are given for progesterone and cortisol. The great differences in the protein concentrations, in some inverse relationship to their steroid-binding affinities are evident; the molar concentration of the specific binder CBG is of the same magnitude as that of the sum of progesterone and cortisol. On the basis of these concentrations of the numbers of binding sites per protein molecule and of the association constants to be discussed, the distribution of progesterone and cortisol among the binding proteins has been calculated (Westphal, 1966). One of the limiting conditions for the calculation is competition of the two steroids for the same binding sites. Columns 2 and 4 in Table VII give the result of the computations which show that progesterone is fairly evenly distributed between the small quantity of CBG and the large amount of HSA. This is an obvious consequence of the fact that the concentration of progesterone-binding sites of HSA in the pregnancy serum (Table VI) is about 1200–1500 times that of CBG, whereas the association constant for the progesterone–HSA complex is approximately 1500 times lower than that of the CBG complex. In contrast, the fraction of cortisol attached to CBG is relatively greater because of the low affinity of the corticosteroids to HSA.

TABLE VI

COMPONENTS OF STEROID–PROTEIN COMPLEXES IN A PREGNANCY SERUM

Component	Molecular weight	Concentration (mg/liter)	$(M \times 10^7)$
HSA	69,000	38,000	5,500
AAG	41,000	750	180
CBG	52,000	74	14
Progesterone	314	0.15	4.8
Cortisol	362	0.30	8.3

TABLE VII

DISTRIBUTION OF PROGESTERONE AND CORTISOL IN PREGNANCY SERUM

Steroid bound to	Progesterone % of total[a]		Cortisol % of total	
	(1)[b]	(2)[c]	(1)[b]	(2)[c]
CBG	48.1	42.8	59.8	79.7
HSA	49.6	} 55.6[d]	32.6	13.1
AAG	1.0		—	—
Unbound	1.3	1.8	7.6	7.8

[a] Numbers in parentheses refer to the following references: (1) Westphal, 1966; (2) Rosenthal *et al.*, 1969.

[b] Calculated for the concentrations given in Table VI.

[c] Determined in a plasma pool from the third trimester, which contained $16.8 \times 10^{-7} M$ CBG, $3.9 \times 10^{-7} M$ progesterone, and $7.4 \times 10^{-7} M$ cortisol.

[d] Bound to HSA and unassigned proteins.

In an extensive analysis of more than sixty sera from different stages of pregnancy, Rosenthal *et al.* (1969) have recently determined experimentally the association of progesterone and cortisol with the binding proteins. Table VII includes some of these results obtained for the third trimester of pregnancy; they show a distribution for progesterone that is similar to that calculated by the equations based on multiple-binding equilibria (Westphal, 1966), if one contrasts binding to CBG and to the total of albumin and "unassigned" proteins (Rosenthal *et al.*, 1969). It should be realized that the distributions assessed by the theoretical and by the experimental procedure (Table VII) are not strictly comparable because the concentrations of the pertinent components are different in the two cases: the plasma pool used for the experimental analysis (Rosenthal *et al.*, 1969) contained a higher CBG concentration, whereas the levels of progesterone and cortisol were lower than those in the "computed" serum (Westphal, 1966). One would expect that such differences result in a higher proportional binding to CBG in relation to HSA binding. This was indeed found for cortisol (Table VII). The somewhat lower proportional CBG binding of progesterone measured experimentally in comparison with the calculated value may be connected with the problem of the unassigned proteins. The percentage concentrations of the unbound hormones are in good agreement.

Another significant result obtained by the group in Buffalo (Rosenthal *et al.*, 1969) is the observation that the actual concentrations of unbound cortisol and progesterone rise during pregnancy. Whereas the percentage fraction of free steroids remained fairly constant from the first to the third trimester, the absolute concentrations increased considerably so that the unbound quantity showed an actual increase of approximately twofold. This finding has an important bearing on our interpretation and understanding of hormonal function in pregnancy since we consider the unbound form the biologically active species.

2. *Suppression of Hormonal Activity*

Ample evidence is available from several laboratories, especially from studies by Sandberg and Slaunwhite, that cortisol bound as CBG complex is biologically inactive (Sandberg *et al.*, 1966). Similarly, only the unbound, not the total level of corticosterone influenced thymus weight in the rat (Gala and Westphal, 1965b) and in the mouse (Gala and Westphal, 1967). Inactivation was likewise observed for deoxycorticosterone associated with albumin (Blecher, 1964).

It was found some years ago (Westphal and Forbes, 1963) that the biological activity of progesterone is suppressed by binding to AAG (Table VIII). This was determined by the Hooker-Forbes test (Hooker and Forbes, 1947) in which a small amount of material is injected into the ligated segment of the uterine horn of the mouse. The technique avoids entrance of the administered solution into the general circulation with the various possibilities of systemic interference, e.g., by metabolism or excretion of the steroid, or by degradation of the protein after dissociation of the complex. The same test system was recently applied to study the influence of CBG and albumin binding on the progestational activity of the pregnancy hormone (Hoffmann *et al.*, 1969). Table IX shows that association with either of these proteins suppresses the biological effects of progesterone. The partially positive responses seen in the uterine horns when the molar ratio of albumin to progesterone in

TABLE VIII

Effect of Binding to α_1-Acid Glycoprotein (AAG) on the Biological Activity of Progesterone[a]

Progesterone[b] ng/horn	AAG[b] μg/horn	Response in uterus horn
None	20.3	$- - - - -$
0.23	None	$+ + + + +$
0.24	None	$+ + + +$
0.23	2.6	$- - - - +$
0.32	3.5	$- - - - - -$
0.24	2.7	$- - - -$

[a] Data from Westphal and Forbes, 1963.

[b] The molar ratio of AAG to progesterone in the experimental solutions is approximately 80:1.

TABLE IX

EFFECT OF BINDING TO CBG OR ALBUMIN ON THE BIOLOGICAL ACTIVITY
OF PROGESTERONE[a]

| Progesterone ng/horn | Rat serum preparation | | | Response in uterus horn |
	CBG μg/horn	Albumin μg/horn	Molar ratio protein/ progesterone	
2.41	None	None	—	+++−
0.60	None	None	—	+[b]+[c]++++(+)−
2.41	59.5	None	1	−−(−)
0.80	19.8	None	1	−−−−−
0.60	14.9	None	1	−[b]−[c]−−−−−−−++
0.60	None	29.8	200	−−−−−−−−−−
0.60	None	14.9	100	+++++++−−−−−−−−−−
0.60	None	1.5	10	+++++−−−−−

[a] From Hoffmann *et al.*, 1969.
[b,c] Identical letters indicate the two horns of the same mouse.

the injected solution was 100 or 10, are caused by dissociation of the complex after dilution with the intrauterine fluid. This has been calculated and discussed in detail (Hoffmann *et al.*, 1969). It should be noted that the recent experiments (Table IX) were performed with a different strain of mice, which has a lower sensitivity to progesterone than the strain used in the study summarized in Table VIII. These results add to the general conclusion, which has now been verified in numerous examples, i.e., that the biological activity of a steroid hormone is given by the unbound form, and that binding to proteins results in inactivation.

B. SERUM ALBUMIN

1. Binding Parameters

Interactions of steroid hormones with serum albumin have been studied extensively. This protein is readily available in relatively pure form and is stable under various experimental conditions. Ever since the ability of albumin was recognized to associate with and thus transport many compounds of different chemical structure (Bennhold, 1932), complexes of this protein with various ligands including steroid hormones have been investigated (Bennhold, 1966). It follows from the multitudinous binding quality that interactions with serum albumin have a poor specificity; the association constants are generally of a low order. Binding affinities of thyroxine and triiodothyronine for HSA, approximately 10^4 times smaller than those for the highly specific TBG, have been discussed

(Table III). The physiological significance of hormone interactions with serum albumin would be very minor were it not for the high concentration of this protein in the circulating blood, which leads to binding of substantial portions of various hormones (Tables IV, V, and VII).

The earlier literature on steroid interactions with serum albumin of bovine and human origin has been reviewed (Roberts and Szego, 1953; Szego and Roberts, 1953; Sandberg et al., 1957; Daughaday, 1959; Westphal, 1961). Some physicochemical parameters of HSA were given in Tables I and II. Affinity constants of the more important steroid hormones with HSA are compiled in Table X as nk, the product of the number of binding sites, n, and the apparent association constant, k. The intrinsic association constants, k, for each binding site may be

TABLE X

NUMBERS OF BINDING SITES, n, APPARENT ASSOCIATION CONSTANTS, nk, AND FREE ENERGY, $\Delta F°$, OF INTERACTIONS BETWEEN STEROID HORMONES AND HUMAN SERUM ALBUMIN

Steroid	Temp. °C	pH	n	nk liter/mole	$\Delta F°$ kcal/mole
1. Estrone	5 (1)[a]	7.0 (1)	1.1 (1)	4.4×10^4 (1)	−5.9 (1)
2. Estradiol	5 (1)	7.0 (1)	— (1)	1.6×10^5 (1)	−6.7 (1)
3. Testosterone	5 (1)	7.0 (1)	— (1)	3.4×10^4 (1)	−5.8 (1)
4. Testosterone	25 (2)	7.6 (2)	2.3 (2)	5.4×10^4 (2)	−6.4 (2)
5. 11β-Hydroxy-androst-4-ene-3,17-dione[b]	4 (3)	7.4 (3)	—	0.8×10^4 (3)	−5.0 (3)
6. Progesterone	4 (4)	7.4 (4)	2.2 (4)	8.9×10^4 (4)	−6.3 (4)
7. Progesterone[b]	4 (4)	7.4 (4)	2.1 (4)	2.1×10^5 (4)	−6.7 (4)
8. Progesterone	25 (2)	7.6 (2)	—	8.9×10^4 (2)	−6.7 (2)
9. Progesterone	37 (5)	7.4 (5)	—	6.1×10^4 (5)	−6.8 (5)
10. Progesterone[b]	37 (3)	7.4 (3)	2.6 (3)	1.2×10^5 (3)	−7.2 (3)
11. Progesterone	45 (5)	7.4 (5)	—	4.3×10^4 (5)	−6.7 (5)
12. Cortexone[b]	4 (3)	7.4 (3)	3.3 (3)	1.9×10^5 (3)	−6.7 (3)
13. Cortexone	25 (2)	7.6 (2)	2.0 (2)	3.6×10^4 (2)	−6.2 (2)
14. Corticosterone	5 (6)	7.0 (6)	2.1 (6)	0.9×10^4 (6)	−5.0 (6)
15. Cortisone	5 (6)	7.0 (6)	—	0.5×10^4 (6)	−4.7 (6)
16. Cortisol	4 (7)	7.4 (7)	—	0.6×10^4 (7)	−4.8 (7)
17. Cortisol[b]	4 (3)	7.4 (3)	—	1.0×10^4 (3)	−5.1 (3)
18. Cortisol	25 (2)	7.6 (2)	—	1.2×10^4 (2)	−5.5 (2)
19. Aldosterone	4 (8)	7.6 (8)	—	2.6×10^3 (8)	−4.3 (8)
20. Aldosterone	37 (8)	7.6 (8)	—	1.7×10^3 (8)	−4.6 (8)
21. Prednisone	20 (9)	6.0 (9)	—	4.6×10^3 (9)	−4.9 (9)

[a] Numbers in parentheses refer to the following references: (1) Sandberg et al., 1957; (2) Westphal et al., 1958, (3) Westphal and Harding, 1969; (4) Westphal, 1966; (5) Westphal, 1964; (6) Sandberg et al., 1957; (7) Daughaday, 1956a; (8) Davidson et al., 1962; (9) Scholtan et al., 1968.

[b] *HSA* delipidated.

calculated for those steroids for which the number of binding sites has been determined. Only primary binding sites are given; they are assumed to be equivalent and independent of each other. In addition to temperature and pH, the apparent free energy values are included, calculated for nk.

It is evident from Table X that the association constants of the HSA–steroid complexes show a systematic decrease with increasing numbers of hydroxy groups introduced into the progesterone molecule. This phenomenon was recognized early in Samuels' laboratory when an inverse relationship was observed between the number of polar groups in the steroid and the strength of binding to bovine serum albumin (Eik-Nes *et al.*, 1954); it is known as the polarity rule. Subsequent studies with some 60 Δ^4-3-ketosteroids (Westphal and Ashley, 1962), using a spectrophotometric method to assess the binding affinity to HSA, have confirmed the basic premise that electron-attracting substituents weaken the steroid–HSA complex, whereas electron-repelling groups strengthen the interaction (Westphal and Ashley, 1958). Binding affinities measured with epimeric steroids suggested that the rear or α-side of the steroid molecule is involved in the association with the protein (Westphal and Ashley, 1959).

Binding behavior in accordance with the polarity rule has also been observed in measurements of binding affinities of various anions to serum albumin (Westphal *et al.*, 1953). The same relationship between hydroxy groups and binding affinity exists in the interaction between hydroxycholanic acids and HSA (Rudman and Kendall, 1957); the association constant decreases in proportion to the number of hydroxyls entering the steroid structure (see Table 9 in Westphal, 1961). This type of interaction is characteristic of hydrophobic bonding; van der Waals' bonds have long been accepted as the dominant forces in the association of small neutral molecules with serum albumin, and certain other proteins (Steinhardt and Beychok, 1964). Recent spectrophotometric studies (Ryan, 1968) have also led to the conclusion that hydrophobic residues may be near the binding site for the less polar steroids in serum albumin.

2. *Influence of Lipids on Steroid Binding*

Most of the binding data given in Table X were obtained with pure serum albumin preparations from commercial sources or of comparable quality. These preparations, often crystalline, contain definite amounts of fatty acids, ranging from near zero up to 2 or 3 mole acid/mole albumin (R. F. Chen, 1967). The most prominent among these contaminating acids are palmitic, stearic, oleic, and linoleic acid (Saifer and Goldman, 1961), lipids that form stable complexes with serum albumin; the association is mediated by the anionic site and by hydrophobic interaction of the aliphatic chain with nonpolar regions in the albumin molecule. Since hydrophobic regions are also involved in binding of steroids to serum albumin it seemed important to test for possible interference of steroid–albumin interaction by the lipid contaminants.

Removal of lipid-soluble material from crystalline HSA by solvent extraction (Therriault and Taylor, 1960) at 0° resulted in a preparation that had a markedly increased binding affinity for progesterone. The affinity constants determined by equilibrium dialysis at 4° and 37° were found to be approximately twice those observed with the nondelipidated HSA (Table X, No. 7 vs 6, No. 10 vs 9). The association constant of the cortisol–HSA complex was also greatly increased when delipidated HSA was used (Table X, No. 17 vs 16). Whereas the number of primary binding sites, n, had mostly a value of 2 for the Δ^4-3-ketosteroid hormones, a delipidated HSA preparation bound cortexone with $n = 3.3$ (Table X, No. 12).

In recent studies on the influence of lipids on steroid binding to HSA (Westphal and Harding, 1969), a delipidated albumin preparation was obtained which formed a progesterone complex (Fig. 1, circles, solid line) with an apparent association constant approximately 4 times that of the progesterone complex with the nondelipidated HSA (circles, broken line). The apparent association constant is given in Fig. 1 by $\bar{v}/[S]$, which

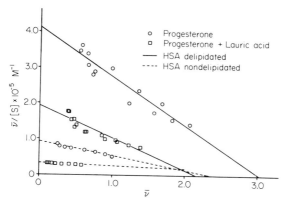

Fig. 1. Effect of delipidation of HSA, and of addition of lauric acid to HSA (molar ratio 5:1) on its progesterone-binding activity, in 0.05 M phosphate, pH 7.4; 4°. For explanation of symbols see text. For simplicity, the Scatchard plots have been evaluated as straight lines, obtained by the method of least squares, although it is realized that there may be different sets of binding sites, especially in the delipidated HSA (Westphal and Harding, 1969).

is equivalent to nk (Westphal, 1969), where $\bar{v}$ equals the average number of steroid molecules bound per molecule protein; [S], the molar concentration of unbound steroid; n, the number of apparent binding sites; and k, the intrinsic association constant. The number of apparent binding sites, n, is increased by the removal of the lipid-soluble contamination from approximately 2 to 3 (Fig. 1).

Addition of lauric acid to the delipidated HSA (5 mole/mole) reduces the $\bar{v}/[S]$ value (nk) to about half (squares, solid line). This inhibition does not appear to be competitive. The number of binding sites is decreased again from $n \cong 3$ to a value of $n \cong 2$. The lower broken line in Fig. 1 indicates that addition of 5 mole lauric acid per nondelipidated HSA molecule results in a progesterone binding affinity less than half its original value. The number of binding sites, $n \cong 2$, does not seem to be affected further by the addition of lauric acid.

The observations on the influence of lipidic substances on the binding affinity and capacity of serum proteins for steroid hormones have an important bearing on our interpretation of binding distribution of given hormones among the different proteins. Under physiological conditions, numerous lipids are present in the blood which may interfere with the albumin binding of a steroid hormone; the proportional associations calculated on the basis of values for k and n established by physiochemical techniques for the isolated, highly purified and possibly lipid-free proteins, may therefore not be valid *in vivo*. These considerations are not unique for serum albumin. Very similar results have been obtained in studies on progesterone interaction with AAG; removal of lipid contaminations increased the affinity constant severalfold as will be discussed in Section III,E,1. The influence of lipids or other inhibitors of steroid binding to proteins seems to play a lesser or insignificant role in the much more specific interactions between certain steroid hormones and their high-affinity binders, such as the complexes between CBG and cortisol or progesterone. This conclusion is based on the finding that the association constants of the complexes between CBG and steroid hormones, measured in whole serum, are approximately the same as those determined after isolation of CBG in pure, homogeneous form (see Table XI vs Table XV).

C. CORTICOSTEROID-BINDING GLOBULIN (CBG)

1. General Properties

Among several proteins present in animal sera in relatively low concentrations and capable of binding certain steroid hormones with high affinity, the corticosteroid-binding globulin (CBG, transcortin) was the first one to be recognized (Daughaday, 1956b; Bush, 1957; Upton and Bondy, 1958; Slaunwhite and Sandberg, 1959) and characterized (Sandberg *et al.*, 1966; Seal and Doe, 1966). Methods for determination of its concentration and steroid-binding affinity have been reviewed (Sandberg *et al.*, 1966; Hoffmann and Westphal, 1969; Westphal, 1969). CBG has been demonstrated in the peripheral or adrenal venous plasma of numerous species, representing all of the vertebrate classes (Seal and Doe, 1966). The ubiquitous occurrence of CBG, in addition to certain characteristic properties, suggested to Seal and Doe (1963) that the fundamental mechanism for binding of corticosteroids to serum protein appeared early in the history of the vertebrates, that it has been retained, including a unique conformation required for the specific tight binding of certain steroid structures.

One characteristic property of the steroid-CBG complexes of all species investigated so far is a marked decrease of the binding affinity with increasing temperature. This is in contrast to the behavior of the associations between serum albumin and steroids which show a very small temperature dependency (Table X; see also Fig. 20). Figure 2 shows the corticosteroid-binding affinity of CBG at different temperatures for the

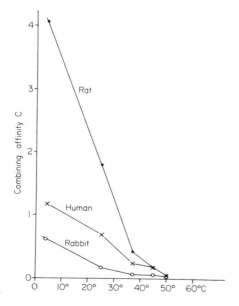

Fig. 2. Corticosterone-binding activity (C-values) of CBG in steroid-stripped sera at different temperatures, in 0.05 *M* phosphate of pH 7.4. From Westphal (1967).

sera of three species whose CBG's have been isolated, as will be discussed.

The binding strength of the steroid–protein complexes in Fig. 2 and in subsequent figures is expressed as combining affinity, C, which is defined (Daughaday, 1958) as

$$C = \frac{S_{\text{bd}}}{S_{\text{unbd}} P_t} \qquad (1)$$

where S_{bd}, S_{unbd}, and P_t indicate concentrations of bound steroid, unbound steroid, and total protein, respectively, in grams per liter. The C-value, which is the resultant of the concentration of binding sites and their intrinsic binding affinity, is a convenient expression for the corticosteroid-binding activity of a serum. In solutions of pure proteins, when the concentrations can be expressed in moles per liter, Eq. (1) becomes

$$\frac{[S]_{\text{bd}}}{[S][P]_t} = \frac{\bar{\nu}}{[S]} \qquad (2)$$

where $[S]_{\text{bd}}$, $[S]$, and $[P]_t$ are the molar concentrations of bound and unbound steroid, and of total protein, respectively, and $\bar{\nu}$ is the average number of steroid molecules bound per molecule of protein present. The dimension is M^{-1}. If one assumes the number of binding sites, $n = 1$, and absence of other binding sites of lower affinity, Eq. (2) is an approximation of the association constant (Edsall and Wyman, 1958),

$$k = \frac{[S]_{\text{bd}}}{[S][P]} \qquad (3)$$

which differs from Eq. (2) only by use of $[P]$, the molar concentration of unbound protein instead of $[P]_t$, the molar concentration of total protein. Evidently, for the approximation to be valid, the condition is $[P] \gg [S]_{\text{bd}}$. For further discussion of use and interpretation of these binding parameters, see Ganguly *et al.* (1967) and Westphal (1969).

The CBG molecule is more labile to heat than serum albumin. Whereas the short exposure to 45° during gel filtration of CBG in serum does not affect the binding affinity (Westphal, 1967), heating for 15 minutes at 60° and above irreversibly denatures human CBG in serum with loss of binding affinity (Daughaday and Mariz, 1961). Studies on heat exposure of CBG in human, rat, and rabbit serum showed that very little recovery of CBG activity was obtained when the equilibrium dialysis solutions, after dialysis at 50° for 48 hours at pH 7.4, were returned to 4° (Westphal, 1969). For comparison, pure HSA does not show any loss of progesterone-binding affinity after exposure to 45° for at least 24 hours, and AAG can be heated as a pure protein in phosphate buffer at pH 7.4 for

24 hours at 60° without significant reduction of progesterone-binding affinity (Ganguly *et al.*, 1967).

Figure 3 shows the pH dependency of the CBG activity of human and rat serum (Westphal, 1969). Maximal association appears to occur at approximately pH 8. The decrease of the binding affinity at this pH to that at pH 9.8 has been found to be completely reversible. Very little reversibility was observed when the serum that had been exposed to pH 2.8 at 4° for 48 hours was readjusted to neutral pH.

It has been demonstrated by various electrophoretic techniques that the CBG of human serum is an α-globulin (Seal and Doe, 1966). The α-globulin nature of CBG has also been reported for serum of rat, rabbit, ox, and horse (Westphal and DeVenuto, 1966). At low pH values, the CBG of rat serum was found to migrate as a prealbumin.

Electrophoretic procedures were also utilized to demonstrate association of aldosterone with CBG by competitive displacement of CBG-bound cortisol by the mineralocorticoid (Westphal and DeVenuto, 1966). The fraction with the highest cortisol-binding affinity (CBG), separated by continuous flow electrophoresis, also showed maximal association with aldosterone. Addition of cortisol to the aldosterone-binding system (molar steroid ratio about 50:1) resulted in a reduction of the amount of bound aldosterone to about 1/6 the value obtained in absence of cortisol. Progesterone and cortisol displaced aldosterone also from the binding sites present in Cohn's Fraction IV-4, a human plasma fraction rich in α-globulins including CBG (Davidson *et al.*, 1962). It was concluded that aldosterone in human blood is associated, besides with albumin

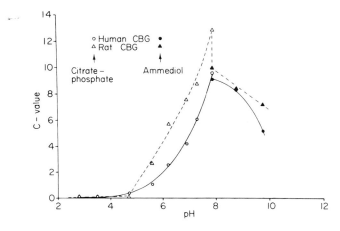

Fig. 3. Corticosterone-binding activity (C-values) of CBG in human and rat serum at different pH values, in 0.05 M buffers; 4°. From data in Westphal (1969).

(Table X), with a protein component indistinguishable from CBG by the electrophoretic method used. These results corroborate earlier suggestions that aldosterone is bound to a serum protein other than albumin, most likely to CBG (Sandberg *et al.*, 1960; Daughaday *et al.*, 1961; Meyer *et al.*, 1961). The question of aldosterone binding to CBG has been raised again recently (Gueriguian *et al.*, 1969) in connection with studies on chromatographic separation of human pregnancy serum. No clear-cut separation was obtained between CBG and the aldosterone-binding activity.

The CBG's in the sera of different mammalian species show considerable differences in their steroid-binding properties. Table XI shows the concentration of CBG binding sites in the sera of five species and their association constants for cortisol, corticosterone, and progesterone at 4° and 37° (Westphal, 1967). These parameters were determined with the sera after removal of the endogenous steroids by gel filtration at 45° to eliminate interference by competitive or noncompetitive binding of related steroids or other small molecules. It is apparent from Table XI that the affinity constant of progesterone to human CBG at 37° is about three times as high as that of cortisol, indicating the validity of the polarity rule. In contrast, the association constant of the progesterone–CBG complex in rabbit serum at 4° is approximately 2.5 times smaller than that of the cortisol complex. The relationship is reversed again and magnified for guinea pig CBG, which seems to bind progesterone with an affinity about 100 times higher than that measured for cortisol; it must

TABLE XI

CONCENTRATION OF BINDING SITES AND ASSOCIATION CONSTANTS, k, OF STEROID–CBG COMPLEXES IN MAMMALIAN SERA[a,b]

| Species | [CBG][c] in $10^{-7} M$ | k in $10^8 M^{-1}$ for | | | | | |
| | | Cortisol | | Corticosterone | | Progesterone | |
		4°	37°	4°	37°	4°	37°
Human	7.2	6	0.3	10	0.3	7	0.9
Monkey	9.3	3	0.3	—	1.4	—	—
Rat	11.3	3	0.1	5	0.3	3	—
Rabbit	3.4	10	0.4	8	0.2	4	—
Guinea pig	5.7	0.5	0.04	1.1	0.14	48	3.9

[a] In 0.05 M phosphate, pH 7.4.

[b] Data from Westphal, 1967.

[c] The concentrations of binding sites for the corticosteroids were approximately the same as those for progesterone.

be remembered, however, that the identity of CBG with the progesterone-binding protein has not been proven (Diamond *et al.*, 1969). These variations in the relative strength of association of the CBG's from different species for the three steroids of increasing polarity suggest a high structural specificity in the CBG molecules at or near the steroid-binding site. This specificity is independent of the chemical nature of the predominant corticosteroid in a given animal species. Elucidation of the chemical structure of the different CBG molecules and their steroid-binding sites in relationship to their affinity for the different steroids evolves as a challenging problem. The first step for its solution is the isolation of the various CBG's in pure, homogeneous form.

2. *Isolation and Properties of CBG's from Serum of Man, Rabbit, and Rat; Observations on Polymerism*

Human CBG was first isolated in pioneering work by Seal and Doe (1962b), followed by later reports from other laboratories (Slaunwhite *et al.*, 1966; Muldoon and Westphal, 1967). Pure homogeneous CBG preparations have also been obtained from rabbit (Chader and Westphal, 1968a) and rat serum (Chader and Westphal, 1968b). In all isolation procedures, serum or plasma was equilibrated with radiolabeled corticosteroid so that exogenous plus added corticoid were in excess of the high-affinity binding sites; it was then fractionated by chromatographic procedures. The purification techniques for human CBG utilized as the first step DEAE-cellulose chromatography initially reported in 1960 (Westphal, 1961). Figure 4 shows this original separation and indicates

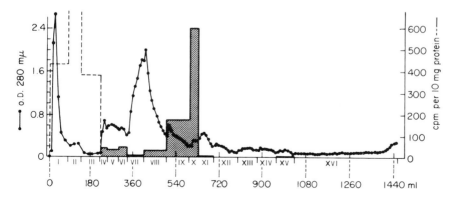

FIG. 4. Partial purification of CBG by chromatography of 10 ml human serum, equilibrated with 2 μg cortisol-4-^{14}C, on DEAE-cellulose. Highest CBG concentration in Fraction X. Trisphosphate gradient prepared from 0.005 M, pH 8.0 to 0.5 M, pH 4.5. Modified from Westphal (1961).

Ulrich Westphal

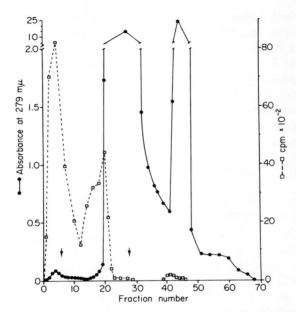

Fig. 5. Hydroxylapatite chromatography at 4° of rat CBG–corticosterone-4-^{14}C complex after Sephadex G-200 filtration. Arrows indicate changes from 0.005 to 0.05 M and to 0.2 M phosphate buffer, pH 6.8. From Chader and Westphal (1968b).

the removal of a high percentage of inactive proteins from the CBG-containing fraction, which is recognized by its association with bound cortisol-4-^{14}C. In the isolation procedures for rat and rabbit CBG, DEAE-Sephadex was used instead of DEAE-cellulose for the initial chromatographic fractionation.

Human CBG was further purified by chromatography on hydroxylapatite. This step, introduced by Seal and Doe (1962b), is particularly efficient because CBG, in contrast to most other proteins, is not adsorbed by this reagent. The high effectiveness of the hydroxylapatite chromatography is evident in Fig. 5, which shows an intermediate stage of the purification of rat CBG (Chader and Westphal, 1968b): practically all of the radiolabeled corticosterone appears in the early fractions in association with a very small portion of the protein, ahead of the bulk of inactive protein. The hydroxylapatite chromatography is repeated until symmetrical coinciding peaks of radioactivity and protein are obtained (Fig. 6).

In the case of the isolation of rat and rabbit CBG, the hydroxylapatite adsorption was preceded by gel filtration over Sephadex G-200. Figure 7 shows this step for rabbit CBG; clearly a substantial portion of inactive

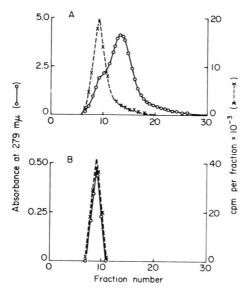

Fig. 6. Hydroxylapatite chromatography of human CBG–cortisol-4-^{14}C complex after separation on DEAE-cellulose. A, first chromatography; B, final chromatography. In 0.001 M phosphate, pH 6.8; 4°. From Muldoon and Westphal (1967).

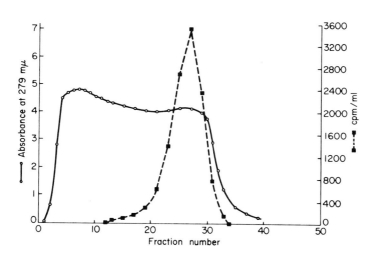

Fig. 7. Sephadex G-200 filtration of rabbit CBG–corticosteroid complex after purification by DEAE-Sephadex chromatography. In 0.05 M phosphate, pH 7.4; 4°. From Chader and Westphal (1968a).

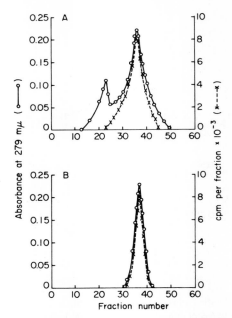

Fɪɢ. 8. Sephadex G-200 filtration of human CBG–cortisol-4-^{14}C complex after final chromatography on hydroxylapatite (see Fig. 6B). A, first gel filtration; B, final gel filtration. In 0.05 M phosphate, pH 7.4; 4°. From Muldoon and Westphal (1967).

protein, free of radioactivity, is removed. As a rule, in all separation steps the fractions of high specific activity (bound radiocorticoid per mg protein) were combined, dialyzed, lyophilized, and applied to the subsequent column. Sephadex G-200 filtration is again applied to advantage after the hydroxylapatite chromatography (Fig. 8), resulting in homogeneous CBG from human serum. In a similar way, the final gel filtration step yielded a pure corticosterone complex with rat CBG (Fig. 9). These filtrations were repeated until symmetrical peaks were obtained, coinciding for protein concentration and radioactivity. The amounts of final CBG preparations obtained per liter of human, rabbit, and rat serum were 14, 6.8, and 29 mg, respectively, representing yields of approximately 50% in each case.

The purified CBG-corticosteroid complexes isolated in our laboratory from normal human, rabbit, and rat serum were found to be homogeneous by several criteria. Immunoelectrophoresis gave single precipitin bands when the pure CBG s were reacted with the antisera against whole serum of the given species; the migration rates were those of α_1-globulins.

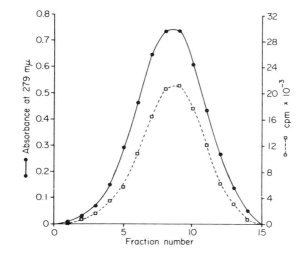

Fig. 9. Final Sephadex G-200 filtration of rat CBG–corticosterone-4-^{14}C complex in 0.05 M phosphate buffer, pH 7.4, 4°. From Chader and Westphal (1968b).

Ultracentrifugation over a range of concentrations resulted in single symmetrical peaks as exemplified in Fig. 10 for rat CBG. Linear relationships between the reciprocal sedimentation coefficients, $s_{20,w}$, and protein concentrations, another indication of homogeneity, were obtained for the CBG's of the three species; this is shown in Fig. 11 for the rabbit protein. Table XII gives the physicochemical properties of human, rabbit, and rat CBG. The general similarity of the three proteins is evident from the various parameters, including molecular weight, sedimentation coefficient, partial specific volume, and spectral properties. The CBG's are glyco-

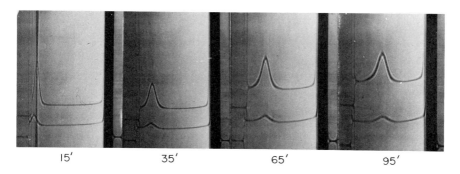

Fig. 10. Ultracentrifugation pattern of 0.9% and 0.2% solutions of rat CBG–corticosterone complex in 0.1 M NaCl, 20°. From Chader and Westphal (1968b).

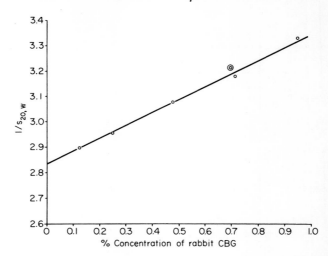

Fɪɢ. 11. Reciprocal $s_{20,w}$ values vs concentration for rabbit CBG–corticosteroid complex in 0.1 M NaCl; 20°. The point circled twice was obtained with a second preparation. From Chader and Westphal (1968a).

TABLE XII

Pʜʏsɪᴄᴏᴄʜᴇᴍɪᴄᴀʟ Pʀᴏᴘᴇʀᴛɪᴇs ᴏғ ᴛʜᴇ Cᴏʀᴛɪᴄᴏsᴛᴇʀᴏɪᴅ Cᴏᴍᴘʟᴇxᴇs ᴏғ Hᴜᴍᴀɴ, Rᴀʙʙɪᴛ, ᴀɴᴅ Rᴀᴛ CBG

Parameter	Human CBG (1)[a]	Rabbit CBG (2)	Rat CBG (3)
Sedimentation coefficient, $s_{20,w}^0$ (S)	3.79	3.55	3.56
Diffusion coefficient, $D_{20,w}$, (cm² sec⁻¹) × 10⁷	6.15	7.02	—
Partial specific volume, $\bar{v}$ (ml/gm)	0.708	0.695	0.711
Molecular weight	51,700[b]	40,700	52,600 ± 3000[c] 61,000 ± 1100[d]
Frictional ratio, f/fo	1.42	1.37	—
$E_{1\,cm}^{1\%}$ at 279 nm	6.45	8.4	6.2
$A_{280}:A_{260}$, corticosteroid complex	1.13	1.38	1.58
$A_{280}:A_{260}$, complex stripped	1.57	—	1.71
Electrophoretic mobility at pH 8.6 (cm² V⁻¹ sec⁻¹) × 10⁵	−4.9	−5.1	—
Carbohydrate (%)	26.1	29.2	27.8
Nitrogen (%)	12.7	12.1	—

[a] Numbers in parentheses refer to the following references: (1) Muldoon and Westphal, 1967; (2) Chader and Westphal, 1968a; (3) Chader and Westphal, 1968b.

[b] Molecular weights reported from other laboratories: 52,000 (Seal and Doe, 1966); 58,500 (Slaunwhite *et al.*, 1966).

[c] From corticosterone content of complex.

[d] From approach to sedimentation equilibrium.

TABLE XIII

AMINO ACID COMPOSITION OF HUMAN, RABBIT, AND RAT CBG

	gm/100 gm CBG Polypeptide		
Amino acid	Human (1)[a]	Rabbit (2)	Rat (3)
Lysine	5.03	4.60	6.64
Histidine	3.29	2.89	2.57
Arginine	3.99	5.22	4.01
Aspartic Acid	9.72	9.84	11.89
Threonine	5.73	6.70	6.13
Serine	6.15	6.21	6.26
Glutamic Acid	12.77	13.33	14.42
Proline	5.48	5.31	4.29
Glycine	2.86	3.67	3.16
Alanine	4.34	5.12	4.26
Cystine/2	0.54	2.10	2.32
Valine	6.66	6.10	5.15
Methionine	3.52	1.51	2.70
Isoleucine	4.76	3.74	3.90
Leucine	11.98	10.05	10.02
Tyrosine	4.22	4.41	4.30
Phenylalanine	7.29	5.80	6.16
Tryptophan	1.49	3.39	1.82

[a] Numbers in parentheses refer to the following references: (1) Muldoon and Westphal, 1967; (2) Chader and Westphal, 1968a; (3) Chader and Westphal, 1968b.

proteins with a relatively high carbohydrate content of the same magnitude for the three species.

The chemical relationship between the CBG's from the three sera is also apparent in the amino acid composition shown in Table XIII. In spite of a general similarity, there are distinct differences in the individual amino acids as for example in cystine/2 and methionine. The same may be said of the carbohydrate composition of the three CBG molecules (Table XIV). Whereas the "backbone" constituents of the glycoproteins, i.e., hexose and hexosamine, are very similar in the three proteins, sialic acid and fucose show greater differences, in analogy to other types of glycoproteins.

The apparent association constants and other thermodynamic parameters of the corticosteroid–CBG complexes may be seen in Table XV. The values for k represent a confirmatory refinement of the data given in Table XI. The number of corticosteroid binding sites, n, equals 1 in each case. It is evident for the three complexes that the affinity constants increase approximately twenty fold when the temperature is reduced from 37° to 4°. The relatively high binding strength of rabbit CBG for

TABLE XIV
CARBOHYDRATE COMPOSITION OF HUMAN, RABBIT, AND RAT CBG

Carbohydrate	Human (1)[a]	Rabbit (2)	Rat (3)
Hexose	11.5%	10.4%	9.8%
Hexosamine	9.0	9.5	9.5
Sialic acid	4.1	8.5	6.4
Fucose	1.5	0.8	2.1
	26.1%	29.2%	27.8%

[a] Numbers in parentheses refer to the following references: (1) Muldoon and Westphal, 1967; (2) Chader and Westphal, 1968a; (3) Chader and Westphal, 1968b.

cortisol is also apparent. The free energy of binding has the high value of 10–11 kcal/mole; it is composed of a very high negative enthalpy change, in association with a negative change of entropy. These thermodynamic data are interpreted as indicative of a very tight fit of the interacting components, so that the enthalpy is drastically reduced; the total order is much increased, so that a negative entropy change results. This is in contrast to the positive entropy changes observed with the steroid complexes of AAG and HSA (see Table XXII and discussion).

In correspondence to the limited data so far available on the chemical characterization of CBG, little is known about the relationship of chemical structure to steroid-binding ability. Complete removal of sialic acid from human CBG by enzymatic hydrolysis at 4° did not affect the cortisol-binding affinity. This is in accordance with observations on TBG, AAG, and the steroid-binding β-globulin, which after removal of sialic

TABLE XV
BINDING PARAMETERS OF CORTICOSTEROID–CBG COMPLEXES

Parameter	Human CBG[a] (1)[c] (2)[c]	Rabbit CBG[a] (2)[c]	Rat CBG[b] (3)[c]
Number of binding sites, n	1	1	1
Association constant, k, 4° (M^{-1})	5.2×10^8	9.0×10^8	5.1×10^8
Association constant, k, 37° (M^{-1})	2.4×10^7	4.7×10^7	2.8×10^7
Free energy, $\Delta F°$, 4° (kcal/mole)	-11.0	-11.3	-11.0
Free energy, $\Delta F°$, 37° (kcal/mole)	-10.5	-10.9	-10.6
Enthalpy, $\Delta H°$, (kcal/mole)	-15.7	-15.0	-14.8
Entropy, $\Delta S°$ (cal mole^{-1} degree^{-1})	-17	-13	-14

[a] Cortisol complex.

[b] Corticosterone complex.

[c] References used in table: (1) Muldoon and Westphal, 1967; (2) Chader and Westphal, 1968a; (3) Chader and Westphal, 1968b.

acid also retain complete binding activity for thyroxine, progesterone, and estradiol, respectively, as reported elsewhere in this article. It may be concluded from these results that sialic acid is not of general significance for the hormone-binding properties of these different types of glycoproteins. It is of interest in this context that enzymatic removal of sialic acid from transferrin does not significantly alter its iron-binding activity (Blumberg and Warren, 1961).

The possible involvement of sulfhydryl in the steroid binding of CBG has not yet been fully investigated. Whereas spectrophotometric determination with p-hydroxymercuribenzoate (HMB) revealed one free thiol group in human CBG (Seal and Doe, 1966; Muldoon and Westphal, 1967), none was detected in rabbit CBG under identical conditions of analysis (Chader and Westphal, 1968a). However, addition of HMB to an equilibrium dialysis system containing rabbit CBG and radiolabeled cortisol resulted in a 27-fold decrease of the association constant at 37° (Chader and Westphal, 1968a).

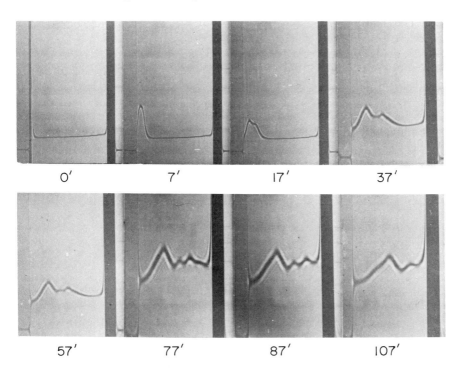

FIG. 12. Ultracentrifugation pattern of rat CBG after removal of 87% of the associated corticosterone at various times (min) after speed of 59,780 rpm was reached. In 0.1 M NaCl; 20°. From Chader and Westphal (1968b).

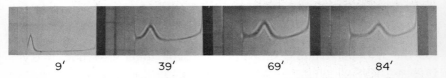

9'   39'   69'   84'

FIG. 13. Ultracentrifugation pattern of rat CBG used for study shown in Fig. 12, after recombination with 1 mole corticosterone/mole CBG. Other conditions as in Fig. 12. From Chader and Westphal (1968b).

Dissociation by gel filtration at 45° of pure human (Muldoon and Westphal, 1967), rabbit (Chader and Westphal, 1968a), or rat CBG (Chader and Westphal, 1968b) leads to complete (human) or partial (rabbit) loss of steroid-binding activity. When rat CBG was subjected to gel filtration under milder conditions, conformational alterations were observed. It has been shown (Fig. 10) that the rat CBG–corticosterone complex sediments in the ultracentrifuge as a homogeneous macromolecule. Removal of 87% of the steroid by Sephadex G-75 filtration at 23° results in the spontaneous formation of at least four molecular species with sedimentation coefficients of 3.4 (= original), 5.4, 6.8, and 8.1, respectively (Fig. 12). When this polymeric material, after recovery from the ultracentrifuge cell, is recombined with 1 mole of corticosterone per 53,000 gm of protein, the sedimentation pattern changes back to that of the original CBG–corticosterone complex (Fig. 13). One homogeneous peak is observed with a sedimentation coefficient of 3.45, a value indistinguishable from that of the original CBG–corticosterone complex under similar conditions. Disc electrophoresis experiments (Chader and Westphal, 1968b) confirmed the appearance of polymeric (dimeric, tetrameric, octameric) forms after corticosterone was removed from the complex by dissociation. This reversible polymerization of the CBG molecule constitutes a first example of the control of the conformational structure of a specific carrier protein by the hormone with which it forms a complex of high affinity.

3. CBG Activity in the Rat as Affected by Age, Sex, and Endocrines; Control by TSH-Thyroid Hormone

The rat has been chosen as the experimental animal to study the influence of various factors on the CBG activity *in vivo*. Figure 14 shows the corticosterone-binding activity in the serum of the developing rat (Gala and Westphal, 1965b). During the first weeks of life, the C-values increase similarly in the male and the female, starting from a low level. At about day 30, the activity in the male rat appears to have reached its highest value, whereas that of the female continues to rise

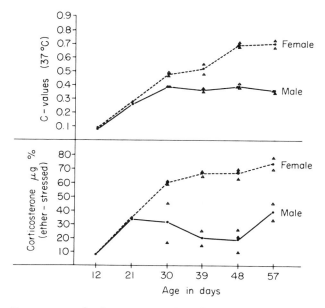

Fɪɢ. 14. Corticosterone-binding activity (C-values) and corticosterone levels in the serum of the developing rat. From Gala and Westphal (1965b).

to a maximum of approximately twice the male value (Keller *et al.*, 1966) at 7 weeks of age. The corticosterone concentration seems to follow a similar pattern although the determinations were made only in ether-stressed animals in this experiment. The observed differences in the CBG level between male and female rats are clearly in contrast to findings in normal adult men and women, who have about the same CBG level (DeMoor *et al.*, 1962).

Gonadectomy resulted in an increased CBG activity in the male rat (Gala and Westphal, 1965b) although the female level was not reached. No significant change was produced by the operation in the female. About the same C-values as in the castrated males were obtained when intact male rats were given estradiol (Fig. 15); again, no significant effect was seen in the female animals after estradiol injection.

The increased CBG activity in the castrated male rat suggested a suppressing influence of the androgenic hormone. This assumption was corroborated when it was found (Gala and Westphal, 1965b) that administration of testosterone to the normal female rat decreased the corticosterone-binding activity significantly (Fig. 16). There was no effect on CBG in the male.

In view of the difference between rats and humans in the female CBG

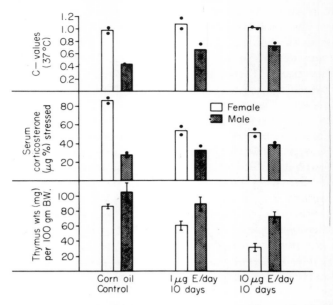

FIG. 15. Effect of estradiol (E) injection on corticosterone-binding activity (C-values) and other parameters in the rat. From data in Gala and Westphal (1965b).

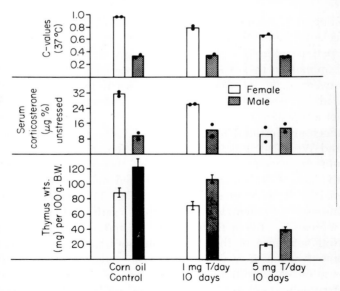

FIG. 16. Effect of testosterone (T) injection on corticosterone-binding activity (C-values) and other parameters in the rat. From data in Gala and Westphal (1965b).

level in relation to that in the male, it seemed of particular interest to measure the corticosterone–binding activity in the pregnant rat. In contrast to the considerable increase observed in the pregnant woman, only a very slight rise was found (Gala and Westphal, 1965a) in the rat during pregnancy. However, a sharp decline of the CBG activity occurred after parturition, and was evident on day 3 of lactation (see Figs. 1 and 2 in Gala and Westphal, 1965a). With the corticosterone level remaining the same or increasing, reduction of CBG would result in increased concentrations of unbound, i.e., physiologically active corticosteroid hormone, which is required in the initiation of lactation. This interpretation (Gala and Westphal, 1965a) would assign a role to CBG in the reproductive processes following parturition. During the subsequent weeks, the C-values returned to normal in the rats suckling four pups whereas the females with twelve pups continued to have low CBG activity. Since the corticosterone levels showed opposite trends in the two groups differing in the number of pups nursed (see Fig. 2 in Gala and Westphal, 1965a), it is apparent that a considerably higher concentration of unbound corticosteroid is present in the rats with the larger litters. This is reflected in the thymus weights, which show a continuous decrease in the mothers nursing twelve pups. Final normalization of all parameters determined takes place after weaning (see Fig. 3 in Gala and Westphal, 1965a).

Contrary to our findings in the rat, a manyfold increase of CBG activity during pregnancy was observed in the mouse, rabbit, and guinea pig (see Figs. 1–3 in Gala and Westphal, 1967). This was measured in all cases with radio-labeled corticosterone as well as cortisol; the differences between the affinities of the two corticosteroids to CBG are in accordance with the apparent association constants determined in these species (Westphal, 1967). Elevation of the corticosteroid-binding capacity during pregnancy has been reported (Seal and Doe, 1963) for mouse, rabbit, guinea pig, and other species. In most sera investigated, the increase in CBG activity is followed by a rise of the endogenous corticosteroid level (Gala and Westphal, 1967), indicating that the negative feedback mechanism controlling corticoid secretion apparently responds to the unbound portion of the corticosteroid hormone (Kawai and Yates, 1966). A particularly high rise was observed for the progesterone-binding activity in the pregnant guinea pig (Fig. 17) as had been independently reported (Seal and Doe, 1967). The investigations of high-affinity binding of steroid hormones during pregnancy in the guinea pig have been extended recently; it was found (Diamond *et al.*, 1969) that the binding activity increased not only for cortisol and progesterone but also for testosterone. Serum of pregnant guinea pigs thus forms a

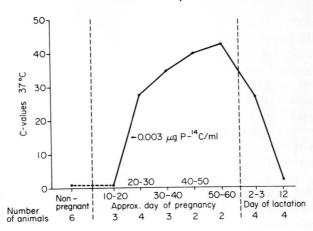

FIG. 17. Progesterone (P)-binding activity (C-values) in the serum of pregnant and lactating guinea pigs. (Gala and Westphal, 1966d.)

rich source for several proteins that interact strongly with certain steroid hormones.

Extirpation of the pituitary gland in the female rat results in a significant decrease of the CBG activity; administration of an anterior pituitary suspension brings the binding back to normal values (Gala and Westphal, 1966b). Systematic testing of pure pituitary hormones in the hypophysectomized female rat showed that growth hormone, prolactin, luteinizing hormone, and follicle-stimulating hormone were unable to restore the C-values to normal (Fig. 18). Only the thyroid-stimulating hormone normalized the corticosteroid-binding activity (Gala and Westphal, 1966b). This result is in accordance with observations from Fortier's laboratory (Labrie *et al.*, 1965), which indicate a decrease of rat CBG activity after thyroidectomy, and an increase by chronic administration of thyroxine. It is assumed that the thyroid-stimulating hormone exerts its effect on the CBG activity through stimulation of the thyroid gland.

On the basis of our observation that estrogen stimulation of CBG activity was abolished by hypophysectomy, and for other reasons, we had concluded that the effect of estradiol was mediated through TSH and the thyroid hormone (Gala and Westphal, 1966c). Experimental confirmation of this mechanism has been obtained recently by Labrie *et al.* (1968), who reported a pronounced rise of plasma TSH and thyroxin levels after estradiol injection, concurrent with increased CBG activity.

Early observations in male and female rats have shown that the CBG activity increases after adrenalectomy (Westphal *et al.*, 1962). Analysis

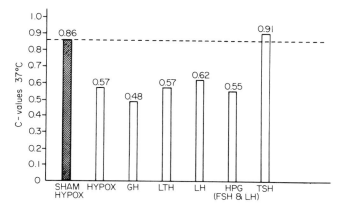

FIG. 18. CBG activity (C-values) in the hypophysectomized (Hypox) female rat treated with growth hormone (GH), prolactin (LTH), luteinizing hormone (LH), human pituitary gonadotropin (HPG), and thyroid-stimulating hormone (TSH). From data in Gala and Westphal (1966b).

of the time dependency of this reaction (Westphal *et al.*, 1963) showed that at least 24 hours passed after the operation before a change in the CBG level could be observed (see Fig. 2 in Westphal *et al.*, 1963). Rising C-values were seen after 48 and 72 hours, for interaction with corticosterone as well as with cortisol. The increase of the corticosterone-binding activity from the 24-hour to the 48-hour value is statistically highly significant as indicated by the fiducial limits (Fig. 19). After 3–4 days, a maximal C-value approximately twice normal is reached; this level remains essentially unchanged for at least 3 weeks. The same trend

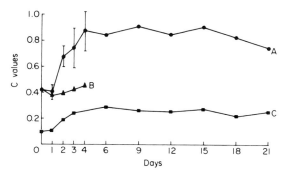

FIG. 19. Binding activity (C-values, 37°) for corticosterone (curve A) and for cortisol (curve C) in the serum of adrenalectomized rats up to 21 days after operation. Curve B shows the corticosterone binding activity for sham-adrenalectomized rats. The vertical lines in Curve A indicate fiducial limits at the 0.99 probability level. From Westphal *et al.* (1963).

obtains for cortisol binding; however, the more polar steroid interacts with a lower affinity (Table XI). Sham-adrenalectomized control rats had normal C-values. The observation of increased CBG activity in the rat after adrenalectomy has been confirmed (Seal and Doe, 1965b; Keller *et al.*, 1966).

The rise of CBG activity in the rat after adrenalectomy can be suppressed and reversed by administration of corticosterone (Westphal *et al.*, 1963). Injection of the massive dose of 5 mg of a microcrystalline suspension of this steroid for 4 days into the adrenalectomized male rat reduced the C-values to about half the normal level. This is the same CBG activity shown by the corticosterone-injected intact rat, which also has about half the corticosterone-binding activity of the normal saline-injected control. Table XVI shows the effect of daily injections of lower amounts of corticosteroids into adrenalectomized female and male rats (Gala and Westphal, 1966a). The CBG activity, which increased after adrenalectomy approximately 50% and 100% in the female and male animal, respectively, is reduced to control levels or lower. Cortisol is clearly more efficient than corticosterone in the suppression of the CBG activity.

The influence of adrenalectomy and of corticosteroid administration can best be interpreted as mediated through TSH and thyroid secretion. Adrenal insufficiency in rat and man has been reported to result in enhanced thyroid activity (Gabrilove and Soffer, 1950; Money, 1955; Grunt and Cunningham, 1965). Observations on depression of thyroid

TABLE XVI

EFFECT OF CORTICOSTERONE (B) AND CORTISOL (F) INJECTION ON CORTICOSTERONE-BINDING ACTIVITY (C-VALUES) OF ADRENALECTOMIZED (ADX) RATS[a]

Experimental group	Sex	Average C-values at 37° after injection of	
		Corticosterone[b]	Cortisol[b]
Control—Sham-adx; corn oil	F	1.04 (8)	0.97 (7)
	M	0.42 (8)	0.40 (8)
Adx—14 days; corn oil last 7 days	F	1.59 (6)	1.46 (8)
	M	0.78 (5)	0.87 (8)
Adx—14 days; 0.4 μg B or F/day last 7 days	F	1.54 (8)	0.99 (8)
	M	0.63 (7)	0.47 (8)
Adx—14 days; 2.0 μg B or F/day last 7 days	F	1.27 (8)	0.30 (7)
	M	0.38 (7)	0.26 (8)

[a] Data from Gala and Westphal, 1966a.
[b] Number of animals in parentheses.

gland secretion by increased corticosteroid levels (Money, 1955) has led to the conclusion (Ingbar and Freinkel, 1956) that corticosteroids decrease thyroid function by inhibiting TSH production. In view of the influence of thyroid hormone on CBG activity discussed previously, this concept of adrenocorticoid–thyroid relationship gives a reasonable explanation for the effects of lacking and of excessive corticosteroid concentration on the CBG level in the rat.

D. HIGH-AFFINITY BINDING OF TESTOSTERONE AND ESTRADIOL

In 1958 Daughaday published his observations on increased steroid binding affinity of serum proteins with decreasing concentration of the steroids. The figure summarizing the results (Fig. 1 in Daughaday, 1958) documented the existence of the specific cortisol or corticosterone-binding protein. The fact that this figure also revealed the presence of binding systems of different affinities for progesterone, as well as for testosterone, was largely ignored at the time. CBG was later identified as the serum protein that bound progesterone with high affinity (Sandberg *et al.*, 1966; Seal and Doe, 1966). The systematic search for a strong testosterone binder began later.

Since testosterone forms a relatively strong complex with serum albumin (see Table X), investigation of this association (Schellman *et al.*, 1954) predominated for many years. Although several observations were published in the literature (Slaunwhite and Sandberg, 1959; P. S. Chen *et al.*, 1961), including gel filtration studies (DeMoor *et al.*, 1962), which indicated testosterone binding to a serum protein other than albumin, it was not until 1965 that Mercier *et al.* (1966) reported results of a systematic investigation of a specific testosterone-binding serum protein with the electrophoretic properties of a β-globulin. Pearlman and Crépy (1967) applied a newly developed Sephadex gel equilibration procedure to the study of testosterone binding in normal and pregnancy serum. The presence of a protein with high binding affinity but low capacity for testosterone was recognized; its relative binding activity increased during pregnancy. A more detailed study (Pearlman *et al.*, 1967) showed that the testosterone-binding activity remained low and relatively constant during the normal menstrual cycle. A marked increase occurred during the first trimester of pregnancy; a gradual rise of the binding activity continued and reached at term 2–3 times the normal level. After delivery a rapid return to nonpregnancy levels was observed. In parallel, the peripheral testosterone level has been found to increase in late pregnancy, and return to normal after delivery (Demisch *et al.*, 1968). Administration of estrogens to patients with prostatic cancer resulted in elevated testosterone binding activity.

The close resemblance of these changes under various physiological conditions with alterations obtained in the CBG levels in comparable situations is obvious. However, the proteins responsible for binding of testosterone and for associating with corticosteroids differ not only in their electrophoretic properties, but can be separated (Guériguian and Pearlman, 1968) by chromatographic techniques; values for the Stokes molecular radius have been assessed by gel filtration to be about 47 Å and 36 Å for the testosterone-binding globulin and CBG, respectively.

Increased binding capacity of the testosterone-binding β-globulin in the pregnant woman has been confirmed (Mercier *et al.*, 1967; Murphy, 1968; Steeno *et al.*, 1968). It seems noteworthy that plasma of male cirrhotic patients had higher binding values than those of pooled male plasma (Murphy, 1968); it would be interesting to test whether this increase of the binding globulin is connected with elevated estrogen levels in these patients. The testosterone-binding affinity declined markedly with increasing temperature (Vermeulen and Verdonck, 1968a). Heating of plasma to 60° (Pearlman and Crépy, 1967; Steeno *et al.*, 1968) or to 57° (Vermeulen and Verdonck, 1968a) was found to destroy the testosterone-binding ability; activity was retained up to 45° (Vermeulen and Verdonck, 1968b). This represents further similarity to the behavior of CBG. Vermeulen and Verdonck (1968a) have reported some approximate data which may serve to assess the order of magnitude of plasma concentration and testosterone-binding affinity in the human (Table XVII).

TABLE XVII

APPROXIMATE CONCENTRATION OF BINDING SITES AND ASSOCIATION CONSTANT
OF THE TESTOSTERONE-BINDING β-GLOBULIN[a]

Subjects	Concentration $M \times 10^8$	Association constant at	
		25° $M^{-1} \times 10^{-8}$	37° $M^{-1} \times 10^{-8}$
Normal[b]	4–6	4–16	—
Estrogen treated[b]	19–31	1–12	—
Pregnant, first trimester	7–14	7–15	—
Pregnant, second trimester	14–36	6–10	—
Pregnant, third trimester	19–30	4–10	—
Plasma pool I	6.3	15	7.8
Plasma pool II	5.9	13	4.5
Plasma pool III	7.1	16	7.4

[a] Data condensed from Vermeulen and Verdonck, 1968a.
[b] No significant difference was observed between males and females.

At approximately the same time when a specific testosterone-binding serum protein was recognized, similar objectives were pursued in other laboratories in studies on nonalbumin binding of estradiol. Tavernetti *et al.* (1967) showed that albumin was not the only serum protein capable of strong association with estrogens. The same group (Rosenbaum *et al.*, 1966) obtained electrophoretic evidence for the presence of an estradiol-binding β-globulin in human plasma. More recent results from several laboratories (Mercier-Bodard and Baulieu, 1968; Murphy, 1968; Steeno *et al.*, 1968; Vermeulen and Verdonck, 1968a) agree in support of the conclusion that the testosterone-binding β-globulin and the estradiol-binding β-globulin are identical molecules to which the term steroid-binding β-globulin has been applied (Steeno *et al.*, 1968). The affinity of this serum protein for the two hormones is in clear distinction from the estradiol-binding receptor proteins of the uterus (see chapter by E. V. Jensen, Volume 2).

Since the steroid-binding β-globulin has not yet been isolated in homogeneous form, the inference of identity of the proteins associating with testosterone and with estradiol was obtained indirectly. Competition experiments (Steeno *et al.*, 1968) showed that testosterone was displaced by estradiol from the specific binding site present in the β-globulin. Estrone also showed competitive inhibition of testosterone binding, although to a lesser degree. Estriol was without influence on the testosterone complex with the steroid binding β-globulin. A number of steroids of similar molecular size, mostly containing a hydroxy group at carbon 17, displaced testosterone. Other steroids with twenty-one carbon atoms such as progesterone, corticosterone, and aldosterone did not interact with the β-globulin; this group also includes a number of reduced steroid metabolites. Murphy (1968) studied various steroids for their testosterone- and estradiol-displacing qualities and obtained generally similar results; she observed a weak effect of cholesterol. Additional displacement studies have been published recently from DeMoor's laboratory (Heyns *et al.*, 1969a). The presence of a 17β-hydroxy group is considered by Vermeulen and Verdonck (1968a) a requirement for association with the testosterone-binding globulin, as concluded from competition experiments with a large number of steroids. The rise of binding activity during pregnancy, which was discussed in relation to the testosterone-binding globulin, logically applies to the steroid-binding β-globulin (DeMoor *et al.*, 1969).

More direct evidence for the dual affinity of the globulin was obtained by Mercier-Bodard and Baulieu (1968) after removal of other binding proteins by DEAE-cellulose and Sephadex G-200 chromatography. Affinity constants were determined by equilibrium dialysis (Table

TABLE XVIII

Affinity of the Steroid-Binding β-Globulin for
Testosterone and Estradiol

| | Association constant | |
| | Testosterone M^{-1} | Estradiol M^{-1} |
Temperature		
4°	1.7×10^9 (1)[a]	0.6×10^9 (1)
—[b]	$\sim 10^8$ (2)	—
25°	4.5×10^8 (3)	1.3×10^8 (3)

[a] Numbers in parentheses refer to the following references: (1) Mercier-Bodard and Baulieu, 1968; (2) Mercier and Baulieu, 1968; (3) Pearlman *et al.*, 1969.

[b] Presumably room temperature.

XVIII). The binding of testosterone and estradiol appeared competitive for the same binding sites; the authors realize that this conclusion is not definite before a homogeneous protein can be studied, but it is considered the most reasonable assumption (Mercier and Baulieu, 1968). Independent work (Van Baelen *et al.*, 1968) on partial purification by similar types of chromatography and by ammonium sulfate precipitation also led to the conclusion of identity of the globulins binding the two hormones; a molecular weight of approximately 100,000 was assumed from elution volume in gel filtration. A value of 52,000 has been determined by Baulieu (1969). Pearlman *et al.* (1969) removed most of the albumin from testosterone-binding globulin; they found the affinity constant for estradiol about one-third that for testosterone (Table XVIII). There is thus agreement that testosterone is bound more strongly to the β-globulin than estradiol.

Preliminary studies on the chemical properties of the steroid-binding β-globulin (Pearlman *et al.*, 1969) suggest the importance of sulfhydryl and disulfide groups for the binding activity: reaction with N-ethyl-maleimide, p-mercuriphenylsulfonate, dithiothreitol, and sodium sulfite resulted in a marked reduction of testosterone-binding activity. Isoelectric focusing experiments (Van Baelen *et al.*, 1969) appeared to indicate microheterogeneity, which has been assumed to be caused by differences in sialic acid content. Enzymatic removal of sialic acid did not affect the estradiol-binding activity. This result is analogous to observations with TBG, CBG, and AAG, proteins in which the sialic acid content is also not necessary for full ability to interact with ligand hormones.

The testosterone-binding globulin has been utilized in several laboratories for sensitive determination of testosterone in plasma or serum by competitive protein binding (Horton *et al.*, 1967; Hallberg *et al.*, 1968; Mayes and Nugent, 1968; Murphy, 1968; Heyns *et al.*, 1969b).

It has been discussed that the CBG activity is under the regulatory control of the thyroid hormone. As an additional analogy between CBG and the steroid binding β-globulin, the testosterone-binding activity has been reported to be significantly increased in the serum of thyrotoxic male and female patients (Crépy *et al.*, 1967). The binding levels decreased or became normal after radical treatment of the hyperthyroid condition.

In view of the extensive observations on the presence of CBG activity in all vertebrate species investigated (Seal and Doe, 1966), it should be mentioned that the steroid binding β-globulin does not seem to be as omnipresent, according to findings by Murphy (1968) and by DeMoor *et al.* (1969). No activity was found in the rat, rabbit, dog, and duck, and no significant steroid association with the β-globulin was noted in seven other species of ruminants. A definite increase of high-affinity testosterone binding to many times normal values has been observed in the serum of pregnant guinea pigs (Diamond *et al.*, 1969).

E. Alpha-1-Acid Glycoprotein (AAG)

1. Properties of AAG Complexes with Progesterone and Other Steroid Hormones; Effect of Lipids

The low concentration of CBG in mammalian sera and the exacting isolation procedure limit the availability of this steroid-binding glycoprotein for intensive investigation of its binding properties in relation to chemical structure. A similar situation obtains for the steroid-binding β-globulin which has not yet been reported as a pure homogeneous protein. It seems of importance, therefore, that another serum glycoprotein, AAG (Gottschalk and Graham, 1966; Jeanloz, 1966), was found to interact fairly strongly with progesterone (Westphal *et al.*, 1961) and other steroids (Westphal, 1964), and that the complexes have considerable similarity with those of CBG. This is shown in Fig. 20 for the temperature dependency of the progesterone affinity to AAG; the resemblance to the binding strength of CBG-corticosteroid complexes at different temperatures (Fig. 2) is evident. Curve B in Fig. 20 illustrates for comparison the influence of temperature on the HSA-progesterone interaction, which is less pronounced. The effect of pH on the association constant of the progesterone-AAG complex (Fig. 21) again resembles closely the corresponding influence on the CBG complexes (Fig. 3); maximal binding occurs in both cases at about pH 8. These and other

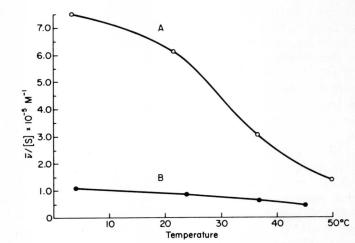

Fɪɢ. 20. Effect of temperature on the progesterone-binding affinity of AAG (curve A) and of HSA (curve B), in 0.05 *M* phosphate, pH 7.4. From Ganguly *et al.* (1967).

properties make AAG a useful protein for the general study of the relationship of chemical structure to steroid binding; the glycoprotein occurs in human serum in approximately 10–20 times the concentration of CBG (Table VI) and can be readily prepared in pure form (Ganguly *et al.*, 1967).

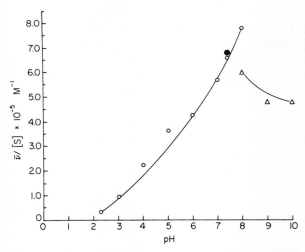

Fɪɢ. 21. Effect of pH on the progesterone-binding affinity of AAG, at 4°. ○ Citrate-phosphate, 0.05 *M*; ● phosphate, 0.05 *M*; Δ 2-amino-2-methyl-1,3-pro-panediol, 0.05 *M*. From Ganguly *et al.* (1967).

TABLE XIX

PHYSICOCHEMICAL PROPERTIES OF HUMAN AAG

Parameter	AAG
Sedimentation coefficient, $s_{20,w}^0$ (S)	3.08 (1)[a]
Diffusion coefficient, $D_{20,w}$ (cm² sec⁻¹ × 10⁷)	5.27 (2)
Partial specific volume, $\bar{v}$ (ml/gm)	0.675 (2)
Molecular weight	41,000 (3)
Frictional ratio, f/fo	1.78 (2)
Electrophoretic mobility at pH 8.6 (cm² V⁻¹ sec⁻¹) × 10⁵	−6.2 (1)
$E_{1\,cm}^{1\%}$ at 278 nm	9.33 (4)
Carbohydrate (%)	41.9[b] (1)
Nitrogen (%)	9.8 (1)

[a] Numbers in parentheses refer to the following references: (1) Ganguly *et al.*, 1967; (2) Schultze and Heremans, 1966; (3) Winzler, 1960; (4) Kerkay and Westphal, 1969.

[b] Hexosamine calculated as acetylhexosamine.

The final AAG preparations obtained from human plasma after a series of fractionation steps (Ganguly *et al.*, 1967) were homogeneous by several criteria applied. The physicochemical properties agreed with those reported in the literature (Table XIX). The amino acid (Table XX) and carbohydrate analysis (Table XXI) gave values compatible with those determined in other laboratories. Despite this degree of purity, which satisfied the usual criteria, it was not possible to obtain consistently high and reproducible affinity constants for the interaction with progesterone. One of the reasons for this behavior was found to be the presence of a lipid soluble contamination, which adhered tenaciously to AAG, and

TABLE XX

AMINO ACID COMPOSITION OF HUMAN AAG[a,b]

Residue	No. per 10⁵ gm	Residue	No. per 10⁵ gm
Asp	63.1	Met	3.7
Thr	47.6	Ile	25.8
Ser	19.7	Leu	42.4
Glu	86.5	Tyr	31.8
Pro	22.6	Phe	27.8
Gly	20.2	Lys	40.1
Ala	26.0	His	8.6
Val	23.3[c]	Arg	25.1
Cys	11.8	Try	9.8[c]

[a] Residues per 100,000 gm.

[b] From Ganguly and Westphal, 1968b. For values from other laboratories see Jeanloz, 1966.

[c] Value from Ganguly *et al.*, 1967.

TABLE XXI
CARBOHYDRATE COMPOSITION OF HUMAN AAG[a]

Carbohydrate	Percent
Hexose	14.5
Acetylhexosamine	14.5
Sialic Acid	11.6
Fucose	1.3
	41.9

[a] Data from Ganguly *et al.*, 1967. For values from other laboratories see Jeanloz, 1966.

which could be removed (Ganguly *et al.*, 1967) by precipitation of the glycoprotein from solution in acetate buffer (pH 4.1) with an alcohol–acetone mixture (9:1, v/v). Another factor that influenced the binding affinity in an unpredictable manner was the presence of small amounts of certain heavy metal ions that inhibited the complex formation (Kerkay and Westphal, 1969). Dialysis of AAG against EDTA solution, or inclusion of EDTA in the equilibrium dialysis system for determination of the binding affinity eliminated the effect. All work with AAG was therefore done with carefully deionized water.

Removal of the lipid contamination from otherwise pure AAG raised the association constant of the progesterone complex three- to eight-fold, depending on the quality of the original preparation. A final reproducible value of $k \cong 10^6 M^{-1}$ at 4° was obtained. The number of binding sites for progesterone rose from a fractional value, e.g., $n = 0.2$ to approximately $n = 1$. This indicated that the primary binding site in about 80% of the molecules was occupied by the lipid material. The influence of the lipid contamination on k and n was reversible (Ganguly *et al.*, 1967).

Table XXII gives the number of binding sites, the apparent association constants at 4° and 37°, and thermodynamic data for the interactions between pure, delipidated AAG and several steroid hormones (Kerkay and Westphal, 1968). It is evident that the number of primary binding sites (see figures in Kerkey and Westphal, 1968) equals approximately one in all complexes with Δ^4-3-ketosteroids, analyzed at both 4° and 37°. The AAG complexes resemble in this respect the steroid associations with CBG. The affinity constants, and consequently the free energies of binding, decrease with increasing number of hydroxy groups in the molecules. The series listed in Table XXII is thus a good example for the validity of the polarity rule; hydrophobic interactions play the predominant role in the associations.

A different type of complex is formed between AAG and estradiol. The

TABLE XXII

NUMBERS OF BINDING SITES, n_1, APPARENT ASSOCIATION CONSTANTS, k_1, AND
THERMODYNAMIC PARAMETERS OF STEROID-α_1-ACID GLYCOPROTEIN COMPLEXES[a,b]

Steroid	Temp.	n_1	$k_1 \times 10^{-5}$ (M^{-1})	$nk \times 10^{-5}$ (M^{-1})	$\Delta F°$ (kcal/ mole)	$\Delta H°$ (kcal/ mole)	$\Delta S°$ (cal/ mole/ degree)
Progesterone	4	0.98	9.0	8.9	−7.5	−4.8	10
	37	1.05	3.5	3.5	−7.9	—	—
Testosterone	4	0.78	7.3	6.0	−7.3	−4.0	12
	37	0.74	3.0	2.4	−7.8	—	—
Cortexone	4	1.12	2.2	2.3	−6.7	−3.4	12
	37	1.11	1.0	0.88	−7.1	—	—
Corticosterone	4	1.27	0.87	1.0	−6.0	−4.8	5
	37	1.35	0.32	0.37	−6.2	—	—
Cortisol	4	1.24	0.16	0.20	−5.5	−1.5	14
	37	—	—	0.15	−5.9	—	—
Estradiol	4	7	0.14	1.0	−6.2	−2.7	13
	37	3	0.19	0.59	−6.8	—	—
Progesterone–HSA[c]	4	2.1	1.0	2.1	−6.3[d]	−4.9	9
	37	2.6	0.46	1.2	−6.6[d]	—	—

[a] 0.05 M phosphate buffer, pH 7.4.

[b] From Kerkay and Westphal, 1968.

[c] Parameters of the progesterone–HSA complex are included for comparison.

[d] Value for k_1.

number of primary binding sites is significantly greater than one (see Fig. 5 in Kerkay and Westphal, 1968) although an accurate value has not been determined because of the limited solubility of the estrogenic hormone. The difference between the Δ^4-3-ketosteroid binding site and the site for estradiol is also evident from competition studies. The Δ^4-3-ketosteroids investigated, i.e., corticosterone and testosterone, compete for the progesterone-binding site. Estradiol does not show competitive inhibition of the association between progesterone and AAG (see Table III in Kerkay and Westphal, 1968).

2. Thermodynamic Data; Effect of Heavy Metals, of Solvent Environment, and of Chemical Modifications of AAG on Steroid Interaction

The free energy changes, $\Delta F°$, of the steroid-AAG complexes listed in Table XXII, and also that of the progesterone–HSA complex, are composed of a negative enthalpy change, $\Delta H°$, and a positive entropy change, $\Delta S°$, according to $\Delta F° = \Delta H° - T\Delta S°$, where T is the absolute temperature. The positive entropy changes may be interpreted by the assumption, first advanced by Klotz (1950), that the highly structured hydration water is displaced and randomized as solvent water in the complex formation. Details of such a mechanism have been discussed elsewhere (Ganguly and Westphal, 1968a).

If one compares the thermodynamic data of Table XXII with corresponding values for the CBG complexes (Table XV), the much higher free energies of the latter are noticeable. The $\Delta F°$ values are composed of a very high negative enthalpy change, in association with a negative change of entropy. These thermodynamic data (Table XV) are interpreted as indicative of a very tight fit of the interacting molecules, so that the enthalpy is drastically reduced. The total order is increased, and a negative entropy change is the consequence. These results provide the thermodynamic basis for an understanding of the different binding affinities of steroid–protein complexes at the level of molecular structure.

Investigation of the inhibitory effect of heavy metal ions on the progesterone–AAG complex showed that out of a large number of metals studied, four cations had very strong activity (Kerkay and Westphal, 1969). When even distribution of the metal ions throughout the dialysis system is assumed, the presence of four ions of Hg^{++}, Ag^+, Cu^+, and Fe^{++} per molecule AAG decreased the association constant (4°) of the progesterone–AAG complex by 81%, 31%, 29%, and 12%, respectively. The effect was clearly reversible by EDTA. A slight reduction of the number of binding sites is indicated in the Scatchard plots when the three more active metals are present (see Figs. 2–5 in Kerkay and Westphal, 1969). For this and other reasons, the inhibition does not appear to be competitive; it is rather assumed that an allosteric mechanism is involved. It is not known whether the metal ions interact with the disulfide groups or with other groupings of the AAG molecule.

Only brief mention will be made of observations (Ganguly and Westphal, 1968a) on the influence of neutral salts and other perturbants on the stability of the steroid–AAG complexes because the phenomena are considered outside the scope of this article. A manyfold increase of the apparent binding affinity of the complexes is obtained by relatively high concentrations of Na_2SO_4, $(NH_4)_2SO_4$, NaCl, or other salts that generally stabilize the conformational structure of globular proteins. Perturbants that are known to destabilize globular proteins, e.g., LiBr, $CaCl_2$, or urea, decrease the apparent stability of the complex. This is reflected in the viscosity of AAG in different solvent environments. For details of these solvent effects on the steroid–AAG interactions see the original publication (Ganguly and Westphal, 1968a).

Our knowledge concerning the relationship of the chemical structure of AAG to its steroid-binding ability is fragmentary. It has been mentioned that complete removal of sialic acid by enzyme action does not affect the association with progesterone (Ganguly and Westphal, 1968a). Reduction of the disulfide linkages results in loss of the progesterone-binding affinity; reoxidation by air oxygen restores the original activity (Ganguly and Westphal, 1968b). Alkylation of the thiol groups of reduced AAG by iodoacetic acid or its amide abolishes progesterone binding while the antigenic properties are maintained. Modification of the ϵ-amino group of lysine leads to virtual disappearance of steroid-binding affinity; partial removal of the modifying substituent causes partial return of the activity. The antigenicity is reduced or completely lost, depending on the nature of the modifying reaction. The results show that antigenicity and steroid-binding affinity are independent properties of the AAG molecule (Ganguly and Westphal, 1968b).

IV. SYNOPSIS

What is the physiological significance of the reversible associations between the circulating hormones and their serum protein binders? Early assumptions had emphasized a transport function inasmuch as the proteins carried the hormones in a water-soluble form even if their concentration would exceed their solubility in water. However, this solubilization principle cannot be of major importance because the hormones occur generally in concentrations far below their aqueous solubility.

The more vital significance of the protein interaction with steroid—and other—hormones is now generally accepted to be control of hormonal distribution and function. The hormone–protein complex is biologically inactive; spontaneous dissociation makes the unbound, active form readily available. Since the major percentages of the hormones discussed are protein-bound, a biologically inert storage system is provided that can deliver the active compounds when and where they are needed. Such a system may be compared to a pH buffer which also carries the neutralizing agent in an inert, "neutral" form.

Suppression of hormonal activity by protein binding results from a reduction of the chemical activity of the low-molecular hormone. Another consequence of the reduced chemical activity is an altered distribution to the various body compartments; metabolism and excretion are decreased. These phenomena may also be interpreted as the result of competition of different types of binding sites for the hormone.

Protein interaction may protect the hormone against chemical or enzymatic attack. For example, some steroid hormones, such as cortisol, are not stable in aqueous solution under ordinary conditions, even if they are not radio-labeled. Cortisol breaks down to several products. The degradation is suppressed by association with serum proteins. Conversely, the corticosteroid hormone will protect the structure of CBG, a protein highly labile to heat denaturation.

There are other possible functions—these more speculative. On the basis of observations on accelerated steroid permeation through dialysis membranes when binding proteins are present on the steroid-free side, it seems possible that the binding proteins facilitate entrance of the hormones from the secretory tissues into the blood capillaries, possibly with participation of the lymph system. On the other hand, macromolecules of molecular weight even larger than the known binding proteins are able to penetrate capillary walls. It must also be considered therefore that the binding proteins fulfill a real carrier function at the secretory organs.

Similar possibilities exist at the other end of the functional pathway, at the receptor tissue. We do not know whether the hormones pass the nuclear membrane to reach the receptor sites after dissociation from the binding protein, or whether the protein carrier interacts with nuclear receptor structures and thus contributes to the specificity of the target site uptake of the hormone. The observed control of the quaternary structure of rat CBG by corticosterone stimulates such speculation. Evidently, the polymeric forms of the CBG would not permeate as readily as the monomeric steroid complex.

REFERENCES

Andreoli, M., Robbins, J., Rall, J. E., and Berman, M. (1965). *In* "Current Topics in Thyroid Research" (C. Cassano and M. Andreoli, eds.), p. 635. Academic Press, New York.

Antoniades, H. N., and Gershoff, S. N. (1966). *Endocrinology* **78**, 1079.

Baulieu, E. E. (1969). Personal communication.

Beigelman, P. M., Antoniades, H. N., Goetz, F. C., Renold, A. E., Oncley, J. L., and Thorn, G. W. (1956). *Metab., Clin. Exptl.* **5**, 44.

Bennhold, H. (1932). *Ergeb. Inn. Med. Kinderheilk.* **42**, 273.

Bennhold, H. (1966). *In* "Transport Function of Plasma Proteins" (P. Desgrez and P. M. DeTraverse, eds.), p. 1. Elsevier, Amsterdam.

Bischoff, F., and Pilhorn, H. R. (1948). *J. Biol. Chem.* **174**, 663.

Blecher, M. (1964). *Biochim. Biophys. Acta* **93**, 158.

Blumberg, B. S., and Warren, L. (1961). *Biochim. Biophys. Acta* **50**, 90.

Braverman, L. E., and Ingbar, S. H. (1965). *Endocrinology* **76**, 547.

Braverman, L. E., and Ingbar, S. H. (1967). *J. Clin. Endocrinol. Metab.* **27**, 389.
Braverman, L. E., Dawber, N. A., and Ingbar, S. H. (1966). *J. Clin. Invest.* **45**, 1273.
Braverman, L. E., Foster, A. E., and Ingbar, S. H. (1967). *J. Clin. Endocrinol. Metab.* **27**, 227.
Brook, A. H., and Share, L. (1966). *Endocrinology* **78**, 779.
Brunelli, B. (1934). *Arch. Intern. Pharmacodyn.* **49**, 262.
Bush, I. E. (1957). *Ciba Found. Colloq. Endocrinol.* **11**, 263.
Chader, G. J., and Westphal, U. (1968a). *J. Biol. Chem.* **243**, 928.
Chader, G. J., and Westphal, U. (1968b). *Biochemistry* **7**, 4272.
Chen, P. S., Mills, I. H., and Bartter, F. C. (1961). *J. Endocrinol.* **23**, 129.
Chen, R. F. (1967). *J. Biol. Chem.* **242**, 173.
Crépy, O., Dray, F., and Sebaoun, J. (1967). *Compt. Rend.* **264**, 2651.
Daughaday, W. H. (1956a). *J. Clin. Invest.* **35**, 1428.
Daughaday, W. H. (1956b). *J. Lab. Clin. Med.* **48**, 799.
Daughaday, W. H. (1958). *J. Clin. Invest.* **37**, 511.
Daughaday, W. H. (1959). *Physiol. Rev.* **39**, 885.
Daughaday, W. H., and Mariz, I. K. (1961). *Metab., Clin. Exptl.* **10**, 936.
Daughaday, W. H., Holloszy, J., and Mariz, I. K. (1961). *J. Clin. Endocrinol. Metab.* **21**, 53.
Davidson, E. T., DeVenuto, F., and Westphal, U. (1962). *Endocrinology* **71**, 893.
Demisch, K., Grant, J. K., and Black, W. (1968). *J. Endocrinol.* **42**, 477.
DeMoor, P., Heirwegh, K., Heremans, J. F., and Declerck-Raskin, M. (1962). *J. Clin. Invest.* **41**, 816.
DeMoor, P., Steeno, O., Heyns, W., and Van Baelen, H. (1969). *Ann. Endocrinol. (Paris)* **30**, 233.
Diamond, M., Rust, N., and Westphal, U. (1969). *Endocrinology* **84**, 1143.
Doe, R. P., Fernandes, R., and Seal, U. S. (1964). *J. Clin. Endocrinol. Metab.* **24**, 1029.
Doe, R. P., Mellinger, G. T., Swaim, W. R., and Seal, U. S. (1967). *J. Clin. Endocrinol. Metab.* **27**, 1081.
Edsall, J. T., and Wyman, J. (1958). "Biophysical Chemistry," Vol. 1, Chap. 11. Academic Press, New York.
Eik-Nes, K., Schellman, J. A., Lumry, R., and Samuels, L. T. (1954). *J. Biol. Chem.* **206**, 411.
Gabrilov, J. L., and Soffer, L. J. (1950). *J. Clin. Invest.* **29**, 814.
Gala, R. R., and Westphal, U. (1965a). *Endocrinology* **76**, 1079.
Gala, R. R., and Westphal, U. (1965b). *Endocrinology* **77**, 841.
Gala, R. R., and Westphal, U. (1966a). *Endocrinology* **78**, 277.
Gala, R. R., and Westphal, U. (1966b). *Endocrinology* **79**, 55.
Gala, R. R., and Westphal, U. (1966c). *Endocrinology* **79**, 67.
Gala, R. R., and Westphal, U. (1966d). Unpublished data.
Gala, R. R., and Westphal, U. (1967). *Acta Endocrinol.* **55**, 47.
Ganguly, M., and Westphal, U. (1968a). *J. Biol. Chem.* **243**, 6130.
Ganguly, M., and Westphal, U. (1968b). *Biochim. Biophys. Acta* **170**, 309.
Ganguly, M., Carnighan, R. H., and Westphal, U. (1967). *Biochemistry* **6**, 2803.
Gershoff, S. N., Huber, A. M., and Antoniades, H. N. (1966). *Metab., Clin. Exptl.* **15**, 325.
Giorgio, N. A., Jr., and Tabachnick, M. (1968). *J. Biol. Chem.* **243**, 2247.
Gjedde, F. (1967a). *Acta Physiol. Scand.* **70**, 57.

Gjedde, F. (1967b). *Acta Physiol. Scand.* **70,** 69.
Goldsmith, R. E., Rauh, J. L., Kloth, R., and Dahlgren, J. (1967). *Acta Endocrinol.* **54,** 494.
Gordon, A. H., Gross, J., O'Connor, D., and Pitt-Rivers, R., (1952). *Nature* **169,** 19.
Gottschalk, A., and Graham, E. R. B. (1966). In "The Proteins" (H. Neurath, ed.), 2nd ed., Vol. 4, p. 95. Academic Press, New York.
Grunt, J. A., and Cunningham, R. D. (1965). *Acta Endocrinol.* **48,** 556.
Guériguian, J. L., and Pearlman, W. H. (1968). *J. Biol. Chem.* **243,** 5226.
Guériguian, J. L., Pavard, J., and Crépy, O. (1969). *Ann. Endocrinol.* (*Paris*) **30,** 211.
Hadden, D. R., and Prout, T. E. (1964). *Nature* **202,** 1342.
Hallberg, M. C., Zorn, E. M., and Wieland, R. G. (1968). *Steroids* **12,** 241.
Heyns, W., Van Baelen, H., and DeMoor, P. (1969a). *J. Endocrinol.* **43,** 67.
Heyns, W., Verhoeven, G., Van Baelen, H., and DeMoor, P. (1969b). *Ann. Endocrinol.* (*Paris*) **30,** 153.
Hoffmann, W., and Westphal, U. (1969). *Anal. Biochem.* **32,** 48.
Hoffmann, W., Forbes, T. R., and Westphal, U. (1969). *Endocrinology* **85,** 778.
Hooker, C. W., and Forbes, T. R. (1947). *Endocrinology* **41,** 158.
Horton, R., Kato, T., and Sherins, R. (1967). *Steroids* **10,** 245.
Ingbar, S. H. (1958). *Endocrinology* **63,** 256.
Ingbar, S. H., and Freinkel, N. (1956). *Metab., Clin. Exptl.* **5,** 652.
Ingbar, S. H., and Freinkel, N. (1960). *Recent Progr. Hormone Res.* **16,** 353.
Jeanloz, R. W. (1966). In "Glycoproteins" (A. Gottschalk, ed.), p. 362. American Elsevier, Amsterdam-London-New York.
Jones, J. E., and Seal, U. S. (1967). *J. Clin. Endocrinol. Metab.* **27,** 1521.
Kawai, A., and Yates, F. E. (1966). *Endocrinology* **79,** 1040.
Keller, N., Sendelbeck, L. R., Richardson, U. I., Moore, C., and Yates, F. E. (1966). *Endocrinology* **79,** 884.
Kerkay, J., and Westphal, U. (1968). *Biochim. Biophys. Acta* **170,** 324.
Kerkay, J., and Westphal, U. (1969). *Arch. Biochem. Biophys.* **129,** 480.
Klotz, I. M. (1950). *Cold Spring Harbor Symp. Quant. Biol.* **14,** 97.
Kripalani, K. J., and Sorby, D. L. (1967). *J. Pharm. Sci.* **56,** 687.
Kumahara, Y., Miyai, K., Itoh, K. F., and Abe, H. (1968). *Proc. 3rd Intern. Congr. Endocrinol., Mexico City, 1968* Intern. Congr. Ser. No. 157, p. 2. Excerpta Med. Found., Amsterdam.
Labrie, F., Raynaud, J. P., and Fortier, C. (1965). *Proc. 6th Pan American Congr. Endocrinol., Mexico City, 1965* Intern. Congr. Ser. No. 99, Abstr. No. 109. Excerpta Med. Found., Amsterdam.
Labrie, F., Pelletier, G., Labrie, R., Ho-Kim, M. A., Delgado, A., MacIntosh, B., and Fortier, C. (1968). *Ann. Endocrinol.* (*Paris*) **29,** 29.
Launay, M. P. (1966). *Can. J. Biochem.* **44,** 1657.
Lutz, J. H., and Gregerman, R. I. (1969). *J. Clin. Endocrinol. Metab.* **29,** 487.
Marshall, J. S., and Pensky, J. (1969). *J. Clin. Invest.* **48,** 508.
Mayes, D., and Nugent, C. A. (1968). *J. Clin. Endocrinol. Metab.* **28,** 1169.
Mercier, C., and Baulieu, E. E. (1968). *Ann. Endocrinol.* (*Paris*) **29,** No. 1 bis, Suppl., 159.
Mercier, C., Alfsen, A., and Baulieu, E. E. (1966). *Proc. 2nd Symp. Steroid Hormones, Ghent, 1965* Intern. Congr. Ser. No. 101, p. 212. Excerpta Med. Found., Amsterdam.
Mercier, C., Alfsen, A., and Baulieu, E. E. (1967). *Compt. Rend.* **264,** 122.

Mercier-Bodard, C., and Baulieu, E. E. (1968). *Compt. Rend.* **267**, 804.
Meyer, C. J., Layne, D. S., Tait, J. F., and Pincus, G. (1961). *J. Clin. Invest.* **40**, 1663.
Money, W. L. (1955). *Brookhaven Symp. Biol.* **7**, 137.
Muldoon, T. G., and Westphal, U. (1967). *J. Biol. Chem.* **242**, 5636.
Murphy, B. E. P. (1968). *Can. J. Biochem.* **46**, 299.
Musa, B. U., Doe, R. P., and Seal, U. S. (1967). *J. Clin. Endocrinol. Metab.* **27**, 1463.
Musa, B. U., Kumar, R. S., and Dowling, J. T. (1969). *J. Clin. Endocrinol. Metab.* **29**, 667.
Nikolai, T. F., and Seal, U. S. (1966). *J. Clin. Endocrinol.* **26**, 835.
Nikolai, T. F., and Seal, U. S. (1967). *J. Clin. Endocrinol.* **27**, 1515.
Oppenheimer, J. H., and Bernstein, G. (1965). In "Current Topics of Thyroid Research" (C. Cassano and M. Andreoli, eds.), p. 674. Academic Press, New York.
Oppenheimer, J. H., and Surks, M. I. (1964). *J. Clin. Endocrinol. Metab.* **24**, 785.
Oppenheimer, J. H., and Werner, S. C. (1966). *J. Clin. Endocrinol. Metab.* **26**, 715.
Oppenheimer, J. H., Squef, R., Surks, M. I., and Hauer, H. (1963). *J. Clin. Invest.* **42**, 1769.
Oppenheimer, J. H., Surks, M. I., Smith, J. C., and Squef, R. (1965). *J. Biol. Chem.* **240**, 173.
Oppenheimer, J. H., Martinez, M., and Bernstein, G. (1966). *J. Lab. Clin. Med.* **67**, 500.
Pearlman, W. H., and Crépy, O. (1967). *J. Biol. Chem.* **242**, 182.
Pearlman, W. H., Crépy, O., and Murphy, M. (1967). *J. Clin. Endocrinol. Metab.* **27**, 1012.
Pearlman, W. H., Fong, I. F. F., and Tou, J. H. (1969). *J. Biol. Chem.* **244**, 1373.
Purdy, R. H., Woeber, K. A., Holloway, M. T., and Ingbar, S. H. (1965). *Biochemistry* **4**, 1888.
Randle, P. J., and Taylor, K. W. (1958). *J. Endocrinol.* **17**, 387.
Robbins, J. (1956). *Arch. Biochem. Biophys.* **63**, 461.
Robbins, J., and Rall, J. E. (1957). *Recent Progr. Hormone Res.* **13**, 161.
Robbins, J., and Rall, J. E. (1960). *Physiol. Rev.* **40**, 415.
Robbins, J., and Rall, J. E. (1967). In "Hormones in Blood" (C. H. Gray and A. L. Bacharach, eds.), 2nd rev. ed., Vol. 1, pp. 383–490. Academic Press, New York.
Robbins, J., Petermann, M. L., and Rall, J. E. (1955). *J. Biol. Chem.* **212**, 403.
Roberts, S., and Szego, C. M. (1953). *Physiol. Rev.* **33**, 593.
Rosenbaum, W., Christy, N. P., and Kelly, W. G. (1966). *J. Clin. Endocrinol. Metab.* **26**, 1399.
Rosenthal, H. E., Slaunwhite, W. R., Jr., and Sandberg, A. A. (1969). *J. Clin. Endocrinol. Metab.* **29**, 352.
Ross, J. E., and Tapley, D. F. (1966). *Endocrinology* **79**, 493.
Rudman, D., and Kendall, F. E. (1957). *J. Clin. Invest.* **36**, 538.
Ryan, M. T. (1968). *Arch. Biochem. Biophys.* **126**, 407.
Saifer, A., and Goldman, L. (1961). *J. Lipid Res.* **2**, 268.
Salvatore, G., Andreoli, M., and Roche, J. (1966). In "Transport Function of Plasma Proteins" (P. Desgrez and P. M. DeTraverse, eds.), p. 57. Elsevier, Amsterdam.
Sandberg, A. A., Slaunwhite, W. R., Jr., and Antoniades, H. N. (1957). *Recent Progr. Hormone Res.* **13**, 209.

Sandberg, A. A., Slaunwhite, W. R., Jr., and Carter, A. C. (1960). *J. Clin. Invest.* **39,** 1914.
Sandberg, A. A., Rosenthal, H., Schneider, S. L., and Slaunwhite, W. R., Jr., (1966). *In* "Steroid Dynamics" (G. Pincus, T. Nakao, and J. F. Tait, eds.), p. 1. Academic Press, New York.
Schellman, J. A., Lumry, R., and Samuels, L. T. (1954). *J. Am. Chem. Soc.* **76,** 2808.
Scholtan, W., Schlossmann, K., and Rosenkranz, H. (1968). *Arzneimittel-Forsch.* **18,** 767.
Schultze, H. E., and Heremans, J. F. (1966). "Molecular Biology of Human Proteins," Vol. 1. Elsevier, Amsterdam.
Seal, U. S., and Doe, R. P. (1962a). *Cancer Chemotherapy Rept.* **16,** 329.
Seal, U. S., and Doe, R. P. (1962b). *J. Biol. Chem.* **237,** 3136.
Seal, U. S., and Doe, R. P. (1963). *Endocrinology* **73,** 371.
Seal, U. S., and Doe, R. P. (1965a). *Proc. 2nd Intern. Congr. Endocrinol., London, 1964* Intern. Congr. Ser. No. 83, p. 325. Excerpta Med. Found., Amsterdam.
Seal, U. S., and Doe, R. P. (1965b). *Steroids* **5,** 827.
Seal, U. S., and Doe, R. P. (1966). *In* "Steroid Dynamics" (G. Pincus, T. Nakao, and J. F. Tait, eds.), p. 63. Academic Press, New York.
Seal, U. S., and Doe, R. P. (1967). *Proc. 2nd Intern. Congr. Hormonal Steroids, Milan, 1966* Internatl. Congr. Ser. No. 132, p. 697. Excerpta Med. Found., Amsterdam.
Slaunwhite, W. R., Jr., and Sandberg, A. A. (1959). *J. Clin. Invest.* **38,** 384.
Slaunwhite, W. R., Jr., Schneider, S., Wissler, F. C., and Sandberg, A. A. (1966). *Biochemistry* **5,** 3527.
Smith, M. W., and Thorn, N. A. (1965). *J. Endocrinol.* **32,** 141.
Steeno, O., Heyns, W., Van Baelen, H., and DeMoor, P. (1968). *Ann. Endocrinol.* (*Paris*) **29,** 141.
Steiner, R. F., Roth, J., and Robbins, J. (1966). *J. Biol. Chem.* **241,** 560.
Steinhardt, J., and Beychok, S. (1964). *In* "The Proteins" (H. Neurath, ed.), 2nd ed., Vol. 2, p. 139. Academic Press, New York.
Sterling, K. (1964a). *Mayo Clin. Proc.* **39,** 586.
Sterling, K. (1964b). *J. Clin. Invest.* **43,** 1721.
Sterling, K., and Brenner, M. A. (1966). *J. Clin. Invest.* **45,** 153.
Sterling, K., and Tabachnick, M. (1961). *J. Biol. Chem.* **236,** 2241.
Sterling, K., Hamada, S., Newman, E. S., Brenner, M. A., and Inada, M. (1967). *Clin. Res.* **15,** 457.
Stouffer, J. E., and Hsu, J. S. (1966). *Biochemistry* **5,** 1195.
Szego, C. M., and Roberts, S. (1953). *Recent Progr. Hormone Res.* **8,** 419.
Tabachnick, M. (1967). *J. Biol. Chem.* **242,** 1646.
Tata, J. R. (1961). *Clin. Chim. Acta* **6,** 819.
Tavernetti, R. R., Rosenbaum, W., Kelly, W. G., Christy, N. P., and Roginsky, M. S. (1967). *J. Clin. Endocrinol. Metab.* **27,** 920.
Taylor, K. W. (1967). *In* "Hormones in Blood" (C. H. Gray and A. L. Bacharach, eds.), 2nd rev. ed., Vol. 1, pp. 47–81. Academic Press, New York.
Therriault, D. G., and Taylor, J. F. (1960). *Biochem. Biophys. Res. Commun.* **3,** 560.
Thorson, S. C., Tauxe, W. N., and Taswell, H. F. (1966). *J. Clin. Endocrinol. Metab.* **26,** 181.
Tritsch, G. L. (1968). *Arch. Biochem. Biophys.* **127,** 384.
Tritsch, G. L., and Tritsch, N. E. (1963). *J. Biol. Chem.* **238,** 138.

Tritsch, G. L., and Tritsch, N. E. (1965). *J. Biol. Chem.* **240**, 3789.

Upton, G. V., and Bondy, P. K. (1958). *Arch. Biochem. Biophys.* **78**, 197.

Van Baelen, H., Heyns, W., Schonne, E., and DeMoor, P. (1968). *Ann. Endocrinol.* (*Paris*) **29**, 153.

Van Baelen, H., Heyns, W., and DeMoor, P. (1969). *Ann. Endocrinol.* (*Paris*) **30**, 199.

Vermeulen, A., and Verdonck, L. (1968a). *Steroids* **11**, 609.

Vermeulen, A., and Verdonck, L. (1968b). *Ann. Endocrinol.* (*Paris*) **29**, *Suppl.*, 149.

von Werder, K., Schwarz, K., and Scriba, P. C. (1968a). *Klin. Wochschr.* **46**, 940.

von Werder, K., Kluge, F., Schwarz, K., and Scriba, P. C. (1968b). *Klin. Wochschr.* **46**, 1028.

Westphal, U. (1961). *In* "Mechanism of Action of Steroid Hormones" (C. A. Villee and L. L. Engel, eds.), p. 33. Pergamon Press, Oxford.

Westphal, U. (1964). *J. Am. Oil Chemists' Soc.* **41**, 481.

Westphal, U. (1966). *Z. Physiol. Chem.* **346**, 243.

Westphal, U. (1967). *Arch. Biochem. Biophys.* **118**, 556.

Westphal, U. (1969). *Methods Enzymol.* **15**, 761.

Westphal, U., and Ashley, B. D. (1958). *J. Biol. Chem.* **233**, 57.

Westphal, U., and Ashley, B. D. (1959). *J. Biol. Chem.* **234**, 2847.

Westphal, U., and Ashley, B. D. (1962). *J. Biol. Chem.* **237**, 2763.

Westphal, U., and DeVenuto, F. (1966). *Biochim. Biophys. Acta* **115**, 187.

Westphal, U., and Forbes, T. R. (1963). *Endocrinology* **73**, 504.

Westphal, U., and Harding, G. B. (1969). Unpublished results.

Westphal, U., Stets, J. F., and Priest, S. G. (1953). *Arch. Biochem Biophys.* **43**, 463.

Westphal, U., Ashley, B. D., and Selden, G. L. (1958). *J. Am. Chem. Soc.* **80**, 5135.

Westphal, U., Ashley, B. D., and Selden, G. L. (1961). *Arch. Biochem. Biophys.* **92**, 441.

Westphal, U., Williams, W. C., Jr., and Ashley, B. D. (1962). *Proc. Soc. Exptl. Biol. Med.* **109**, 926.

Westphal, U., Williams, W. C., Jr., Ashley, B. D., and DeVenuto, F. (1963). *Z. Physiol. Chem.* **332**, 54.

Westphal, U., Chader, G. J., and Harding, G. B. (1967). *Steroids* **10**, 155.

Winzler, R. J. (1960). *In* "The Plasma Proteins" (F. W. Putnam, ed.), Vol. 1, p. 309. Academic Press, New York.

Woeber, K. A., and Ingbar, S. H. (1968). *J. Clin. Invest.* **47**, 1710.

CHAPTER 7

Insulin and Protein Synthesis

K. L. Manchester

I. INTRODUCTION

The details of the precise mechanism of the action of insulin are still unsolved, but interest in its actions remains of concern as the continuing volume of published papers on the subject attests. That the effects of the hormone so frequently crop up is indicative of the fact that its actions are widely observable on all aspects of metabolism, namely of carbohydrates, fats, proteins, and nucleic acids. The question obviously arises as to whether all the effects of the hormone result from one primary action. This would be the most aesthetically satisfying situation. In the absence of knowledge of the answer to this question however we must reckon with the alternative possibility that insulin exerts its manifold effects by several quite separate mechanisms. The author would not wish to feel committed to one or other point of view.

This chapter is concerned with the influence of insulin on protein and nucleic acid metabolism. We shall treat with the subject in its own right, but clearly too we must look to see to what extent there are parallels with effects of the hormone on carbohydrate and fat metabolism and to what extent the various effects are interdependent. We need to decide whether stimulation of protein synthesis is or is not dependent on a simultaneous stimulation of glucose utilization/transport and to what extent inhibition of specific facets of metabolism do or do not prevent manifestation of the various other effects of the hormone. Thus we can ask to what extent the transport hypothesis, which has been of such value in understanding the effects of the hormone on sugar uptake, is equally applicable to consideration of the uptake of amino acids, to what extent insulinlike effects of various enzymes manifest these properties in respect to protein synthesis, and to what extent the activity of adenyl cyclase contributes to the actions of insulin.

Although the wastage of nitrogen resulting from insulin insufficiency and the importance of availability of the hormone for adequate protein deposition has been realized for many years, systematic consideration of the numerous aspects of action of the hormone in nitrogen metabolism has been appreciated only more recently thanks initially to pioneering observations of Krahl (1952, 1953) and Hastings and colleagues (Sinex et al., 1952). Several authors have reviewed the literature in this field (Krahl, 1961; Manchester and Young, 1961; Manchester, 1965a, 1970a; Rieser, 1967), and a systematic account will not be presented here.

II. GENERAL EFFECTS OF INSULIN ON NITROGEN METABOLISM

In general terms, as well as influencing nitrogen balance, there are three series of phenomena that point to the importance of the action of insulin on protein and amino acid metabolism. They are (1) the lowering by insulin of the blood amino acid level, (2) promotion by the hormone of the incorporation of labeled amino acids into the protein of isolated tissues, and (3) stimulation by the hormone of the synthesis of various specific enzymes that play important roles in regulating the direction of metabolism. These last effects are seen largely in the liver and also in adipose tissue, but do not appear to occur in kidney and have not been demonstrated for identifiable enzymes in muscle. The lowering of the blood amino acid content by insulin occurs rapidly following administration of the hormone (Forker et al., 1951; Sanders and Riggs, 1967;

Manchester, 1970a) but the significance of the change is complicated (1) by the role of other hormones in simultaneously affecting the same parameter (London and Prenton, 1968) and (2) (unlike with glucose) by lack of obvious elevation of the plasma amino acid content in diabetes (Ivy *et al.*, 1951; Gray and Illing, 1952; Müting, 1964; Scharff and Wool, 1966; Zinneman *et al.*, 1966). Clearly, however, in the diabetic animal there is a draining of amino acids away from the protein of muscle (probably accentuated by glucocorticoids) to degradation in the liver and this movement is reversed on administration of insulin. That insulin stems the release of amino acids by muscle is most strikingly demonstrated in recent studies of forearm metabolism carried out by Pozefsky *et al.* (1968).

In the normal animal, secretion of insulin is induced by a carbohydrate load (and of course by amino acids). Administration of glucose as a means of stimulating insulin secretion has the advantage of not resulting in hypoglycemia and it is interesting to note that the emphasis under these conditions is on nitrogen deposition in the carcass rather than in the viscera (Munro, 1964). Thus feeding glucose to otherwise fasting rats, as would be expected, reduced urinary nitrogen loss, but none of the nitrogen spared was deposited in the liver, which paradoxically, underwent a significant loss of protein (Munro *et al.*, 1959). Conversely, when rats on a protein-free diet of carbohydrate are fasted, the liver gains protein although the overall loss of nitrogen increases (Rosenthal and Vars, 1954). Steiner (1966) has also emphasized that in the chronic diabetic the liver and viscera constitute a larger than usual fraction of the total body weight. Thus though insulin in many ways affects the liver, its role in anabolism is more in evidence in the metabolism of extrahepatic tissue. This is again demonstrated inter alia by the increased uptake by muscle of labeled amino acid from plasma on administration of insulin (Forker *et al.*, 1951) and on feeding carbohydrate to fasting animals (Munro *et al.*, 1959). This chapter will therefore deal mainly with the influence of insulin on protein synthesis in muscle.

III. PROTEIN SYNTHESIS IN MUSCLE

A. Stimulation by Insulin of Incorporation of Amino Acids

An observation that has proved of crucial importance in the development of the concept of a direct control by insulin of protein synthesis was first made by Krahl (1952, 1953) and by Sinex *et al.* (1952). They found that when the isolated rat diaphragm is incubated in a medium containing insulin the capacity of this tissue to incorporate added labeled amino acids into its protein is raised. This stimulation of incorporation of label into protein is observable for all the naturally occurring amino acids; it occurs when the labeled amino acid is presented at concentrations ranging from trace levels up to 20 mM and the size of the stimulation is usually of the order of 50–100%, though there is some variation (Manchester and Young, 1958; Wool and Krahl, 1959a,b; Manchester, 1961a; Parrish and Kipnis, 1964). Stimulation of incorporation is seen with a variety of other muscles and with other tissue preparations (listed in Manchester, 1970a).

When Krahl and others first made these observations it was of course well established that insulin stimulated the uptake of glucose by diaphragm and it was not unreasonable to conclude that these two effects were in some way related. The question still remains as to how. Since the stimulating influence of insulin is as clearly demonstrable in the absence of added glucose in the supporting medium as in its presence (Manchester and Young, 1958; Wool and Krahl, 1959a) the action of insulin on amino acid incorporation does not appear to depend on a stimulation by the hormone of glucose uptake. Moreover, the presence of glucose in the medium does not result in consistent enhancement of incorporation or affect the response of incorporation to insulin. This indicates that availability of energy derived from glucose catabolism is not specifically important for protein synthesis or more importantly its enhancement by insulin. The lowest level at which a consistent stimulation of incorporation is seen (50 μunit/ml) is comparable to the amounts of insulin stimulating glucose uptake though the dose response curve is rather more shallow (Krahl and Park, 1948; Manchester and Young, 1959; Manchester et $al.$, 1959). 50 μunit/ml is within the range of what is at present believed to be the insulin content of plasma of the normal fed rat or man (Morgan and Lazarow, 1965). However under the conditions in which diaphragm muscle is usually incubated there may be appreciable absorption of the hormone to the glassware and certainly is rapid breakdown (Antoniades and Gershoff, 1966). Avoidance of these hazards would be likely to enhance the sensitivity of the diaphragm system. The potentiation of insulin action by certain other protein hormones may result from their capacity to spare insulin from binding or destruction (Manchester et $al.$, 1959). Like glucose uptake, amino acid incorporation is enhanced in muscle briefly dipped in an insulin-containing solution (Manchester and Young, 1959). There is no stimulation by the separated chains of the insulin molecule though the possibility that synthetic A chain is active has been suggested (Volfin et $al.$, 1964).

With adipose tissue cells where the rate of insulin destruction is low (Crofford, 1968) a stimulation of incorporation is seen with 10 μunits/ml of insulin and is maximal with 800 μunits/ml (Miller and Beigelman, 1967)—a response curve very similar to that observed by several authors for influence on glucose metabolism of adipose tissue (Ball *et al.*, 1959; Beigelman, 1962) though greater sensitivity—from 1 to 25 μunits/ml has been observed for the dispersed cells (Crofford, 1968).

Thus we can see here an example of the parallel between effects of insulin on carbohydrate and protein metabolism, on the one hand increased uptake of sugar and its conversion to a macromolecule, namely glycogen, and on the other increased uptake of amino acid as reflected in increased incorporation into protein, which takes place independent of enhancement of sugar metabolism. Moreover inhibition of glucose uptake by phloridzin is without effect on glycine incorporation into protein (Battaglia *et al.*, 1960). Are the two effects really independently mediated or do they contain common actions different from or more fundamental than those usually measured? The converse observation of the independence of insulin action on glucose uptake from effects on protein metabolism is impossible to make by excluding amino acids altogether because they are bound to be present in the tissue. However inhibition of protein synthesis by the presence of puromycin does not prevent enhancement of sugar entry by insulin (Eboué-Bonis *et al.*, 1963; Burrow and Bondy, 1964; Carlin and Hechter, 1964). Disconcertingly the presence of puromycin interferes with stimulation by insulin of glycogen synthesis (Søvik and Walaas, 1964; Søvik, 1965) but probably for reasons quite different than through inhibition of protein synthesis, namely through inhibition of cyclic AMP phosphodiesterase and elevation of the concentration of the nucleotide with consequent phosphorylase activation (Søvik, 1966, 1967; Appleman and Kemp, 1966).

A similar problem does not arise with cycloheximide and in its presence a clear stimulation by insulin of glycogen synthesis as well as of glucose uptake is seen under conditions where amino acid incorporation is negligible (Table I). In a different context we may note here that inhibition of nucleic acid synthesis by addition of actinomycin does not interfere with stimulation by insulin of uptake of glucose, synthesis of glycogen, or incorporation of amino acids into protein (Eboué-Bonis *et al.*, 1963; Wool and Moyer, 1964; Søvik, 1966). It is important to remember too that although puromycin and cycloheximide inhibit amino acid incorporation they do not specifically inhibit the sensitivity of these processes to insulin if we look at the response in proportional terms (Søvik, 1965; Wool *et al.*, 1965; Manchester, 1967a). Obviously if incorporation is reduced to unmeasurable levels its enhancement by insulin

TABLE I

EFFECT OF CYCLOHEXIMIDE ON THE UPTAKE OF GLUCOSE AND SYNTHESIS OF
GLYCOGEN BY ISOLATED RAT DIAPHRAGM[a]

Additions to the medium	Uptake of glucose (mg/gm)	Synthesis of glycogen (mg/gm)	Proportion of uptake converted to glycogen (%)
No addition	2.52 ± 0.32	1.10 ± 0.07	44
Cycloheximide	2.78 ± 0.32	0.94 ± 0.06	34
Insulin	6.70 ± 0.37	3.40 ± 0.44	51
Cycloheximide ± insulin	6.10 ± 0.25	3.29 ± 0.12	54

[a] Each figure is the mean ±S.E. of the mean of six observations. Incubation was for 1.5 hours. Concentration of insulin 0.1 unit/ml, cycloheximide 100 μg/ml.

cannot be seen, but for intermediate degrees of inhibition the response to insulin persists.

Quite apart from nonspecific toxic effects of inhibitors, interference with protein synthesis must be expected to influence cellular metabolism if only by virtue of reducing the demand for energy for its accomplishment. Calculation suggests that in diaphragm muscle protein synthesis consumes 5–10% of the energy liberated by respiration. Inhibition of protein synthesis might on these grounds decrease respiration, or as seen with ouabain, depress glucose uptake or enhance glycogen formation (Clausen, 1965, 1966; Manchester, 1969a). These expectations have not been fully realized with diaphragm muscle (unpublished observations of the author), but inhibition of respiration when protein synthesis is stopped can be seen with a more slowly respiring tissue such as costal cartilage (Salmon *et al.*, 1967). It is possible that the capacity of puromycin to prevent the normal stimulation by insulin of respiration in frog muscle also results from a similar economy in the tissue's demand for energy for protein synthesis (Gourley and Brunton, 1969).

The enhancement of glucose uptake by insulin obviously provides a boost to glycogen synthesis even if it is not the entire explanation (Villar-Palasi and Larner, 1968). To what extent is enhancement of amino acid entry into the cellular space of muscle the cause of increased incorporation of amino acids into protein? Undoubtedly insulin can increase the uptake of certain amino acids by muscle both *in vitro* and *in vivo*, but despite intensive investigation the significance of this observation is very confused and, as discussed further on, for only a few amino acids is increased accumulation readily observable. In trying to trace a parallel between glycogen and protein synthesis there are obviously very important differences. For example in muscle the intracellular free glucose level is normally low (Randle and Morgan, 1962) and the rate of transport of glucose into the cell is thus a potentially rate-limiting step in allowing glycogen synthesis to proceed. Moreover, stimulation of glycogen synthesis is chemically measurable and not dependent on use of isotopes. With amino acids and protein synthesis, since there is a pool of amino acids in the cell as concentrated as in plasma, there is no reason to suppose that protein synthesis is limited in short periods by the transport of amino acids into the cell (though of the twenty amino acids it is possible that one or two are present in more limiting quantities than the others), and obviously when only one labeled amino acid is added to the medium this will not alone support protein synthesis but truly act only as a tracer. Assuming that this amino acid itself is present chemically in more than limiting quantity, then its increased incorporation into protein in the presence of insulin arises either (1) because its rate of entry into the cell is increased and it therefore labels the amino acids of the cell pool to a higher specific activity than in the absence of the hormone—a constant rate of protein synthesis would thus enhance the incorporation of label, (2) because the cell pool of amino acids shrinks under the influence of insulin and a given quantity of label assumes a higher specific activity, or (3) because there is a real increase in the rate of protein formation.

B. Rate of Protein Synthesis

Unlike the situation with glycogen, for several reasons it is not possible to measure directly the rate of protein synthesis. First, the quantity of synthesis is small, particularly as a proportion of the quantity of protein already present. Second, there is not necessarily any net synthesis of protein. The rate of breakdown, particularly in an isolated tissue preparation is likely to be as fast as the rate of synthesis; that is we are dealing essentially with turnover rather than net synthesis of protein (and one extra source of amino acids for synthesis will be those liberated in protein breakdown). The actual rate of peptide bond synthesis can be calculated from assumptions as to the specific activity of the label entering protein, the frequency of the amino acid in protein, and the amount of label incorporated. Figures presented by several authors give a value of about 500 μg/gm diaphragm muscle/hour (Manchester and Young, 1961; Hechter and Halkerston, 1964; Buse and Buse, 1967). Such a figure indicates an average rate of turnover of about 0.2%/hour and is consistent with observations that if after incubation for a period with radioactive amino acids the tissue is incubated for a further period with unlabeled material, the label incorporated remains in the protein and is not lost (Manchester, 1961b; Hider *et al.*, 1969a). The bulk of the incorporation is thus not into a few proteins with a very rapid rate of turnover, nor does the picture change substantially on addition of insulin (Goldstein and Reddy, 1967). By mixing proteins labelled with ^{14}C-amino acid in the presence of insulin with protein labeled with ^{3}H-amino acid in its absence Kurihara and Wool (1968) found by acrylamide gel fractionation little evidence of any change in the relative proportions or types of proteins taking up the isotopes as a result of the hormonal treatment.

An indirect procedure for estimating the rate of protein synthesis is to measure changes in the levels of free amino acids in the incubation system, that is in both tissue and medium in the presence and absence of insulin, since an increase in protein synthesis might manifest itself in a decrease in the amount of free amino acid and vice versa. The results of such experiments are shown in Fig. 1. The rate of protein synthesis calculable from these figures agrees well with that estimated from incorporation experiments and provides support for the belief that insulin is inducing a real increase in the rate of protein synthesis. Some suppression of amino acid release by adductor muscle fibers (R. H. Peterson *et al.*, 1963) (and by isolated hepatic mitochondria; Alberti and Bartley, 1965) is seen in the presence of insulin, but no change was reported to be observed with the perfused heart (Scharff and Wool, 1965a). It has

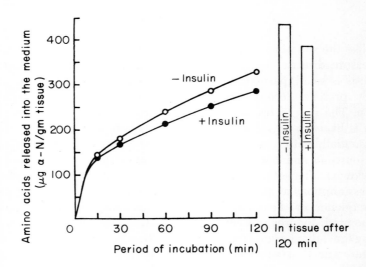

Fig. 1. Time course of the concentration of amino acids and other ninhydrin reacting materials liberated by diaphragm and retained by it during incubation in the presence and absence of insulin. (From Manchester, 1961a,b.)

7. *Insulin and Protein Synthesis* 275

TABLE II
THE FREE AMINO ACID CONTENT OF VARIOUS RAT MUSCLES

Amino acid	Heart[a]	Diaphragm[b]	Extensor[c] digitorum longus	Thigh[d]
	μmole/100 ml Tissue water			μmole/100 gm
Alanine	295	430	475	173
Arginine	35	38	32	18
Aspartate	364	260	105	20
Citrulline	21	63	82	19
Glutamate	513	463	206	146
Glycine	92	293	797	451
Histidine	16	65	81	16
Hydroxyproline				27
Isoleucine	10	10	10	11
Leucine	20	16	13	14
Lysine	87	77	24	68
Methionine	9	13	11	5
Ornithine	8	12	21	4
Phenylalanine	10	18	9	7
Proline	41		51	20
Serine	88	237		64
Threonine	55	64	46	44
Tryptophan	5			
Tyrosine	12	17	16	8
Valine	20	19	18	17
Ammonia	1556	461		440
Glutathione	493			
Taurine	4000	1800	1400	229

[a] Scharff and Wool (1964).
[b] L. V. Turner and K. L. Manchester, unpublished observations.
[c] Pain and Manchester (1970).
[d] Ryan and Carver (1963).

to be remembered too that a large proportion of the free amino acid content of muscle (ninhydrin reacting material) is taurine and other compounds not involved in protein metabolism (Table II). However close examination of the figures of Scharff and Wool (1965a) shows that, although with the given number of samples analyzed, the variability of results precluded demonstration of statistically significant changes in the levels of amino acids in hearts with and without insulin, they did observe a smaller concentration in the tissue in the presence of insulin after 60 minutes of perfusion for aspartate, alanine, isoleucine, tyrosine, phenylalanine, lysine, histidine, tryptophan, and arginine. But equally they found a fall in taurine, glutathione, and ammonia, and as the authors concluded, they did not find any clear or meaningful changes. However, the recent studies of Pozefsky *et al.* (1968), showing suppression by insulin of release of amino acids from forearm muscle, provide striking confirmation of the result shown in Fig. 1. In the experiments of Scharff and Wool (1965a), the greater total quantity of amino acid present in the perfusate as against that in the tissue would tend to minimize the size of any change that metabolism in the tissue could make to the total amino acid concentration.

It is interesting to note that to support the measured rates of protein synthesis each ribosome of diaphragm muscle, given a content of rRNA of about 1 mg/gm tissue, will synthesise on average 300 peptide bonds a minute—comparable with values found for other tissues (Manchester, 1970c). Red fibers incorporate amino acid faster than white partly because of greater content of RNA (Citoler *et al.*, 1967; A. L. Goldberg, 1967). A rate of protein synthesis of 5 μmole amino acid incorporated per hour means a requirement of about 0.25 μmole/gm for each of the amino acids. This is equivalent to 50 μmole/100 ml of intracellular water. Since the intracellular concentration is lower than this for many of the amino acids (Table II) the rate of their provision could well be of significance. On the other hand unless there is net synthesis the same quantity of amino acids will presumably be returning continually to the pool for recycling.

Clearly, figures derived *in vitro* for rates of protein synthesis may not reflect those *in vivo*—the classic instance being the very low activity of cell-free systems by comparison with cellular rates. Estimates of the rate of protein synthesis from isotope incorporation in short incubations are likely to err on the low side because of incomplete equilibration of the added label with intracellular amino acid and because such procedures fail to take into account the continual return to the intracellular pool of amino acids arising from protein breakdown (Gan and Jeffay, 1967). The rates of incorporation noted in the diaphragm would indicate turnover rates of muscle proteins somewhat faster than some long standing *in vivo* observations, but more recent estimates (Waterlow and Stephen, 1968; Garlick, 1969), in which the problems of isotope recycling have been taken into account, give an average turnover rate for rat muscle of about 7–10 days, which is in fact appreciably faster than the *in vitro* figures suggest. Several amino acids appear to be oxidized rapidly by muscle (Manchester, 1965b), including the essential branched chain acids whose intracellular concentration is comparatively small. In conditions of fasting or protein malnutrition it seems possible that their availability could become crucially limiting. On the other hand, McFarlane and von Holt (1969) found that in the fasting rat the rate of leucine oxidation progressively diminished—though in preliminary experiments in this laboratory there was no reduction in the oxidation of exogenously added leucine by rat diaphragm from rats fasted 48 hours. That there must be a mechanism *in vivo* for conserving amino acids in prolonged fasting has been suggested by Felig *et al.* (1969) and the reduced plasma alanine in such a condition may be indicative of reduced carriage of ammonia as alanine from extrahepatic tissues to the liver for conversion to urea.

As pointed out, increased incorporation of label could arise if insulin were to decrease the size of the endogenous pool of amino acids, so lessening the extent of dilution of the entering labeled amino acid. This would result in maintenance of a higher specific activity of precursor to protein synthesis. This could occur without a change in the amount of labeled amino acid accumulated in the tissue. It is of interest to note that on several occasions, for amino acids whose uptake is not observed to be raised by insulin, there actually appears to be a diminution in the size of the cell pool as observed by radioactive measurement in the presence of insulin (Manchester and Young, 1960a; Wool *et al.*, 1965; Arvill and Ahren, 1967b; Guidotti *et al.*, 1968a). These differences are not clearly substantiated by chemical measurements with cardiac muscle (Scharff and Wool, 1965a) and a diminution in uptake of label would not be likely to presage an increase in specific activity in the cell pool.

IV. ACCUMULATION OF AMINO ACIDS BY MUSCLE

A. Nature of Compartmentation of Amino Acid Pool

Although the total amount of measurable amino acid does not change, alteration in the size of the pool from which amino acids entering protein are taken for protein synthesis can still occur if there is some form of compartmentation. Compartmentation and separate pools have been suggested to explain the anomalous behavior of metabolites in labeling experiments (Shaw and Stadie, 1959; Sims and Landau, 1966; Landau and Sims, 1967; Antony *et al.*, 1969), but the cytological basis is often obscure.

With amino acids compartmentation of the cell pool has been postulated from observations of the constancy of the rate of incorporation of amino acids into protein under conditions when the specific activity of the cell pool is changing. Thus Kipnis *et al.* (1961) found a linear rate of incorporation of proline by diaphragm and lymph node cells under conditions in which the specific activity of free amino acid extracted from the cells was rising rapidly. Rosenberg *et al.* (1963) found with kidney slices a linear rate of incorporation, whereas the rate of oxidation of the amino acid increased with the increase in specific activity of the cell pool. Manchester and Wool (1963) observed a lack of linearity in the rate of incorporation of labeled glycine and proline by diaphragm, though this was not seen with arginine and leucine. A delay in linear incorporation of glycine, though not for leucine, is also seen with extensor digitorum longus muscle (Hider *et al.,* 1969a). A linear rate of incorporation when radioactivity is accumulating in the cell pool is certainly indicative that the pool from which the amino acids are going into protein is not co-extensive with and rapidly mixing with the total free amino acid pool. One has to recognize therefore that measurement of the size or specific activity of the total pool of the tissue does not necessarily tell us much about the parameters of the effective pool from which amino acids go into protein in the type of experiment normally carried out.

The significance or the explanation of these observations is not certain. Evidence points to the "ordering" of water in muscle (Hazlewood *et al.,* 1969). E. J. Harris (1960) has emphasized that it is a mistake to regard the cell interior as a homogeneous unit where mixing is instantaneous, and he cites several instances in which measurement of intracellular ion fluxes fit a two- or multicompartment model (Mudge, 1953; Schreiber, 1955; Solomon and Gold, 1955; Tosteson and Robertson, 1956). Guroff and Udenfriend (1960) found that for amino acids only a small fraction of the tyrosine of isolated diaphragm was readily available for isotopic

TABLE III

The Extent of Uptake of Labeled Amino Acids by Extensor Digitorum Longus Muscle Compared with the Concentration of the Unlabeled Material in the Cell[a]

Amino acid	Medium (μM)	Chemical concentration ratio	Radioactive concentration ratio	Radioactive: chemical ratio
Glycine	455	23.4	1.8	0.08
Leucine	110	1.5	0.6	0.45
Phenylalanine	39	1.9	0.5	0.52
Proline	27	4.1	1.0	0.30

[a] The muscle was incubated for 1 hour in medium containing amino acids at their plasma concentration with one of the amino acids appropriately labeled. After incubation the medium and tissue concentrations were determined by both chemical analysis and distribution of radioactivity. (From Pain and Manchester, 1970.)

exchange (though this did not appear to apply with brain *in vivo;* Chirigos *et al.,* 1960). The authors noted that the ratio of total amino acid in the diaphragm to that in the medium was greater than the isotopic ratio established. In more detailed experiments with extensor digitorum longus we have also found for several amino acids that radioactive species appear within 1 hour to have penetrated only a fraction of the total amino acid pool (Table III). The extent of penetration is particularly low for glycine and proline, two amino acids whose uptake is raised by insulin.

In a different manner Hider *et al.* (1969a) have noted additional evidence that labeled amino acids entering muscle (extensor digitorum) are incorporated into protein before mixing with the total cell pool. They found that if the tissue was first incubated with ^{14}C-amino acid and then transferred to medium containing the same amino acid labeled with tritium, incorporation of ^{14}C ceased virtually at once before there had been appreciable efflux of the amino acid from the tissue, whereas incorporation of tritium into protein began immediately, before much accumulation in the cell pool had occurred (Fig. 2). Though they suggest

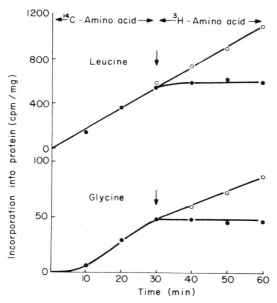

FIG. 2. The sequential incorporation of ^{14}C and ^{3}H-amino acid by extensor digitorum muscle. The muscle was incubated for the indicated periods first with ^{14}C-amino acid then transferred to fresh medium containing ^{3}H-amino acid and the speed with which incorporation of ^{14}C ceased and ^{3}H began observed. (Based on data of Hider *et al.,* 1969a.)

that incorporation of incoming amino acids may take place in the membrane, their results do not preclude the possibility of a pool of amino acids close to the membrane not in rapid equilibrium with the bulk of the pool in the tissue. The latter possibility, suggested for potassium movements in heart (Schreiber, 1955), has been advocated by the author previously (Manchester, 1965a), namely that there may be amino acids dissolved in water associated with the myofibrils of muscle whose rate of exchange with amino acids in the fluid between the fibrils and the membrane is slow (Fig. 3). The myofibrils occupy the bulk of the muscle cell, and the quantity of amino acid in the myofibrillar water if uniformly distributed would be correspondingly great. For example the greater concentration of glycine and alanine in muscle may be related to their size and/or their charge to size ratio in this respect. [London *et al.* (1965) have suggested, on the basis of the steady release of amino acids from muscle under normal conditions, that extrahepatic pools may actually constitute a means of storing amino acids.] Obviously if the rate of movement of the labeled amino acid within the cell is slow, the spatial location of the ribosomes in the muscle cell will affect how soon they

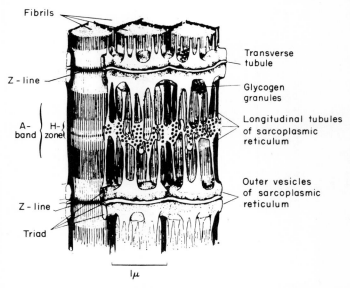

Fig. 3. Diagrammatic representation of the structure of a muscle cell, showing fibers, sarcoplasmic reticulum, and tubular system. Note also the spaces between the fibers constituting the sarcoplasm. It is suggested in the text that there is likely to be more rapid movement of solutes into these spaces than into the center of the fibers. (From Peachey, 1965.)

begin to use entering labeled amino acids. Although some ribosomes may be attached to membranes (Muscatello *et al.,* 1962; Ezerman and Ishikawa, 1967), it is a more common observation that on homogenization of the tissue much of the RNA remains with the debris but can be detached in medium of high ionic strength (Breuer *et al.,* 1964; Heywood *et al.,* 1967, 1968; Chen and Young, 1968). Though these facts suggest the association of ribosomes with the myofibrils (Mihalyi *et al.,* 1957; Perry and Zydowo, 1959; Zak *et al.,* 1967; Heywood and Rich, 1968), the ribosomes are more likely to be around the fibers than within, and where polysomes are visible in election micrographs they are found either in the open sarcoplasm or alongside the fibrils (Anderson-Cedergren and Karlsson, 1967; Shimada *et al.,* 1967; Ishikawa *et al.,* 1968; Staley and Benson, 1968; Schiaffino and Margreth, 1969). Thus the ribosomes, even if within the cell, may still come into contact with entering labeled amino

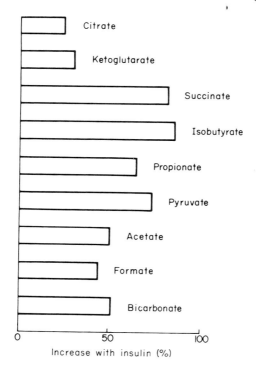

FIG. 4. The stimulation by insulin of the incorporation of ^{14}C from the various precursors into the protein of isolated rat diaphragm. From the data of Manchester and Krahl (1959). The amino acids into which the ^{14}C becomes incorporated are indicated in Manchester (1960).

acids much sooner than the time it takes for equilibration throughout the cell volume (Fig. 3). The fact that some delay of commencement of linear incorporation of both glycine and proline is observed (Manchester and Wool, 1963; Hider *et al.*, 1969a) suggests that the site of their incorporation is intracellular rather than in the membrane.

The capacity, moreover, of diaphragm to incorporate into protein amino acids already accumulated (Wool and Krahl, 1959c) and to incorporate into protein amino acids synthesized in the cell from nonamino acid precursors (Manchester and Krahl, 1959; Manchester, 1960; and Fig. 4) again argues in favor of an intracellular site for protein synthesis. If in this instance the amino acids are formed inside the cell, it is to be expected that the rate of their incorporation will reflect the rate of change of their specific activity in the cell. However an attempt to verify this point revealed a possible difficulty in experiments studying amino acid incorporation in short time periods, namely that the smaller the actual amount of incorporation the more likely it is that errors may arise if the washing procedure for preparation of protein samples is not 100% efficient. Figure 5a shows an experiment in which a time course of incorporation of ^{14}C from ^{14}C-acetate was studied. [The ^{14}C enters the protein mainly as glutamate and to a lesser extent aspartate (Manchester, 1960).] As a control, diaphragms that had been preincubated with cycloheximide to stop protein synthesis were also incubated with the ^{14}C-acetate and the protein prepared as usual. It will be seen that the actual

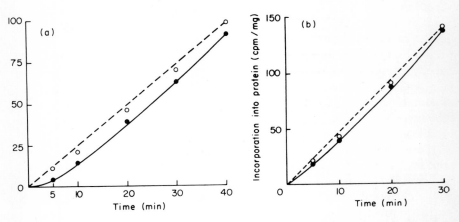

FIG. 5. Time course of incorporation of ^{14}C from (a) ^{14}C-acetate and (b) ^{14}C-leucine into protein of rat diaphragm muscle. The open circles are the actual incorporation values observed; the closed circles are the corrected figures for the incorporation obtained by substracting the counts found in tissue incubated with the same amount of radioactivity but in the presence of cycloheximide (100 μg/ml).

incorporation of ^{14}C in the absence of cycloheximide gives a linear time course, but that if we substract from these figures the amount of radio-activity also found in the tissue incubated with cycloheximide, which is assumed to constitute nonspecific contamination, then the shape of the curve changes to show an initial lag. With acetate, where the proportion of added label that enters protein is minimal, the danger of nonspecific contamination of low activity samples is likely to be greatest, but similar considerations can apply to some extent even with ^{14}C-leucine (Fig. 5b).

B. INSULIN AND AMINO ACID ACCUMULATION

In summary, of the three possible interpretations of the significance of the observation of stimulation by insulin of incorporation of amino acids into protein, there is circumstantial evidence of an increase in the actual rate of protein formation, though direct proof for the intact tissue is lacking. There is no clear evidence for a diminution in the size of the pool from which amino acids are taken, which results in a substantial elevation of the specific activity of the precursor. We must now consider the evidence for stimulation by insulin of amino acid uptake. This on the face of it appears the most obvious approach to this question; however the results of such investigations have proved inconclusive. Obviously measurement of amino acid transport is most easily carried out with a structure that is not incorporated into protein or utilized or degraded in other ways. The two amino acids α-aminoisobutyric acid and cycloleucine fulfil these criteria and we find that their entry into muscle is stimulated by insulin (Kipnis and Noall, 1958; Manchester and Young, 1960a; Akedo and Christensen, 1962; Manchester and Wool, 1963; Arvill and Ahren, 1967a,b; Guidotti et al., 1968b). However the uptake of another unutilized analogue α-methyltyrosine is not enhanced; r.ither is that of the species β-alanine, γ-aminobutyric acid, ornithine, norleucine, α,γ-diaminobutyric acid or α-aminobicyclo[2,2,1]heptene-2-carboxylic acid though that of ethionine, isovaline and sarcosine is (see Table IV for references).

Turning to the natural amino acids, the accumulation of glycine, proline, and methionine is enhanced by insulin, but, with the possible exception of serine, threonine, histidine, and alanine, accumulation of none of the others is observable (Table IV). This, it is important to note, is by contrast to their incorporation into protein, which insulin enhances in every case. Enhanced accumulation of histidine by chicken embryo hearts has recently been shown by Guidotti et al. (1969).

Accumulation of serine and threonine were found by Wool to be enhanced by insulin (Wool, 1964; Wool et al., 1965). Akedo and Christen-

TABLE IV

THE ENHANCEMENT OF ACCUMULATION OF ^{14}C-AMINO ACIDS IN MUSCLE BY INSULIN

Uptake enhanced by insulin

Alanine[a,i]	Aminoisobutyric acid[b,c,e]
Glycine[b,c,e]	Cycloleucine[c,h]
Histidine[a,i]	Ethionine[a]
Methionine[c]	Isovaline[c]
Proline[c,e,f]	Sarcosine[c]
(Hydroxyproline[f])	
Serine[f,g]	
Threonine[f,i]	

Not enhanced by insulin

Alanine[b,c,e,i]	β-Alanine[a]
Arginine[f,g]	γ-Aminobutyric acid[a]
Aspartic acid[b]	α,γ-Diaminobutyric acid[h]
Cystine[f]	α-Methyltyrosine[d]
Glutamic acid[b,e]	Norleucine[c]
Histidine[c,f,i]	Ornithine[b]
Isoleucine[f,g]	α-Aminobicyclo[2,2,1]heptene-2-carboxylic
Leucine[b,c,f,g]	acid[i]
Lysine[b,e]	
Phenylalanine[b,e,f]	
Threonine[a,i]	
Tryptophan[f]	
Tyrosine[d,f]	
Valine[c,e]	

[a] Table V and Manchester (1970b).
[b] Manchester and Young (1960a).
[c] Akedo and Christensen (1962).
[d] Guroff and Udenfriend (1961)
[e] Manchester and Wool (1963).
[f] Wool (1964).
[g] Wool et al. (1965).
[h] Elsas et al. (1968).
[i] Christensen and Cullen (1969).
[j] Amino acids which have been found by different workers to give different responses.
A more complete bibliography is given in Manchester (1970a).

sen (1962) recorded negative results for serine but my results suggest a positive response. In my experience and that of Hider *et al.* (1969b) uptake of threonine is not affected either with the isolated hemidiaphragm or intact diaphragm preparation (Table V), but increased uptake by chicken embryo hearts is reported (Guidotti *et al.*, 1969). The reasons for these discrepancies are not clear. The concentration of added amino acid may be critical in order to observe stimulation (e.g., one has to use a concentration low enough not to saturate the uptake process) but in this context Wool (1964) has shown that even at added concentrations as low as 10^{-9} M no effect of insulin on uptake of leucine could be observed. Though possessing an OH group, threonine on occasion interchanges with leucine in variants of protein structure (E. L. Smith, 1967), which suggests that it is functionally hydrophobic. We might therefore expect it to behave in a manner comparable to that of leucine, isoleucine, and valine in regard to response to insulin. However, there is no obvious feature that explains why uptake of glycine, proline, alanine, serine, histidine, and methionine is influenced by insulin whereas uptake of other amino acids is not. They bear no close structural resemblance, their frequency of appearance in proteins is not especially similar, and whereas the amount of free glycine in muscle is comparatively large, that of proline and methionine is low (some comparative figures for the concentration of amino acids in rat muscle are given in Table II). Methionine does not share exclusively with glycine and proline entry into cells via the "alanine preferring" site (Oxender and Christensen, 1963; Christensen, 1964). Alanine was not found in earlier experiments to be one of the amino acids whose uptake was enhanced by insulin (Manchester and Young, 1960a; Akedo and Christensen, 1962) but closer inspection of the figures suggests that there was indeed a tendency for its uptake to be enhanced. More recent experiments again show a slight response to insulin (Table V), which makes more feasible the concept that those amino acids which respond to insulin belong to the group taken up by the alanine preferring site on the membrane.

Castles and Wool (1964) and Wool *et al.* (1965) found that when puromycin was added to incubating diaphragm muscle in sufficient amount to inhibit protein synthesis, insulin enhanced the accumulation of a larger number of amino acids than normally observed. Although these observations suggest the possibility that in stimulating protein formation insulin causes the use of so many of the amino acids of the cell pool as to preclude their accumulation in the pool to an enhanced extent, the author does not feel that this is the full explanation—for several reasons. First, since the proportion of labeled amino acid entering the tissue that is incorporated into protein declines as the external concentration is raised (e.g., figures in Wool and Weinshelbaum, 1959; Manchester, 1961a; Riggs and Walker, 1963) it might be expected that the effect of insulin on transport would become more readily apparent at these higher concentrations when the proportion of the uptake going into protein is less, but this is not so, though there is still stimulation of incorporation even when the labeled amino acid is presented at 20 mM (Manchester, 1965a). Alternatively, if transport processes were to be-

TABLE V

INFLUENCE OF INSULIN ON THE ACCUMULATION OF VARIOUS AMINO ACIDS BY THE ISOLATED RAT DIAPHRAGM IN THE PRESENCE AND ABSENCE OF PUROMYCIN AND CYCLOHEXIMIDE[a]

Experiment	Amino acid	Concentration in medium (μM)	Ratio $\dfrac{\text{Concentration of amino acid in tissue water}}{\text{Concentration of amino acid in medium}}$	
			No insulin	Insulin added
1	Threonine[d]	40	2.14 ± 0.09 (6)[b]	2.25 ± 0.04
2	Threonine[d,f]	8	1.73 ± 0.05 (6)	1.68 ± 0.03
3	Alanine[c,g]	16	1.38 ± 0.07 (6)	1.60 ± 0.08[g]
4	Histidine[d]	1000	2.97 ± 0.15	3.36 ± 0.09
				($P = 0.05$)
5	p-Fluorophenylalanine[d,h]	1000	1.54 ± 0.08 (6)	1.46 ± 0.06
6	β-Alanine[e]	15	0.84 ± 0.02 (6)	0.83 ± 0.07
7	Ethionine[d]	120	1.66 ± 0.05	2.24 ± 0.12
				($P < 0.01$)
8	γ-Aminobutyrate[d]	32	0.82 ± 0.013 (6)	0.82 ± 0.017
9	Tyrosine[d] (cycloheximide present)	1000	2.05 ± 0.048 (6)	2.20 ± 0.049 ($P = 0.05$)
10	β-Alanine[e] (cycloheximide present)	15	0.79 ± 0.016 (6)	0.86 ± 0.014 ($P = 0.01$)
11	α-Methyltyrosine[e] (cycloheximide present)	1000	1.81 ± 0.050 (12)	1.76 ± 0.037

[a] Significant stimulation of incorporation of label into protein was observed in the experiment with threonine, alanine, histidine and p-fluorophenylalanine. There was no incorporation into protein of ^{14}C from β-alanine, γ-aminobutyrate, and ethionine. Tyrosine and α-methyltyrosine were not radioactive and were estimated chemically by the method of Udenfriend and Cooper (1952), otherwise accumulation of the radioactive forms was measured as in Manchester and Young (1960a). For a fuller account see Manchester (1970b).

[b] Each figure is the mean ±S.E. of the mean of the number of observations in parentheses. The differences when significant are indicated.

[c] Incubation was for 0.5 hour.

[d] Incubation for 1 hour.

[e] Incubation for 1.5 hour.

[f] Intact diaphragm preparation.

[g] [The paired difference 0.217 ± 0.031 was highly significant ($P_1 = 0.001$).

[h] DL form.

come saturated by these higher concentrations of amino acid we should expect that the influence of puromycin to make manifest the stimulating effect of insulin would be lost, but this does not appear to be so since the stimulation of alanine accumulation, one of the species more sensitive to this test, is readily seen when at 1 mM (Manchester, 1970b). The inhibitor used in this experiment was cycloheximide instead of puromycin to demonstrate that it appears to be inhibition of protein synthesis *per se* as opposed to any action peculiar to puromycin, such as formation of peptidyl fragments, that is the essential feature (Allen and Zamecnik, 1962; Rabinovitz and Fisher, 1962; Morris *et al.*, 1963; Nathans, 1964; Williamson and Schweet, 1964). Curiously, however, cessation of protein synthesis in the absence of insulin does not lead to enhancement of accumulation of label to any great extent as might be expected from the sparing of amino acid going into protein but rather the inhibitor emphasizes the endocrine response. The inhibitors appear to induce a small stimulation of uptake of the nonutilizable amino acids, cycloleucine, ethionine, and α-methyltyrosine and possibly also induce a response to insulin of β-alanine (Table V). Treatment of the perfused heart with puromycin (Scharff and Wool, 1965b) was found to raise the concentration of ornithine and taurine as well as of alanine, and these observations all suggest that the explanation of the effects of the inhibitors is complex. In fact, since it now seems likely that uptake of alanine and histidine, the two amino acids which appeared to show the largest response to insulin in the presence of puromycin (Castles and Wool, 1964), is responsive to the hormone in the absence of inhibitor (Table V, and Guidotti *et al.*, 1969; Manchester, 1970b), the influence of the inhibitors is perhaps less striking than formerly thought.

Although there are no specific claims of toxicity of cycloheximide to mammalian cells other than as an inhibitor of protein synthesis, there are a number of curious observations concerned with amino acid transport in muscle to which the actions of the two antibiotics may be related. First, there are the facts that aminobutyrate uptake by the intact diaphragm is very much slower than that carried out by the hemi-diaphragm (Manchester, 1966) and that the capacity for concentrative uptake can be enhanced by, for example, crushing the tissue with a glass rod (Peckham and Knobil, 1962). Second, diaphragm from acutely diabetic animals appears to accumulate aminoisobutyrate and proline at an enhanced rate and exhibits a greater than normal response to insulin (Castles *et al.*, 1965). Third, trypsin treatment of muscle reportedly enhances proline uptake (Rieser and Rieser, 1964) and phloridzin enhances aminoisobutyrate uptake by kidney slices (Segal *et al.*, 1961). The enhanced entry of sugars into muscle induced by anoxia has suggested the possibility that the cell normally limits the rate of glucose entry (G. H. Smith *et al.*, 1961). It is possible that with amino acids there is again a mechanism imposing a limitation on their rate of entry, for example to minimize expenditure of energy, but that inhibitors of protein synthesis and other agents overcome this mechanism and allow accumulation to occur more rapidly and to respond to insulin. It is interesting that incubation of diaphragm with puromycin or cycloheximide for several hours eventually depresses the uptake of amino acids (Elsas *et al.*, 1967; Manchester, 1967a). In this case it is postulated that the carrier has a fairly short half-life and its availability therefore declines in the absence of protein synthesis. There seems to be no loss of capacity though to take up glucose or to maintain potassium ions (Burrow and Bondy, 1964; Carlin and Hechter, 1964; Elsas and Rosenberg, 1967). Alternatively, if inhibition of protein synthesis allows breakdown to proceed at the usual rate, one might expect an enhanced intracellular pool of amino acid. A larger intracellular pool would enable more exchange to occur and so lead to enhancement of uptake of the labeled form. But both these explanations, along with the original observations, do not explain why the inhibition primarily facilitates the action of insulin rather than inducing changes itself. Since puromycin can enhance glycogenolysis (p. 271) it is possible that its presence increases the energy available for amino acid accumulation. By contrast Gourley and Brunton (1969) have found that puromycin can enhance the respiration of frog muscle and stimulate the conversion of lactate to glycogen, demonstrating in fact an insulin-like action. The mechanism of this is not clear.

C. Influence of Insulin on Kinetics of Accumulation of Amino Acids

Although we do not know the identity of the membrane components responsible for carrying amino acids across the cell membrane, it is possible to study their capacity and, by analogy with enzyme kinetics, make measurements of kinetic parameters. That transport can be demonstrated to be active and to be subject to saturation suggests the applicability of the Michaelis-Menten formulation. Thus the rate of energy of an amino acid into the cell (with special applicability in this case to a nonutilizable amino acid that is not already present) will be equal to $VS/(K_t + S)$, where V is the maximal velocity of the saturable process, S is the concentration of solute outside the cell and K_t the apparent Michaelis constant. In addition to the saturable process diffusion will play a part so that the initial rate of entry of amino acid will be

$$\frac{VS}{(K_t + S)} + K_D S \tag{1}$$

where K_D is the rate constant for diffusion. Akedo and Christensen (1962) were the first to attempt to evaluate the values of K_t and V_{max} for uptake of aminoisobutyrate by diaphragm and the effect of insulin on these figures. With the intact diaphragm they found that insulin did not appreciably affect the value of V_{max} but that K_t fell from about 16 to 1.6 mM. The value of K_D did not change appreciably. Similar figures were obtained by Elsas *et al.* (1968). With the chicken embryo heart Guidotti *et al.* (1968b), using the same procedure, found a different situation, namely that insulin raised the V_{max} for aminoisobutyrate entry, lowered the value of K_D from 0.37 to 0.25 hr^{-1} but had no effect on K_t (2.34 mM). It is interesting to note a similar variety of results have been obtained measuring K_t for glucose uptake by muscle and fat tissue (Post *et al.*, 1961; Froesch and Ginsberg, 1962; Narahara and Özand, 1963; Baker and Rutter, 1964; Morgan *et al.*, 1964; Crofford and Renold, 1965; Denton *et al.*, 1966; Guidotti *et al.*, 1966; Kuo *et al.*, 1967; Chaudry and Gould, 1969). Riggs *et al.* (1968) found that estradiol promoted uptake of several amino acids by the uterus and that with aminoisobutyrate the hormone promoted primarily a rise in V_{max} rather than change of K_m.

As the concentration of amino acid in the cell (C) increases, when $C > S$ diffusion will allow the escape of the amino acid rather than its accumulation. Eventually a steady state may be reached at which we can write

$$\frac{VS}{(K_t + S)} = K_D(C - S) \tag{2}$$

from which with sufficient values of C and S, K_t can be determined. However we have also to reckon with the possibility that efflux of amino acid is mediated and is proportional to $VC/(K_c + C)$ where K_c is the apparent Michaelis constant for the saturable efflux. Thus at steady state

$$\frac{VS}{(K_s + S)} = \frac{VC}{(K_c + C)} + K_D(C - S) \tag{3}$$

where K_t for uptake is now K_s. Given sufficient values of C and S it should again be possible to find suitable values of K_s and K_c and V/K_D to fit the equation. Note that the equation can be written

$$\frac{V}{K_D} \cdot \frac{S}{(K_s + S)} = \frac{V}{K_D} \cdot \frac{C}{(K_c + C)} + (C - S) \tag{4}$$

indicating that V and K_D cannot from this be independently determined, as is to be expected—absolute rates cannot be evaluated from steady-state figures.

The results of experiments of this sort are shown in Fig. 6, in which the steady state concentrations for aminoisobutyrate and cycloleucine in isolated diaphragm muscle have been determined. The figures show the concentration (C) finally attained in the tissue for various concentrations of amino acid in the incubation medium (S). Because of the range of

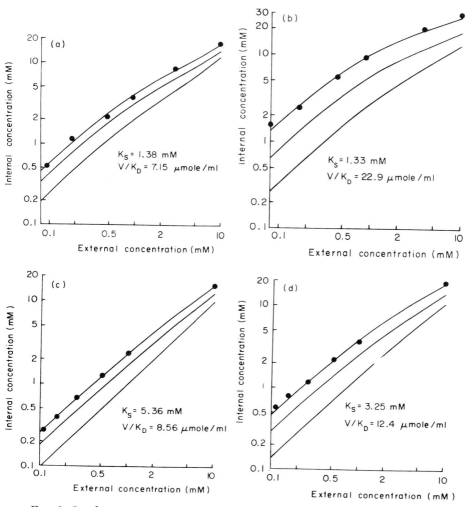

FIG. 6. Steady state concentrations of aminoisobutyrate (a) and (b) and cyclo-leucine (c) and (d) in isolated diaphragms in the absence (a) and (c) and presence (b) and (d) of insulin. The circles are the experimental values, the line passing through them that calculated from Eq. (4) with the values of K_s and V/K_D indicated. The two successively lower lines result from substitution of the same values of K_s and V/K_D in Eq. (4) with $K_c = 20$ mM and 5 mM.

concentrations covered a logarithmic scale is necessary. It is interesting to note that in the presence of insulin the intracellular concentration of aminoisobutyrate rises as high as 30 mM—far in excess of the concentration of any amino acid normally present. What consequences if any accumulation of so much charged solute have on the metabolism of the cell or for what purpose uptake to this extent occurs is not known. Although stimulation of sodium flux rates during amino acid uptake is observed with avian erythrocytes (Wheeler and Christensen, 1967), neither in these cells nor in isolated diaphragm do the levels of sodium and potassium appear to change.

The lines drawn through the experimental points in Fig. 6 are a best fit derived from the data by computer analysis. In these experiments a best fit was found with values of K_c so high (in excess of 10^{10} mM) such as to reduce Eq. (3) to the simpler Eq. (2) which has the advantage that K_s and V/K_D can be readily assessed by graphical means for, on rearrangement,

$$\Delta = V/K_D - K_s(\Delta/S) \tag{5}$$

where $\Delta = C - S$, the concentration difference established. Under these circumstances the apparent K_m of uptake of aminoisobutyrate came to about 1.3 mM both in the presence and absence of insulin, the value of V/K_D showing a threefold rise with insulin (Fig. 6a and b). For cycloleucine K_s fell from around 5.2 mM to 2.75 mM with insulin and ratio V/K_D again showed a rise (Fig. 6c and d). The additional curves show the change in amount of accumulation that would result if, with the values of V/K_D of the best fit, K_c was either 20 mM or 5 mM. The difference is substantial.

The value of K_s for aminoisobutyrate are similar to other determinations (Akedo and Christensen, 1962; Maio and Rickenberg, 1962; Kuchler and Marlowe-Kuchler, 1965; Bombara and Bergamini, 1968; Elsas et al., 1968; Guidotti et al., 1968b) with a variety of tissues. Fewer figures are available for cycloleucine (Oxender and Christensen, 1963; Eavenson and Christensen, 1967; Cutler and Lorenzo, 1968). The results in Fig. 6 suggest that the steady state concentrations finally attained are consistent with a model in which a saturable uptake process is balanced by outward movement with kinetics similar to diffusion. Guidotti et al. (1968b) have data for the chicken embryo heart, which are again explicable on this model. These results are particularly interesting in the light of Cohen (1967), in which published data of steady state concentrations for histidine uptake by intestine (Agar et al., 1954) and aminoisobutyrate and cycloleucine uptake by mouse brain (Lahiri and Lajtha, 1964) were analyzed. In both cases the data would not fit Eq. (2)

but were consistent with a suitable process operative in both directions and negligible diffusion, i.e.,

$$\frac{VS}{(K_s + S)} = \frac{VC}{(K_c + C)} \tag{6}$$

which on taking logarithms becomes

$$\log C = \log S + \log (K_c/K_s) \tag{7}$$

Cohen (1967) found a linear relationship for $\log C$ vs $\log S$. Likewise the figures provided by Lembach and Charalampous (1967) for steady state levels of aminoisobutyrate and serine in KB cells give a linear $\log C$ and $\log S$ relationship—a situation not encountered in the data of Fig. 6.

However, it seems possible that although the data of Fig. 6 fit well to Eq. (2) there may be several alternative values for V/K_D, K_s and K_c which will give very similar fitting to the experimental data. Some of these alternative values are given in Table VI. The high but finite values of K_c will still mean that a saturable efflux process plays only a small part. Where K_s and K_c are very low both systems are likely to be saturated and to operate maximally at low solute concentrations.

As pointed out earlier, attempts at measuring kinetic parameters of glucose uptake by muscle have given confusing results. It seems that

TABLE VI
ALTERNATIVE VALUES FOR KINETIC PARAMETERS[a,b]

	K_s (mM)	K_c (mM)	V/K_D (μmole/ml)
Aminoisobutyrate			
− insulin	1.38	∞	7.15
	1.64	208	8.11
+ insulin	1.33	∞	22.9
	0.074	0.98	852
Cycloleucine			
− insulin	5.36	∞	8.56
	6.62	64.4	13.8
	0.017	0.041	6280
+ insulin	3.23	∞	12.4
	4.11	64.1	19.7
	0.0178	0.0703	5124

[a] Giving suitable fits to the data for steady state concentrations of aminoisobutyrate and cycloleucine shown in Fig. 6 for isolated rat diaphragm.

[b] The first set of figures in each case are the values employed in Fig. 6.

similar measurements for amino acids may give similar diversity of result. Whether insulin acts by lowering the apparent K_m of uptake or the maximum rate of transport still leaves open the question of what in fact these changes mean in terms of the functioning of the membrane carrier for the amino acids. For example a change in V_{max} could indicate either the bringing into play of extra carrier molecules or may arise from an enhanced rate of operation of those already in use. Likewise, a lowering of K_m by insulin can be conceived of in enzymic terms as a raising of the affinity of the solute for the carrier and implies that the action of the hormone will be more apparent at low solute concentrations. The ability of insulin to stimulate incorporation of amino acid presented to the tissue in high concentrations suggests therefore that the influence of

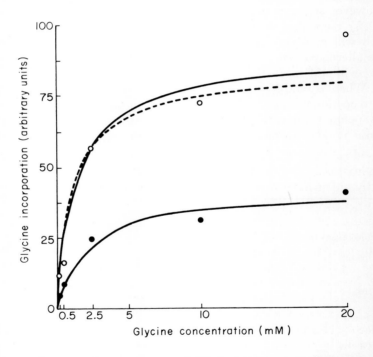

FIG. 7. The rate of incorporation of ^{14}C-glycine into protein of isolated rat diaphragm at various glycine concentrations. The circles are the data of Hechter and Halkerston (1964) in the presence ○ and absence ● of insulin. The solid lines are extrapolated Michaelis-Menten curves with values of $K_m = 1.43$ mM, $V = 88.4$ and $K_m = 1.73$, $V = 40$, obtained by treating the data by the procedure of Barber *et al.* (1967). The broken line is from $K_m = 1.24$, $V = 83.4$, obtained by conventional treatment of the data; in the absence of insulin the solid and broken lines superimpose.

the hormone on incorporation is not solely through stimulation of transport processes.

The facility with which the Michaelis-Menten formulation can be fitted to appropriate curves has been commented on previously and is illustrated in Fig. 7 in which data of Hechter and Halkerston (1964) have been analyzed to give a K_m for the incorporation of ^{14}C-glycine into protein, a process that is manifestly made up of several quite separate reactions. However, if it can be shown that the K_m for glycine entry into the tissue is considerably higher than that of glycine activation or transfer to glycyl-tRNA, presumably the procedure is valid for measurement of the parameters of accumulation. A similar argument is implicit in experiments measuring kinetics of glucose uptake from the rate of $^{14}CO_2$ output (Froesch and Ginsberg, 1962; Kuo *et al.*, 1967) and in those of E. J. Harris and Manger (1968) measuring succinate penetration into mitochondria.

V. EFFECT OF INSULIN ON LABELING OF AMINOACYL-tRNA

If indeed there is effective compartmentation of the pool of free amino acids in muscle (see Section IV,A), it is of course impossible to measure directly either the size, or in the case of labeled amino acids the specific activity, of the pool that functions as the source of amino acids entering protein. An indirect procedure that has been attempted in the author's laboratory (Davey and Manchester, 1969) is to take advantage of the fact that in the course of protein synthesis amino acids are first activated by the appropriate activating enzymes and then become linked to transfer RNA. Measurements of the specific activity of amino acids attached to tRNA should be an indication of the specific activity of the pool from which these amino acids are drawn. The procedure however is not without technical difficulties.

Because of the greater content of tRNA in cardiac muscle than diaphragm and the greater weight of tissue, we employed hearts in these experiments. After perfusion of the hearts for a period with labeled amino acid, the hearts were homogenized, the transfer RNA extracted and purified from protein by treatment with bentonite, and separated and identified from other cellular components by gradient centrifugation. It was hoped to study labeling of the tRNA with glycine, proline, and methionine (amino acids whose accumulation is enhanced by insulin), and with leucine and tyrosine (amino acids whose accumulation is not observably affected by insulin). However, though in gradient centrifugation there was good correlation of radioactivity and optical density when leucine or tyrosine were employed, with the other three amino acids the radioactivity lagged behind the optical density profile. These findings, though disappointing, are not unexpected in that there is a surprising variation in stability for the different aminoacyl-tRNA species, some values of which are noted in Table VII. It is interesting to observe that hydrolysis is enhanced by tris (Sarin and Zamecnik, 1964; Heredia and Halvorson, 1966) and also interesting to realize that certain amino acid species may be expected to decay very rapidly under the conditions of *in vitro* incorporating systems when these are used as the source of activated amino acid for protein synthesis.

The results of the perfusion studies are shown in Table VIII and the specific activity of the aminoacyl-tRNA is compared with that calculated for the free amino acid in the total system, adding the content of muscle and perfusate together. However, it has to be remembered that only a portion of the total tRNA in the cell accepts any one particular amino acid. Quite how much constitutes the specific acceptor capacity, the values of which for cardiac tRNA are not known. Acceptor capacities have been determined for tRNA from rabbit liver, yeast, *E. coli,* and *Neurospora* and the figures so obtained are contained in Table IX. Apart from the obvious variations from one amino acid to another and between

TABLE VII

THE HALF-LIFE OF VARIOUS AMINOACYL-tRNA ESTERS[a]

Amino acid	$t\frac{1}{2}$ (min) at 37° at pH of								
	7.0	7.25	7.5	7.65	8.0	8.15	8.5	8.65	9
Alanine	—	—	15[b]	—	—	—	—	—	—
Aspartic acid	27	17	—	5.3	—	2.5	—	0.63	—
Arginine	—	11	—	—	—	—	—	—	—
Glutamic acid	17	12.5	—	5.1	—	1.5	—	0.53	—
Glycine	—	9	—	—	—	—	—	—	—
Histidine	54	—	37	—	22	—	18	—	16
Methionine	—	—	13[b]	—	—	—	—	—	—
Phenylalanine	60	55[b]	30	—	20	—	16	—	15
Proline	15	—	9	—	3	—	2	—	1.8
Threonine	130	—	65	—	35	—	30	—	25
Valine	—	65	—	—	—	—	—	—	—

[a] Compiled from data of Coles *et al.* (1962), Gilbert (1963), Wolfenden (1963), Gatica *et al.* (1966) and Shearn and Horowitz (1969).

[b] At 30°.

TABLE VIII

THE SPECIFIC ACTIVITY OF AMINOACYL-tRNA ISOLATED FROM RAT HEART
MUSCLE AFTER PERFUSION WITH LABELED AMINO ACIDS

Labeled amino acid in perfusate	Concentration (μM)	Specific activity (Ci/mole)	Specific activity of acyl-tRNA		specific aminoacyl-tRNA (Ci/mole)[b]
			total aminoacyl-tRNA		
			(dpm/O.D. unit)	(Ci/mole)[a]	
Tyrosine	0.24	3,900	41,500	10.3	1,290
Tyrosine	90	130	6,100	1.52	190
Tyrosine[c]	90	130	4,300	1.06	133
Leucine[c]	144	45	9,000	2.24	41
Glycine[c]	268	11	c. 700	c. 0.15	c. 7
Methionine[c]	54	166	<10,000	<2.4	<150
Proline[c]	277	27	<200	<0.05	<2

[a] Calculated from dpm/O.D. unit on the basis of 1 O.D. unit = 1.82 mμmole tRNA.

[b] Calculated from acceptor capacities given by Cantoni *et al.* (1962).

[c] Amino acids added at plasma levels.

organisms it is interesting to note that the total acceptor capacity falls considerably short of 1000 mmole/mole tRNA. Novelli (1967) and Shearn and Horowitz (1969) have recently emphasized that different amino acids appear to have different requirements for optimal attachment to tRNA so that it may well be that the quoted figures are an underestimate of true acceptor capacities. However, equally it is not known whether tRNA *in vivo* is fully loaded with amino acid or whether the degree of esterification is substantially short of 100%, and if the latter, the extent to which unesterified tRNA can affect the rate of protein synthesis through abortive binding to messenger (Levin and Nirenberg, 1968).

With these reservations, and using the acceptor capacities for liver, the determined specific activities of the individual amino acids come remarkably close to the values calculated for the free amino acids (Table VIII). This is particularly so when the perfusate contains amino acids at the concentrations normally found in plasma—under these conditions the total quantity of amino acid present in the perfusate was much greater than that in the heart so that the perfusate amino acid would not be expected to undergo much dilution if there were complete equilibration with the pool in the tissue. When the perfusate contained only a trace quantity of tyrosine the amount of amino acid in the heart was considerably greater than that added to the perfusate. The specific activity calculated on the basis of complete equilibration therefore represents a

TABLE IX

AMINO ACID ACCEPTOR CAPACITY FOR tRNA FROM VARIOUS SOURCES[a]

	Rat liver[b]	E. coli[c] (mmole/mole tRNA)	Yeast[d]	Neurospora[e]
Alanine	34	70	6	43
Arginine		73	36	55
Aspartic acid		22	22	35
Cysteine				8
Glutamic acid	12	65	11	50
Glycine	22	89	5	27
Histidine	9	24	10	10
Isoleucine	60	13	22	47
Leucine	54	78	41	57
Lysine	19	69	29	21
Methionine	16	24	19	42
Phenylalanine	18	22	19	12
Proline	26	36	7	18
Serine	43	37	44	61
Threonine	13	48	35	37
Tryptophan	7			29
Tyrosine	8	21	18	25
Valine	29	67	35	57
	370	768	359	634

[a] For conversion of figures expressed in terms of O.D. units it has been assumed that 1 O.D. $_{260}$ unit = 1.82 mμmole tRNA.

[b] Cantoni *et al.* (1962).

[c] Yegian and Stent (1969).

[d] Cantoni and Richards (1966).

[e] Shearn and Horowitz (1969).

minimum value but is nonetheless three times that of the extracted tRNA. This arises possibly because when only one amino acid is added, and that in trace concentration, there is a substantial net efflux of amino acid from the tissue. Insofar as with an appreciable concentration of amino acid in the perfusate the specific activity of the aminoacyl-tRNA approaches that of the medium, the results are consistent with the suggestion (p. 278) of entry of amino acids into protein before they have mixed much with the cell pool.

Heart muscle has a tRNA content of 30 to 80 mg/100 gm tissue (Earl and Korner, 1966; Wool *et al.*, 1968a; Davey and Manchester, 1969), which represents a maximal acceptor capacity of 1.2 to 3.2 μmole/100 gm. This is very small by comparison with the size of the amino acid pool of muscle (Table II). For diaphragm the potential acceptor capacity is about 0.5 μmole/100 gm (Margreth and Novello, 1964; Davey and Manchester, 1969) and for liver probably about 5 μmole/100 gm. Calculations (Manchester, 1970d) suggest that the rate of synthesis of protein in isolated diaphragm is not less than 5 μmole amino acid incorporated in peptide linkage per gram of tissue per hour. Assuming full esterification 5 mμmole tRNA ester must be turning over on average 1000 times an hour. In liver with a rate of protein synthesis of 12 mg/gm/hr (Richmond *et al.*, 1963) the figure will be approximately 2400.

An interesting feature of the labeling of the heart muscle tRNA for tyrosine and leucine was an apparent increase in the uptake of ^{14}C in the presence of insulin (Fig. 8). This could arise in several ways. First, an increased incorporation of label into protein means an increased transfer of radioactivity through tRNA, but this would more likely explain an increase in the speed of its labeling rather than an increase in the extent. Second, if insulin does increase the entry of label into a limited amino acid pool in the tissue, hence increasing its specific activity, this would reflect in extra radioactivity attached to the tRNA. A third possibility would be for insulin to affect the extent of esterification of the tRNA, that is tRNA may not at all times be fully loaded with amino acid but depending inter alia on the availability of amino acids and/or hormonal influences the extent of esterification may change.

In muscle probably about 65% of the total RNA is ribosomal (Wool

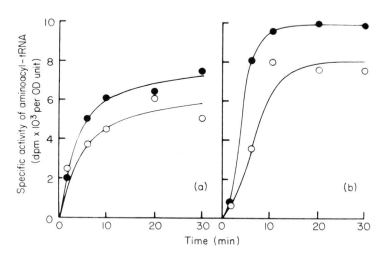

Fɪɢ. 8. Incorporation of ^{3}H-amino acids into aminoacyl-tRNA in heart muscle. The hearts were perfused for the periods stated with (a) tyrosine and (b) leucine and then the aminoacyl-tRNA extracted. ●, Insulin present in the perfusate; ○, insulin absent. (From Davey and Manchester, 1969.)

et al., 1968a) and 15–20% transfer. Expressed in molar terms this is a ratio of about 20 transfer molecules to each ribosome. It is not possible to say *in vivo* what constitutes the optimal ratio, whether availability of tRNA is more limiting than the number of ribosomes or vice versa; that is, whether the rate of movement of the ribosome along the messenger is limited by the availability of the appropriate tRNA species or by other factors. Increase particularly of tRNA has been noted as one of the early responses of the uterus to estrogen (J. D. Wilson, 1963; O'Malley *et al.,* 1968), suggesting its importance in extra protein synthesis. On the other hand increased synthesis of rRNA is a frequently observed response to endocrine stimulation and there are observations suggesting that a primary defect in insulin deficiency lies in the ribosome, as discussed in the next section.

Incorporation of phenylalanine by poly U primed ribosomes of *E. coli* appears to rise as the concentration of the phe-tRNA is raised until the ratio of the phe-tRNA to ribosomes is 7:1 (Anderson, 1969). Thereafter further phe-tRNA begins to inhibit. With muscle ribosomes a molar ratio of tRNA to ribosomes of over 400:1 was found to be necessary to saturate the capacity of the ribosomes for incorporation (Wool and Cavicchi, 1967). Although we can hardly extrapolate from these figures to the whole cell, if we have around sixty forms of tRNA the average ratio of any particular species to the number of ribosomes is going to be 1:3 and for any rare form it will of course be lower (Yang and Novelli, 1968). We thus have in the availability of charged tRNA of the right codon recognition form a powerful potential for modulation of the rate of growth of the peptide chain, some codons being capable of translation more rapidly than others (Stent, 1964). Moreover, if we have appreciable tRNA not loaded with amino acid we have a potential competitive inhibitor for binding to the ribosome, which could prevent access of the appropriate amino acid bearing form (Seeds and Conway, 1966; Levin and Nirenberg, 1968; Ikemura and Fukutome, 1969). Affecting the availability of amino acids may therefore exert a controlling influence both on the supply of substrate in itself and by reducing the amount of unchanged tRNA. Though at present unproven, these proposals offer a potential explanation of the way the effects of insulin on both protein synthesis and amino acid accumulation may be linked. Bacteria can in fact alter the activity of their t-RNA according to circumstances (Sueoka and Kano-Sueoka, 1964; Kaneko and Doi, 1966). The extent of methylation of tRNA appears to change in different growth phases in yeast (Kjellin-Straby and Phillips, 1968) and affects amino acid acceptor function (Shugart *et al.,* 1968). In mammary gland explants, insulin has recently been reported to increase methylating activity towards RNA as well as preferentially increasing tRNA synthesis (Turkington, 1969).

The concentration of tRNA in skeletal muscle is of the order of 250 μg/gm. If all of this is in the intracellular space, the concentration rises to 500 μg/ml of fluid, which is 2×10^{-6} M. This of course constitutes at least twenty varieties so that individual tRNA's are likely to be present at concentrations less than 10^{-7} M. The K_m values for several activating enzymes towards their appropriate tRNA's have been given as 2–4×10^{-7} M (Makman and Cantoni, 1966; Baldwin and Berg, 1966; Peterkofsky et al., 1966; Stulberg, 1967) though a value as low as 3×10^{-8} has been reported (Clark and Eyzaguirre, 1962). Thus the activating enzymes are unlikely to be saturated with tRNA, though this may have the virtue of assisting the aminoacyl-tRNA to detach from the enzyme. With respect to free amino acids K_m values for various activating enzymes range from 10^{-7} M to 10^{-2} M (summarized in P. J. Peterson, 1967; also Heinrikson and Hartley, 1967). If values similar to these are applicable to the activating enzymes of muscle, several amino acids will be present in concentrations substantially below the K_m for the appropriate enzymes and variations in the availability of these amino acids could be of consequence if the overall activity of the activating enzymes is not present in appreciable excess of potential amino acyl-tRNA requirements. Wool et al. (1968b) noted a decline in cardiac activating enzymes in diabetes, and Germanyuk and Mironenko (1969) have noted a defect in the functioning of both hepatic tRNA and activating enzymes of diabetic rabbit liver. Charging of limiting species of tRNA may be the explanation of the findings of Earl et al. (1967), who observed that increasing the concentration of amino acids supplied to perfused hearts above the normal plasma level increased the rate of incorporation but diminished the response to insulin. This suggested that even in the presence of normal concentrations of amino acids the rate of protein synthesis may be limited by the supply of amino acids or some factor relating to this which can be regulated by increasing their availability. In fact under their conditions the hearts only retained their *in vivo* amino acid content during perfusion when amino acids were present in the perfusate at above-plasma concentrations. Similarly, with liver slices the rate of protein synthesis appears to be enhanced by addition of increasing concentrations of certain amino acids (Hanking and Roberts, 1965) and a comparable phenomenon is seen with the perfused liver (Jefferson and Korner, 1969). They found that stability of polysome profile and ability of ribosome preparations to incorporate amino acids was dependent on the presence of eleven amino acids: arginine, asparagine, isoleucine, leucine, lysine, methionine, phenylalanine, proline, threonine, tryptophan, and valine. They suggested that availability of amino acid in some way regulated binding of ribosomes to messenger. Similar considerations may explain the toxic influence of certain amino acids (Hardin and Hove, 1951) and the interference of various amino acids with the activation or incorporation of other species (Kovačević, 1967; Roscoe et al., 1968).

VI. INSULIN AND RNA METABOLISM IN MUSCLE

It was noted earlier (p. 271) that insulin stimulates both glucose uptake by muscle and incorporation of amino acids into protein in the presence of sufficient actinomycin to give virtually complete inhibition of nucleic acid synthesis (Eboué-Bonis et al., 1963; Wool and Moyer, 1964). Though this observation suggests that the immediately apparent actions of the hormone on muscle are not dependent on or mediated through synthesis of any particular species of RNA, in the longer term the protein synthetic activity of a tissue will depend in part on its content of RNA (A. L. Goldberg, 1967), which may be subject to regulation by insulin. Heart muscle of alloxan-diabetic rats was found to have only 60% of the RNA content of controls (Wool et al., 1968a) though the amount of DNA was unchanged. This would suggest that directly or indirectly the availability of insulin controls the level of RNA, though it is important to note that RNA content was affected by fasting and in this condition even the amount of DNA declined. Analysis of the RNA showed comparable proportions of ribosomal material in each case. Several workers have shown enhanced incorporation of various precursors into extractable RNA of muscle in the presence of insulin (Wool, 1963; Davidson and Goodner, 1966) but the author has had difficulty in fully confirming this action of the hormone (Manchester, 1967b). The reason for the difference in result is not clear. The efficiency of the procedure used for extraction of the RNA may be of consequence and there is a wide variation in published figures for muscle (compare Wool, 1963, and A. L. Goldberg, 1967). The choice of precursor may also have a bearing in that in the author's experiments there appeared to be some stimulation of incorporation of ^{14}C from orotic acid and uracil but not from adenine. [The variability in response with different precursors is not unique to this problem, but is also observed in studies of RNA metabolism following denervation (Manchester and Harris, 1968) and also of dietary influence (Wannemacher et al., 1968).] Clearly, as with incorporation of labeled amino acids into protein, the extent of dilution of the precursor on entry into the tissue will influence the rate of entry of radioactivity into nucleic acid. Since the adenine nucleotides are the most plentiful it might be expected that use of ^{14}C-adenine would lead to least incorporation of label, but the converse appears to be the case. Presumably the greater incorporation of ^{14}C must be indicative of a very much more rapid conversion of adenine to ATP than of the other precursors to their triphosphate forms and this can be seen in the very much greater concentration gradient established between soluble adenine derivatives in the cell by comparison with other precursors (Table X). It is possible that insulin in its general stimulation of anabolic reactions in muscle can lead to circumstances that promote the enzymic interconversions of the nucleotide bases to their triphosphate forms and that this is more noticeable experimentally for the slower reactions. RNA synthesis is largely limited to the cell nucleus, and this factor could also complicate its response to insulin. Wool (1963) claimed that diaphragm muscle incubated in the presence of insulin increased its content of nucleic acid to a measurable extent. Though these figures are probably incorrect, the presence of insulin does appear to maintain a slightly greater content of extractable RNA than in its absence (Manchester, 1967b).

Though actinomycin does not prevent the stimulation of protein synthesis by insulin, its presence does eventually interfere with incorporation (Manchester, 1964; Wool and Moyer, 1964). On the assumption that the decline in incorporation results from loss of some crucial species of RNA (e.g., messenger) the fall-off in incorporation suggests it has a half-life of around 2.5 hours, a value that fits in well with many other estimates of mRNA turnover in animal tissues (listed in Manchester, 1968a). If indeed ^{14}C-adenine rapidly equilibrates with the cell adenine nucleotide pool we can from the rate of adenine incorporation calculate

TABLE X

CONCENTRATION RATIOS ESTABLISHED FOR VARIOUS NUCLEOTIDE PRECURSORS
BY ISOLATED RAT DIAPHRAGM DURING INCUBATION

Precursor	Concentration added to medium (μM)	Concentration ratio established[a]
Adenine	13	19.4
Uracil	7	0.89
Orotic acid	9	0.85
Thymine	10	0.83
Thymidine	4	0.91

[a] Ratio of radioactivity extracted from tissue by boiling in water, expressed for a unit of tissue water divided by radioactivity in the same volume of medium at the end of the incubation. Each figure is the mean of three observations. Thymidine was ^3H-labeled, the others contained ^{14}C. Incubation was for 2 hours.

the rate of RNA synthesis. Assuming that the RNA synthesized contains roughly 25% adenine, then on the basis of published figures (Manchester, 1967b) RNA formation occurs at a rate of about 0.22 μmole nucleotide joined up/gm tissue/hour. This is about 1/25 of the rate of peptide bond synthesis on a molar basis, but a much greater fractional rate of 4% per hour. A half-life for rRNA of 5 days (Loeb et al., 1965; S. H. Wilson and Hoagland, 1967) represents a turnover of 0.6% per hour, though Hadjiolov (1966) found a more rapid turnover. If we assume the quantity of messenger to be in the proportion of 90 nucleotides per ribosome, then the mRNA content of diaphragm muscle (at least that attached to ribosomes) would be not more than 25 μg/gm tissue. Since it is unlikely that turnover of messenger occurs twice an hour, a large part of the observed incorporation is presumably into material that breaks down again before leaving the nucleus (H. Harris, 1968).

VII. PROTEIN SYNTHESIS IN SUBCELLULAR SYSTEMS

The measurement of protein synthesis in subcellular preparations clearly offers a valuable approach to the manner in which insulin controls this process. Muscle has the disadvantage by comparison with several other tissues in being difficult to homogenize and in possessing less RNA. However, ribosomes and polysomes have been prepared from cardiac and skeletal muscle from a variety of animals (Florini, 1964; Earl and Korner, 1965; Rampersad et al., 1965; Moraz, 1967; Schreiber et al., 1968) and from chicken embryo muscle (Heywood et al., 1967; Heywood and Rich, 1968). In the latter case high concentrations of KCl are incorporated in the initial extraction medium to dissolve myosin and increase the yield of polysomes, which is otherwise very low (Heywood et al., 1968) and a similar procedure has been used by Chen and Young (1968). Since the molecular weights of the filbrillar proteins are relatively high, their synthesis will employ large polysomes and classes of polysomes suitable for synthesis of myosin (50–60 ribosomes) and for actin and tropomyosin have been isolated by Heywood and Rich (1968).

The majority of the work to be described in this section is concerned with the difference in function between ribosomes from diabetic and from normal animals. This is in distinction to the major part of the work in the previous sections, for whereas insulin added to diabetic muscle preparations undoubtedly restores their activity toward normal, the action of the hormone is indubitable in enhancing protein synthesis and many other functions when added to tissue from normal animals. It is not clear whether the same mechanisms are operative in the two situations. We may therefore have to distinguish between a defect in the capacity for protein synthesis that exists in insulin deficient tissues, as opposed to an alternative or additional mechanism that marks the response of the otherwise healthy tissue. The following paragraphs are largely a summary of the elegant studies of Wool and his colleagues (reviewed in Wool *et al.*, 1968b).

Ribosomes isolated from cardiac muscle of diabetic animals possess about 70% of the ability of ribosomes from normal tissue to incorporate amino acids (Rampersad and Wool, 1965). Particles from both sources incorporate a great deal more phenylalanine in the presence of poly U, but whereas cardiac particles retain the differential between normal and diabetic in the presence of poly U, skeletal muscle ribosomes, though starting from different activities, seem to reach a common ceiling or even in the diabetic exceed the incorporating capacity of normal particles (Wool and Cavicchi, 1967). The concentration of magnesium ions present however has a marked influence on the response to poly U and in part determines the relative responses to the synthetic polynucleotide. The ability of poly U to raise incorporation to similar levels irrespective of the origin of the ribosomes could be interpreted to mean that diabetic preparations possess essentially normal ribosomes but that fewer are contained in polysomes (say because of shortage of messenger-RNA) and this conclusion might be supported from the sucrose gradient profiles, which show many fewer polysomes and more monomers and complexes in diabetic preparations (Stirewalt *et al.*, 1967). That poly U does not raise the rate of incorporation of diabetic cardiac ribosomes to the level of controls suggests the possibility that diabetic ribosomes have an impaired functional capacity. In point of fact if there were simply more ribosomes and fewer polysomes in diabetic preparations we might have expected poly U to raise incorporation by the diabetic material to greater than control values because of the greater number of single ribosomes available, and this indeed seems to happen with skeletal muscle preparations. However it is questionable whether the results with poly U are to be taken at their face value since saturating concentrations are 20-fold the amount of rRNA (to be compared with the usual 2% for mRNA in a polysome) and an additional function of synthetic nucleotides, namely to detach nonfunctioning ribosomes from polysomes where the former are inhibiting translation, has recently been proposed (Hunter and Korner, 1969).

From the gradient profiles about 70% of ribosomes are in polysomes in normal muscle (Stirewalt *et al.*, 1967) but a substantially lower percentage were in polysomes in diabetic tissue. As stated, the presence of single ribosomes may indicate lack of messenger but it may also indicate lack of initiation factor or translocase required for ribosomal subunits to rejoin polysomes and for the ribosome to proceed along the messenger (Leder et al., 1969). That many ribosomal subunits are present would be consistent with a failure of initiation (Brawerman and Eisenstadt, 1966; Kaempfer, 1969) but for what cause it is not possible to say. One of the most striking features of the gradient profiles is the speed of return of the diabetic profile to normal—0.1 unit of insulin per animal 5 minutes before sacrifice is sufficient to produce a significant change (Stirewalt et al., 1967). [Ketosis of fasting it is interesting to note is apparently also reversed equally rapidly on administration of insulin (Foster, 1967).] Particles from fasting rat muscle show impaired protein synthesis, which is restored towards normal on treatment with insulin but administration of the hormone to fed animals had no effect (Wool et al., 1968b). This is of interest since Young et al. (1968) found that administration of insulin to normal rats did raise the proportion of heavier polysomes.

Puromycin inhibits protein synthesis because it inserts itself between the ribosome and the growing peptide chain to which it links, and the peptidyl puromycin is then liberated (Allen and Zamecnik, 1962; Rabinovitz and Fisher, 1962; Morris et al., 1963; Nathans, 1964; Williamson and Schweet, 1964). By measuring the number of labeled puromycin molecules that become incorporated into peptides, Wool and Kurihara (1967) attempted to determine how many ribosomes were actually synthesizing peptide bonds in their preparations. In systems of normal origin they found about 25% of the ribosomes functional, in diabetics 8%—a striking difference—and for both figures a considerably lower percentage than the number of ribosomes contained in polysomes, but consistent with the idea that one factor limiting the rate of protein synthesis in cell-free preparations is the blockage of messenger with nonfunctional ribosomes (Hunter and Korner, 1969). It is of course open to question whether gradient profiles are an accurate measure of what existed in the cell prior to homogenization. For one thing the yield of RNA on extraction is low and therefore not necessarily representative, and because of the relatively lengthy procedure involved in preparation some breakdown may have occurred. Equally it would seem improbable that so few ribosomes are functional in vivo. However this may be one of the factors that explains why amino acid incorporation by cell-free systems is two orders of magnitude slower than in situ (Hendler, 1962). From the rates of phenylalanine incorporation it is possible to calculate that each active ribosome, assuming that it is incorporating an equal quantity of each of the other amino acids, forms about 27 peptide bonds in the course of the lifetime of the system. Thirty peptide units is supposed to be about the spacing of the ribosomes in mammalian polysomes. If only 25% of the ribosomes are active it seems possible that at least some of the other 75% will be bound to messenger and lead to translation arrest, but if so they might be expected to inhibit movement of the active ribosomes along the messenger before they have moved 27 codons. On the other hand if puromycin can bring about liberation of inactive ribosomes (Hunter and Korner, 1969) the significance of the number of active ribosomes estimated with puromycin becomes less clear. For puromycin to be able to bring about release of the peptide chain, the peptide must be in the peptide binding site in order that puromycin can attach to the amino acid binding site on the ribosome. The distribution of the nascent peptide chains between the two sites existing in the ribosomal preparations will obviously affect their reactivity with puromycin in the absence of adequate transferase activity.

Treatment of normal animals with puromycin or cycloheximide 30 minutes before death leads to breakdown of polysomes to give patterns similar to those in the diabetic state, that is a large proportion of monomers and dimers and fewer larger units (Stirewalt *et al.*, 1967). The incorporating capacity of the particles is also substantially below normal (Wool and Cavicchi, 1966). In this instance administration of insulin is without effect on the profile, nor does its administration enhance the capacity of the particles to incorporate amino acids or bring about restoration of the diabetic state to normal. The disappearance of polysomes on administration of cycloheximide is somewhat unexpected since in several systems the antibiotic seems to "freeze" polysomes and hinder their breakdown (Wettstein *et al.*, 1964; Colombo *et al.*, 1965; Trakatellis *et al.*, 1965, Stanners, 1966) but presumably in the cell other mechanisms come into play, and the high concentration used by Wool and Cavicchi (1966) may have been significant in this respect—lower concentrations can indeed lead to more polysome formation (Jondorf *et al.*, 1966). Because administration of insulin is without effect in animals dosed with cycloheximide, Wool *et al.* (1968b) proposed that the action of insulin in restoring the defect in diabetic ribosomes results from the hormone's stimulation of the synthesis of a rapidly turning over protein component, which is necessary for the effective functioning of the ribosomes and clearly is not being made in the presence of an inhibitor of protein formation. From the rate of decay of incorporating capacity following administration of cycloheximide it was concluded that the postulated protein has a half-life of about 30 minutes.

Whether these deductions are correct or not remains to be determined. In view of the decay of the polysome pattern following injection of cycloheximide it is not surprising that the cell-free system has reduced incorporating capacity Moreover, if cycloheximide leads to breakdown of polysomes in normal animals that already possess sufficient insulin it is hardly surprising that insulin administration to the diabetic in the presence of inhibitor has little effect. The nub of the question is what in fact the cycloheximide does that leads to breakdown of the polysome profile —does it inhibit synthesis of a protein specifically required for ribosomal functioning or does inhibition of protein synthesis lead to liberation of degrading enzymes that break up the polysomes? It has been claimed that polysomes isolated from regenerating liver possess greater stability than those from controls (Tsukada and Lieberman, 1965), and more recently it has been suggested that liver from hypophysectomized rats contains more active and latent ribonuclease, the level of these activities correlating with the degree of disaggregation of the gradient profiles (Brewer *et al.*, 1969). Whether a similar situation is responsible for the different profiles of diabetics and inhibitor-treated animals is at present not known. Inhibition by cycloheximide of chain initiation (Lin *et al.*, 1966; Baliga *et al.*, 1969) would in time presumably also bring about polysome disaggregation and under these circumstances failure to respond to insulin is hardly surprising.

Obviously if a tissue is incubated with sufficient inhibitor such that no protein synthesis occurs it is not possible to see whether insulin is still capable of influencing the process. If, however, inhibitor is present at levels such that protein synthesis in the tissue as judged by amino acid incorporation is much reduced, an influence of insulin on incorporation is still observable (Wool *et al.*, 1965; Manchester, 1967a; and Fig. 9). Of course the amount of extra incorporation induced by insulin will be much less, but proportionally the stimulation may be similar; e.g., if (Fig. 9) the scale is expanded the effect of insulin appears more obvious. These observations do not suggest that the action of insulin in stimulating incorporation in normal muscle results from the production by insulin of a specific protein unless we assume that synthesis of this particular protein is more than averagely resistant to inhibition by cycloheximide or puromycin.

That ribosomes of diabetic origin may have impaired capacity is more directly demonstrated in the work of Martin and Wool (1968) in which they dissociated ribosomes into their constituent large and small (60 S and 40 S) subunits. These they then recombined with appropriate subunits derived from normal ribosomes to give hybrids, one subunit coming from normal sources and the other from diabetic. The capacity for incorporation of these new ribosomes in the presence of poly U depended

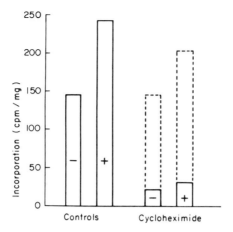

Fig. 9. The effect of cycloheximide on the capacity of insulin to enhance incorporation of ^{14}C-glycine into protein of rat diaphragm. The two columns on the left show the influence of insulin on incorporation in the absence of inhibitor; for those on the right the tissue was preincubated for 30 minutes with cycloheximide at 2 μg/ml before addition of ^{14}C-glycine. The columns with solid lines were the actual results obtained, the broken lines show these figures expanded to the same scale as the tissue incubated without inhibitor. (Based on data of Manchester, 1967a.)

on the concentration of magnesium ions employed. At 9 mM the hybrid containing the 60 S subunit of diabetic origin was less efficient than controls, whereas in 15 mM magnesium both hybrids were equally efficient. Elucidation of whether there is a particular ribosomal protein, whose synthesis is enhanced by the presence of insulin, has been sought by Kurihara and Wool (1968) by acrylamide gel analysis of ribosomal proteins labeled in diabetic and insulin-treated animals. Though they claim to have found evidence of a particular peak of activity present after insulin treatment but absent before, the figures are not very convincing.

In liver, as is to be expected, fasting or diabetes cause breakdown of polysomes but it is interesting to note comparatively little change in the profile in the first week or so of the diabetic condition (Wittman *et al.*, 1969). Administration of insulin to the diabetics brought about a prompt appearance of heavier polysomes but was without much effect when given to starving animals. It has been suggested (Wunner *et al.*, 1966; Baliga *et al.*, 1968; Sidransky *et al.*, 1968) that the availability of certain amino acids, particularly tryptophan, may play a key role in regulating hepatic ribosomal activity, but Wittman *et al.* (1969) point out that hepatic levels of amino acids do not change very much during fasting and that under their conditions feeding glucose to otherwise fasting animals, which causes a decrease in hepatic amino acid concentration (Thomson *et al.*, 1953), restores the number of polysomes. As pointed out earlier, in diabetes the liver may enlarge relative to the rest of the body and its content of a number of enzymes concerned with gluconeogenesis, ketosis, and amino acid metabolism increases so clearly synthesis of specific proteins proceeds rapidly even if the overall activity and that of cell-free preparations is below normal (Green and Miller, 1960; Marsh, 1961; Korner, 1960; Robinson, 1961). Under the circumstances it is interesting that the concentration of activating enzymes appears to rise in fasting (Mariani *et al.*, 1966), perhaps reflecting a need for increased capacity to abstract amino acids for protein synthesis in the face of their enhanced rate of degradation.

VIII. SUMMARY AND CONCLUSIONS

The results of the previous section leave no doubt that insulin exerts a powerful role in enhancing the capacity of muscle to synthesize protein. In the diabetic, either by virtue of lack of insulin alone or of the action of the glucocorticoids unopposed by insulin, muscle will lose protein at least in part through lack of synthesis, and the movements of amino acids either complement or augment the change of rate. The results at the molecular level also fully complement the changes that we observe in clinical or physiological studies. Yet the question remains of what, at the molecular level, insulin actually does, and to this we have as yet no answer. As Wool *et al.* (1968b) emphasized, direct addition of insulin to ribosomes is without effect and, with diaphragm muscle, as the tissue is cut into progressively smaller pieces so is the influence on incorporation lost (Manchester, 1966). Addition of insulin to homogenates or even study of incorporation by homogenates from insulin-treated animals has been found to give negative results (Manchester, 1965c) though it is difficult in such preparations to know how much autolysis is taking place. That the hormone promotes so many other processes in muscle, glucose uptake, glycogen synthesis, precursor incorporation into fat, and even oxidation of amino acids (Manchester, 1963, 1965b), as well as influencing ion movements (Zierler, 1966; Creese, 1968), raises the problem of how we can link together these various effects and show them to stem from a common action. Clearly the movement of amino acids into the cell may be related to the action of the sodium pump and in this way we may see a common influence. In fact the rate of incorporation of glycine is influenced by the availability of potassium ions (Figure 10), both its accumulation and entry into protein being enhanced at 5–10 mM external potassium as opposed to 0 and 20 mM, but the uptake and incorporation of leucine are unaffected (E. J. Harris and Manchester, 1966). That the influence of insulin on leucine incorporation is readily demonstrable argues against any influence of the hormone being operative through regulation of potassium movements. The distinction of enhancement of accumulation and incorporation for glycine responding to potassium and that of leucine not doing so again divides the amino acids into those whose transport appears to be active and possibly using Christensen's A preferring site as opposed to those of the L group (Oxender and Christensen, 1963). Such a division probably characterizes those amino acids whose accumulation is influenced by insulin as opposed to those unresponsive to the hormone (Table IV).

That the extent of penetration of labeled amino acids into the cell pool

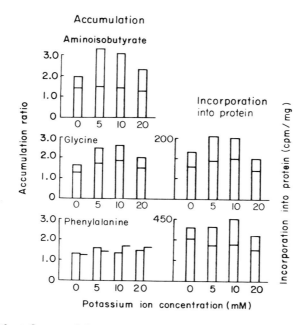

Fig. 10. The influence of the concentration of potassium in the incubation medium on the accumulation and incorporation into protein of ^{14}C-glycine and leucine. The tissue was preincubated for 30 minutes in a large volume of medium of the appropriate potassium concentration then transferred to fresh medium containing ^{14}C-amino acid. (From data of E. J. Harris and Manchester, 1966.)

may be a factor controlled by the functioning of the cell membrane is suggested by some rather strange results found by the author (Manchester, 1966). When diaphragm is incubated in buffer in which sodium has been replaced by potassium then insulin can still enhance incorporation when the labeled amino acid is presented at a low concentration (i.e., less than the plasma level) but when the concentration of added amino acid is raised to 1 mM the effect of the hormone ceases. In other words, with low concentrations of amino acid, the membrane and through it, insulin, can still exert a discriminating influence on amino acid movements, but when amino acid is provided in high concentration the membrane under these conditions is swamped and no longer exerts control. When sodium is replaced by choline rather than potassium the disturbance of membrane function is less severe and insulin continues to exert an influence on incorporation, though not on transport, at all concentrations of amino acids tested.

Clearly it is possible that the rate of protein synthesis could be regulated by the concentrations of ions in the cells as well as outside. The variation in incorporating capacity of ribosomal systems is very sensitive to the amount of magnesium present. Novelli (1967) and Shearn and Horowitz (1969) have emphasized how the efficiency of charging of tRNA is dependent on the ratio of Mg/ATP and that the optimal ratio is different for different amino acids, being quite outside the possible range of *in vivo* conditions for several species. Some of the activating enzymes, moreover, are influenced by potassium levels (Fraser, 1963; Peterson, 1967). Changes in ion concentrations and ATP could therefore readily modify the rate of protein anabolism. It is probably unlikely that under normal conditions *in vivo* that there are gross changes in ion content, but it could be that activation of one or two particular amino acids occurs under suboptimal conditions and that the rate is very sensitive to small fluctuations in the intracellular state.

It is still not established where in or on the cell insulin first acts. Autoradiography of iodine-labeled insulin does not give very clear-cut pictures and a large portion of the hormone appears *in vivo* to be abstracted by the kidneys (Maggi *et al.*, 1969; Mahler and Szabo, 1968). The influence of insulin on transport processes would obviously be consistent with a membrane site of action, though of course is not definitive proof of this and it is less clear how the hormone could influence glycogen synthetase and ribosomal function from this locus. Several hormones are believed to bring about their physiological effects by activating adenyl cyclase in the cell membrane, the intracellular mediator of their effects being cAMP (Robison *et al.*, 1968). Although insulin may suppress the rise in adenyl cyclase activity in adipose tissue following treatment with epinephrine (Jungas, 1966), such action or change in cAMP concentration has not been readily demonstrated in muscle (N. D. Goldberg *et al.*, 1967; Laraia and Reddy, 1969; Craig *et al.*, 1969; Walaas *et al.*, 1969). Addition of cAMP or the dibutyryl derivative is without effect on amino acid incorporation by ribosomal preparations (Wool *et al.*, 1968b) or by diaphragm muscle, and in the author's experience epinephrine in amounts such as to enhance glycogen breakdown etc. is likewise without effect on incorporation (Manchester and Young, 1960b), though inhibition has also been noted (Wool, 1960). Certainly in the presence of epinephrine insulin can enhance incorporation without suppressing the elevated level of lactate formation, which would imply lack of interference with presumed promotion of cAMP formation. Theophylline and caffeine, it is interesting to note, in concentrations often used with other tissue (1 mg/ml) inhibit incorporation, induce rigor, and substantially promote respiration by muscle (Manchester, 1970d) by a mechanism that is not clear (Bianchi, 1961).

In conclusion, therefore, we remain as far from knowing the details at the molecular level of how insulin first interacts with responsive tissues, what is the nature of the insulin receptor, what is the structural feature of the molecule that confers on it its biological properties, and what the first intracellular changes are following contact with insulin, as we were in 1957, when Krahl first proposed the concept of insulin-induced conformational changes in the structure of responsive cells. Such changes, which would facilitate anabolic reactions by enhancing access of appropriate components to each other, imply the role of compartmentation in control and are clearly applicable to many aspects of metabolism, but by virtue of their generality are devoid of specific detail. Unfortunately electron microscopy does not show any visible change in structure with insulin (Orth and Morgan, 1962). There is, however, a difference in change in weight of tissues during incubation or perfusion induced by the hormone, which is consistent with these conformational postulates (Mortimore, 1961; Manchester, 1969b). The author has also proposed that a possible action of insulin of wide influence would be to induce a shift in intracellular pH since so many cellular enzymes appear to have pH optima more alkaline than the intracellular figure. Preliminary measurements seem to suggest that this might be so as judged by relative levels of uptake of the pH indicator DMO (5,5-dimethyloxazolidine-2,4-dione) (Manchester, 1968b) but the problem of discriminating between cytoplasmic and mitochondrial accumulation of the indicator make interpretation difficult, since any hydrogen ion gradient between intra- and extramitochondrial fluid leaving the mitochondria more alkaline would lead to disproportionate accumulation of the indicator by the mitochondria. That insulin might directly or indirectly influence respiratory control is suggested by observations of lack of influence in mammalian muscle of the hormone on respiration even when turnover and demand for ATP (as judged for example by increased protein synthesis) must be increased. However the ability of the hormone to enhance sugar uptake under anerobic conditions (Randle and Smith, 1958) precludes the mitochondria from being the prime site of insulin action. Elucidation of this prime site of action therefore remains a problem wide open to solution.

REFERENCES

Antoniades, H. N., and Gershoff, S. N. (1966). *Diabetes* **15**, 655.

Agar, W. T., Hird, F. J. R., and Sidhu, G. S. (1954). *Biochim. Biophys. Acta* **14**, 80.

Akedo, K., and Christensen, H. N. (1962). *J. Biol. Chem.* **237**, 118.

Alberti, K. G. M. M., and Bartley, W. (1965). *Biochem. J.* **95**, 641.

Allen, D. W., and Zamecnik, P. C. (1962). *Biochim. Biophys. Acta* **55**, 865.

Anderson, W. F. (1969). *Proc. Natl. Acad. Sci. U. S.* **62**, 566.

Anderson-Cedergren, E., and Karlsson, U. (1967). *J. Ultrastruct. Res.* **19**, 409.

Antony, G. J., Srinivasan, I., Williams, H. R., and Landau, B. R. (1969). *Biochem. J.* **111**, 453.

Appleman, M. M., and Kemp, R. G. (1966). *Biochim. Biophys. Res. Commun.* **24**, 564.

Arvill, A., and Ahrén, K. (1967a). *Acta Endocrinol.* **56**, 279.

Arvill, A., and Ahrén, K. (1967b). *Acta Endocrinol.* **56**, 295.

Baker, W. K., and Rutter, W. J. (1964). *Arch. Biochem. Biophys.* **105**, 68.

Baldwin, A. N., and Berg, P. (1966). *J. Biol. Chem.* **241**, 831.

Baliga, B. S., Pronczuk, A. W., and Munro, H. N. (1968). *J. Mol. Biol.* **34**, 199.

Baliga, B. S., Pronczuk, A. W., and Munro, H. N. (1969). *J. Biol. Chem.* **244**, 4480.

Ball, E. G., Martin, D. B., and Cooper, O. (1959). *J. Biol. Chem.* **234**, 774.

Barber, H. E., Welch, B. L., and MacKay, D. (1967). *Biochem. J.* **103**, 251.

Battaglia, F. C., Manchester, K. L., and Randle, P. J. (1960). *Biochim. Biophys. Acta* **43**, 50.

Beigelman, P. M. (1962). *Metab., Clin. Exptl.* **11**, 1315.

Bianchi, C. P. (1961). *J. Gen. Physiol.* **44**, 845.

Bombara, C., and Bergamini, E. (1968). *Biochim. Biophys. Acta* **150**, 226.

Brawerman, G., and Eisenstadt, J. M. (1966). *Biochemistry* **5**, 2784.

Breuer, C. B., Davies, M. C., and Florini, J. R. (1964). *Biochemistry* **3**, 1713.

Brewer, E. N., Foster, L. B., and Sells, B. H. (1969). *J. Biol. Chem.* **244**, 1389.

Burrow, G. N., and Bondy, P. K. (1964). *Endocrinology* **75**, 455.

Buse, M. G., and Buse, J. (1967). *Diabetes* **16**, 735.

Cantoni, G. L., and Richards, H. H. (1966). *Procedures Nucleic Acid Res.* **1**, 624.

Cantoni, G. L., Gelboin, H. V., Luborsky, S. W., Richards, H. H., and Singer, M. F. (1962). *Biochim. Biophys. Acta* **61**, 354.

Carlin, H., and Hechter, O. (1964). *Proc. Soc. Exptl. Biol. Med.* **115**, 127.

Castles, J. J., and Wool, I. G. (1964). *Biochem. J.* **91**, 11C.

Castles, J. J., Wool, I. G., and Moyer, A. N. (1965). *Biochim. Biophys. Acta* **100**, 609.
Chaudry, I. H., and Gould, M. K. (1969). *Biochim. Biophys. Acta* **177**, 527.
Chen, S. C., and Young, V. R. (1968). *Biochem. J.* **106**, 61.
Chirigos, M., Greengard, P., and Udenfriend, S. (1960). *J. Biol. Chem.* **235**, 2075.
Christensen, H. N. (1964). *Proc. Natl. Acad. Sci. U. S.* **51**, 337.
Christensen, H. N., and Cullen, A. M. (1969). *J. Biol. Chem.* **244**, 1521.
Citoler, P., Benitez, L., and Maurer, W. (1967). *Exptl. Cell Res.* **45**, 195.
Clark, J. M., and Eyzaguirre, J. P. (1962). *J. Biol. Chem.* **237**, 3698.
Clausen, T. (1965). *Biochim. Biophys. Acta* **109**, 164.
Clausen, T. (1966). *Biochim. Biophys. Acta* **120**, 361.
Cohen, S. R. (1967). *Experientia* **23**, 712.
Coles, N., Bukenberger, M. W., and Meister, A. (1962). *Biochemistry* **1**, 317.
Colombo, B., Felicetti, L., and Baglioni, C. (1965). *Biochem. Biophys. Res. Commun.* **18**, 389.
Craig, J. W., Rall, T. W., and Larner, J. (1969). *Biochim. Biophys. Acta* **177**, 213.
Creese, R. (1968). *J. Physiol. (London)* **197**, 255.
Crofford, O. B. (1968). *J. Biol. Chem.* **243**, 362.
Crofford, O. B., and Renold, A. E. (1965). *J. Biol. Chem.* **240**, 3237.
Cutler, R. W. P., and Lorenzo, A. V. (1968). *Science* **161**, 1363.
Davey, P. J., and Manchester, K. L. (1969). *Biochim. Biophys. Acta* **182**, 85.
Davidson, M. B., and Goodner, C. J. (1966). *Diabetes* **15**, 835.
Denton, R. M., Yorke, R. E., and Randle, P. J. (1966). *Biochem. J.* **100**, 407.
Earl, D. C. N., and Korner, A. (1965). *Biochem. J.* **94**, 721.
Earl, D. C. N., and Korner, A. (1966). *Arch. Biochem. Biophys.* **115**, 437.
Earl, D. C. N., Broadus, A. E., and Morgan, H. E. (1967). *Fed. European Biochem. Soc. Meeting 1967*, Abstr. 5. Universitetsforlaget, Oslo.
Eavenson, E., and Christensen, H. N. (1967). *J. Biol. Chem.* **242**, 5386.
Eboué-Bonis, D., Chambaut, A. M., Volfin, P., and Clauser, H. (1963). *Nature* **199**, 1183.
Eichhorn, J., Scully, E., Halkerston, I. D. K., and Hechter, O. (1961). *Proc. Soc. Exptl. Biol. Med.* **106**, 153.
Elsas, L. J., and Rosenberg, L. E. (1967). *Proc. Natl. Acad. Sci. U. S.* **57**, 371.
Elsas, L. J., Albrecht, I., Koehne, W., and Rosenberg, L. E. (1967). *Nature* **214**, 916.
Elsas, L. J., Albrecht, I., and Rosenberg, L. E. (1968). *J. Biol. Chem.* **243**, 1846.
Ezerman, E. B., and Ishikawa, H. (1967). *J. Cell Biol.* **35**, 405.
Felig, P., Owen, O. E., Wahren, J., and Cahill, G. F. (1969). *J. Clin. Invest.* **48**, 584.
Florini, J. R. (1964). *Biochemistry* **3**, 209.
Forker, L. L., Chaikoff, I. L., Entenman, C., and Tarver, H. (1951). *J. Biol. Chem.* **188**, 37.
Foster, D. W. (1967). *J. Clin. Invest.* **46**, 1283.
Fraser, M. J. (1963). *Can. J. Biochem. Physiol.* **41**, 1123.
Froesch, E. R., and Ginsberg, J. L. (1962). *J. Biol. Chem.* **237**, 3317.
Gan, J. G., and Jeffay, H. (1967). *Biochim. Biophys. Acta* **148**, 448.
Garlick, P. J. (1969). *Nature* **223**, 61.
Gatica, M., Allende, C. C., Mora, G., Allende, J. E., and Medina, J. (1966). *Biochim. Biophys. Acta* **129**, 201.
Germanyuk, Y. L., and Mironenko, V. I. (1969). *Nature* **222**, 486.
Gilbert, W. (1963). *J. Mol. Biol.* **6**, 389.
Goldberg, A. L. (1967). *Nature* **216**, 1219.

Goldberg, N. D., Villar-Palasi, C., Sasko, H., and Larner, J. (1967). *Biochim. Biophys. Acta* **148**, 665.

Goldstein, S., and Reddy, W. J. (1967). *Biochim. Biophys. Acta* **141**, 310.

Gourley, D. R. H., and Brunton, L. L. (1969). *Biochim. Biophys. Acta* **184**, 43.

Gray, C. H., and Illing, E. K. B. (1952). *J. Endocrinol.* **8**, 44.

Green, M., and Miller, L. L. (1960). *J. Biol. Chem.* **235**, 3202.

Guidotti, G. G., Loreti, L., Gaja, G., and Foà, P. P. (1966). *Am. J. Physiol.* **211**, 981.

Guidotti, G. G., Gaja, G., Loreti, L., Ragnotti, G., Rottenberg, D. A., and Borghetti, A. F. (1968a). *Biochem. J.* **107**, 575.

Guidotti, G. G., Borghetti, A. F., Gaja, G., Loreti, L., Ragnotti, G., and Foà, P. P. (1968b). *Biochem. J.* **107**, 565.

Guidotti, G. G., Luneburg, B., and Borghetti, A. F. (1969). *Biochem. J.* **114**, 97.

Guroff, G., and Udenfriend, S. (1960). *J. Biol. Chem.* **235**, 3518.

Guroff, G., Udenfriend, S. (1961). *Biochim. Biophys. Acta* **46**, 386.

Hadjiolov, A. A. (1966). *Biochim. Biophys. Acta* **119**, 547.

Hanking, B. M., and Roberts, S. (1965). *Biochim. Biophys. Acta* **104**, 427.

Hardin, J. D., and Hove, E. L. (1951). *Proc. Soc. Exptl. Biol. Med.* **78**, 728.

Harris, E. J. (1960). "Transport and Accumulation in Biological Systems," 2nd ed. Butterworth, London and Washington, D. C.

Harris, E. J., and Manchester, K. L. (1966). *Biochem. J.* **101**, 135.

Harris, E. J., and Manger, J. R. (1968). *Biochem. J.* **109**, 239.

Harris, H. (1968). "Nucleus and Cytoplasm." Oxford Univ. Press (Clarendon), London and New York.

Hazlewood, C. F., Nichols, B. L., and Chamberlain, N. F. (1969). *Nature* **222**, 747.

Hechter, O., and Halkerston, I. D. K. (1964). *Hormones* **5**, 697.

Heinrikson, R. L., and Hartley, B. S. (1967). *Biochem. J.* **105**, 17.

Hendler, R. W. (1962). *Nature* **193**, 821.

Heredia, C. F., and Halvorson, H. O. (1966). *Biochemistry* **5**, 946.

Heywood, S. M., and Rich, A. (1968). *Proc. Natl. Acad. Sci. U. S.* **59**, 590.

Heywood, S. M., Dowben, R. M., and Rich, A. (1967). *Proc. Natl. Acad. Sci. U. S.* **57**, 1002.

Heywood, S. M., Dowben, R. M., and Rich, A. (1968). *Biochemistry* **7**, 3289.

Hider, R. C., Fern, E. B., and London, D. R. (1969a). *Biochem. J.* **114**, 171.

Hider, R. C., Fern, E. B., and London, D. R. (1969b). Personal communication.

Hunter, A. R., and Korner, A. (1969). *Biochim. Biophys. Acta* **179**, 115.

Ikemura, T., and Fukutome, H. (1969). *Biochim. Biophys. Acta* **182**, 98.

Ishikawa, H., Bischoff, R., and Holtzer, H. (1968). *J. Cell Biol.* **38**, 538.

Ivy, J. H., Svec, M., and Freeman, S. (1951). *Am. J. Physiol.* **167**, 182.

Jefferson, L. S., and Korner, A. (1969). *Biochem. J.* **111**, 703.

Jondorf, W. R., Simon, D. C., and Avnilmelech, M. (1966). *Mol. Pharmacol.* **2**, 506.

Jungas, R. L. (1966). *Proc. Natl. Acad. Sci. U. S.* **56**, 757.

Kaempfer, R. (1969). *Nature* **222**, 950.

Kaneko, I., and Doi, R. H. (1966). *Proc. Natl. Acad. Sci. U. S.* **55**, 564.

Kipnis, D. M., and Noall, M. W. (1958). *Biochim. Biophys. Acta* **28**, 226.

Kipnis, D. M., Reiss, E., and Helmreich, E. (1961). *Biochim. Biophys. Acta* **51**, 519.

Kjellin-Straby, K., and Phillips, J. H. (1968). *J. Bacteriol.* **96**, 760.

Korner, A. (1960). *J. Endocrinol.* **20**, 256.

Kovačević, A. (1967). *Biochem. J.* **103**, 535.

Krahl, M. E. (1952). *Science* **116**, 524.

Krahl, M. E. (1953). *J. Biol. Chem.* **200**, 99.

Krahl, M. E. (1957). *Perspectives Biol. Med.* 1, 69.
Krahl, M. E. (1961). "The Action of Insulin on Cells." Academic Press, New York.
Krahl, M. E., and Park, C. R. (1948). *J. Biol. Chem.* 174, 939.
Kuchler, R. J., and Marlowe-Kuchler, M. (1965). *Biochim. Biophys. Acta* 102, 226.
Kuo, J. F., Dill, I. K., and Holmlund, C. E. (1967). *Biochim. Biophys. Acta* 144, 252.
Kurihara, K., and Wool, I. G. (1968). *Nature* 219, 721.
Lahiri, S., and Lajtha, A. (1964). *J. Neurochem.* 11, 77.
Landau, B. R., and Sims, E. A. H. (1967). *J. Biol. Chem.* 242, 163.
Laraia, P. J., and Reddy, W. J. (1969). *Biochim. Biophys. Acta* 177, 189.
Larson, P. F., Hudgson, P., and Walton, J. N. (1969). *Nature* 222, 1168.
Leder, P., Skogerson, L. E., and Nau, M. M. (1969). *Proc. Natl. Acad. Sci. U. S.* 62, 454.
Lembach, K., and Charalampous, F. C. (1967). *J. Biol. Chem.* 242, 2606.
Levin, J. G., and Nirenberg, M. (1968). *J. Mol. Biol.* 34, 467.
Lin, S.-Y., Mosteller, R. D., and Hardesty, B. (1966). *J. Mol. Biol.* 21, 51.
Loeb, J. N., Howell, R. R., and Tomkins, G. M. (1965). *Science* 149, 1093.
London, D. R., and Prenton, M. A. (1968). *Clin. Sci.* 35, 55.
London, D. R. Foley, T. H., and Webb, C. G. (1965). *Nature* 208, 588.
McFarlane, I. G., and von Holt, C. (1969). *Biochem. J.* 111, 557.
Maggi, V., Franks, L. M., Wilson, P. D., and Carbonell, A. W. (1969). *Diabetologia* 5, 67.
Mahler, R. J., and Szabo, O. (1968). *Endocrinology* 83, 1166.
Maio, J. J., and Rickenberg, H. V. (1962). *Exptl. Cell Res.* 27, 31.
Makman, M. H., and Cantoni, G. L. (1966). *Biochemistry* 5, 2246.
Manchester, K. L. (1960). *Biochim. Biophys. Acta* 38, 555.
Manchester, K. L. (1961a). *Biochem. J.* 81, 135.
Manchester, K. L. (1961b). *Mem. Soc. Endocrinol.* 11, 113.
Manchester, K. L. (1963). *Biochim. Biophys. Acta* 70, 208.
Manchester, K. L. (1964). *Biochem. J.* 90, 5C.
Manchester, K. L. (1965a). *In* "On the Nature and Treatment of Diabetes" (E. S. Leibel and G. A. Wrenshall, eds.), Intern. Congr. Ser. No. 84, p. 101. Excerpta Med. Found., Amsterdam.
Manchester, K. L. (1965b). *Biochim. Biophys. Acta* 100, 295.
Manchester, K. L. (1965c). *Diabetologia* 1, 72.
Manchester, K. L. (1966). *Biochem. J.* 98, 711.
Manchester, K. L. (1967a). *Nature* 216, 394.
Manchester, K. L. (1967b). *Biochem. J.* 105, 13C.
Manchester, K. L. (1968a). *In* "The Biological Basis of Medicine" (E. E. Bittar, ed.), Vol. 2, p. 221. Academic Press, New York.
Manchester, K. L. (1968b). *Diabetologia* 4, 375.
Manchester, K. L. (1969a). *Nature* 221, 188.
Manchester, K. L. (1969b). *In* "Protein and Polypeptide Hormones," Intern. Congr. Ser. No. 161, p. 828. Excerpta Med. Found. Amsterdam.
Manchester, K. L. (1970a). *In* "Diabetes: Theory and Practice" (M. Ellenberg and H. Rifkin, eds.) McGraw-Hill, New York (in press).
Manchester, K. L. (1970b). *Biochem. J.* 117, 457.
Manchester, K. L. (1970c). *Nature,* in press.
Manchester, K. L. (1970d). *Biochem. J.* 39 P.
Manchester, K. L., and Harris, E. J. (1968). *Biochem. J.* 108, 177.
Manchester, K. L., and Krahl, M. E. (1959). *J. Biol. Chem.* 234, 2938.

Manchester, K. L., and Wool, I. G. (1963). *Biochem. J.* **89**, 202.
Manchester, K. L., and Young, F. G. (1958). *Biochem. J.* **70**, 353.
Manchester, K. L., and Young, F. G. (1959). *J. Endocrinol.* **18**, 381.
Manchester, K. L., and Young, F. G. (1960a). *Biochem. J.* **75**, 487.
Manchester, K. L., and Young, F. G. (1960b). *Biochem. J.* **77**, 386.
Manchester, K. L., Randle, P. J., and Young, F. G. (1959). *J. Endocrinol.* **19**, 259.
Manchester, K. L., and Young, F. G. (1961). *Vitamins Hormones* **19**, 95.
Margreth, A., and Novello, F. (1964). *Exptl. Cell Res.* **35**, 38.
Mariani, P., Migliaccio, P. A., Spadoni, M. A., and Ticca, M. (1966). *J. Nutr.* **90**, 25.
Marsh, J. B. (1961). *Am. J. Physiol.* **201**, 55.
Martin, T. E., and Wool, I. G. (1968). *Proc. Natl. Acad. Sci. U.S.* **60**, 569.
Mihalyi, E., Laki, K., and Knoller, M. I. (1957). *Arch. Biochem. Biophys.* **68**, 130.
Miller, L. V., and Beigelman, P. M. (1967). *Endocrinology* **81**, 386.
Moraz, L. A. (1967). *Circulation Res.* **21**, 449.
Morgan, C. R., and Lazarow, A. (1965). *Diabetes* **14**, 669.
Morgan, H. E., Regen, D. M., and Park, C. R. (1964). *J. Biol. Chem.* **239**, 369.
Morris, A., Arlinghaus, R., Flavelukes, S., and Schweet, R. (1963). *Biochemistry* **2**, 1084.
Mortimore, G. E. (1961). *Am. J. Physiol.* **200**, 1315.
Mudge, G. H. (1953). *Am. J. Physiol.* **173**, 511.
Munro, H. N. (1964). *In* "Mammalian Protein Metabolism" (H. N. Munro and J. B. Alisson, eds.), Vol. 1, p. 381. Academic Press, New York.
Munro, H. N., Black, J. G., and Thomson, W. S. T. (1959). *Brit. J. Nutr.* **13**, 475.
Muscatello, U., Anderson-Cedergren, E., and Azzone, G. F. (1962). *Biochim. Biophys. Acta* **63**, 55.
Müting, D. (1964). *Diabetes* **13**, 14.
Narahara, H. T., and Özand, P. (1963). *J. Biol. Chem.* **238**, 40.
Nathans, D. (1964). *Proc. Natl. Acad. Sci. U. S.* **51**, 585.
Novelli, G. D. (1967). *Ann. Rev. Biochem.* **36**, 449.
O'Malley, B. W., Aronow, A., Peacock, A. C., and Dingman, C. W. (1968). *Science* **162**, 567.
Orth, D. N., and Morgan, H. E. (1962). *J. Cell. Biol.* **15**, 509.
Oxender, D. L., and Christensen, H. N. (1963). *J. Biol. Chem.* **238**, 3686.
Pain, V. R., and Manchester, K. L. (1970). *Biochem. J.* in press.
Parrish, J. E., and Kipnis, D. M. (1964). *J. Clin. Invest.* **43**, 1994.
Peachey, L. D. (1965). *Intern. Congr. Ser. No. 87*, p. 391. Excerpta Med. Found., Amsterdam.
Peckham, W. D., and Knobil, E. (1962). *Biochim. Biophys. Acta* **63**, 207.
Perry, S. V., and Zydowo, M. (1959). *Biochem. J.* **72**, 682.
Peterkofsky, A., Gee, S. J., and Jesensky, C. (1966). *Biochemistry* **5**, 2789.
Peterson, P. J. (1967). *Biol. Rev.* **42**, 552.
Peterson, R. H., Beatty, C. H., and Bocek, H. M. (1963). *Endocrinology* **72**, 71.
Post, R. L., Morgan, H. E., and Park, C. R. (1961). *J. Biol. Chem.* **236**, 269.
Pozefsky, T., Felig, P., Soeldner, J. S., and Cahill, G. F. (1968). *Trans. Assoc. Am. Physicians* **81**, 258.
Rabinovitz, M., and Fisher, J. M. (1962). *J. Biol. Chem.* **237**, 477.
Rampersad, O. R., and Wool, I. G. (1965). *Science* **149**, 1102.
Rampersad, O. R., Zak, R., Rabinowitz, M., Wool, I. G., and DeSalle, L. (1965). *Biochim. Biophys. Acta* **108**, 95.
Randle, P. J., and Morgan, H. E. (1962). *Vitamins Hormones* **20**, 199.

Randle, P. J., and Smith, G. H. (1958). *Biochem. J.* **70**, 490.

Richmond, J. E., Shoemaker, W. C., and Elwyn, D. H. (1963). *Am. J. Physiol.* **205**, 848.

Rieser, P. (1967). "Insulin, Membranes and Metabolism." Williams & Wilkins, Baltimore, Maryland.

Rieser, P., and Rieser, C. H. (1964). *Proc. Soc. Exptl. Biol. Med.* **116**, 669.

Riggs, T. R., and Walker, L. M. (1963). *J. Biol. Chem.* **238**, 2663.

Riggs, T. R., Pan, M. W., and Feng, H. W. (1968). *Biochim. Biophys. Acta* **150**, 92.

Robinson, W. S. (1961). *Proc. Soc. Exptl. Biol. Med.* **106**, 115.

Robison, G. A., Butcher, R. W., and Sutherland, E. W. (1968). *Ann. Rev. Biochem.* **37**, 149.

Roscoe, J. P., Eaton, M. D., and Chin Choy, G. (1968). *Biochem. J.* **109**, 507.

Rosenberg, L. E., Berman, M., and Segal, S. (1963). *Biochim. Biophys. Acta* **71**, 664.

Rosenthal, O., and Vars, H. M. (1954). *Proc. Soc. Exptl. Biol. Med.* **86**, 555.

Ryan, W. L., and Carver, M. J. (1963). *Proc. Soc. Exptl. Biol. Med.* **114**, 816.

Salmon, W. D., von Hagen, M. J., and Thompson, E. Y. (1967). *Endocrinology* **80**, 999.

Sanders, R. B., and Riggs, T. R. (1967). *Endocrinology* **80**, 29.

Sarin, P. S., and Zamecnik, P. C. (1964). *Biochim. Biophys. Acta* **91**, 653.

Scharff, R., and Wool, I. G. (1964). *Nature* **202**, 603.

Scharff, R., and Wool, I. G. (1965a). *Biochem. J.* **97**, 257.

Scharff, R., and Wool, I. G. (1965b). *Biochem. J.* **97**, 272.

Scharff, R., and Wool, I. G. (1966). *Biochem. J.* **99**, 173.

Schiaffino, S., and Margreth, A. (1969). *J. Cell Biol.* **41**, 855.

Schreiber, S. S. (1955). *Am. J. Physiol.* **185**, 337.

Schreiber, S. S., Oratz, M., Evans, C., Silver, E., and Rothchild, M. A. (1968). *Am. J. Physiol.* **215**, 1250.

Seeds, N. W., and Conway, T. W. (1966). *Biochem. Biophys. Res. Commun.* **23**, 111.

Segal, S., Blair, A., and Rosenberg, L. E. (1961). *Nature* **192**, 1085.

Shaw, W. N., and Stadie, W. C. (1959). *J. Biol. Chem.* **234**, 2491.

Shearn, A., and Horowitz, N. H. (1969). *Biochemistry* **8**, 295.

Shimada, Y., Fischman, D. A., and Moscona, A. A. (1967). *J. Cell Biol.* **35**, 445.

Shugart, L., Novelli, G. D., and Stulberg, M. P. (1968). *Biochim. Biophys. Acta* **157**, 83.

Sidransky, H., Sarma, D. S. R., Bongiorno, M., and Verney, E. (1968). *J. Biol. Chem.* **243**, 1123.

Sims, E. A. H., and Landau, B. R. (1966). *Federation Proc.* **25**, 835.

Sinex, F. M., MacMullen, J., and Hastings, A. B. (1952). *J. Biol. Chem.* **198**, 615.

Smith, E. L. (1967). *Harvey Lectures* **62**, 63.

Smith, G. H., Randle, P. J., and Battaglia, F. C. (1961). *Mem. Soc. Endocrinol.* **11**, 124.

Solomon, A. K., and Gold, G. L. (1955). *J. Gen. Physiol.* **38**, 371.

Søvik, O. (1965). *Acta. Physiol. Scand.* **63**, 325.

Søvik, O. (1966). *Acta Physiol. Scand.* **66**, 307.

Søvik, O. (1967). *Biochim. Biophys. Acta* **141**, 190.

Søvik, O., and Walaas, O. (1964). *Nature* **202**, 396.

Staley, N. A., and Benson, E. S. (1968). *J. Cell Biol.* **38**, 99.

Stanners, C. P. (1966). *Biochem. Biophys. Res. Commun.* **24**, 758

Steiner, D. F. (1966). *Vitamins Hormones* **24**, 1.

Stent, G. S. (1964). *Science* **144**, 816.

Stirewalt, W. S., Wool, I. G., and Cavicchi, P. (1967). Proc. Natl. Acad. Sci. U. S. 57, 1885.
Stulberg, M. P. (1967). J. Biol. Chem. 242, 1060.
Sueoka, N., and Kano-Sueoka, T. (1964). Proc. Natl. Acad. Sci. U. S. 52, 1535.
Thomson, R. Y., Heagy, F. C., Hutchison, W. C., and Davidson, J. N. (1953). Biochem. J. 53, 460.
Tosteson, D. C., and Robertson, J. S. (1956). J. Cellular Comp. Physiol. 47, 147.
Trakatellis, A. C., Montjar, M., and Axelrod, A. E. (1965). Biochemistry 4, 2065.
Tsukada, K., and Lieberman, I. (1965). Biochem. Biophys. Res. Commun. 19, 702.
Turkington, R. W. (1969). J. Biol. Chem. 244, 5140.
Udenfriend, S., and Cooper, J. R. (1952). J. Biol. Chem. 196, 227.
Villar-Palasi, C., and Larner, J. (1968). Vitamins Hormones 26, 65.
Volfin, P., Chambaut, A. M., Eboué-Bonis, D., Clauser, H., Brinkhoff, O., Brember, H., Meienhofer, J., and Zahn, H. (1964). Nature 203, 408.
Walaas, O., Walaas, E., and Wick, A. N. (1969). Diabetologia 5, 79.
Wannemacher, R. W., Cooper, W. K., and Yatvin, M. B. (1968). Biochem. J. 107, 615.
Waterlow, J. C., and Stephen, J. M. L. (1968). Clin. Sci. 35, 449.
Wettstein, F. O., Noll, H., and Penman, S. (1964). Biochim. Biophys. Acta 87, 525.
Wheeler, K. P., and Christensen, H. N. (1967). J. Biol. Chem. 242, 3782.
Williamson, A. R., and Schweet, R. (1964). Nature 202, 435.
Wilson, J. D. (1963). Proc. Natl. Acad. Sci. U. S. 50, 93.
Wilson, S. H., and Hoagland, M. H. (1967). Biochem. J. 103, 556.
Winter, C. G., and Christensen, H. N. (1964). J. Biol. Chem. 239, 872.
Wittman, J. S., Lee, K.-L., and Miller, O. N. (1969). Biochim. Biophys. Acta 174, 536.
Wolfenden, R. (1963). Biochemistry 2, 1090.
Wool, I. G. (1960). Am. J. Physiol. 198, 357.
Wool, I. G. (1963). Biochim. Biophys. Acta 68, 28.
Wool, I. G. (1964). Nature 202, 196.
Wool, I. G., Castles, J. J., and Moyer, A. N. (1965). Biochim. Biophys. Acta 107, 333.
Wool, I. G., and Cavicchi, P. (1966). Proc. Natl. Acad. Sci. U. S. 56, 991.
Wool, I. G., and Cavicchi, P. (1967). Biochemistry 6, 1231.
Woll, I. G., and Krahl, M. E. (1959a). Am. J. Physiol. 196, 961.
Wool, I. G., and Krahl, M. E. (1959b). Am. J. Physiol. 197, 367.
Wool, I. G., and Krahl, M. E. (1959c). Nature 183, 1399.
Wool, I. G., and Kurihara, K. (1967). Proc. Natl. Acad. Sci. U. S. 58, 2401.
Wool, I. G., and Moyer, A. N. (1964). Biochim. Biophys. Acta 91, 248.
Wool, I. G., and Weinshelbaum, E. I. (1959). Am. J. Physiol. 197, 1089.
Wool, I. G., Stirewalt, W. S., and Moyer, A. N. (1968a). Am. J. Physiol. 214, 825.
Wool, I. G., Stirewalt, W. S., Kurihara, K., Low, R. B., Bailey, P., and Øyer, D. (1968b). Recent Progr. Hormone Res. 24, 139.
Wunner, E. H., Bell, J., and Munro, H. N. (1966). Biochem. J. 101, 417.
Yang, W.-K., and Novelli, G. D. (1968). Proc. Natl. Acad. Sci. U. S. 59, 208.
Yegian, C. D., and Stent, G. S. (1969). J. Mol. Biol. 39, 45.
Young, V. R., Chen, S. C., and MacDonald, J. (1968). Biochem. J. 106, 913.
Zak, R., Rabinowitz, M., and Platt, C. (1967). Biochemistry 6, 2493.
Zierler, K. L. (1966). Am. J. Med. 40, 735.
Zinneman, H. H., Nuttal, F. Q., and Goetz, F. C. (1966). Diabetes 15, 5.

CHAPTER 8

Mineralocorticoids

Isidore S. Edelman and Darrell D. Fanestil

I. HISTORICAL BACKGROUND

The first indication of adrenal cortical regulation of mineral metabolism was obtained 70 years after Addison's discovery (1855) of the vital function of the adrenal gland. Lucas (1926) noted that adrenalectomy in the dog resulted in hypochloremia, uremia, and hemoconcentration. Shortly thereafter, Baumann and Kurland (1927) added a set of key observations: adrenalectomy in the cat lowered plasma sodium and chloride concentrations and raised plasma potassium and magnesium concentrations. A primary target in mineralocorticoid action was defined by the finding of renal losses of NaCl that coincided with the fall in plasma concentrations of these ions (Loeb *et al.*, 1933). Identification of the salt-active steroids began with the isolation and characterization of corticosterone (de Fremery *et al.*, 1937) and the synthesis of deoxy-corticosterone (Steiger and Reichstein, 1937). The discovery, isolation, and synthesis of aldosterone in the 1950's (100 years after Addison) soon led to its characterization as the principal and most potent mineralo-corticoid in vertebrates (Grundy *et al.*, 1952; Simpson *et al.*, 1954; Schmidlin *et al.*, 1957). Aldosterone is a normal secretory product of the adrenal cortex or its analog, the interrenal gland, in anurans, reptiles, birds, and mammals (Ganong and van Brunt, 1968). In anurans and mammals, aldosterone regulates active sodium transport or sodium–potassium-linked transport across most, and perhaps all, epithelial structures specialized to carry out transepithelial sodium transport. Regulation of salt transport, however, is not a unique property of aldos-terone. The other secretory products of the adrenal, cortisol and corticos-terone, have significant effects on sodium transport in anurans and mammals (Edelman, 1968).

II. COMPARATIVE PHYSIOLOGY

A. Target Tissues in Various Species

Loeb and his associates (1933) established that the effect of adrenal steroids on salt balance in mammals is determined predominantly by the response of the kidney. In fact, the renal effects of the corticosteroids led to the discovery of aldosterone and was used as the basis for a bio-assay (Luetscher and Deming, 1951; Grundy *et al.*, 1952). The relative effects of aldosterone on renal conservation of sodium and excretion of potassium depend on the experimental conditions. In the adrenalecto-mized dog (Barger *et al.*, 1958) and rat (Fimognari *et al.*, 1967a) on low potassium diets, aldosterone produced coordinate antinatriuresis and kaliuresis. On routine diets, however, the only effect observed in the adrenalectomized rat was on sodium excretion. Conversely, aldosterone had no effect on sodium excretion but promoted potassium excretion in normal and in salt-loaded adrenalectomized dogs (Barger *et al.*, 1958; Share and Hall, 1958). The intrarenal sites of action of aldosterone has recently come under study by micropuncture techniques (Hierholzer *et al.*, 1965; Wiederholt *et al.*, 1966). Movement of potassium into and movement of sodium from the lumen of the distal tubule were impaired by adrenalectomy in the rat and aldosterone corrected these defects. Additional actions of aldosterone on sodium reabsorption by proximal segments and by collecting ducts have also been noted (Wiederholt, 1966; Uhlich *et al.*, 1969).

Extrarenal sites of action of mineralocorticoids have been identified in a variety of vertebrates, including the sweat glands, salivary glands, and the gastrointestinal tract (Shuster, 1962; Ross, 1959). The characteristic effect is to enhance sodium transport inward, from the lumen to the subepithelial space, and potassium transport outward, from the subepithelial space into the lumen. These effects have been well documented in studies on the parotid glands of sheep (Denton, 1957) and rat (Mangos and McSherry, 1968), and the small intestine (Moll and Koczorek, 1962) and colon (Edmonds and Marriott, 1967) of rats. Essentially no progress, however, was made on the biochemical determinants of the action of mineralocorticoids until studies on isolated anuran tissues were introduced.

B. Aldosterone Action in Anurans

The principal steroids produced by the interrenal gland of anurans are D-aldosterone and corticosterone (Carstensen *et al.*, 1961; Crabbé, 1963a; Ulick and Feinholtz, 1968). Maetz *et al.* (1958), Morel and Maetz (1958), and Scheer *et al.* (1961) found that salt balance in anurans is regulated by the rates of secretion of D-aldosterone. Toads (*Bufo marinus*) kept in distilled water maintained plasma aldosterone concentrations of 1.2 μg/100 ml; the levels fell to 0.7 μg/100 ml on transfer of the toads into saline (Crabbé, 1963a). Similar results were obtained in bullfrogs (*Rana catesbeiana*) (Ulick and Feinholtz, 1968). In the anurans, three sites of action have been identified: the ventral skin, urinary bladder, and colon. Thus, sodium transport across isolated ventral skin of frogs adapted to 0.125 *M* NaCl (isotonic with frog plasma) or to 0.150 *M* NaCl was much less than skins taken from frogs kept in fresh water (Maetz *et al.*, 1958; Scheer *et al.*, 1961). This effect is probably mediated by the level of aldosterone in the plasma as interrenalectomy mimicked the effects of the high salt environment. To complete the logic of the argument, it was shown that injection of aldosterone into the donor frogs reversed the effects of the high salt environment and of adrenalectomy (Bishop *et al.*, 1961; Maetz *et al.*, 1958). In the early 1960's McAfee and Locke (1961), using frog skin, and Crabbé (1961), using toad urinary bladder and skin, obtained significant steroidal stimulation of active sodium transport after direct addition of cortisol or aldosterone to the bathing media *in vitro*. Cofré and Crabbé (1965) also reported that administration of aldosterone, either *in vivo* or *in vitro* stimulated active sodium transport across the isolated toad colon. The use of *in vitro* systems simplified considerably the approach to the mechanism of mineralocorticoid action. Crabbé (1963a) exploited the *in vitro* system with toad skin and urinary bladder to ask specific questions on mechanism. He established that aldosterone rather than any of its metabolites was responsible for the effect on sodium transport as all of the ^{3}H-aldosterone in the isolated toad bladder was recovered as the unmodified compound. This finding was confirmed by Kliman (1966). In considering the significance of this result, Crabbé (1963a) directed attention to the possible molecular basis of the latent period in the time course of action of aldosterone.

III. THE INDUCTION HYPOTHESIS

A. The Significance of the Latent Period

After intravenous injection of aldosterone in mammals, a latent period of about 1 hour is generally seen in both the renal and extrarenal effects on sodium transport (Barger *et al.*, 1958; Edmonds and Marriott, 1967; Fimognari *et al.*, 1967a; Liddle *et al.*, 1955). The pattern of the response is illustrated in Fig. 1, taken from the work of Fimognari *et al.* (1967a). Compared to the control levels, the differences in urinary sodium and potassium concentrations at 1 hour did not achieve statistical significance. Similar results were obtained by Castles and Williamson (1967). Crabbé (1963a) noted a 1–2-hour latent period even after the direct addition of aldosterone to the media in the isolated toad bladder system and found that the duration of the delay time was independent of the concentration of the steroid. Subsequent studies confirmed these results (Edelman, 1968; Sharp and Leaf, 1966). On the expectation that a diffusion-limited process would be concentration-dependent, Crabbé inferred that the latent period was the time needed to synthesize or activate an intermediate involved in active sodium transport.

The inference that the latent period is not determined by the rate of

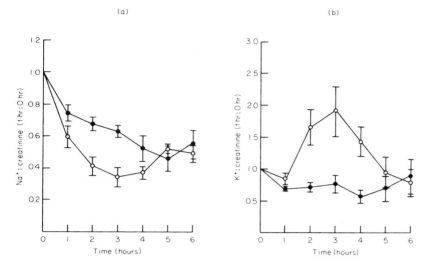

Fig. 1. Time course of response to *d*-aldosterone by the kidney of the adrenal-ectomized rat eating a low-potassium chow. The ordinates are sodium: creatinine ratio (A) and potassium: creatinine (B) expressed as the ratio of the hourly collection periods divided by that of the −2 to 0 hour collection period. The rats injected with 2 μg *d*-aldosterone at time zero are denoted by —○— and the saline controls by —●—. The vertical line is ±1 SEM. From Fimognari *et al.* (1967a).

uptake of the steroid—or slow penetration to the target sites—was tested with labeled aldosterone in the isolated toad bladder system (Edelman *et al.*, 1963). Intracellular accumulation of aldosterone reached a steady, maximal level 30–75 minutes before the onset of the effect on sodium transport. These results are in accord with Crabbé's inference that the latent period is determined by the generation time of intermediates. A general scheme for such a process is given by

$$A + R \rightleftharpoons AR \tag{1}$$

$$X \overset{(AR)}{\rightleftharpoons} I \tag{2}$$

$$S \overset{(I)}{\rightleftharpoons} \Delta S \tag{3}$$

where A is aldosterone, R the specific physiologic receptor, I the active intermediate, S the rate of sodium transport, and ΔS the increase in active sodium transport. One implication of this scheme is that the duration of the effect on sodium transport after removal of aldosterone from the system would depend on the turnover time of the intermediate. To test this prediction, the rate of release of aldosterone from tissue binding sites must be known. It was found that in toad bladders, preloaded with ³H-aldosterone, 90% of the steroid was eluted after 1 hour in steroid-free media and 95% in 6 hours (Edelman *et al.*, 1963). Removal of aldosterone from the bathing media during the latent period did not alter the duration of the latent period nor the initial rate of increase in sodium transport (Edelman *et al.*, 1963; Sharp and Leaf, 1963; Sharp *et al.* 1966b). Sharp and Leaf (1966) estimated that the residual tissue aldosterone content in these experiments was 10^{-12} mole/gm. They concluded that direct attachment of the steroid to the lipids of the plasma membrane, thereby altering the sodium transport system as proposed by Willmer (1961), was not a valid concept. Similar observations have also been made in the adrenalectomized rat *in vivo*. After a single sub-cutaneous injection of ³H-aldosterone, plasma and kidney attained maximum levels in 30 minutes; less than 10% of the accumulated steroid was in the kidney at 2 hours (Fanestil and Edelman, 1966c). The peak effect on electrolyte excretion is at 3–4 hours when little steroid remains in the kidney (Fig. 1). This triggerlike effect in both the toad bladder and rat kidney is consistent with the concept of steroid action via the generation of an intermediate. This effect, however, could be a result of a small amount of aldosterone bound firmly to specific receptor sites as the tissues contained a residual, slowly released quantity of steroid at the time of the increase in sodium transport.

B. Subcellular Site of the Mineralocorticoid Receptors

1. Toad Bladder Studies

High resolution radioautographs provided the first clue to the sub-cellular site of binding of aldosterone. As shown in Fig. 2, ³H-aldosterone is preferentially localized to the nuclear and perinuclear areas of the target epithelial cells of the toad bladder. In contrast, the inactive steroid, ³H-progesterone is randomly distributed between the nuclear and cytoplasmic areas of these cells (Porter *et al.*, 1964). These results suggest that nuclear accumulation of aldosterone is not a result of indiscriminate binding of steroids. Sharp *et al.* (1966b) used a displacement technique to distinguish specifically bound aldosterone from unbound or nonspecifically adsorbed steroid. Toad bladders were exposed to tracer concentrations of labeled aldosterone, followed by the addition of higher concentrations of unlabeled steroids. The displacement curves indicated that the saturable component of aldosterone binding involved two sets of sites with two characteristic affinities for aldosterone. With one exception, the ability of a steroid to displace aldosterone correlated with the activity of the test steroid on active sodium transport. At con-

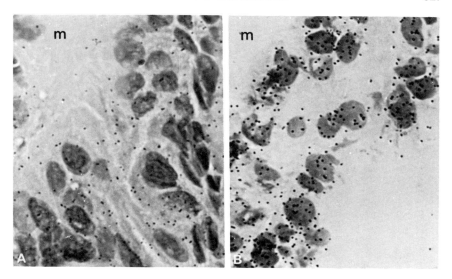

FIG. 2. Phase contrast photomicrographs of sections of toad bladder and over-lying radioautographs. Toad bladder exposed to ³H-progesterone for 1.5 hour is shown in (A). Toad bladder exposed to ³H-aldosterone for 1.5 hour is shown in (B). The magnification is 980 ×. The mucosal surface is denoted by m. From Porter *et al.* (1964).

centrations of ∼5 × 10⁻⁷ M, progesterone and aldosterone displaced equal quantities of ³H-aldosterone, although progesterone at this concentration does not inhibit the response to aldosterone nor does it activate sodium transport (Porter and Edelman, 1964; Porter *et al.*, 1964). From recent cell fractionation studies, Ausiello and Sharp (1968) inferred that the nuclei of the toad bladder epithelial cells contain ∼60% of the aldosterone-binding sites of the intact bladder. Active mineralocorticoids (9α-fluorocortisol, DOC, cortisol) and spirolactone displaced ³H-aldosterone from the nuclear binding sites but inactive steroids (testosterone and cholesterol) did not.

2. Rat Kidney Studies

Similar criteria were used to identify the subcellular site of binding of aldosterone in the rat kidney (Fanestil and Edelman, 1966b). Adrenalectomized rats were injected with varying amounts of aldosterone (i.e., from 2.3 × 10⁻¹¹ to 2.8 × 10⁻⁷ moles of aldosterone/rat) 30 minutes before removal of the kidneys. Conventional cell fractions were prepared by differential centrifugation, and the quantity of native aldosterone and aldosterone-metabolites determined by extraction with CH₂Cl₂. The aldosterone-metabolites, physiologically inert analogs of the native steroid, were used as markers for nonspecific uptake of steroid. The metabolite content of all cell fractions was directly proportional to plasma aldosterone concentrations and conformed to the prediction of a simple, nonspecific partition between the organelles and plasma. Similar results were obtained in the binding of native aldosterone to the mitochondrial, microsomal, and supernatant fractions. In contrast, the uptake of aldosterone by the nuclear fraction consisted of saturable and nonsaturable compartments. Thus, at plasma aldosterone concentrations below the limit for maximum antinatriuresis (i.e., $5 \times 10^{-9} M$), the nuclear fraction had the highest ^{3}H-aldosterone and the lowest metabolite contents. Moreover, 9α-fluorocortisol inhibited nuclear accumulation of ^{3}H-aldosterone but the inactive steroids, 6α-methylprednisolone and 17β-estradiol had no effect. These results are shown in Fig. 3 and support the inference that the renal nuclei contain a unique set of binding

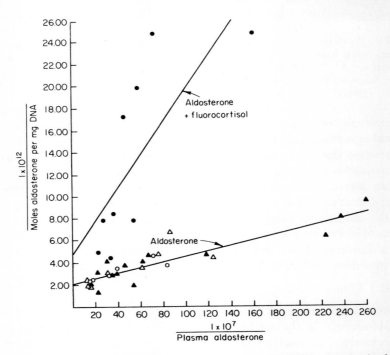

FIG. 3. Double-reciprocal plot of aldosterone content of rat kidney nuclei (isolated in $2.2 M$ sucrose) versus plasma aldosterone concentration. Adrenalectomized rats injected only with ^{3}H-aldosterone are denoted by $\triangle$; rats injected with ^{3}H-aldosterone and 2.1×10^{-8} mole estradiol-17β by $\bigcirc$; rats injected with ^{3}H-aldosterone and 2.1×10^{-8} mole 9α-fluorocortisol by $\bullet$; rats injected with ^{3}H-aldosterone and 2.1×10^{-8} mole 6α-methylprednisolone by $\blacktriangle$. From Fanestil and Edelman (1966b).

sites that are specific for mineralocorticoids. Additional evidence in support of this inference was obtained with spirolactone, a pharmacological antagonist of aldosterone (Fanestil, 1968a). Injection of excess spirolactone (SC 14266) in the adrenalectomized rat inhibited uptake of ^{3}H-aldosterone by the nuclear and cytosol fractions but had no effect on mitochondrial or microsomal binding (Table I). The kinetics of inhibition of nuclear uptake was characteristic of competitive displacement of aldosterone.

Additional progress was made recently on the isolation and characterization of the aldosterone-binding substances in the nuclear and cytosol fraction of the rat kidney (Herman *et al.*, 1968). The binding substances were identified as proteins by the following criteria: (1) chemical analysis of tris-extracts of renal nuclei; (2) dissociation of the ^{3}H-aldosterone-macromolecular complexes from the nuclear and cytosol fractions by wide-spectrum proteolytic enzymes but not by nucleases, lipase or phospholipase; (3) precipitation of the ^{3}H-aldosterone complexes by 50% $(NH_4)_2SO_4$; and (4) loss of aldosterone-binding activity on treatment of the complexes with sulfhydryl reagents. The steroidal specificity of the aldosterone-binding proteins (ABP) was indicated by the finding that 9α-fluorocortisol, DOC, 6α-methylprednisolone, and 17β-estradiol competed with ^{3}H-aldosterone for the binding sites in direct proportion to their respective potencies in the regulation of renal tubular transport of sodium. In addition, spirolactone inhibited aldosterone binding to the isolated nuclear and cytosol ABP's at concentration ratios equivalent to those needed to inhibit the mineralocorticoid effect in the intact rat.

TABLE I

EFFECT OF SPIROLACTONE SC14266 ON INTRACELLULAR DISTRIBUTION OF ^{3}H-ALDOSTERONE[a,b]

Fraction	Aldosterone	Aldosterone + SC14266[c]	p Value
Plasma[d]	1.24 ± 0.19	1.39 ± 0.28	>0.50
Nuclei	5.39 ± 0.52	1.89 ± 0.54	<0.005
Supernatant	9.39 ± 0.52	5.61 ± 0.65	<0.005
Mitochondria	3.13 ± 0.73	2.43 ± 0.34	>0.40
Microsomes	2.77 ± 0.63	1.67 ± 0.22	<0.05

[a] Reprinted from Fanestil (1968a).

[b] Values are means $\pm$ SEM. of five animals in each group. All animals received 2.8×10^{-9} mole ^{3}H-aldosterone.

[c] These animals received, in addition, 2.8×10^{-5} mole SC14266.

[d] Plasma values are moles of aldosterone/liter $\times 10^{-9}$. All other values are mole aldosterone/mg protein $\times 10^{-14}$.

Both nuclear and cytosol ABP's proved to be stereospecific as 17α-iso-aldosterone did not bind nor did it compete with aldosterone for the binding sites. These findings correlate well with the observation that this stereoisomer had no effect on urinary electrolyte excretion in the adrenalectomized rat at five times the dose of aldosterone needed for maximal antinatriuresis (Swaneck *et al.*, 1969).

Additional direct evidence has been obtained that the ^{3}H-aldosterone-binding mechanism in renal nuclei is saturable and aldosterone-specific (Edelman, 1969). Adrenalectomized rats were injected with ^{3}H-aldosterone and 10 or 100 times more carrier aldosterone. Thirty minutes after these injections, the kidneys were removed and purified nuclear fractions prepared by differential centrifugation. The quantity of ^{3}H-aldosterone bound to nuclear binding proteins was determined by preparing 50% $(NH_4)_2SO_4$ precipitates of tris-$CaCl_2$ extracts of the nuclear fractions. The results in Table II indicate parallel and proportional displacement of ^{3}H-aldosterone from both nuclear and ABP binding sites by cold aldosterone (Herman and Edelman, 1969).

Specific binding of aldosterone to the nuclei of target tissue does not, of course, imply direct involvement of the binding process in the mechanism of action on sodium transport. It is possible, for example, that the binding mechanism provides a means of prolonging the action of the hormone during periods of falling concentrations in circulating plasma. In view of the striking correlation between mineralocorticoid potency and affinity for binding to ABP, however, it is reasonable to examine the possibility that mineralocorticoid action is actually initiated by the binding of the steroid to specific receptors probably in the nucleus of target cells.

TABLE II

COMPETITION FOR ^{3}H-ALDOSTERONE BINDING SITES BY
d-ALDOSTERONE IN RENAL NUCLEI[a]

Fraction	*d*-Aldosterone (moles injected)	Specific activity (moles $\times 10^{14}$/mg protein)	% Bound
Purified nuclei	0	4.3 ± 0.3	100
	2.6×10^{-9}	1.1 ± 0.2	25.5
	2.6×10^{-8}	0.41 ± 0.06	9.5
50% $(NH_4)_2SO_4$	0	18.4 ± 1.1	100
	2.6×10^{-9}	3.9 ± 0.3	21.1
	2.6×10^{-8}	0.97 ± 0.06	5.3

[a] Results are given as mean $\pm$SEM. All rats were injected with 2.6×10^{-10} mole ^{3}H-aldosterone with or without added *d*-aldosterone. The rats were killed 30 minutes after injection. Results are from Herman and Edelman (1969).

C. Nucleic Acid and Protein Synthesis; Effects of Inhibitors
and Incorporation Studies

The latent period, the discrepancy between aldosterone uptake and
time of appearance of the effect on sodium transport, the triggerlike
properties, and the nuclear localization of mineralocorticoids suggest that
nuclear biosynthetic events may mediate the effect. As the two primary
nuclear functions are DNA-dependent DNA synthesis and DNA-dependent RNA synthesis, tests have been made of the relevance of these pathways to mineralocorticoid action. At the moment it appears unlikely
that DNA-dependent DNA synthesis is involved in the action of aldosterone as Fanestil (1968b) found no inhibitory effect on the response
of the isolated toad bladder to aldosterone with inhibitors of DNA synthesis (i.e., phleomycin and hydroxyurea).

A considerable body of evidence has been obtained implicating DNA-
dependent RNA synthesis and *de novo* synthesis of proteins in mineralocorticoid action. The induction hypothesis was proposed simultaneously by Edelman *et al.* (1963) and Williamson (1963). The evidence
in support of the induction hypothesis may be summarized briefly as
follows.

(1) In the toad bladder system, actinomycin D, an inhibitor of RNA
synthesis at the transcriptional level, and puromycin and cycloheximide,
inhibitors of ribosomal assembly of proteins, inhibit the response to
aldosterone at concentrations that have a lesser or no effect on the baseline rate of sodium transport (Edelman *et al.*, 1963; Crabbé and De Weer
(1964) Fanestil and Edelman, 1966a).

(2) Stimulation of sodium transport by vasopressin or by glucose (in
substrate-depleted toad bladders) was not significantly impaired by
actinomycin D or puromycin (Edelman *et al.*, 1963).

(3) That these inhibitors might act by displacing aldosterone from
the specific receptor sites was negated by the findings of Sharp and Leaf
(1966) that actinomycin D and puromycin did not compete for binding
sites in the intact toad bladder.

(4) Incorporation of ^{3}H-uridine into RNA was enhanced by aldosterone prior to the onset of the effect on sodium transport (Porter *et al.*,
1964). That the observed effect is not secondary to altered rates of electrolyte transport was substantiated by the observation that aldosterone
also increased ^{3}H-uridine incorporation into RNA in toad bladders
incubated in mucosal media devoid of sodium (De Weer and Crabbé,
1968).

Similar evidence in support of the induction hypothesis has also been provided by studies in adrenalectomized rats. Actinomycin D significantly inhibited the antinatriuretic effect of aldosterone (Williamson, 1963; Fimognari *et al.*, 1967a). A curious collateral finding reported by Williamson (1963) and confirmed by Fimognari *et al.* (1967a) is that actinomycin D did not inhibit the kaliuretic response to aldosterone despite the similarity in the time course of the effects on sodium and potassium excretion. Wiederholt (1966) extended these observations using micropuncture techniques and reported that actinomycin D blocked only the aldosterone-stimulated fraction of distal tubular transport of sodium. A number of reports have also appeared on the effects of aldosterone on renal nuclear synthesis of RNA (Castles and Williamson, 1965, 1967; Fimognari *et al.*, 1967a). Although some inconsistencies in the results remain to be elucidated, the general effect seems clear. Incorporation of precursors of RNA into renal nuclear RNA is enhanced by aldosterone before the maximum effect on urinary sodium is achieved. Moreover, this enhancement is inhibited by actinomycin D (Fimognari *et al.*, 1967a). In view of the body of evidence cited, it is reasonable to formulate a more detailed hypothesis of the mechanism of action of aldosterone:

$$A + ABP \rightleftharpoons C^* \tag{4}$$

$$\text{Precursor Bases} \xrightarrow{\text{(C*)(DNA)}} mRNA^* \tag{5}$$

$$\text{a-a} + tRNA \xrightarrow{\text{(Ribosomes)(mRNA)*}} AIP \tag{6}$$

$$S \xrightarrow{\text{(AIP)}} \Delta S \tag{7}$$

where A denotes aldosterone, ABP the nuclear aldosterone-binding protein, C^* the activated complex, a-a the precursor amino acids, tRNA the transfer RNA, mRNA* the aldosterone-specific messenger RNA, AIP the specific aldosterone-induced protein(s) and S is the rate of transepithelial sodium transport.

IV. ROLE OF ALDOSTERONE-INDUCED PROTEIN (AIP) IN MINERALOCORTICOID ACTION

A. Ussing-Skou Model of Sodium Transport

Current concepts of the basic components of active steroidal regulation of transepithelial sodium transport are derived almost exclusively from studies on the isolated urinary bladder of the toad, *Bufo marinus*.

Leaf and his co-workers (1958) pioneered the exploitation of this system based on the short-circuit current technique (scc) of Ussing and Zerahn (1951). The scc provides a convenient and accurate method for measuring active sodium transport across the toad bladder. Double isotope flux studies showed that net sodium flux and scc were equivalent in the basal state and after stimulation by aldosterone (Crabbé, 1961). In further studies, aldosterone had no effect on serosal to mucosal unidirectional flux of sodium and the increase in mucosal to serosal unidirectional flux matched the increase in scc produced by the steroid (Porter and Edelman, 1964). The effect of aldosterone on scc in the toad bladder is shown in Fig. 4. The scc pattern on exposure to progesterone illustrates the contrasting effects of an inactive steroid (Edelman *et al.*, 1964).

To analyze the means by which AIP may regulate sodium transport, a model incorporating the primary features of the transport system is needed. A currently popular model of transepithelial sodium transport, given in Fig. 5, has been deduced from electrophysiological, isotopic flux and biochemical studies (Koefoed-Johnsen and Ussing, 1958; Frazier, 1962; Bricker *et al.*, 1963; Skou, 1965). The rate-limiting steps are placed at membrane boundaries, in series. Thus, sodium enters the epithelial

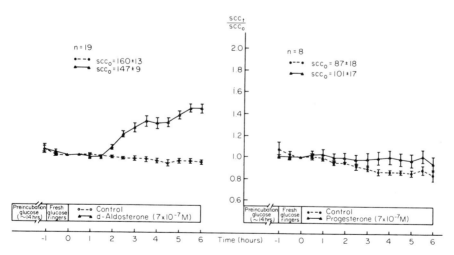

FIG. 4. A comparison of the relative effects of aldosterone and of progesterone on active Na^+ transport. The ordinate is the ratio of the short-circuit current at time t after the addition of the steroid (scc_t) to the value recorded at the time of addition of the steroid (scc_0). The length of the vertical bar equals 1 standard error of the mean. The number of paired observations is denoted by n. From Edelman *et al.* (1964).

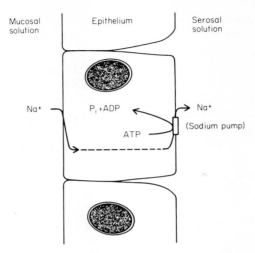

FIG. 5. A model of transepithelial active sodium transport. The mucosal solution is in contact with the apical surface and the serosal solution the lateral-basal surfaces of the plasma membrane.

cell from the lumen, driven by the electrochemical gradient across the apical boundary and is extruded from the interior of the cell into the subepithelial spaces across the basal-lateral side of the plasma membrane against an electrochemical gradient. ATP is the proximate energy donor and provides the energy substrate for the sodium pump located in the basal-lateral plasma membrane. The magnesium-dependent, sodium–potassium activated ATPase described by Skou (1965) is probably a principal component of the sodium pump.

This model predicts three ways by which a hormonal regulator could accelerate sodium transport: (1) by increasing the permeability of the apical boundary to sodium, thereby facilitating access of sodium to the pump; (2) by increasing activity of the sodium pump [e.g., increased synthesis or activation of the (Na + K)-activated ATPase]; (3) by increasing the activity of one or several metabolic steps resulting in increased synthesis of ATP and as a result an increased concentration of ATP at the pump site. Experimental evidence is available to indicate that these are plausible pathways in hormonal regulation. The effect of an increase in apical entry of sodium may be tested by raising the electrochemical gradient for inward movement of sodium. Frazier *et al.* (1962) found that sodium transport across the toad bladder and the sodium content of the tissue increased proportionately (but not linearly) with increasing concentrations of sodium in the mucosal media up to ~50 mEq/liter. They also concluded that entry of sodium across the apical boundary involves a saturable interaction with a membrane component that constitutes the major determinant of the rate of transepithelial sodium transport. Hormonal regulation at the apical entry site has been dubbed the "permease" theory. The plausibility of the second pathway, activation of the sodium pump, has not been assessed directly. The converse of pump activation, however, inhibition of the $(Na + K)$-ATPase with ouabain inhibits sodium transport in the toad bladder system (Sharp and Leaf, 1965). In principle, therefore, activation of the transport ATPase should increase sodium transport. The plausibility of the third pathway, increased synthesis of ATP, is indicated by the finding that addition of a variety of substrates to the media (i.e., glucose, lactate, pyruvate) produced prompt and sustained elevations in the rate of sodium transport in substrate-depleted toad bladders (Maffly and Edelman, 1963). This effect is illustrated in Fig. 6. The inference that

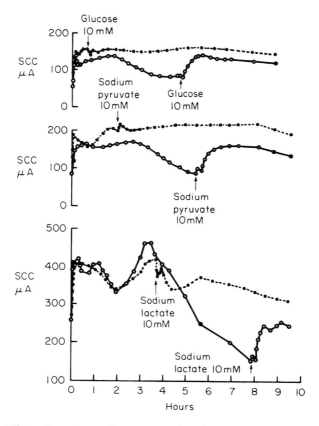

FIG. 6. Effect of various substrates on the short-circuit current (scc) of the urinary bladder of the toad. The additions were made to the serosal solutions. From Maffly and Edelman (1963).

the substrate effect is mediated by ATP synthesis is reinforced by the
observation that inhibitors of oxidative metabolism eliminated the response to substrates.

In addition to the pathways for regulating sodium transport implicit
in the Ussing-Skou model, a physicochemical regulatory mechanism not
predicted by the model has been described. In 1963, Maffly and Edelman
reported that hypoosmotic solutions stimulated sodium transport and
hyperosmotic solutions were inhibitory in the isolated toad bladder system. The effect is shown in Fig. 7 (Lipton and Edelman, 1968). Ussing
(1965) studied the effect of osmotic shifts on sodium transport across
frog skin extensively and concluded that the critical process was the
change in epithelial cell volume. An increase in cell volume stimulated
active sodium transport and a decrease inhibited the transport process.
It is conceivable, therefore, that the mineralocorticoid effect might be

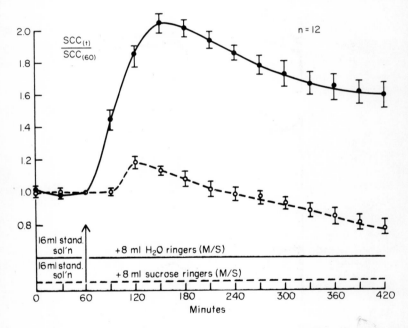

Fig. 7. The effect of decreasing the osmolarity of the bathing media on the
scc across the isolated toad bladder. Bladders were incubated overnight in standard
solutions (225 mOsmolal). Fresh standard solution was added at $t = 1$ hour. At the
time shown by the arrow H$_2$O-Ringers (diluted standard Ringers) was added to one
hemibladder and sucrose-Ringers was added to the other. The final osmolarity of
the bathing media were 155 mOsmolal and 225 mOsmolal after the addition of the
H$_2$O and sucrose-Ringers, respectively. $n = 12$ experiments. Bars are ± one SEM.
From Lipton and Edelman (1968).

mediated by osmotic shifts resulting in expansion of the surface epithelial cells. The results shown in Fig. 7 indicate that the magnitude of the osmotic effect is sufficient to account for mineralocorticoid action. Evaluation of this possibility awaits further experimental study. The Ussing-Skou model predicts that the osmotic or cell volume effect would have to be mediated by one of the three rate-limiting steps outlined previously.

B. The Sodium Pump Hypothesis

To date, no one has derived a method to evaluate the possibility of a direct action of AIP on the sodium pump in intact epithelial systems. Such an effect can be visualized in three ways: (1) activation of one or more of the components of the sodium pump at the basal-lateral borders by AIP or an intermediate generated by the action of AIP on some synthetic process; (2) derepression of the sodium pump by neutralization of an inhibitor with ouabain-like properties; or (3) an increase in the total number of operating pumps (e.g., synthesis of new pumps or recruiting of inactive epithelial cells into some sodium transport activity). Attempts to show an aldosterone-dependent effect on the enzymatic equivalent of the sodium pump, the $(Na^+ + K^+)$-activated ATPase, in broken cell or isolated membrane preparations have been consistently negative thus far (Bonting and Canady, 1964; Chignell *et al.*, 1965; Lichtenstein and Hagopian, 1966; Turakolov *et al.*, 1968). These negative results do not, of course, exclude the possibility of an action by AIP or its deputy on the sodium pump, as all of the components of the pump have not yet been identified. Moreover, an activation effect could easily be lost in the preparation of the enzyme. The possibility of an action on the sodium pump is supported (albeit tenuously) by two pieces of evidence. Landon *et al.* (1966) found that dialyzed membrane preparations prepared from adrenalectomized rats or rats treated with spirolactone had diminished $(Na^+ + K^+)$-activated ATPase activity, which was restored toward normal by treatment with aldosterone, DOC, or triamcinolone. The discrepancy between the dosage required for the electrolyte effect and the enzyme effect led to the conclusion that there was no direct relation between mineralocorticoid and enzyme-maintenance activity. The possibility remains, however, that the active intermediate may be damaged in preparation for enzyme assay, necessitating higher levels for detection. Another suggestive piece of evidence is provided by studies with ouabain, a specific inhibitor of $(Na^+ + K^+)$ ATPase activity (Skou, 1965). At a concentration of $10^{-5} M$, ouabain eliminated the increment in sodium transport produced by aldosterone but had no effect on the steroid-independent baseline rate of sodium transport (Sharp and Leaf, 1966). The inhibitory effect of ouabain on the response to aldosterone is shown in Fig. 8 from the work of Porter (1968). At a concentration of $2.5 \times 10^{-5} M$, ouabain had no effect on basal sodium transport. At a concentration of $10^{-4} M$, however, steroid-independent sodium transport was inhibited by about 50% (Table III). The differential sensitivity of steroid-dependent sodium transport to ouabain raises the question of modification of the pump by AIP (i.e., that aldosterone sensitizes one class of $(Na^+ + K^+)$-ATPase to ouabain). It is apparent, therefore, that the "sodium pump hypothesis" remains an open question.

C. The Permease Hypothesis

The concept that aldosterone (or AIP) accelerates sodium transport by facilitating the entry of sodium across the apical plasma membrane was first advanced by Sharp and Leaf (1963, 1964) and Crabbé (1963b) based on the radiosodium tissue-labeling technique. It is now recognized, however, that these results do not provide valid evidence in support of the permease hypothesis (Sharp and Leaf, 1966). The technique

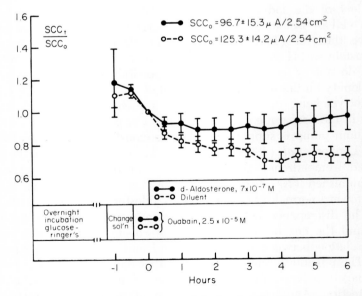

Fig. 8. The effects of ouabain on steroid-depleted and aldosterone-treated hemi-bladders of *Bufo marinus*. See legend of Fig. 4 for definition of symbols. Number of paired hemibladders = 9. From Porter (1968).

TABLE III

EFFECT OF OUABAIN ON BASAL Na$^+$ TRANSPORT IN TOAD BLADDER[a]

Ouabain (molar)	No. Expts.	0 scc_0[b]	15	30	45	60
				scc_t/scc_0		
0	6	83 ± 19	0.810 ± 0.024	0.727 ± 0.046	0.702 ± 0.056	0.697 ± 0.066
2.5 × 10^{-5}		68 ± 12	0.846 ± 0.080	0.752 ± 0.094	0.716 ± 0.106	0.693 ± 0.093
p		>0.4	>0.5	>0.8	>0.9	>0.9
0	9	37 ± 6	0.961 ± 0.020	0.934 ± 0.051	0.888 ± 0.050	0.818 ± 0.058
1.25 × 10^{-4}		46 ± 10	0.778 ± 0.028	0.574 ± 0.066	0.439 ± 0.051	0.422 ± 0.060
p		>0.5	<0.0001	<0.001	<0.00001	<0.001

[a] Paired hemibladders from *Bufo marinus* were preincubated for 16 hours in glucose (10 mM)—frog-Ringer's solutions. Ouabain was added to the concentrations indicated in the table to both serosal and mucosal bathing media. scc_t/scc_0 denotes the ratio of the short-circuit currents at time t to that recorded at time zero in each hemibladder. All values are given as mean ±SEM.

[b] Short-circuit current at time zero (i.e., time of addition of ouabain to the media) in μA/2.54 cm^2. From Porter (1968).

provides no information on the distribution of the radiosodium among the various cell types of the toad bladder or on trapping by nonepithelial elements. In a recent study, Leaf (1967) reported that the efflux of ^{24}Na across the serosal surface of toad bladders preloaded with the isotope, was not depressed by inhibitors of sodium transport, indicating that most of the ^{24}Na in the tissue had been discharged from the epithelial cells and was on the serosal side of the sodium pump. The radiosodium labeling technique, therefore, is invalid as a means of estimating specific effects at the apical or mucosal permeability barrier.

Recently five other lines of evidence have been advanced in support of the permease hypothesis.

1. Oxidation of ^{14}C-pyruvate and ^{14}C-acetoacetate by the toad bladder was enhanced by aldosterone in parallel with the increase in sodium transport (Sharp *et al.*, 1966a). Removal of sodium from the mucosal bathing medium, which eliminates active sodium transport, abolished the aldosterone-dependent increase in substrate oxidation. Sharp *et al.* (1966a) concluded that this result is in accord with the permease hypothesis but at the same time granted that this evidence is not conclusive. In our judgment, these findings are equally compatible with an action of AIP on production of ATP or a direct action on the sodium pump and is, therefore, essentially noninformative. Substrate oxidation in intact, coupled mitochondria is limited by the local concentration of ADP and inorganic phosphate (P_i). Active sodium transport consumes between 20% and 40% of the ATP synthesized aerobically in toad bladder (Leaf *et al.*, 1959; Lipton and Edelman, 1969). Even if aldosterone acted primarily on oxidative phosphorylation, in sodium-free media, a small and probably undetectable increase in respiration would increase ATP concentration sufficiently to lower the ADP and P_i concentrations to limiting values. The result would be no change in steady-state respiration in aldosterone-treated tissue. In sodium-rich media, however, a rise in ATP concentration produced by the action of AIP would stimulate active sodium transport and further hydrolysis of ATP. The increase in ADP and P_i production would maintain a sustained increase in respiration and substrate oxidation.

2. Amphotericin B, a polyene antibiotic, stimulates sodium transport when applied to the mucosal but not the serosal surface of the toad bladder (Lichtenstein and Leaf, 1965). Amphotericin B also increases the permeability of artificial lipid monolayer and bilayer membranes to ions (Kinsky *et al.*, 1966; Van Zutphen and Van Deenen, 1966). This antibiotic increased the radiosodium pool size and permeability to urea of the toad bladder (Lichtenstein and Leaf, 1965). These effects could be explained by a direct attack of amphotericin B on the integrity of the

apical permeability barrier. It had previously been observed that aldosterone enhanced the sodium transport response to specific substrates (i.e., glucose, pyruvate, lactate, acetoacetate, oxaloacetate) in substrate-depleted toad bladders (Edelman *et al.*, 1963; Sharp and Leaf, 1965; Fimognari *et al.*, 1967b). Under similar conditions, amphotericin B also enhanced the sodium transport response to pyruvate and acetoacetate (Sharp *et al.*, 1966a). By analogy, therefore, it was concluded that aldosterone and amphotericin B act at the same site, namely the apical permeability barrier. Because pretreatment with aldosterone significantly attenuated the response of the toad bladder to amphotericin B (Fanestil, 1966; Crabbé, 1967), Crabbé (1967) supported the argument presented by Sharp *et al.* (1966a). These arguments, however, are open to serious question. In substrate-depleted hemibladders, amphotericin B produced highly significant increases in sodium transport but no response to aldosterone was found in the paired hemibladders (Fanestil *et al.*, 1968). Thus it can not be inferred that both agents are equally dependent on exogenous substrate. As shown in Table IV, the dependence on adequate supply of substrate is unique to aldosterone. Evidence was also presented to show that the synthesis of AIP was not substrate-dependent. Moreover, inhibition of NADH dehydrogenase activity with rotenone or sodium amytal abolished the sodium transport response to aldosterone but had virtually no effect on the response to amphotericin B. These results contradict the inference that AIP and amphotericin B both have direct actions on the apical permeability barriers. We will return to this argu-

TABLE IV

COMPARISON OF THE RESPONSE OF SUBSTRATE-DEPRIVED TOAD BLADDERS TO
ALDOSTERONE VS VASOPRESSIN AND AMPHOTERICIN B[a,b]

No. of Pairs	Additions	scc_0[c]	scc_{max}[d]	p
6	Aldosterone (7×10^{-8} *M*)	35 ± 14	36 ± 14	n.s.[e]
	Vasopressin (100 mU/ml)	24 ± 6	42 ± 7	<0.001
10	Aldosterone (7×10^{-8} *M*)	40 ± 10	40 ± 6	n.s.
	Amphotericin B ($18 \mu g/ml$)	30 ± 7	83 ± 7	<0.001

[a] From Fanestil *et al.* 1968.

[b] $\mu A/2.54$ cm² as mean $\pm$ SEM.

[c] scc_0 denotes the short-circuit current recorded at the time of addition of aldosterone, vasopressin, or amphotericin B to the media.

[d] scc_{max} denotes the short-circuit current at the peak of the response which was about 30 minutes after the addition of vasopressin or amphotericin B and about 3 hours after the addition of aldosterone. The rate of active sodium transport is assumed to be equivalent to the short-circuit current.

[e] n.s. denotes not significant or $p > .05$.

ment again when we consider the evidence of an action of AIP on oxidative phosphorylation (Section IV,F,3).

3. Sharp *et al.* (1966a) presented a theoretical argument in favor of the permease hypothesis as follows: sodium transport is usually limited by the rate of entry of sodium across the saturable mucosal permeability barrier and the sodium concentration in the active transport pool is maintained at a low level by efficient active extrusion of sodium by the pump in the basal-lateral plasma membranes. Any mechanism that stimulated the sodium pump would be ineffective as a further drop in sodium concentration in a low-level pool could contribute only a small percentage increase in the gradient for sodium entry which is required to restore the steady-state relationships between entry and exit. This argument, however, is inconclusive and suppositious. It assumes that the permeability properties of the apical boundary are independent of the concentration gradient by analogy to simple, artificial membranes. Complex, living membranes are known to be sensitive to ion gradients (e.g., axonal membranes). There is the further assumption, which is by no means proved, that sodium transport is ordinarily limited by the rate of entry. This inference is based on the curvilinear dependence of the transport rate on mucosal sodium concentrations and the simultaneous measurement of the sodium transport pool size (Frazier *et al.*, 1962). As no accurate method for measuring the transport pool size has yet been developed, the concept that sodium transport is uniquely controlled by the permeability of the apical boundary is still hypothetical.

4. Dalton and Snart (1967) noted that an increase in the temperature of the bathing media from 8°–20° C, increased active sodium transport across the toad bladder and that aldosterone enhanced this effect. They attributed the aldosterone effect to enhancement of a temperature-dependent change in the permeability of the apical plasma membrane to sodium. This interpretation, however, was based on the assumption that the apical boundary uniquely determines the rate of sodium transport and that the temperature jump had no effect on either ATP synthesis or the activity of the sodium pump. The first of these assumptions is open to question, as indicated in our foregoing argument, and the second is entirely without experimental support.

5. Ehrlich and Crabbé (1968) studied the inhibitory effects of amiloride on sodium transport across the isolated toad bladder and skin, and inferred that this agent impairs the binding of sodium to hypothetical specific carriers in the apical plasma membrane. This inference was based primarily on measurements of the sodium transport pool and the combined effects of amphotericin B and the inhibitor. As pretreatment with aldosterone decreased the percentage inhibition of sodium transport

produced by amiloride, Crabbé and Ehrlich (1968) concluded that AIP increased the density of the specific carriers (or permeases) in the apical boundary and thereby facilitated sodium entry. As we indicated above, the method for measuring the sodium transport pool has not been validated and our knowledge of the mechanism of action of amphotericin B is still incomplete. Thus, additional studies are needed to validate the conclusion that amiloride is a specific inhibitor of an apical "permease" system. If amiloride is to serve as a reliable means of analyzing the mechanism of action of aldosterone, it will first be necessary to define the site of action of this interesting agent unequivocally.

D. PHYSIOLOGICAL ANALYSIS OF THE PERMEASE HYPOTHESIS

Because of the limitations in the evidence offered in defense of the permease hypothesis, we sought a physiological test of the effects of aldosterone on the apical boundary. The test we devised made use of the relationship between the flux ratio and the forces involved in the transport process. The argument is as follows: the Na^+ flux ratio (f) measured by determining the simultaneous unidirectional fluxes with ^{22}Na and ^{24}Na may be related to the driving forces by a modification of the Kedem and Essig (1965) equation:

$$RT \ln f = -X_{ec} + \sum_i X_i + X_m \tag{8}$$

where X_{ec} denotes the difference in electrochemical potential of Na^+ in the external bathing media, X_i the contribution of all transepithelial flows to sodium transport (e.g., solvent drag), X_m the driving force provided by the sodium pump (i.e., the direct contribution of metabolic energy to sodium transport), R the gas constant and T the absolute temperature. When X_{ec} is kept constant at any arbitrary level by fixing the electrical potential difference with a voltage clamp and maintaining the sodium concentration in the bathing media at a constant level, then

$$RT(df/f) = dX_m \tag{9}$$

provided that there is no significant change in coupled transepithelial transport of species other than sodium ($d\Sigma_i X_i = 0$). In the isolated toad bladder bathed by identical solutions, $[Na^+] = 115$ mEq/liter, and the potential difference (p.d.) clamped at zero (i.e., $X_{ec} = 0$), aldosterone increased the sodium flux ratio by 52%, indicating an increase in the activity of the sodium pump (Porter *et al.*, 1964). This effect, however, could be attributed to an action on the apical boundary as an increase in intracellular sodium concentration would be expected to stimulate the sodium pump in the same way that sodium activates the transport ATPase. If, however, the driving force for sodium transport across the apical boundary were reversed, an action on the apical barrier could not lead to an increase in sodium entry or a sodium-dependent increase in the activity of the sodium pump. Accordingly, in another set of experiments, we clamped the p.d. at $+100$ mV (serosal side positive) and diluted the mucosal sodium concentration to $1/5$ that of the serosal solution (Fanestil *et al.*, 1967). At this fixed electrochemical gradient, net sodium transport was maintained in the reverse direction (i.e., from serosa to mucosa). Under these conditions, aldosterone produced a more than 60% increase in the sodium flux ratio (Table V). The time course of the increase in the sodium flux ratio was the same as that of the increase in net sodium transport measured by the scc method. These results support the inference of an effect of AIP on sodium transport independent of an effect on the permeability of the apical boundary. The validity of this inference is based on the assumption that net flow of sodium across the apical boundary is reversed when net transepithelial sodium transport is reversed. This assumption depends on the quantitative relationship between the amounts of sodium moving between the epithelial cells compared to the amounts moving through the epithelial cell bodies. If the bulk of the reversed flow of sodium was via low resistance, intercellular shunts application of the voltage clamp should have no effect on the intracellular sodium concentration. In bladders, clamped at $+100$ mV, intracellular sodium concentration was significantly higher than in the bladders maintained under open-circuit conditions, indicating that a significant fraction of the serosal to mucosal flux of sodium was via the transcellular path.

TABLE V

EFFECT OF ALDOSTERONE ON THE NA^+ FLUX RATIO[a]

Aldosterone (μM)	Na^+ flux ratio			
	1st hour	6th hour	Δ	p
0	0.164 ± 0.05	0.117 ± 0.03	-0.046 ± 0.03	n.s.
0.7	0.159 ± 0.09	0.263 ± 0.13	$+0.104 \pm 0.04$	0.05

[a] Pairs of steroid-depleted hemibladders from *Bufo marinus* were incubated in standard frog-Ringer's solution ($Na^+ = 114$ mEq/liter) on the serosal side and choline-frog Ringer's solution ($Na^+ = 23$ mEq/liter and $Choline^+ = 91$ mEq/liter) on the mucosal side. At time zero, d-aldosterone ($7 \times 10^{-7}\ M$) was added to the serosal media of one of each pair of hemibladders and the transepithelial electrical p.d. was clamped at $+100$ mV (serosal side positive). The Na^+ flux ratio was calculated from simultaneous bidirectional flux measurements made with ^{22}Na and ^{24}Na. Data are given as the mean $\pm$ standard error of the mean for six pairs of hemibladders. From Fanestil *et al.* (1967).

E. Extrarenal Action of Mineralocorticoids

That aldosterone may modify the activity of the sodium pump independent of effects on the permeability properties of the plasma membrane has also been suggested by results obtained with a variety of tissues in which the sodium pump is symmetrically distributed in the plasma membrane. Significant extrarenal effects were observed by Losert *et al.* (1964) following administration of 0.5 μg/rat of D-aldosterone daily for 4 days to adrenalectomized rats. Steroid administration lowered intracellular sodium concentration in liver, heart, skeletal muscle, and erythrocytes; simultaneous administration of 1.5 mg of spirolactone (SC-8109) diminished this effect in liver, heart, and erythrocytes. As these studies were carried out in rats with intact kidneys, however, the observed extrarenal effects may be attributable to changes in Na^+/K^+ balance rather than direct effects of the steroid at the target cell level. This reservation, however, does not apply to their subsequent studies on adrenalectomized–nephrectomized rats. Administration of a single physiological dose of aldosterone to adrenalectomized–nephrectomized rats decreased hepatic sodium concentration from 17.2 ± 1.9 to 10.1 ± 1.3 μEq/ml of cell water (Bartelheimer *et al.*, 1967). The latent period in the hepatic response and inhibition of the effect by actinomycin D suggested that equivalent mechanisms were operative in the kidney and liver. Similar results were obtained with human carcinoma cells grown in tissue culture (Richards *et al.*, 1966). Addition of aldosterone to the culture medium (2.8×10^{-8} M final concentration) lowered the sodium content from 33.1 ± 1.2 to 29.4 ± 1.0 mEq/kg wet weight of cells. The effect was small but statistically significant. These results obviously imply an action of AIP on the sodium extrusion process rather than sodium entry. Some support for this conclusion may also be deduced from studies on skeletal muscle. In skeletal muscle incubated *in vitro* for 4–6 hours, addition of aldosterone prevented the spontaneous decline in transmembrane p.d. in rat and frog muscle suggesting steroidal support of the sodium pump (Galand and Ildefonse, 1965; Schottelius and Schottelius, 1967). Contradictory results, however, were obtained by Lim and Webster (1967), who reported that addition of aldosterone (2.8×10^{-7} M) to diaphragms from adrenalectomized rats, incubated *in vitro*, increased intracellular sodium and potassium concentrations. A puzzling feature of this effect was the finding of no accompanying change in the volume of intracellular water. To explain these unusual findings, it was necessary to postulate osmotic inactivation of the newly acquired cations. Further studies on extrarenal, nonepithelial systems may aid in resolving the question of an action of aldosterone on the sodium extrusion process.

F. Effects of AIP on Intermediary Metabolism

In the substrate-depleted state, the response of the isolated toad bladder to aldosterone is virtually nil (Edelman *et al.*, 1963). Subsequent addition of glucose or pyruvate to the aldosterone pretreated bladder elicited the mineralocorticoid response without an appreciable latent period. The synergistic effects of aldosterone and substrates on active sodium transport led to the proposal that ATP synthesis coupled with oxidation of pyruvate mediated the mineralocorticoid action of AIP. In the last 5 years, a variety of studies have been made on the effects of aldosterone on metabolic pathways and the relationship of these effects to mineralocorticoid action. These studies will be reviewed in three categories: (1) glycolysis; (2) the phosphogluconate oxidation pathway; and (3) mitochondrial oxidative phosphorylation.

1. Aldosterone and Glycolysis

In a preliminary communication, Handler *et al.* (1968) reported that in aldosterone-treated isolated toad bladders, sodium transport remained at a higher level than in controls even under anaerobic conditions. A comparison of the concentrations of various glycolytic intermediates in these bladders indicated that the activities of phosphofructokinase and pyruvate kinase were increased by the steroid. Ouabain, which abolished the mineralocorticoid effect, also abolished the aldosterone-dependent changes in the glycolytic intermediates. These results imply that stimulation of glycolysis, therefore, is an indirect consequence of a primary effect of AIP on sodium transport.

2. Aldosterone and Phosphogluconate Oxidation

Mineralocorticoid effects on the phosphogluconate oxidation pathway (HMP shunt) have also been reported. The activity of the HMP shunt has been evaluated in the toad bladder by measuring the relative rates of oxidation of C-1 and C-6 of labeled glucose (Kirchberger *et al.*, 1968). Aldosterone significantly reduced oxidation of $1\text{-}^{14}C$ and increased oxidation of $6\text{-}^{14}C$. As the increase in $6\text{-}^{14}C$ oxidation depended on the presence of sodium in the medium, it was concluded that the steroid-dependent increase in sodium transport activated glycolysis. In contrast, the aldosterone-dependent decrease in HMP shunt activity (i.e., the fall in the ratio of $1\text{-}^{14}C$ to $6\text{-}^{14}C$ oxidation) occurred in the absence of sodium in the medium and had the same time course as the effect on active sodium transport. That this effect could be attributed to the generation of AIP was indicated by the elimination of the fall in $1\text{-}^{14}C$ oxidation by inhibitors of RNA or protein synthesis. The relationship between the action of aldosterone on sodium transport and inhibition of the HMP shunt has not yet been defined, but Handler *et al.* (1969) have offered evidence that the effect on the HMP shunt may be glucocorticoid rather than a mineralocorticoid property of aldosterone.

3. Aldosterone and Oxidative Phosphorylation

The first direct evidence implicating an effect of aldosterone on mitochondrial enzymes was reported by Feldman *et al.* (1961, 1963). They injected normal and adrenalectomized rats with 100 μg of aldosterone and assayed the kidneys for succinate dehydrogenase and cytochrome oxidase activity. There was no change in the enzyme patterns at 1 hour and a 40% increase in succinate dehydrogenase and 60% increase in cytochrome oxidase activities at 3 hours. The enzyme levels returned toward the control value 5 hours after injection. The time course of these enzyme changes, therefore, parallels the changes in urinary electrolyte excretion. Nevertheless, the relevance of these findings to physiological action on electrolyte transport is doubtful as the dosage of aldosterone used in these studies was 100-fold greater than that required for maximal effects on sodium excretion. It is significant that Domjan and Fazekas (1961) found no increase in renal succinate dehydrogenase activity after 4 days of administration of physiological amounts (i.e., 1 μg/kg body weight) of aldosterone to adrenalectomized rats. Fimognari (1965) studied the issue of dose dependence in aldosterone activation of succinate dehydrogenase from adrenalectomized rat kidneys. She confirmed the findings of Feldman *et al.* (1963) in that 100 μg of aldosterone per rat provoked a 57% increase in enzyme activity (Table VI). At a dose level of 2 μg/rat, however, no change in activity was found; thus no role can be assigned to activation of succinate dehydrogenase (and by implication

TABLE VI

EFFECT OF *d*-ALDOSTERONE ON SUCCINIC DEHYDROGENASE OF
ADRENALECTOMIZED RAT KIDNEY[a]

No. of rats	μg of Aldosterone[b]	Enzyme activity[c]	p
10	0	0.42 ± 0.02	
10	2	0.45 ± 0.02	n.s.
6	100	0.66 ± 0.02	<0.001

[a] From Fimognari and Edelman (1965).

[b] Injected subcutaneously, kidneys removed 3 hours later.

[c] Milligrams of formazan/15 min/mg protein. Assay of 1:100 dilution of whole kidney homogenate after 700 $\times$ g centrifugation. Mean $\pm$ standard error of the mean.

cytochrome oxidase) in mediating mineralocorticoid action at this time.

Attempts to detect a direct or *in vitro* action of aldosterone on mitochondrial enzymes have been either unsuccessful or of questionable physiological significance. Liljeroot and Hall (1965) found that mitochondria prepared from adrenalectomized rat liver were partially uncoupled and that addition of aldosterone to the media improved the P:O ratios. The effect was relatively nonspecific, however, as insulin, cortisone, or epinephrine exerted the same influence. Moreover, Bedrak and Samoiloff (1966) obtained contradictory results; at concentrations of $10^{-4}\,M$, $10^{-7}\,M$, and $10^{-10}\,M$, aldosterone added to rat liver mitochondria inhibited P:O ratios. The changes noted in rat liver and kidney mitochondrial enzymes after *in vivo* injection of aldosterone by Bedrak and Samoiloff (1967) may be relevant to stress situations but may not be relevant to the physiological issues, as they used 200 μg aldosterone/100 gm body weight in their studies.

V. THE OXIDATIVE PHOSPHORYLATION HYPOTHESIS

A. MITOCHONDRIAL ENZYMES

Recent evidence does implicate changes in mitochondrial enzyme activity in mineralocorticoid action. Kinne and Kirsten (1968) reported that adrenalectomy decreased the activities of mitochondrial citrate synthetase, glutamate dehydrogenase, and NADP-isocitrate dehydrogenase of rat kidney. Administration of 80 μg of *d*-aldosterone/100 gm rat restored normal activities. These dose levels, however, are about ten-fold greater than the physiological requirement for regulation of renal Na^+ and K^+ excretion (Wiederholt *et al.*, 1966). Nevertheless, additional studies have tended to confirm the relevance of these findings to regulation of ion transport. A single injection of 15 μg/rat of d-aldosterone reversed the adrenalectomy-induced decrease in mitochondrial NADP-isocitrate dehydrogenase but had no effect on the extramitochondrial enzyme (Senft, 1968). An extensive study by Kirsten *et al.* (1968) in the isolated toad bladder system yielded impressive results. Addition of *d*-aldosterone ($10^{-7}\,M$) increased the activities of citrate synthetase, NADP-isocitrate dehydrogenase, glutamate dehydrogenase and malate dehydrogenase of toad bladder mucosal epithelial cells in 2 hours. In contrast, no change in the activities of the extramitochondrial enzymes, lactate dehydrogenase, aldolase, and pyruvate kinase were noted. This

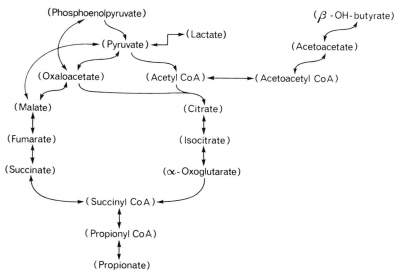

FIG. 9. Outline of the tricarboxylic acid cycle.

latter result agrees with the findings of Handler *et al.* (1968). The possible significance of these results may be seen by reference to Fig. 9 and 10, which summarize the mitochondrial tricarboxylic acid cycle and oxidative phosphorylation. Activation of the citrate synthetase, isocitrate dehydrogenase, and malate dehydrogenase pathways will promote substrate utilization and production of reduced pyridine nucleotides (i.e.,

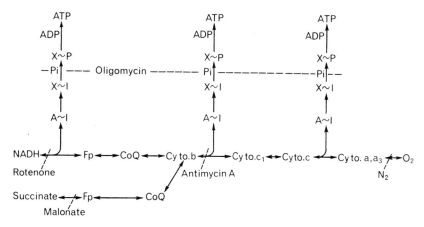

FIG. 10. Outline of mitochondrial electron transport, oxidative phosphorylation and sites of inhibition. (From D. R. Sanadi (1965). *Ann. Rev. Biochem. 34*, 21.)

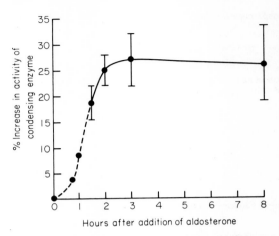

Fig. 11. Time course of increments in condensing enzyme activity in toad bladder mucosa. The bars represent standard errors of the means. d-Aldosterone was added to the medium bathing the serosal side of one quarter bladder at zero time to give a final concentration of 10^{-7} mole/liter, the other quarter served as the control. Enzyme activity was significantly greater in the aldosterone treated tissues at 1.5 hours ($p < 0.01$, $n = 6$), at 2 hours ($p < 0.001$, $n = 7$), at 3 hours ($p < 0.001$, $n = 10$) and at 8 hours ($p < 0.05$, $n = 6$). From Kirsten *et al.* (1968).

$NADH_2$). This in turn will provide substrate for ATP synthesis coupled to $NADH_2$ oxidation in proportion to the available supply of phosphate acceptor-ADP. Kirsten *et al.* (1968) also found that the time course of the increase in citrate synthetase activity produced by aldosterone was approximately the same as the time course of the increase in rate of sodium transport (Figs. 11 and 12). Moreover, as shown in Fig. 12, there was a significant, positive correlation between the relative steady-state increases in sodium transport and in citrate synthetase activity. Inhibitors of RNA and protein synthesis (actinomycin D and puromycin) abolished both the sodium transport and enzyme activation effects of aldosterone. The possibility that the changes in mitochondrial enzyme activity could be a secondary, nonspecific consequence of a primary effect on sodium transport was excluded by the finding of similar enzyme changes in toad bladders incubated in sodium-free mucosal solutions. Moreover, there is striking agreement between these enzymatic findings and our physiological studies, which will now be described.

B. INHIBITORS AND SUBSTRATES OF OXIDATIVE METABOLISM

It has been clearly established that steroids possess multifunctional properties. Thus, glucocorticoids, such as cortisol, have significant miner-

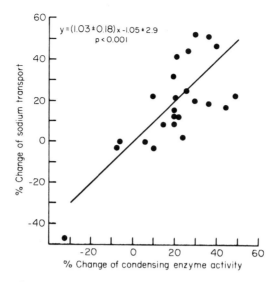

FIG. 12. The relationship of increased sodium transport to increased activity of condensing enzyme with aldosterone. The percent change in sodium transport is plotted as a function of the percent change in activity of condensing enzyme with aldosterone. The regression line was obtained from a least-mean-square analysis of the 24 experiments. From Kirsten *et al.* (1968).

alocorticoid effects and mineralocorticoids, including aldosterone, have significant glucocorticoid effects. The distinction is primarily one of dosage needed to elicit the effect. Thus, an unknown portion of the effect of aldosterone on RNA and protein synthesis, or on mitochondrial enzyme activities may be an expression of a glucocorticoid rather than an ion transport type of effect. It is essential, therefore, that criteria for a cause and effect relationship be established between biochemical changes and physiological action.

The toad bladder system has been exploited to test the role of oxidative phosphorylation in steroidal stimulation of sodium transport. Implicit in the hypothesis that AIP increases sodium transport by increasing the rate of supply of ATP to the sodium pump is the assumption that the sodium pump is not saturated with ATP in steroid-depleted tissue (i.e., that changes in ATP concentration change the activity of the sodium pump). Experimental evidence in support of this assumption was provided by Maffly and Edelman (1963) in that addition of substrates (e.g., glucose or pyruvate) to bladders preincubated for several hours in substrate-free media produced significant increases in sodium transport (Fig. 6). Subsequently, Edelman *et al.* (1963) noted that the response to aldosterone is nil in substrate-depleted bladders but is elicited without a measurable

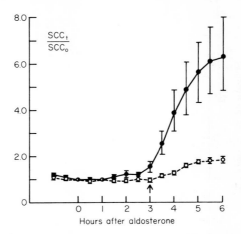

FIG. 13. Synergistic effects of oxaloacetate and $(+)$-aldosterone on the rate of active Na^+ transport across toad bladders. Paired hemibladders were incubated 16 hours prior to time zero in frog-Ringer solution. At time zero, 0.7 μM aldosterone was added to one hemibladder (●—●) and diluent to the other (○ - - - ○). The arrow at $t = 3$ hours indicates the addition of 4.8 mM sodium oxaloacetate to both hemibladders. The ratio scc_t/scc_0 denoted the short-circuit current at time t divided by that observed in the same hemibladder at time zero. The points and vertical lines represent the mean ± 1 standard error of the mean. $n = 6$ pairs of hemibladders. The absolute scc's at time zero were 37 ± 10 and 38 ± 9, $\mu A/2.54$ cm^2 for the aldosterone-treated and control hemibladders, respectively. From Fimognari *et al.* (1967b).

latent period by the subsequent addition of substrates to the media (Fig. 13) (Edelman *et al.*, 1963; Fimognari *et al.*, 1967b). These results prompted us to propose that enhanced oxidation of pyruvate and coupled generation of ATP mediated the action on sodium transport. Support for this proposal was provided by the findings that oxaloacetate and acetyl CoA or their precursors, pyruvate, glucose, β-OH butyrate, and acetoacetate, were synergistic with aldosterone in the regulation of sodium transport, but tricarboxylic acid cycle intermediates, α-ketoglutarate, succinate, and fumurate were ineffective (Sharp and Leaf, 1965; Fimognari *et al.*, 1967b). Oxythiamine, an inhibitor of the conversion of pyruvate to acetyl CoA blocked the pyruvate-dependent effect of aldosterone but not that of acetoacetate or β-OH butyrate (Fimognari *et al.*, 1967b). The inference that AIP may regulate the metabolic steps between acetyl CoA and succinate (Fig. 9) was supported by two additional observations:

1. Propionate, a precursor of succinyl CoA, stimulated sodium transport to the same extent in steroid-depleted and aldosterone-treated toad bladders (Fig. 14) and subsequent addition of glucose to the steroid-depleted bladders produced only a small rise in sodium transport

(Fanestil, 1967). These results suggest that propionate corrected most of the substrate deficiency. The failure to support the aldosterone response, however, was not a consequence of limitations in the responsiveness of the propionate–aldosterone-treated bladders as the subsequent addition of glucose promptly elicited the steroid-dependent rise in sodium transport. These results suggested that aldosterone activated only the steps prior to the formation of succinate.

2. Malonate, a competitive inhibitor of succinate dehydrogenase activity blocked the response of substrate-depleted bladders to propionate, indicating that propionate supported sodium transport via conversion to succinyl CoA (Fanestil *et al.*, 1968). In addition, malonate had no significant effect on aldosterone–pyruvate synergism (Fig. 15).

These inhibitor–substrate studies led to the proposal that aldosterone stimulates sodium transport either by increasing the rate of NADH production by modifying the steps between citrate synthetase and α-ketoglutarate dehydrogenase, or by increasing the rate of flavoprotein dependent NADH oxidation coupled to ATP synthesis (Edelman and Fimognari, 1967). The findings of Kirsten *et al.* (1968) of significant increases in citrate synthetase and isocitrate dehydrogenase activity after exposure to physiological levels of aldosterone provide direct support for the former inference.

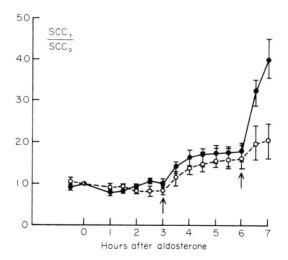

FIG. 14. Comparison of the synergistic effects of propionate vs glucose with aldosterone on scc. At time zero, 0.7 μM aldosterone was added to one of each pair of hemibladders (—●—) and diluent to the other (- - -○- - -). The arrow at $t = 3$ indicates addition of 4.25 mM sodium propionate and the arrow at $t = 6$ addition of 10 mM glucose to all hemibladders. From Fanestil (1967).

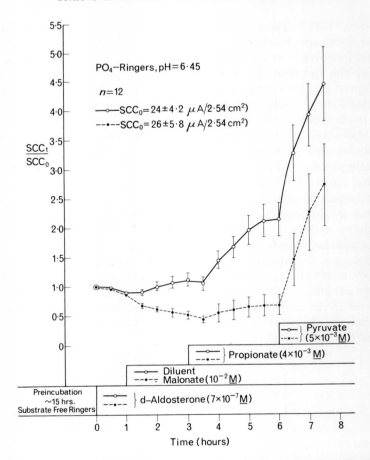

FIG. 15. Effect of malonate on propionate and pyruvate synergism with aldosterone on short-circuit current of the toad bladder. Duration of preincubation and additions are as indicated on the figure. From Fanestil *et al.* (1968).

Falchuck and Sharp (1968) contested this hypothesis and concluded that "available evidence does not support the theory that aldosterone stimulates sodium transport by enhancing the activity of the tricarboxylic acid cycle at some point between condensing enzyme and α-oxoglutarate. Rather, the functioning of an intact tricarboxylic acid cycle is necessary for the full expression of the action of aldosterone." This conclusion was based on two findings that contradicted our results with propionate and malonate: (1) in their studies, propionate was synergistic with aldosterone in support of the effect on sodium transport; and (2) malonate inhibited the aldosterone effect elicited by pyruvate in substrate-depleted bladders. The finding of propionate–aldosterone synergism, however, was obtained in a subspecies of *Bufo marinus* indigenous to the Dominican Republic. Davies *et al.* (1968) showed that in this subspecies, no substrate effect is obtained in the aldosterone-depleted state despite preincubation in substrate-free media for many hours. As aldosterone reverses the block to substrate utilization in support of sodium transport, the propionate effect may have been obtained by conversion of propionate → succinate → malate → oxaloacetate or pyruvate. In the subspecies used in our studies obtained from South America, the steroid-depleted, substrate-depleted bladders responded significantly to propionate. As the South American toads responded significantly to propionate, the failure to obtain augmentation of the response with aldosterone constitutes a significant result. The second contradiction, malonate inhibition of pyruvate-aldosterone synergism, is a result, we believe, of a failure to distinguish between the effects of malonate on the basal rate of sodium transport versus those on the aldosterone-dependent rate. Falchuck and Sharp (1968) noted that malonate + aldosterone gave a lower rate of sodium transport than aldosterone alone. In our studies, however, we found that this difference is entirely attributable to malonate inhibition of the basal, steroid-independent rate of sodium transport (Fanestil *et al.*, 1968). This is shown by the equivalent degrees of inhibition in the presence and absence of aldosterone in the right-hand panel of Fig. 16.

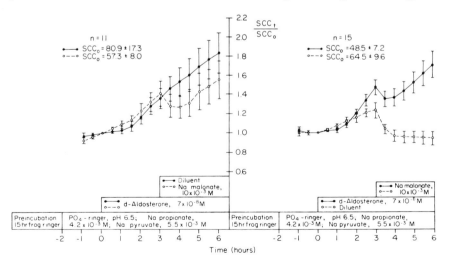

FIG. 16. Effect of malonate on the response of the toad bladder to aldosterone. Preincubation was in bicarbonate-Ringers, pH = 8.2. All solutions were exchanged with phosphate-Ringers, pH = 6.5 and all additions were made to both the serosal and mucosal media at the indicated times. From Fanestil *et al.* (1968).

This inference is also supported by studies of the effects of sequential addition of malonate, propionate and pyruvate shown in Fig. 15. In substrate-depleted hemibladders pretreated with aldosterone, malonate inhibited sodium transport by about 50%. Addition of propionate stimulated sodium transport only in the malonate-free system but subsequent addition of pyruvate produced the same increase in sodium transport in the presence and absence of malonate. Malonate, therefore, inhibited only the basal rate of sodium transport. The magnitude of the malonate "gap" was unchanged by the addition of pyruvate, suggesting that malonate inhibition of succinate dehydrogenase activity remained effective during pyruvate stimulation of sodium transport. It appears, therefore, that mineralocorticoid action is neither coupled to nor dependent on succinate oxidation.

The products of mitochondrial conversion of pyruvate to succinate are NADH, GTP, and succinate. To obtain additional evidence on the role of NADH oxidation (or production) in the action of aldosterone we used rotenone and amobarbital, inhibitors of flavoprotein-dependent NADH dehydrogenase activity. These inhibitors block NADH oxidation

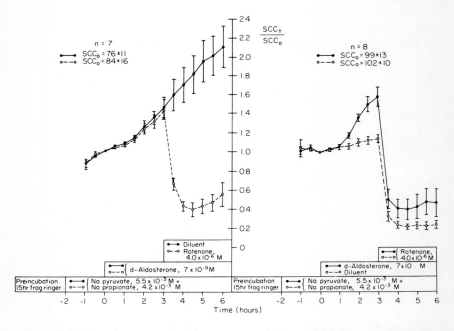

FIG. 17. Effect of rotenone on the response of the toad bladder to aldosterone. All additions were made to both the serosal and mucosal solutions at the indicated times. From Fanestil *et al.* (1968).

prior to the point where succinate and NADH generated reducing equivalents join in a common final electron transport path (Fig. 10). As shown in Fig. 17, rotenone promptly inhibited sodium transport in the aldosterone-treated hemibladders to about 40% of the control level (Fanestil *et al.*, 1968). Furthermore, rotenone virtually eliminated the aldosterone effect; the sodium transport rate was nearly the same in the presence or absence of aldosterone (Fig. 17, right). Similar results were obtained with sodium amobarbital (Karl and Edelman, 1968). These differential effects of inhibition of succinate oxidation versus inhibition of NADH oxidation on the response to aldosterone are difficult to reconcile with the permease theory. If oxidative metabolism were stimulated by aldosterone as a secondary effect of facilitated sodium entry, both succinate- and NADH-linked oxidative phosphorylation should be capable of supporting the action of aldosterone on sodium transport.

C. COMPARATIVE RESPONSES TO VASOPRESSIN AND AMPHOTERICIN B

As a test of the inference that the metabolic requirements for mineralo-corticoid action are secondary to a primary effect on the permeability of the apical surface to sodium, we used vasopressin and amphotericin B in parallel studies. Evidence has been presented suggesting that these agents act at the apical permeability barrier (i.e., pharmacological "permeases") (Frazier *et al.*, 1962; Lichtenstein and Leaf, 1965). As noted, aldosterone is ineffective in substrate-deprived hemibladders. A comparison of the response of these bladders to vasopressin and amphotericin B is given in Table IV. In contrast to the results with aldosterone, highly significant increases in sodium transport were obtained with vasopressin and amphotericin B. It is unlikely, therefore, that all three agents act at a common point in the regulation of sodium transport. The degree of metabolic dependence of the response to vasopressin and amphotericin B was also assessed with rotenone and sodium amobarbital. The results obtained with rotenone are given in Table VII. Rotenone only partially inhibited the response to vasopressin and had no effect on the response to amphotericin B. Moreover, amobarbital had no significant effect on the responses to either vasopressin or amphotericin B (Karl and Edelman, 1968). These results indicate that of these three agents, only aldosterone has a critical requirement for an intact pathway for NADH oxidation.

An additional test of independent sites of action of aldosterone versus vasopressin or amphotericin B is provided by studies on the effects of combinations of these agents. Crabbé (1967) found that amphotericin B and aldosterone gave the same rise in sodium transport as amphotericin B

TABLE VII

EFFECT OF ROTENONE ON THE RESPONSE TO VASOPRESSIN AND AMPHOTERICIN B[a]

No. of Pairs	Rotenone (4 μM)	Vasopressin (100 mU/ml)	Amphotericin B (15 μg/ml)	scc_B	scc_M	Δscc[b]	p
				(μA/2.54 cm^2)[c]			
7	0	+	0	83 ± 7	158 ± 33	75 ± 27	0.05
	+	+	0	32 ± 2	79 ± 11	49 ± 9	
11	0	0	+	105 ± 9	143 ± 12	38 ± 3	n.s.
	+	0	+	39 ± 6	80 ± 9	41 ± 3	

[a] From Fanestil et al. (1968).

[b] Δscc denotes the rise in short-circuit current after the addition of vasopressin or amphotericin B to the media and is the difference between the maximal short-circuit current (scc_M) and the base-line value (scc_B) recorded just before the additions.

[c] Mean ± SEM.

alone in the toad bladder system and concluded that both agents facilitated sodium entry or apical permeation. In toad bladders preincubated in steroid-free solutions, however, the increase in sodium transport produced by vasopressin was enhanced by pretreatment with aldosterone (Fanestil *et al.*, 1967; Handler *et al.*, 1969).

VI. MODEL OF THE MECHANISM OF MINERALOCORTICOID ACTION

The available evidence is consistent with the inference that AIP acts via effects on NADH production or NADH-linked electron transport coupled to phosphorylation of ADP. The results obtained with specific substrates (e.g., pyruvate, oxaloacetate, and propionate) and specific inhibitors (e.g., oxythiamine, malonate, rotenone, and amobarbital) and those on assays of mitochondrial enzyme activity implicate activation of citrate synthetase and isocitrate dehydrogenase in the action of AIP (Fimognari *et al.*, 1967b; Fanestil *et al.*, 1968; Kirsten *et al.*, 1968). The induction-metabolic pathway hypotheses may be combined into a single more comprehensive scheme:

$$A + ABP \rightleftharpoons C^* \tag{10}$$

$$\text{Precursor bases} \xrightarrow{(C^*),\ (DNA)} mRNA^* \tag{11}$$

$$\text{a-a} + tRNA \xrightarrow{(\text{Ribosomes (mRNA*)})} AIP \tag{12}$$

$$CS,\ IDH,\ (?E) \xrightarrow{(AIP)} CS^*,\ IDH^*,\ (?E^*) \tag{13}$$

$$\text{Pyruvate} + O_2 \xrightarrow{(CS^*),\ (IDH^*),\ (?E^*)} CO_2 + H_2O \tag{14}$$
$$ADP + P_i \qquad\qquad\qquad\qquad ATP$$

$$ATP + S \rightarrow \Delta S + ADP + P_i \tag{15}$$

where CS, IDH, E denote the basal state of citrate synthetase, isocitrate dehydrogenase and unspecified metabolic enzymes, respectively. CS*, IDH*, and E* denote the corresponding activated enzymes.

VII. FUTURE DIRECTIONS

Although a plausible hypothesis of the mechanism of action of aldosterone has been constructed, until all of the components in the process are explicitly defined the hypothesis will remain inferential and unproven. Thus, efforts are now being directed to the purification of ABP and to elucidation of its relationship to steroid-dependent induction of RNA synthesis.

The role of ABP in mineralocorticoid action may fall into one of three classes: (1) ABP may provide a carrier mechanism for transporting aldosterone from the plasma membrane to an intra-nuclear site of action; (2) ABP may provide an intracellular storage mechanism to prolong the action of the steroid during fluctuations in plasma levels, or (3) ABP may be directly involved in the regulation of DNA-dependent RNA synthesis (e.g., as a repressor whose function is altered by binding of the steroid or as an inactive regulator of transcription which is activated by the steroid). Isolation, purification, and molecular characterization of ABP may clarify these issues.

The conflicting views on the role of AIP in the regulation of sodium transport (i.e., permease vs NADH theories) will probably not be resolved definitively until AIP is isolated and its biochemical functions defined directly. Among the criteria that may be applied to the identification of AIP in addition to the conventional means of identifying a newly synthesized intermediate, e.g., increased incorporation of labeled amino acids and inhibition of physiological action by specific inhibitors of the intermediate, are the following: (1) corresponding time courses in the appearance of AIP and the effect on sodium transport; (2) biosynthesis of the intermediate protein should not be inhibited by anoxia or substrate-depletion; (3) spirolactone should prevent the formation of the suspected intermediate; and (4) steroids lacking mineralocorticoid activity should be incapable of promoting the synthesis of the suspected intermediate.

The concept that isolation and identification of ABP and AIP will elucidate the mechanism of action of aldosterone is based on the assumption that current concepts of the organization of the system for transepithelial sodium transport are correct. If the Ussing-Skou model should prove to be seriously mistaken, definition of the regulatory role of AIP may require an entirely new approach to the problem. Thus, an important goal of future research is a further analysis of the nature of the basic components of the sodium transport system itself.

REFERENCES

Addison, T. (1855). "On the Constitutional and Local Effects of Disease of the Supra-Renal Capsules." Highley, London.

Ausiello, D. A., and Sharp, G. W. G. (1968). *Endocrinology* **82**, 1163.

Barger, A. C., Berlin, R. D., and Tulenko, J. F. (1958). *Endocrinology* **62**, 804.

Bartelheimer, H. K., Losert, W., Senft, G., and Sitt, R. (1967). *Arch. Exptl. Pathol. Pharmakol.* **258**, 372.

Baumann, E. J., and Kurland, J. (1927). *J. Biol. Chem.* **71**, 281.

Bedrak, E., and Samoiloff, V. (1966). *J. Endocrinol.* **36**, 63.

Bedrak, E., and Samoiloff, V. (1967). *Can. J. Physiol. Pharmacol.* **45**, 717.

Bishop, W. R., Mumbach, M. W., and Scheer, B. T. (1961). *Am. J. Physiol.* **200**, 451.

Bonting, S. L., and Canady, M. R. (1964). *Am. J. Physiol.* **207**, 1005.

Bricker, N. S., Biber, T., and Ussing, H. H. (1963). *J. Clin. Invest.* **42**, 88.

Carstensen, H., Burgers, A. C. J., and Li, C. H. (1961). *Gen. Comp. Endocrinol.* **1**, 37.

Castles, T. R., and Williamson, H. E. (1965). *Proc. Soc. Exptl. Biol. Med.* **119**, 308.

Castles, T. R., and Williamson, H. E. (1967). *Proc. Soc. Exptl. Biol. Med.* **124**, 717.

Chignell, C. F., Roddy, P. M., and Titus, E. O. (1965). *Life Sci.* **4**, 559.

Cofré, G., and Crabbé, J. (1965). *Nature* **207**, 1299.

Crabbé, J. (1961). *J. Clin. Invest.* **40**, 2103.

Crabbé, J. (1963a). "The Sodium-Retaining Action of Aldosterone." Presses Acad. Européennes S. C., Editions Arscia, Brussels.

Crabbé, J. (1963b). *Nature* **200**, 787.

Crabbé, J. (1967). *Arch. Intern. Physiol. Biochim.* **75**, 342.

Crabbé, J., and De Weer, P. (1964). *Nature* **202**, 298.

Crabbé, J., and Ehrlich, E. N. (1968). *Arch. Ges. Physiol.* **304**, 284.

Dalton, T., and Snart, R. S. (1967). *Biochim. Biophys. Acta* **135**, 1059.

Davies, H. E. F., Martin, D. G., and Sharp, G. W. G. (1968). *Biochim. Biophys. Acta* **150**, 315.

de Fremery, P., Lacqueur, E., Reichstein, T., Spanhoff, R. W., and Uyldert, I. E. (1937). *Nature* **139**, 26.

Denton, D. A. (1957). *Quart J. Exptl. Physiol.* **42**, 72.

De Weer, P., and Crabbé, J. (1968). *Biochim. Biophys. Acta* **155**, 280.

Domjan, G., and Fazekas, A. G. (1961). *Enzymologia* **23**, 281.

Edelman, I. S. (1968). *In* "Functions of the Adrenal Cortex" (K. W. McKerns, ed.), Vol. 1, p. 80. Appleton, New York.

Edelman, I. S. (1969). *In* "Renal Transport and Diuretics" (K. Thurau and J. Jahrmärker, eds.), p. 139. Springer, Berlin.

Edelman, I. S., and Fimognari, G. M. (1967). *Proc. 3rd Intern. Congr. Nephrol., Wash. D. C. 1966* Vol. 1, p. 27. Karger, Basel.

Edelman, I. S., Bogoroch, R., and Porter, G. A. (1963). *Proc. Natl. Acad. Sci. U. S.* **50**, 1169.

Edelman, I. S., Bogoroch, R., and Porter, G. A. (1964). *Trans. Assoc. Am. Physicians* **77**, 307.

Edmonds, C. J., and Marriott, J. C. (1967). *J. Endocrinol.* **39**, 517.

Ehrlich, E. N., and Crabbé, J. (1968). *Arch. Ges. Physiol.* **304**, 284.

Falchuk, M. Z., and Sharp, G. W. G. (1968). *Biochim. Biophys. Acta* **153**, 706.

Fanestil, D. D. (1966). *Abstr. 3rd Intern. Congr. Nephrol., 1966* p. 188. Secretariat, 3rd Int. Congr. Nephrol. Wash. D. C.

Fanestil, D. D. (1967). Quoted in Fimognari *et al.* (1967b).

Fanestil, D. D. (1968a). *Biochem. Pharmacol.* **17**, 2240.

Fanestil, D. D. (1968b). *Life Sci.* **7**, 191.

Fanestil, D. D., and Edelman, I. S. (1966a). *Federation Proc.* **25**, 912.

Fanestil, D. D., and Edelman, I. S. (1966b). *Proc. Natl. Acad. Sci. U. S.* **56**, 872.

Fanestil, D. D., and Edelman, I. S. (1966c). Unpublished observations.

Fanestil, D. D., Porter, G. A., and Edelman, I. S. (1967). *Biochim. Biophys. Acta* **135**, 74.

Fanestil, D. D., Herman, T. S., Fimognari, G. M., and Edelman, I. S. (1968). *In* "Regulatory Functions of Biological Membranes" (J. Jarnefelt, ed.), p. 177. Elsevier, Amsterdam.

Feldman, D., Vander Wende, C., and Kessler, E. (1961). *Biochim. Biophys. Acta* **51**, 401.

Feldman, D., Brenner, M., and Fleisher, M. B. (1963). *Biochim. Biophys. Acta* **78**, 775.

Fimognari, G. M. (1965). Unpublished observations.

Fimognari, G. M., and Edelman, I. S. (1965). Unpublished observations.

Fimognari, G. M., Fanestil, D. D., and Edelman, I. S. (1967a). *Am. J. Physiol.* **213**, 954.

Fimognari, G. M., Porter, G. A., and Edelman, I. S. (1967b). *Biochim. Biophys. Acta* **135**, 89.

Frazier, H. S. (1962). *J. Gen. Physiol.* **45**, 515.

Frazier, H. S., Dempsey, E. F., and Leaf, A. (1962). *J. Gen. Physiol.* **45**, 529.

Galand, G., and Ildefonse, M. (1965). *J. Physiol. (Paris)* **57**, 612.

Ganong, W. F., and van Brunt, E. E. (1968). *In* "Handbuch der experimentellen Pharmakologie" (H. W. Deane and B. Rubin, eds. p. 3), Vol. 14, p. 4. Springer, Berlin.

Grundy, H. M., Simpson, S. A., and Tait, J. F. (1952). *Nature* **169**, 795.

Handler, J. S., Preston, A. S., and Orloff, J. (1968). *Federation Proc.* **27**, 234.

Handler, J. S., Preston, A. S., and Orloff, J. (1969). *J. Clin. Invest.* **48**, 823.

Herman, T. S., and Edelman, I. S. (1969). Quoted in Edelman (1969).

Herman, T. S., Fimognari, G. M., and Edelman, I. S. (1968). *J. Biol. Chem.* **243**, 3849.

Hierholzer, K., Wiederholt, M., Holzgreve, H., Giebisch, G., Klose, R. M., and Windhager, E. E. (1965). *Arch. Ges. Physiol.* **285**, 193.

Karl, R. J., and Edelman, I. S. (1968). Quoted Fanestil *et al.* (1968).

Kedem, O., and Essig, A. (1965). *J. Gen. Physiol.* **48**, 1047.

Kinne, R., and Kirsten, R. (1968). *Arch. Ges. Physiol.* **300**, 244.

Kinsky, S. C., Luse, S. A., and Van Deenen, L. L. M. (1966). *Federation Proc.* **25**, 1503.

Kirchberger, M. A., Martin, D. G., Leaf, A., and Sharp, G. W. G. (1968). *Biochim. Biophys. Acta* **165**, 22.

Kirsten, E., Kirsten, R., Leaf, A., and Sharp, G. W. G. (1968). *Arch. Ges. Physiol.* **300**, 213.

Kliman, B. (1966). Quoted in Sharp and Leaf (1966, p. 601).

Koefoed-Johnsen, V., and Ussing, H. H. (1958). *Acta Physiol. Scand.* **42**, 298.

Landon, E. J., Jazeb, N., and Forte, L. (1966). *Am. J. Physiol.* **211**, 1050.

Leaf, A. (1967). *Proc. 3rd Intern. Congr. Nephrol., 1966* Vol. 1, p. 18. Karger, Basel.

Leaf, A., Anderson, J., and Page, L. B. (1958). *J. Gen. Physiol.* **41**, 657.

Leaf, A., Page, L. B., and Anderson, J. (1959). *J. Biol. Chem.* **234**, 1625.

Lichtenstein, N. S., and Hagopian, L. (1966). Quoted in Sharp and Leaf (1966).

Lichtenstein, N. S., and Leaf, A. (1965). *J. Clin. Invest.* **44**, 1328.

Liddle, G. W., Cornfield, J., Casper, A. G. T., and Bartter, F. C. (1955). *J. Clin. Invest.* **34**, 1410.

Liljeroot, B. S., and Hall, J. C. (1965). *J. Biol. Chem.* **240,** 1446.

Lim, V. S., and Webster, G. D. (1967). *Clin. Sci.* **33,** 261.

Lipton, P., and Edelman, I. S. (1968). Unpublished observations.

Lipton, P., and Edelman, I. S. (1969). *Biophys. J.* **9,** A-164 (Soc. Abstr.).

Loeb, R. F., Atchley, D. W., Benedict, E. M., and Leland, L. (1933). *J. Exptl. Med.* **57,** 775.

Losert, W., Senft, C., and Senft, G. (1964). *Arch. Exptl. Pathol. Pharmakol.* **248,** 450.

Lucas, G. H. W. (1926). *Am. J. Physiol.* **77,** 114.

Luetscher, J. A., Jr., and Deming, Q. B. (1951). *2nd Conf. on Renal Function 1950, Josiah Macy, Jr. Found.,* p. 155.

McAfee, R. D., and Locke, W. (1961). *Am. J. Physiol.* **200,** 797.

Maetz, J., Jard, S., and Morel, F. (1958). *Compt. Rend.* **247,** 516.

Maffly, R. H., and Edelman, I. S. (1963). *J. Gen. Physiol.* **46,** 733.

Mangos, J. A., and McSherry, N. R. (1968). *Am. Soc. Nephrol.* p. 40 (abstr.).

Moll, H. Ch., and Koczorek, Kh. R. (1962). *Klin. Wochschr.* **40,** 825.

Morel, R., and Maetz, J. (1958). *J. Med. Bordeaux Sud-Ouest,* 13.

Porter, G. A. (1968). Unpublished observations.

Porter, G. A., and Edelman, I. S. (1964). *J. Clin. Invest.* **43,** 611.

Porter, G. A., Bogoroch, R., and Edelman, I. S. (1964). *Proc. Natl. Acad. Sci. U. S.* **52,** 1326.

Richards, P., Smith, K., Metcalfe-Gibson, A., and Wrong, O. (1966). *Lancet* **II,** 1099.

Ross, E. J. (1959). "Aldosterone in Clinical and Experimental Medicine." Blackwell, Oxford.

Scheer, B. T., Mumbach, M. W., and Cox, B. L. (1961). *Federation Proc.* **20,** 177.

Schmidlin, J., Anner, G., Billeter, J. R., Heusler, K., Ueberwasser, H., Wieland, P., and Wettstein, A. (1957). *Helv. Chim. Acta* **40,** 2291.

Schottelius, B. A., and Schottelius, D. D. (1967). *Proc. Soc. Exptl. Biol. Med.* **125,** 898.

Senft, G. (1968). *Arch. Exptl. Pathol. Pharmakol.* **259,** 117.

Share, L., and Hall, P. W. (1958). *Am. J. Physiol.* **183,** 291.

Sharp, G. W. G., and Leaf, A. (1963). *J. Clin. Invest.* **42,** 978.

Sharp, G. W. G., and Leaf, A. (1964). *Nature* **202,** 1185.

Sharp, G. W. G., and Leaf, A. (1965). *J. Biol. Chem.* **240,** 4816.

Sharp, G. W. G., and Leaf, A. (1966). *Physiol. Rev.* **46,** 593.

Sharp, G. W. G., Coggins, C. H., Lichtenstein, N. S., and Leaf, A. (1966a). *J. Clin. Invest.* **45,** 1640.

Sharp, G. W. G., Komack, C. L., and Leaf, A. (1966b). *J. Clin. Invest.* **45,** 450.

Shuster, S. (1962). *Proc. Roy. Soc. Med.* **55,** 719.

Simpson, S. A., Tait, J. F., Wettstein, A., Neher, R., von Euw, J., Schindler, O., and Reichstein, T. (1954). *Experientia* **10,** 132.

Skou, J. C. (1965). *Physiol. Rev.* **45,** 596.

Steiger, M., and Reichstein, T. (1937). *Nature* **139,** 925.

Swaneck, G. E., Highland, E., and Edelman, I. S. (1969). *Nephron* **6,** 297.

Turakolov, Y. X., Tashmohamedov, B. A., Ilyasov, D., and Bekmohamedova, Z. U. (1968). *Rept. Acad. Sci. USSR* **178,** 977.

Uhlich, E., Baldamus, C. A., and Ullrich, K. J. (1969). *Arch. Ges. Physiol.* **308,** 111.

Ulick, S., and Feinholtz, E. (1968). *J. Clin. Invest.* **47,** 2523.

Ussing, H. H. (1965). *Acta Physiol. Scand.* **63,** 141.

Ussing, H. H., and Zerahn, K. (1951). *Acta Physiol. Scand.* **23**, 110.
Van Zutphen, H., and Van Deenen, L. L. M. (1966). *Biochem. Biophys. Res. Commun.* **22**, 393.
Wiederholt, M. (1966). *Arch. Ges. Physiol.* **292**, 334.
Wiederholt, M., Stolte, H., Brecht, J. P., and Hierholzer, K. (1966). *Arch. Ges. Physiol.* **292**, 316.
Williamson, H. E. (1963). *Biochem. Pharmacol.* **12**, 1449.
Willmer, E. N. (1961). *Biol. Rev.* **36**, 368.

CHAPTER 9

Parathyroid
Hormone and Calcitonin

Howard Rasmussen and Alan Tenenhouse

I. INTRODUCTION

The major functions of both parathyroid hormone and calcitonin are to regulate plasma calcium concentration, and the related activities of calcium transport and excretion, and bone accretion and resorption (Arnaud *et al.*, 1967; Tenenhouse *et al.*, 1968; Copp, 1969). Parathyroid hormone acts upon at least three major organs: gut, kidney, and bone (Rasmussen, 1961). Calcitonin acts primarily on bone and may have an additional effect upon kidney, although this is a matter of continuing controversy (Rasmussen *et al.*, 1967b; Robinson *et al.*, 1966; Clark and Kenny, 1969). This chapter will consider primarily the biochemical aspects of the subject. The proceedings of two recent symposia can be consulted for a more detailed knowledge of the physiological, anatomical, and clinical aspects of this subject ("Calcitonin and the C Cell," published by Heineman, 1968; "Parathyroid Hormone and Calcitonin," published by Excerpta Medica Foundation, 1968).

The critical question to be examined in this review is the biochemical basis of the effects of these two peptide hormones. Experimental evidence from morphological, physiological, and biochemical studies has accumulated at a remarkable rate in the past 5 years, and a consideration of these data allows one to construct a rather satisfactory model of how these two hormones act.

The first important aspect of this model is that extracellular calcium homeostasis is achieved by the adaptation of the fundamental mechanisms involved in intracellular calcium homeostasis. In other words, nature evolved mechanisms for regulating cellular calcium influx and efflux long before a boney skeleton appeared with its associated demands of control of calcium movements into and out of this calcified mass. When this later need arose, these ancient mechanisms were adapted to subserve this new need. Furthermore, the regulation of calcium influx and efflux is as fundamental a property of the plasma membrane as the regulation of Na^+ fluxes. Hence before presenting a model of hormone action, we shall review our present knowledge of intracellular calcium homeostasis (Borle, 1967; Ebashi and Endo, 1969; Hagiwara and Nakajima, 1966; Rasmussen, 1966; Portzehl *et al.*, 1964; Weber, 1966; Politoff *et al.*, 1969; Maizels, 1956; Baker *et al.*, 1967, 1969; Adelman and Moore, 1961; Hasselbach, 1964; Wallach *et al.*, 1966). This subject falls naturally into two parts: (1) the regulation of calcium fluxes across the plasma membrane of the cells, and (2) the uptake and release of calcium by subcellular organelles, primarily mitochondria and microsomes.

II. CALCIUM EXCHANGE IN CELLS AND SUBCELLULAR COMPARTMENTS

Calcium is one of the essential ions required for most forms of life. Its functions are varied. It is a key regulator of the activity of extracellular enzymes, e.g., in blood clotting; of membrane function; of excitation–

contraction coupling in all forms of muscle; of excitation–secretion coupling in both exocrine and endocrine glands; and of the activity of key intracellular enzymes, e.g., phosphorylase b kinase. In order to subserve these functions, the concentration of this ion, in the extracellular fluid compartment as well as the several intracellular fluid compartments, is closely regulated primarily by three systems, or calcium pumps, respectively in the cell or plasma membrane, the inner mitochondrial membrane, and the sarcoplasmic or endoplasmic reticulum.

A. Exchange of Calcium in Cells

An analysis of calcium exchange in cellular systems is complicated by the fact that changes in extracellular calcium ion concentration greatly affect the permeability properties of the cell membrane (Curran and Gill, 1962; Herrera and Curran, 1963), and that calcium binds to many organic ions both inside and outside the cell (Hasselbach, 1964; Nanninga, 1961). The first problem is that of obtaining an accurate estimate of calcium ion concentration within the cell (Schoffeniels, 1963). Based upon total cell calcium and H_2O content, and assuming uniform distribution in cell water, the concentration of intracellular calcium is between 0.4 and 2.0 mM. However, studies of ionophoretic mobility of calcium within nerve (Keynes and Lewis, 1956; Hodgkin and Keynes, 1957) the minimal calcium concentration required for contraction of isolated myofibrils (Nanninga, 1961; Hasselbach, 1964), the free calcium in red blood cells (Schatzmann, 1966), and the K_m for calcium binding in mitochondria (Chance, 1965) and sarcoplasmic reticulum (Hasselbach, 1961), indicate that the ionized calcium concentration within the cytosol of most cells is below 10^{-5} M or 0.01 mM. In contrast, the calcium ion concentration in mammalian extracellular fluid is approximately 10^{-3} M or 1 mM (Rasmussen, 1968). This means that the actual ratio of $[Ca^{++}]_i/[Ca^{++}]_o$ is $> 10^{-2}$, and the predicted ratio calculated on the basis of the Nernst diffusion equilibrium and the membrane potential of -80 mV, is approximately 10^2. Thus, calcium ion distribution does not follow a simple passive distribution based upon the electrochemical gradients of the other major ions across the cell membrane. These facts have led to the conclusion that a "calcium pump" is an operational part of the plasma membrane of most mammalian cells (Borle, 1967; Hodgkin and Keynes, 1955; Schatzmann, 1966).

For some time there had been some confusion about the existence of such a pump, and particularly whether or not calcium efflux was driven by the same ATPase involved in Na^+ extrustion. The situation has now been resolved by the clear demonstration of a Ca^{++}-activated ATPase in the red blood cell membrane (Schatzmann, 1966; Olson and Cazort, 1969; Wins and Scoffeneils, 1966a) which is ouabain-insensitive and Na⁺-insensitive, and by the discovery that changes in Na^+ distribution across the cell membrane alter the distribution of calcium across the membrane (Baker *et al.*, 1967, 1969).

The complicated nature of the ionic interrelationships at the level of the plasma membrane is well illustrated by the fact that a change in extracellular calcium ion concentration leads to a very significant change in the Na^+ leak or sodium permeability of the membrane: a fall in extra-cellular Ca^{++} leads to an increase in Na^+ leak (Maizels, 1956; Adelman and Moore, 1961). Conversely, as mentioned, a rise in intracellular Na^+ leads to an increase in intracellular Ca^{++} (Baker *et al.*, 1967, 1969). Hence the net change in intracellular Ca^{++} following a decrease in extracellular calcium will depend upon two opposing forces: (1) a decreased rate of Ca^{++} entry because of a fall in extracellular Ca^{++}, and (2) an increased entry and/or decreased efflux because of an increased intracellular Na^+ secondary to the Ca^{++}-dependent change in Na^+ permeability of the cell membrane. Finally, a significant increase in external K^+ concentration leads to an increase in calcium influx across the plasma membrane of many cells.

There is an additional important feature of the relationship between Ca^{++} and the plasma membrane. An increase in ionized calcium within the cell alters the properties of the plasma membrane in at least four ways: (1) a decreased membrane deformability (Weed *et al.*, 1969); (2) a decreased ionic permeability of cell membrane junction in epithelial cell layers (Lowenstein *et al.*, 1967); (3) a decrease in water permeability (Manery, 1966); and (4) a "hardening" of the membrane as judged in several ways, e.g., breaking pressure (Manery, 1966). These effects of calcium can be inhibited or reversed by the addition of ATP or Mg^{++} (Politoff *et al.*, 1969). The ATP is thought to function in two ways: (1) to chelate free Ca^{++}, and (2) to increase the activity of the calcium-dependent ATPase and thereby lower Ca^{++} concentration. The mechanism by which Mg^{++} acts is not clear, but it is presumed that this ion competes with calcium for sites in or on the membrane. The mechanism by which intracellular calcium brings about these effects is not completely established. One of two mechanisms may be responsible: (1) Ca^{++}-phospholipid interactions (Papahadjapoulos and Ohki, 1969), or (2) Ca^{++}-dependent sol–gel transformations in actomysinlike proteins within or beneath the cell membrane (Weed *et al.*, 1969; Wins and Schoffeniels, 1966a,b; Ohnishi, 1962).

It has recently been shown that artificial bilayers of phosphatidylserine are unstable under conditions of asymmetric distribution of calcium and hydrogen ions (Papahadjapoulos and Ohki, 1969), and that redistribution of these ions may greatly increase membrane stability and resistance. This behavior might be of considerable biologic significance. However, this Ca^{++} effect is inhibited if the bilayer contains considerable cholesterol. Cholesterol is a normal constituent of the plasma membrane; hence, it is not clear how significant these calcium-dependent changes in bilayer properties are to the situation in the cell.

Since Ohnishi (1962) first reported the isolation of actinomysinlike proteins from the erythrocyte membrane, considerable evidence has been obtained to support the view that actinomysinlike (or possibly only actinlike) myofilaments on the inner aspects of the plasma membrane are present in nearly all cells. This evidence consists of (1) the demonstration by V. T. Marchesi and Palade (1967) and F. T. Marchesi *et al.* (1968) of such filaments on the inner aspects of the red blood cell membrane by electron microscopy, and more recently the demonstration by electron microscopy of such filaments capable of binding heavy meromyosin in many cell types (Ishikawa, 1966b); (2) ATP-dependent changes in the shape of cell and ghosts by Nakao *et al.* (1960, 1961); (3) the calcium-ATP-dependent "contraction" of red cell ghosts (Wins and Schoffeniels, 1966b); and (4) the demonstration by Weed and associates (1969) of the metabolic dependence of red cell deformability.

A summary of our present knowledge of cellular calcium exchange is presented in Fig. 1. Basically, it appears that calcium enters the cell passively down a steep electrochemical gradient, a calcium "leak." This passive influx undoubtedly involves interaction with some component(s) in the plasma membrane and is estimated to be in the range of 0.01–0.08 pmole $cm^{-2}sec^{-1}$. It is not yet clear whether this component is the same as that involved in Na^+ entry or is a separate and unique calcium carrier, but the latter appears more likely. Calcium efflux is controlled by the activity of a calcium-dependent ATPase, which is distinct from the better characterized Na^+/K^+ activated ATPase. If this basic model accounts for the exchange of calcium between the intra- and extracellular fluids, it is immediately clear that an increase in intracellular calcium can result from one of three changes: (1) an increase in rate of passive entry; (2) a direct decrease in the activity of the pump by some intrinsic change in its properties, e.g., a change in K_m for Ca^{++}; or (3) a decrease in the effective concentration of ATP at the membrane by changes in the activity of other membrane bound ATPases. However, before discussing these mechanisms in more detail, mention must be made of another major mechanism for regulating calcium ion content of the cell cytosol, namely, the exchange of calcium between this and the other intracellular compartments.

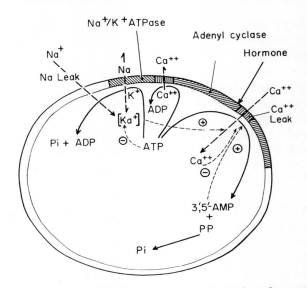

Fig. 1. The possible interrelationships between adenyl cyclase, calcium entry, sodium entry, and the Ca^{++}-activated and Na$^+$–K$^+$-activated ATPases of the plasma membrane. Either adenyl cyclase activation is accompanied by or leads, via 3′,5′-AMP, to increased Ca^{++} entry. The competition for a pool of ATP near the membrane might lead to a fall in ATP level, when adenyl cyclase is activated, with a decreased activity of both ATPases. A decrease in the activity of the Ca^{++}-activated enzyme would lead to increased intracellular calcium. Also, the inhibition of the Na$^+$–K$^+$-activated ATPase would lead to an increase in intracellular Na$^+$, which would in turn lead to an increased Ca^{++} entry. Finally, a rise in intracellular Ca^{++} would lead to an inhibition of adenyl cyclase activity, thus secondarily limiting the hormonal activation of the cyclase.

B. Subcellular Calcium Exchange

Two major intracellular calcium exchange systems have been recognized, the mitochondria, and the sarcoplasmic reticulum most prominently developed in muscle. These two subcellular compartments contain by far the bulk of intracellular calcium. However, much of this calcium is probably not in solution. The bulk of this intracellular calcium is bound either to membrane components or organic anions. Of possible great physiologic import is the fact that calcium influx into these compartments is several orders of magnitude greater than across the cell membrane, 200–2000 pmole cm^{-2}sec^{-1} compared with 0.01–0.08 for the cell membrane; and that uptake or influx into these two compartments are both energy-dependent reactions (Chance, 1965; Borle, 1967; Rasmussen, 1966; Ebashi and Endo, 1969).

A determination of the physiologic significance of these two systems has been highly successful in the case of the sarcoplasmic reticulum, which is now recognized as the major subcellular system involved in regulating calcium ion concentration in muscle cytosol (Ebashi and Endo, 1969), i.e., an integral part of excitation–contraction coupling and relaxation in muscle. However, the physiologic role of mitochondrial calcium exchange is still a matter of controversy, and is not as yet completely defined. It may play an important role in transcellular calcium transport in those tissues in which such transport is of significant magnitude, e.g., kidney, intestine, and bone. It may merely be a mechanism for maintaining a low and stable concentration of calcium ion within the cytosol of the cell, or calcium exchange and its regulation between mitochondria and cytosol may be of importance in controlling intracellular metabolic events. However, it is clear that the great ability and capacity of these intracellular membrane systems to take up calcium rapidly, means that they both play major roles in regulating calcium ion content in the cytosol.

Both calcium uptake by sarcoplasmic reticulum and mitochondria are energy-dependent reactions. The uptake by sarcoplasmic reticulum requires ATP hydrolysis and has many properties similar to the calcium ATPase of the plasma membrane. On the other hand, the mitochondrial calcium pump is clearly different being driven either by energy derived by ATP hydrolysis, or electron transport, being inhibited by lanthanum (Mela, 1968), and by agents that inhibit electron transport but not oxidative phosphorylation.

The relationship between calcium ion content of the cell cytosol and energy metabolism is a complex one because of the foregoing relationships and the fact that ATP, ADP, and AMP are chelators of Ca^{++} as well as Mg^{++} in the order $ATP > ADP \gg AMP$ (Nanninga, 1961). Thus, when increased ATP hydrolysis leads to an increased energy demand on mitochondria, less Ca^{++} will be taken up because Ca^{++} uptake and ADP phosphorylation are competing processes. In addition, a decrease of the ratio $ATP/AMP + ADP$ will lead to a greater calcium ion activity. Both these changes could lead to increased calcium ion content in the cytosol. Unfortunately, because of the technical problems involved, it has not been possible to examine these possibilities in intact cells.

C. Unique Functions of Ca^{++} Binding and Ca^{++} Influx in Plasma Membrane

Returning to the regulation of cellular calcium exchange, as noted, the calcium ion concentration of the cytosol could be altered either by changes in inward calcium leak or outward calcium pumping.

TABLE I

POLYPEPTIDE AND AMINE HORMONES THAT HAVE BEEN SHOWN TO INFLUENCE
CELLULAR CALCIUM EXCHANGE AND THE INTRACELLULAR EVENT PRESUMED
TO BE CONTROLLED BY CHANGES IN INTRACELLULAR CALCIUM

Hormone	Cell	Physiologic event
Oxytocin (1)	Myometrium	Contraction[a]
Angiotensin (2)	Adrenal glomerulosa	Steroidogenesis
LHRF (3)	Adenohypophysis	LH release
TRF (4)	Adenohypophysis	TSH release
Epinephrine (5)	Heart	Inotropic response
Acetylcholine (6)	Salivary gland	Enzyme release
Acetycholine (7)	Adrenal medulla	Epinephrine release
Vasopressin (8)	Toad bladder	H_2O permeability
MSH (9)	Melanocytes	Melanin dispersal
Leucocidin (10)	Leucocyte	Granule release
PTH (11)	Renal tubule	Gluconeogenesis
Acetylcholine (12)	Exocrine pancreas	Enzyme release
Glucagon (13)	Liver	Gluconeogenesis

[a] References in order of table: (1) Csapo, 1959; (2) Daniels *et al.*, 1967; (3) Samli and Geschwind, 1968; (4) Vale *et al.*, 1967; (5) Namm *et al.*, 1968; (6) Douglas and Poisner, 1962; (7) Douglas and Rubin, 1961; (8) Schwartz and Walter, 1968; (9) Dikstein *et al.*, 1963; (10) Woodin and Wieneke, 1964; (11) Nagata and Rasmussen, 1968; (12) Hokin, 1966; (13) Friedmann and Park, 1968.

A change in calcium entry is apparently of great physiologic significance. Calcium ions are clearly involved in excitation–contraction coupling in most if not all forms of muscle (Ebashi and Endo, 1969; Bianchi, 1961); in excitation–secretion coupling in exocrine glands (Douglas and Poisner, 1962; Douglas and Rubin, 1961); in excitation–secretion coupling in many endocrine glands (Milner and Hales, 1967; Samli and Geschwind, 1968; Vale *et al.*, 1967; Zor *et al.*, 1968; Rasmussen and Nagata, 1969); and in the regulation of metabolism in several different cell types. Many of the peptide hormones, one site of whose action is the plasma membrane, bring about one or more of these calcium-dependent changes in cellular activity (Table I).

1. Calcium and Cyclic AMP

Of particular interest is the increasing number of such systems in which both Ca^{++} and cyclic 3′,5′-AMP are involved in the cellular response to the hormonal or other stimulus (Table II). In most of these systems, the evidence is of the following nature: (1) extracellular Ca^{++} is required for the physiologic response; (2) an increase in intracellular 3′,5′-AMP is a very early consequence of the stimulus; and (3) 3′,5′-AMP increases whether or not extracellular calcium is present. In many of these systems excess Mg^{++} has an effect similar to Ca^{++} lack, and is some a marked increase in extracellular K^+ is a nonspecific stimulus to the calcium-dependent process. Finally, in the few instances in which such studies have been carried out, the stimulus is followed by an increased rate of entry of labeled calcium into the responsive cells. The changes in Ca^{++}

TABLE II

THE RELATIONSHIP BETWEEN Ca^{++} AND 3',5'-AMP IN PHYSIOLOGIC SYSTEMS

System	Ca^{++}	3',5'-AMP	Stimulus
Neurotransmission	+	+ (?)	Electrical, KCl[a]
Amylase (SG)	+ (?)	+	Epinephrine, KCl[b]
Growth hormone release	+	+	GHRF[c]
Insulin release	+	+	Glucose; tolbutamide[d]
LH release	+	+	LHRF; KCl[e]
TSH release	+	+	TRF; KCl[f]
Steroid release	+	+	ACTH[g]
Glucose release	+ (?)	+	Glucagon[h]
Thyroxine release	+ (?)	+	TSH[i]
Heart			
Glycogenolysis	+	+	Epinephrine[j]
Intropy	+	+ (?)	
H_2O permeability	+	+	AVP[k]
Renal tubule			
Gluconeogenesis	+	+	PTH[l]
Ca^{++} transport	+	+	
Melanin dispersal	+	+	MSH[m]
Slime mold aggregation	+ (?)	+	?[n]
Sea urchin egg	+	+	Fertilization[o]

[a] Eccles, 1964; DeRobertis *et al.*, 1967.

[b] Rasmussen and Tenenhouse, 1968; Bdolah and Schramm, 1965.

[c] Schofield, 1967.

[d] Grodsky and Bennett, 1966; Hales and Milner, 1968; Turtle *et al.*, 1967; Malaisse *et al.*, 1967.

[e] Samli and Geschwind, 1968.

[f] Vale and Guillemin, 1967; Vale *et al.*, 1967.

[g] Birmingham *et al.*, 1953; Sutherland *et al.*, 1965.

[h] Sutherland *et al.*, 1965; Friedmann and Park, 1968.

[i] Zor *et al.*, 1968; Gilman and Rall, 1966.

[j] Sutherland *et al.*, 1965; Cheung and Williamson, 1965; Namm *et al.*, 1968; Ozawa and Ebashi, 1967; Meyer *et al.*, 1964.

[k] Orloff and Handler, 1962; Schwartz and Walter, 1968; Thorn, 1961.

[l] Chase and Aurbach, 1967; Nagata and Rasmussen, 1968; Wells and Lloyd, 1967.

[m] Abe *et al.*, 1969; Dikstein *et al.*, 1963.

[n] Konijn *et al.*, 1967; Gingell and Garrod, 1969.

[o] Castañeda and Tyler, 1968.

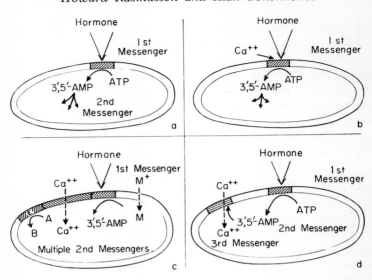

Fig. 2. The role of Ca^{++} in the physiological response of cells to many peptides and its relationship to adenyl cyclase and 3′,5′-AMP. (a) The second messenger concept of Sutherland, in which the hormone interacts with the adenyl cyclase in the cell membrane and leads to an increase in 3′,5′-AMP within the cell. The rise in 3′,5′-AMP leads in turn to the activation of many different processes resulting in the physiological response. (b) (c), and (d) Possible interrelations between Ca^{++} binding and/or permeability, adenyl cyclase, and 3′,5′-AMP. (b) Ca^{++} might be required either in the binding of hormone to receptor, or in the activation of the cyclase. (c) A change in Ca^{++} permeability and an activation of adenyl cyclase might be simultaneous consequences of hormone–receptor interaction, i.e., multiple second messengers. (d) A change in Ca^{++} permeability might be the consequence of the rise in intracellular 3′,5′-AMP and represent a third-stage messenger.

influx and/or binding and in 3′,5′-AMP concentrations may be related in one of three ways (Fig. 2): (1) the change in adenyl cyclase activity and the change in calcium entry may be simultaneous but independent results of hormone–receptor interaction; (2) the change in calcium entry or binding could alter the activity of adenyl cyclase; or (3) an initial increase in 3′,5′-AMP could lead to a change in calcium entry.

It has not yet been possible to decide between these alternatives. However, in the case of epinephrine action on the heart (Namm *et al.*, 1968), releasing factors on the pituitary (Vale *et al.*, 1967), and parathyroid hormone on the kidney (Nagata and Rasmussen, 1969), 3′,5′-AMP increases upon hormone addition even when extracellular calcium is absent. These data imply that calcium entry is not necessary for adenyl cyclase activation. However, they do not exclude the possibility that adenyl cyclase activity is determined by the amount and/or type of calcium bound to the membrane, and that the appropriate stimulus acts by altering calcium binding at key sites within the membrane. In this regard, it is worthwhile indicating that the assumption has been made, on rather incomplete evidence, that adenyl cyclase is located solely in the plasma membrane of cells. However, adenyl cyclase has been found in the sarcoplasmic reticulum of muscle cells (Rabinowitz *et al.*, 1965). If this location is confirmed, the immediate possible relevance of adenyl cyclase to excitation–contraction coupling in muscle becomes apparent.

A possible direct effect of cyclic AMP upon membrane calcium permeability is supported by the fact that dibutyryl 3′,5′-AMP mimics the effects of many of these agents (Sutherland *et al.*, 1965). This is also consistent with the fact that theophylline, a competetive inhibitor of the phosphodiesterase responsible for the hydrolysis of 3′,5′-AMP to 5-AMP, is capable of changing calcium binding or permeability of cellular and subcellular membranes (Bianchi, 1968). On the other hand, a major assumption of the studies with dibutyryl 3′,5′-AMP is that 10^{-3}–10^{-2} M 3′,5′-AMP on the outside of the cell brings about the identical changes in cellular metabolism as 10^{-7}–10^{-6} M 3′,5′-AMP generated within the cell. This assumption may not be valid.

The best that can be done at present is to summarize the possible relationships of Ca^{++} and 3′,5′-AMP, as illustrated in Fig. 2, and state that the weight of this evidence favors the view that 3′,5′-AMP and Ca^{++} permeability are intimately related events at the plasma membrane of the cell when activated by specific stimuli. In the scheme depicted in Fig. 2, several additional aspects of calcium, 3′,5′-AMP, adenyl cyclase interactions are indicated. When ATP is converted to 3′,5′-AMP at the membrane it could cause an increase in Ca^{++} in three ways: (1) a change in the chelated calcium: the affinity constant for the calcium–ATP complex is at least 10,000-fold greater than that for 3′,5′-AMP-calcium; (2) a decrease in the ATP concentration of the membrane could decrease the activity of the calcium-activated ATPase; and (3) a decrease in ATP concentration of the membrane could decrease the activity of the Na^+/K^+-activated ATPase with a resultant increase in intracellular Na^+, which would in turn alter Ca^{++} exchange across the membrane.

An additional aspect of this relationship is that Ca^{++} is an inhibitor of adenyl cyclase (Chase *et al.*, 1969). Thus one could envision that Ca^{++} bound to the membrane is the natural inhibitor of the enzyme and the effect of the specific stimulus is to cause exchange of this Ca^{++} with Mg^{++}, an activator of the enzyme, with resultant enhanced activity. On the other hand, the rise in intracellular calcium following stimulation may normally limit the degree of adenyl cyclase activation by a negative feedback effect. This effect may well account for the commonly observed time course of 3′,5′-AMP changes following stimulation consisting of a very prompt rise, then a fall to a steady state level significantly less than the peak rise, but more than the control value.

2. Second Messengers—One or Many

One current model of the role of the adenyl cyclase system is that articulated by Sutherland and his colleagues (1965) in the second messenger concept. In this formulation the specific second messenger, 3′,5′-AMP, rises when the first messenger, the specific hormone, activates adenyl cyclase in the cell membrane. This second messenger is then responsible for the multiple changes in cell metabolism expressed finally as the specific physiologic response of the cell to the particular hormonal stimulus. However, we believe that this system is more complex in view of the widespread association between changes in calcium permeability and adenyl cyclase activation in the response of both simple and highly differentiated cells to appropriate stimuli (Rasmussen and Tenenhouse, 1968; Rasmussen and Nagata, 1969). In our view there are nearly always multiple membrane events and multiple second messengers when a specific stimulus interacts with a responsive cell. We envision that these multiple membrane events are all integral parts of coordinated response of the cell. For example, in several cells 3′,5′-AMP generation is one consequence of cell activation and leads to the activation of glycogenolysis (Sutherland *et al.*, 1965). It was once believed that this effect was the major mechanism by which 3′,5′-AMP regulated the specific response of the cell (Haynes *et al.*, 1960; Orloff and Handler, 1962). However, in most instances it is now clear that this particular role of 3′,5′-AMP in the cell plays an anticipatory role, in mobilizing energy reverses in anticipation of need, in a fashion similar to the role of epinephrine in the organism.

Control and specificity of response by any tissue resides at two distinct levels. The most obvious is the enzymatic capability of the cell as determined by the genetic expression of the cell, i.e., its state of differentiation or specialization. The second is the cell membrane, which selectively discriminates between stimuli, this selectively also being genetically determined. The types of response by the plasma membrane of any cell to an effective stimulus are limited. In simplest (electrical) terms they can be considered to be only two, either depolarization or hyperpolarization. There is considerable evidence that the consequence of the activation of many cells by specific peptide hormones or small molecules (Table II) leads to activation of adenyl cyclase, membrane depolarization, and an increase in calcium permeability. To our knowledge, adenyl cyclase activation and membrane hyperpolarization never occur together. In other words the depolarization of cells is associated in many instances with adenyl cyclase activation. It also appears that in many cases the net result of this combination of changes is the secretion of the specific product of the tissue, e.g., hormones from pituitary, thyroid, β-cells of islets of Langerhans, adrenal cortex; glucose from the liver; free fatty acids from adipose tissue; and acetylcholine from neuromuscular junction or synapse. The depolarization–secretion sequence is well known in ganglion and neuromuscular junctions. Depolarization of adrenal cortex in response to ACTH (Matthews and Saffran, 1968) and β-cells of islets of Langerhans in response to glucose have also been demonstrated (Dean and Matthews, 1968). In all these cell types only the stimulus required to depolarize the membrane and the product finally secreted differ; the sequence of events that translate stimulus into ultimate response appear to be very similar if not identical. However, in other cells the same biochemical events, i.e., increased $3',5'$-AMP and change in Ca^{++} permeability, do not lead to elaboration of an extracellular product. In these cases it is not yet clear whether membrane depolarization is associated with such interactions as vasopressin with toad bladder, PTH with renal tubule, and MSH with melanocytes. However, in terms of the present discussion, one would predict that depolarization is an integral part of the response. Stated in another way, it would appear that adenyl cyclase activation is one of the biochemical events associated with depolarization of many cell membranes by specific stimuli.

The most impressive evidence in favor of the view that hormone–membrane interaction leads to multiple and simutaneous membrane events comes from the study of insulin action (Krahl, 1961; Levine, 1966; Schwartz and Hechter, 1966). In this case the following changes in membrane properties have been observed: (1) increased glucose transport; (2) increased amino acid transport; (3) membrane hyperpolarization; (4) decreased adenyl cyclase activity; and (5) a redistribution of K^+ across the membrane.

Thus it would appear possible to differentiate between those stimuli that lead to hyperpolarization and those to depolarization of plasma membrane. Viewed from the perspective of function, hyperpolarization makes a cell more efficient in serving its own nutritive and anabolic functions; depolarization activates a cell to serve the organism and leads to activation of catabolic functions. It would appear that the adenyl cyclase system always functions in the latter context, and that the interaction of a peptide hormone with a responsive cell is often associated with multiple changes in membrane function. In the context of the present discussion, the important need is to examine the evidence concerning the nature of cell–hormone interaction in the case of parathyroid hormone and calcitonin, and in particular the possible importance of the relationship between 3′,5′-AMP and Ca^{++} in the actions of parathyroid hormone, calcitonin, and vitamin D. Before doing so, it is necessary to review briefly our current concepts of bone cell function and calcium homeostasis.

D. Possible Additional Effects of 3′,5′-AMP upon Transport Processes

The foregoing discussion has concentrated attention upon the relationship between 3′,5′-AMP and calcium transport across the plasma membrane. This attention is primarily because it is a relationship that has recently received considerable investigative attention. However, there are other data that clearly show that 3′,5′-AMP may influence the distribution or transport of other ions, and possibly the binding and/or transport of calcium in subcellular membranes (Friedmann and Park, 1968). For example, in the case of the liver, Friedmann and Park (1968) have shown that during the stimulation of gluconeogenesis in the isolated perfused liver by either glucagon or 3′,5′-AMP, there is an initial release of calcium from cells and a later change in K^+ distribution. In another case listed in Table II, e.g., the release of insulin (Hales and Milner, 1968), extracellular Na^+ as well as Ca^{++} is required. These data indicate that adenyl cyclase activation may be related to changes in the transport or binding of monovalent cations as well. Of equal interest, the data of Friedmann and Park (1968) raise the possibility that 3′,5′-AMP may alter Ca^{++} binding or transport in subcellular membranes, and that in some cells this might be the predominant fashion in which 3′,5′-AMP alters the intracellular concentration and distribution of Ca^{++}. Further support for the concept that 3′,5′-AMP alters subcellular Ca^{++} distribution comes from the observation of Nagata and Rasmussen (1968) who showed that Ca^{++} infusion and PTH infusion into parathyroidectomized rats led to similar metabolic changes in animals treated with hydrocortisone or made vitamin D-deficient, but to different changes in control animals. As discussed by these authors (Nagata and Rasmussen, 1968; Rasmussen and Tenenhouse, 1968), there is considerable evidence that both vitamin D and cortisone have marked effects upon mitochondrial calcium transport (see also Rasmussen, 1966). Thus it is possible that 3′,5′-AMP alters calcium transport and distribution across the mitochondrial membrane.

A final point of interest are the observations (Bianchi, 1968) that caffeine and theophylline alter calcium binding to membranes, and this is thought to be the basis of their pharmacologic effects on muscle. In view of the similarity of structure between these xanthines and 3′,5′-AMP, and the fact that the xanthines are inhibitors of the enzyme, phosphodiesterase, it seems possible that 3′,5′-AMP binds to sites on membranes similar to the ones with which the xanthines interact.

III. BONE CELLS AND THEIR FUNCTION

Classically, the cells in bone have been classified into five types: (1) active osteoblasts; (2) resting osteoblasts; (3) osteoclasts; (4) osteocytes; and (5) precursor or mesenchymal cells. The functions of these were considered to be (1) active osteoblasts were responsible for bone formation, i.e., collagen synthesis; (2) osteoclasts were responsible for bone resorption; (3) the mesenchymal cells gave rise to bone osteoblasts and osteoclasts; and (4) osteocytes and resting osteoblasts were metabolically inactive, and contributed little to the normal metabolism or mineral exchange of bone.

A very significant and important change in this viewpoint has taken place in recent years. First, both the active and resting osteoblasts form a curtain of cells covering the entire bone surface, and thereby serve as a functional membrane that regulates the exchange of ions and small molecules between the bulk extracellular fluids and those in bone (Rasmussen, 1968; Howell *et al.*, 1968). Furthermore, in bone it is safe to predict that there are two specialized extracellular fluid compartments: one on the bone side of the curtain of active osteoblasts, and the other on the bone side of the resting osteoblasts. The major difference is the fact that collagen synthesis leads to areas of partially calcified and uncalcified matrix, which interact with the ions in this solution, whereas in the area of resting osteoblasts new collagen is no longer being produced (Fig. 3).

The resting osteoblasts do not appear to function in isolation. There is now considerable histochemical, morphological, biochemical, and microradiographic evidence that these cells form a functional syncytium with the osteocytes, that this syncytium is vitally concerned with calcium homeostasis, and that all these cells are metabolically active. In an adult organism, they represent by far the majority of bone cells, and are in contact with a vast area of bone surface. Present evidence supports the view that the syncytium of resting osteoblasts and osteocytes are the ones that respond first to changes in the concentrations of parathyroid hor-

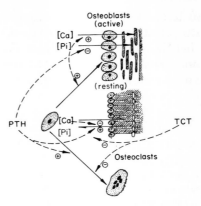

FIG. 3. Bone cells, their exchange of mineral with the bulk extracellular fluids, and the influence of PTH and TCT upon them. Resting osteoblasts are joined in a syncytium with osteocytes.

mone and calcitonin in circulating blood, and it seems likely that these cells are responsible for the minute-to-minute regulation of plasma calcium concentration. In this view, the regulation of calcium transport is similar in intestine, bone and kidney because in each instance a membrane system regulates the exchange of calcium between a specialized compartment(s) of extracellular fluid (gastrointestinal fluids, bone extracellular fluids, and glomerular filtrate) from the bulk extracellular fluid phase (Fig. 4). In this figure only a single bone extracellular fluid phase

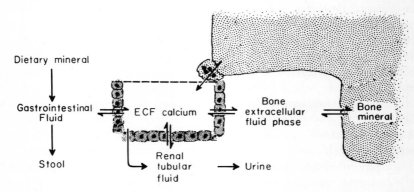

FIG. 4. Calcium homeostasis. The level of calcium in the extracellular fluids is normally regulated by controlling the exchange of calcium between the bulk extracellular fluids and three specialized extracellular fluid compartments: gastrointestinal fluids, renal tubular fluid, and bone extracellular fluid. Each of these specialized compartments is separated from the bulk phase by a functional membrane. In times of prolonged calcium deficiency osteoclasts activity also contributes directly to mineral homeostasis.

is represented. This is the one beneath the syncytium of resting osteo-blasts and osteocytes. A second much smaller fluid phase of different composition exists in the area of active bone formation. Finally, in this view osteoclasts are primarily involved in skeletal homeostasis or re-modeling, but become involved in mineral homeostasis when significant and sustained aberrations of mineral metabolism occur.

IV. PARATHYROID HORMONE, 3',5'-AMP, AND INTRACELLULAR CALCIUM

Two independent lines of current research on the mechanism of action of parathyroid hormone can be brought together quite logically in the light of the preceding discussion. On the one hand is the evidence that the hormone stimulates adenyl cyclase in responsive tissues, and on the other, the evidence that PTH increases calcium uptake and calcium content of responsive cells.

A. PTH AND 3',5'-AMP

The first suggestion for a role of 3',5'-AMP in PTH action was made by Wells and Lloyd (1967) on the basis of their observation that large doses of theophylline cause a rise in plasma calcium in parathyroid-ectomized animals. This interpretation was based upon the known fact that one of the biochemical effects of this drug is the inhibition of the phosphodiesterase responsible for 3',5'-AMP hydrolysis (Fig. 5). How-ever, this interpretation ignored completely the fact that theophylline has a direct effect upon calcium transport and/or membrane binding (Bianchi, 1968). Furthermore, the data of Wells and Lloyd were clearly far from convincing because the combination of PTH plus theophylline did not exert a synergistic effects even though this is one of the usual criteria employed to establish the fact that 3',5'-AMP is an intermediate in the action of a hormone.

The first substantial evidence of a relationship between PTH and 3',5'-AMP was presented by Chase and Aurbach (1967). They found a rapid and significant increase in urinary 3',5'-AMP after the infusion of PTH. This was followed by their demonstration of a PTH-sensitive membrane-bound adenyl cyclase in both renal cortex and bone (Chase and Aurbach, 1967), and by their finding that the 3',5'-AMP levels in both renal and bone tissue increase after PTH administration (Chase *et al.*, 1969). Further confirmation of a role of 3',5'-AMP in PTH action was obtained from comparative studies of 3′,5′-AMP, dibutyryl 3′,5′-AMP, and PTH upon calcium and phosphate metabolism and bone resorption *in vivo* (Rasmussen *et al.,* 1968). This latter study showed that dibutyryl 3′,5′-AMP produces most of the changes in calcium and phosphate excretion and bone resorption that one sees after PTH infusion (Fig. 6). Two striking aspects of this study were the findings that theophylline did not enhance the effect of submaximal doses of PTH, but did enhance the effect of dibutyryl 3′,5′-AMP. This latter result is of particular interest because dibutyryl 3′,5′-AMP is not hydrolyzed rapidly by phosphodiesterase; hence a phosphodiesterase inhibitor, such as theophylline, would not be expected to potentiate the effect of the dibutyryl analog unless, of course, dibutyryl 3′,5′-AMP exerted effects other than simply increasing its own concentration within the cell. That such may be the case is apparent from unpublished observations (Rasmussen) showing that dibutyryl 3′,5′-AMP has at least two effects upon the concentration of 3′,5′-AMP within isolated cells, and it is clear that these effects cannot be explained by a conversion of dibutyryl 3′,5′-AMP to 3′,5′-AMP.

A particularly convincing demonstration of the probable key importance of 3′,5′-AMP in the action of PTH is the finding of Nagata and Rasmussen (1968) that 3′,5′-AMP is elevated in renal cortical tissue after PTH administration to thyroparathyroidectomized rats whether maintained on a normal diet, a vitamin D deficient diet, or one supplemented with cortisone (Fig. 7). Most noteworthy, they found the level of 3′,5′-AMP in the renal cortex of sham-operated vitamin D-deficient animals with hypocalcemia and presumed secondary hyperparathyroidism to be

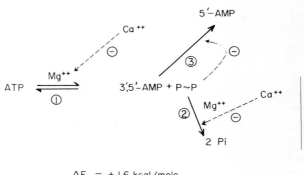

$$\Delta F_1 = + 1.6 \ \text{kcal/mole}$$

$$\Delta F_2 = - 6 \ \text{kcal/mole}$$

$$\Delta F_3 = - 11 \ \text{kcal/mole}$$

Fig. 5. The interrelationships between ATP, 3′,5′-AMP, P ∼ P, 5′-AMP, Pi, Mg^{++}, Ca^{++}, and the enzymes adenyl cyclase 1, pyrophosphatase 2, and phosphodiesterase 3. Also listed are the free energy changes, ΔF, of each reaction.

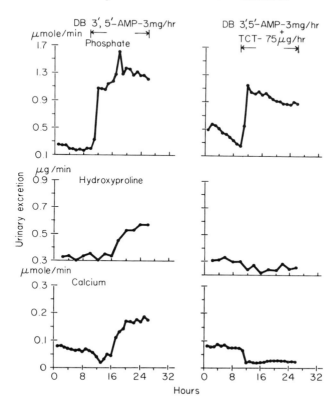

FIG. 6. The changes in the rates of the urinary excretion of phosphate, hydroxyproline, and calcium in thyroparathyroidectomized rats infused with dibutyryl 3',5'-AMP (left), or dibutyryl 3',5'-AMP and thyrocalcitonin (right). Note the inhibition of the mobilization of calcium and hydroxyproline by DB 3',5'-AMP when TCT was given simultaneously.

significantly greater than normal. The obvious conclusion is that chronic secondary hyperparathyroidism leads to a chronic elevation of intracellular 3',5'-AMP.

In summary, there is convincing evidence that a rise in 3',5'-AMP occurs in responsive tissues after PTH administration, that 3',5'-AMP or its dibutyryl analog can mimic the physiologic effects of PTH, but that theophylline does not potentiate the effects of PTH.

B. PTH AND CELL CALCIUM

The second line of research concerning PTH action began with the observation that PTH altered calcium transport or accumulation in isolated mitochondria (Rasmussen, 1966). This initial observation was

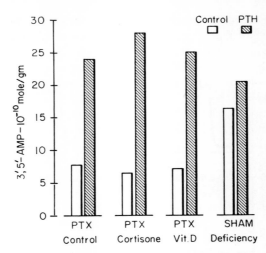

FIG. 7. The concentration of 3′,5′-AMP in renal tissue removed from parathyroidectomized (PTX) or sham-operated (sham) rats, 3 minutes after they were given a saline (control) or parathyroid hormone infusion (PTH). Some of the animals were either vitamin D deficient or treated with cortisone for several days before the experiment.

followed by an extensive investigation of this membrane effect of PTH. It was shown to have the requisite specificity and sensitivity to be of possible physiologic significance (Rasmussen *et al.,* 1967a; Goodman and Rasmussen, 1968). However, with the discovery of adenyl cyclase activation by PTH, most attention has been directed toward the hypothesis that PTH acts upon the plasma membrane of the cell, and not on subcellular membranes. Nevertheless, there is experimental evidence that implies either a direct or indirect effect of PTH upon mitochondrial ion exchange *in vivo* (Nagata and Rasmussen, 1968). At present it is not possible to decide, nor for that matter to determine by direct experimental means, the possible role that a direct effect of PTH upon mitochondrial ion exchange might play in the overall physiologic response of the cell to this hormone. However, it is noteworthy that activation of adenyl cyclase *in vitro,* and the activation of ion-dependent respiration by PTH in isolated mitochondria have nearly identical dose-response characteristics (Fig. 8). Also, it is noteworthy that the primary effect of parathyroid hormone upon the mitochondrial membrane is to change Mg^{++} permeability (Rasmussen *et al.,* 1967a). A similar effect upon the cell membrane could lead to an activation of adenyl cyclase, a magnesium-dependent enzyme.

These mitochondrial studies were followed by a series of increasingly more convincing experiments by Borle (1967, 1968a,b, 1969a,b) showing that PTH increases calcium uptake in isolated tissue culture cells. The design and techniques employed in some of his earlier studies were open to considerable criticism, but his more recent studies of calcium exchange in isolated HeLa and kidney cells grown in monolayer culture are more elegant and clear-cut. Four important conclusions have come from these studies: (1) calcium influx is a passive process: (2) calcium efflux is an energy-dependent process; (3) the intracellular calcium content increases as a function of extracellular calcium concentration; and (4) PTH increases the passive influx and intracellular calcium content of these cells (Fig. 9). The doses of PTH required to produce these effects are similar to those required for renal adenyl cyclase activation *in vitro*.

The questions that need to be answered in relationship to these observations are (1) is this a specific hormonal effect or only a pharmacologic effect of this hormone upon an abnormal cell? (2) is adenyl cyclase activation part of the response to PTH in these isolated cells? and (3) is the increased intracellular calcium of any metabolic significance? Borle assumes a single intracellular compartment, which is clearly not the case (see foregoing discussion), and it is thus possible that all the extra calcium taken up by the cell is sequestered within the mitochondria or other subcellular compartment and as such is not exerting

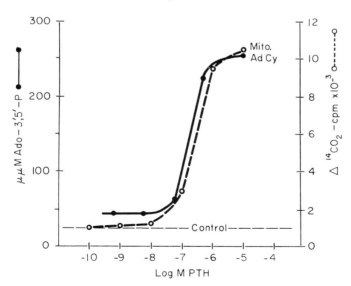

FIG. 8. The change in 3',5'-AMP produced (●—●) by a preparation of renal adenyl cyclase, and the rate of $^{14}CO_2$ production from succinate (○--○) by isolated rat kidney mitochondria as a function of the log dose of parathyroid hormone.

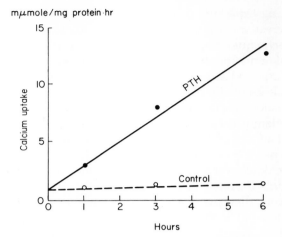

FIG. 9. The accumulation of calcium by tissue culture cells derived from monkey kidney as a function of time in the presence of 1.0 m*M* Ca and with (PTH) or without (control) parathyroid hormone. Modified from Borle (1969b).

any control function. In addition, it is of interest to inquire whether there is any evidence that the calcium content of normal PTH-responsive cells changes under physiologic conditions.

Concerning the first point, Borle has presented some evidence of specificity in regard to this PTH effect, but more extensive evidence is clearly needed, and no evidence is presently available concerning the third point.

At present there are no published data concerning the relationship between adenyl cyclase activation and this change in cellular calcium exchange. However, in preliminary studies with Borle (unpublished), it has been found that PTH, at concentrations sufficient to induce Ca^{++} influx, produces no significant change in 3',5'-AMP concentration in isolated tissue culture cells derived from monkey kidney, but an increase can be observed if theophylline is present. This is in rather striking contrast to the effects of PTH upon isolated renal tubules. A similar dose of PTH causes a rapid and significant increase in 3',5'-AMP within this tissue. Thus in terms of one important biochemical criterion, there is a striking difference between the response to PTH of normal kidney cells, and of tissue culture cells derived from kidney. More extensive studies of the adenyl cyclase system and its response to PTH in these tissue culture cells are clearly needed before making a final judgment as to the physiologic relevance and importance of this model *in vitro* system. Parenthetically, it is worth pointing out that if the interaction of PTH with its receptor on the cell surface leads simultaneously to an activation of adenyl cyclase, and a change in the calcium permeability of the membrane, then one of these changes, e.g., an activation of adenyl cyclase, might well become less pronounced in a cell cultivated *in vitro* without altering the response of the cell in terms of a second parameter, calcium permeability.

Some evidence has been produced in support of the notion that Ca^{++} increases within normal cells in response to parathyroid hormone. Cameron *et al.* (1967) have described an increase in the number of electron dense granules in the mitochondria of resting osteoblasts following parathyroid hormone administration (Fig. 10). These granules are thought to be the morphologic equivalent of calcium phosphate salts accumulated within the mitochondria. Kashiwa (1968) has described

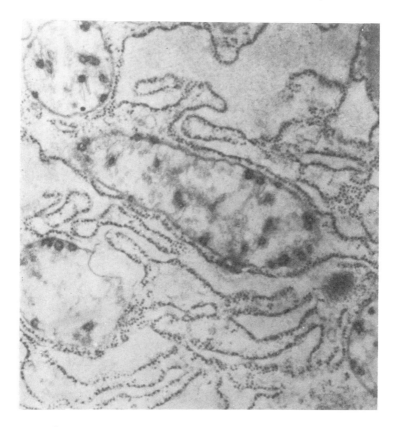

Fɪɢ. 10. Electron dense granules in the mitochondria of resting osteoblasts several hours after the administration of PTH *in vivo*. From Cameron *et al.* (1967).

a histochemical stain for intracellular calcium, and reported that this increases in osteocytes after parathyroid hormone treatment. In addition to this morphologic evidence certain metabolic effects of calcium administration are similar to those seen after PTH administration. Park and Talmage (1968) have shown that both PTH and Ca^{++} increase RNA synthesis and decrease protein synthesis in the bone cells of parathyroidectomized animals. Also, parathyroid hormone administration leads to an increased citrate and lactate production (Neuman and Neuman, 1958; Nichols, 1963; Schartum and Nichols, 1962).

All of these morphologic and metabolic effects can be interpreted in one of two ways: (1) PTH causes a primary effect on metabolism, which leads to changes in calcium transport, and thus eventually to an increase in intracellular calcium; or (2) PTH causes a primary effect upon the uptake and redistribution of calcium within the cell, which leads in turn to the metabolic effects. It has not been possible to test this alternative in bone systems, but recent studies on the renal effects of PTH have helped to distinguish between them.

C. PTH and Renal Gluconeogenesis

The first studies carried out by Nagata and Rasmussen (1968) were done in thyroparathyroidectomized rats *in vivo*. The experiments were designed to determine whether either PTH or Ca^{++} infusion had immediate metabolic effects upon the kidney. Krebs cycle and glycolytic intermediates were determined by sensitive fluorometric enzyme assays. The results showed that both PTH and calcium infusion caused an increase in the concentration of phosphoenol pyruvate (PEP) and a fall in that of pyruvate (PYR) and all Krebs cycle intermediates in animals that were vitamin D deficient or treated with excess cortisone, but that PTH infusion had the additional effect of increasing isocitrate and decreasing α-ketoglutarate in normal animals. These effects were observed within a few minutes after the infusion of PTH or Ca^{++}. It was also found that changes in HCO_3^-, Mg^{++}, or phosphate did not produce similar effects, and that PTH, but not Ca^{++}, caused a rise in 3',5'-AMP. However, because of the complexities involved, this *in vivo* system was not useful in defining further the possible relationship between PTH, 3',5'-AMP. and Ca^{++} in regulating renal function.

In order to examine this relationship in a critical fashion an *in vitro* system was developed employing isolated renal tubules prepared by digestion of kidney cortex with hyaluronidase and collagenase. The disadvantage of using tubules is the obvious loss of the most unique and important physiologic parameters of renal cell function, i.e., its excretory and secretory functions. However, it has been known from the work of Krebs and others that the kidney is capable of gluconeogenesis, and renal cortical slices possess similar functional capabilities. Furthermore, Rutman *et al.* (1965) had shown that in kidney slices, in contrast to the perfused liver, changes in extracellular Ca^{++} lead to changes in rates of renal gluconeogenesis.

These isolated renal tubules were capable of converting malate, pyruvate, glutamate, lactate, glycerol, and other Krebs cycle intermediates to glucose. The rate of glucoenogenesis was linear for at least 30 minutes and often longer. The rate was a function of extracellular calcium concentration, and was enhanced by the addition of parathyroid hormone (Fig. 11). Parathyroid hormone, but not increasing extracellular Ca^{++} led to an increase in 3′,5′-AMP. In the absence of external calcium,

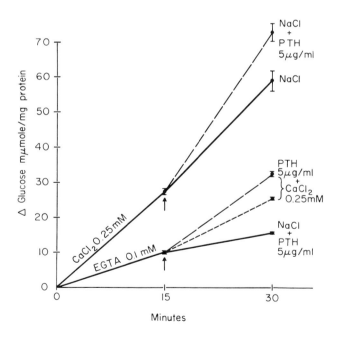

Fig. 11. Glucose production from lactate as a function of time in a preparation of isolated segments of rat renal tubule incubated in modified Krebs-Ringer containing either 0.1 mM EGTA, lower lines, or 0.25 mM calcium, upper lines. After 15 minutes of incubation, either PTH dissolved in saline, CaCl$_2$ to a final concentration of 0.25 mM, or both PTH and CaCl$_2$ were added to separate flasks incubated previously with 0.1 mM EGTA; and in those flasks incubated initially in 0.25 mM CaCl$_2$ medium either saline or PTH dissolved in saline were added.

i.e., less than 10^{-7} M, parathyroid hormone no longer caused an increase in the rate of gluconeogenesis, but still caused the same increase in 3′,5′-AMP concentration. It was clear that the lack of enhanced gluconeogenesis, seen when PTH was added in the absence of calcium, was not due to an irreversible or nonspecific change in cell function because if PTH was added to tubules in the absence of calcium no change in rate of gluconeogenesis occurred, but the subsequent addition of calcium led to the same rate of glucose production as that seen when PTH was added to tubules preincubated in the same concentration of Ca++ (Rasmussen and Nagata, 1969).

Dibutyryl 3′,5′-AMP, 0.5 mM, also caused an increased rate of gluconeogenesis, and this effect depended upon calcium (Fig. 12). There were some differences in the response of the tubules to PTH and to dibutyryl 3′,5′-AMP, but differences in response of the intact kidney *in vivo* were also seen (Rasmussen *et al.*, 1968).

The separate metabolic effects of changing external calcium concentration or adding PTH at a fixed calcium concentration were compared (Nagata and Rasmussen, 1969). It was found that a change in external calcium concentration from 0.25 to 2.5 mM produced nearly the same stimulation in gluconeogenesis as that seen when PTH was added to tubules incubated in 0.25 mM calcium (Fig. 13). Metabolite concentrations were determined under these four conditions, and the changes

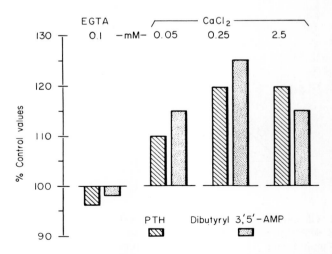

FIG. 12. The effect of PTH and dibutyryl 3′,5′-AMP upon gluconeogenesis in rat renal tubules as a function of the calcium content of the medium. The results are recorded as percentage of the control value (in the absence of hormone or nucleotide) at each concentration of calcium.

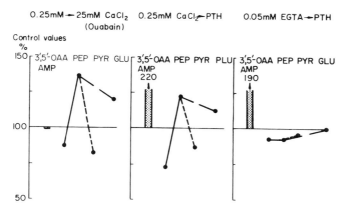

FIG. 13. Metabolite profiles derived by comparing the concentrations of oxalacetate (OAA), phosphoenolpyruvate (PEP), pyruvate (PYR), glucose (GLU), and 3',5'-AMP measured in rat renal tubules incubated in modified Krebs-Ringer containing malate as substrate, 0.25 or 2.5 mM CaCl₂, 0.05 mM EGTA, 0.25 mM CaCl₂ with 5 μg/ml PTH, and 0.05 mM EGTA with 5 μg/ml PTH. On the left are plotted the relative changes in metabolite levels seen when medium calcium concentration was changed from 0.25 to 2.5 mM in the presence of ouabain; in the center when PTH was added to tubules in a medium containing 0.25 mM Ca⁺⁺; and on the right when PTH was added to tubules in a medium containing 0.05 mM EGTA. Control values in each instance refer to the values measured in the initial condition, i.e., left to right, 0.25 mM Ca⁺⁺, 0.25 mM Ca⁺⁺, and 0.05 mM EGTA.

in metabolite levels that were induced by PTH addition were compared to those seen by changing external calcium concentration. This was done in an effort to define if possible the sites of interaction or intracellular regulation affected by the two different changes. The results, shown in Fig. 13, show that either change, increasing external Ca⁺⁺ or adding PTH, led to nearly identical metabolic changes, a rise in PEP, fall in OAA, and a fall in PYR. However, only PTH caused a rise in 3',5'-AMP. Also, as shown in this same figure, PTH added to tubules incubated in the absence of Ca⁺⁺ had no striking effects on the concentrations of these three metabolites, but did cause a rise in 3',5'-AMP. The other important difference between PTH treatment and a change in external Ca⁺⁺ was that an increase in external Ca⁺⁺ caused an increase in ATP, but PTH addition did not. Part of this rise in ATP could be prevented by ouabain and was interpreted as resulting from an effect of Ca⁺⁺ on the cell membrane, that of decreasing Na⁺ permeability and thereby decreasing the energy needed for Na⁺ extrusion by the Na⁺/K⁺-activated ATPase. An increase in external calcium caused an increase in gluconeogenesis in either the presence or absence of ouabain, indicating that the change in ATP was not a crucial factor in controlling intracellular events.

D. Acidosis and Renal Gluconeogenesis

The other known stimulus of renal gluconeogenesis is metabolic acidosis (A. D. Goodman *et al.,* 1966; Simpson, 1967; Alleyne and Scullard, 1969; Goorno and Rector, 1967). The possible similarities and differences between enhanced gluconeogenesis brought about by an increase in extracellular Ca^{++} and extracellular H^+ have been studied (Nagata and Rasmussen, 1969). The changes in renal cell metabolites seen by Alleyne (1968) after acid administration to rats *in vivo* were similar to the pattern seen by Nagata and Rasmussen (1968) when they infused calcium into thyroparathyroidectomized rats. The complexities of these *in vivo* studies make them difficult to interpret. However, when changes in the Ca^{++} or H^+ concentration in the media bathing isolated renal tubules were induced *in vitro*, the resulting changes in metabolite profiles were also strikingly similar (Fig. 14). Both ionic changes brought similar

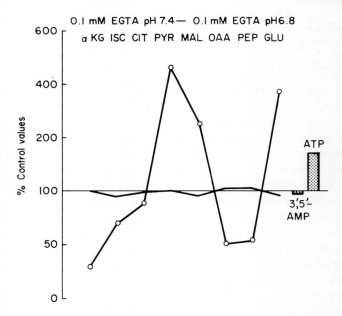

Fig. 14. Metabolite profile derived by comparing the concentrations of α-ketoglutarate (αKG), isocitrate (ISC), citrate (CIT), pyruvate (PYR), malate (MAL), oxaloacetate (OAA), phosphoenol pyruvate (PEP), glucose (GLU), 3',5'-AMP, and ATP measured in rat renal tubules utilizing lactate as substrate when the pH of the medium containing 0.1 mM EGTA was changed from 7.4 to 6.8. The light line represents, for comparison, the metabolite profile derived by comparing the metabolite levels when PTH was added to tubules incubated in a medium containing 0.1 mM EGTA, pH 7.4.

changes in metabolite levels, and both enhanced gluconeogenesis from a wide variety of substrates except glycerol and fructose. It is possible that the two act by regulating a common third factor, or that either an increase in intracellular Ca^{++} influences intracellular pH, or an increase in intracellular H^+ enhances intracellular calcium ion activity. Of the three alternatives, it is simpler to consider one of the latter two more seriously than to postulate a third unknown factor. Of the latter alternatives, there is quite good evidence upon which to propose that an uptake of calcium into the cell could increase the H^+ concentration within the cytosol of the cell. This is based upon the mitochondrial studies *in vitro*, in which it has been clearly shown that the uptake of calcium by isolated liver or kidney mitochondria, in the presence of phosphate, leads to the simultaneous uptake of phosphate into the mitochondria and the ejection of H^+ (Chance, 1965; Rasmussen, 1966). The stoichiometry of 0.67 H^+/Ca^{++} has led to the suggestion that the Ca^{++} and $HPO_4^{=}$ react within the mitochondria to form calcium phosphate with the release of H^+: $3\ Ca^{++} + 2\ HPO_4 \rightleftharpoons Ca_3(PO_4)_2 + 2H^+$. If a similar reaction takes place within the cell, it would lead to an increase in the H^+ concentration within the cytosol and bring about the same changes in activities of enzymes in this compartment as an increase in external H^+ concentration. If this is the mechanism, one might expect some differences in the metabolism of mitochondrial metabolites under the two different conditions. Nagata and Rasmussen (1969) have found differences in the effects of H^+ and Ca^{++} upon citrate oxidation by isolated renal tubules, Ca^{++} inhibited and H^+ stimulated C^{-6}-citrate oxidation. This finding would be consistent with uptake of calcium into mitochondria. However, when pyruvate oxidation was compared, H^+ led to an inhibition whereas Ca^{++} led to either no change or enhanced pyruvate oxidation. These differences are not readily accounted for by any simple known relationship between Ca^{++}, H^+, and pyruvate oxidation. Hence some data are consistent with the concept that a major means by which changes in extracellular Ca^{++} regulate renal gluconeogenesis is by changing intracellular, or more specifically cytoplasmic, H^+ concentration. Conversely, it is possible to envision that a rise in H^+ concentration could bring about a change in the stability of many calcium chelates or complexes with organic anions and lead thereby to an increase in Ca^{++} activity within the cell. Hence, the best that can be said at present is that a change in either external H^+ or Ca^{++} brings about changes in renal gluconeogenesis by regulating the activities of key cytoplasmic enzymes, PEPCK and PK (Fig. 15) but it is not known whether they do so by a common mechanism.

One additional point of some interest in regard to the question of

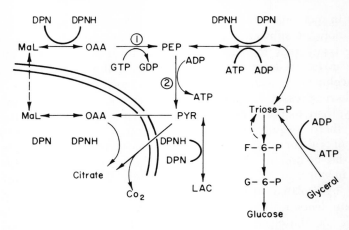

FIG. 15. The pathways of carbon during gluconeogenesis 1 and 2 represent respectively the enzymes PEP carboxykinase and pyruvate kinase.

intracellular distribution of accumulated calcium is the nature of the cell being stimulated. In cells rich in mitochondria, such as those in the renal cortex, the predominant change might well be a rise in cytoplasmic H^+, whereas in cells that are more dependent upon anaerobic metabolism such as the bone cells, the predominant change might be a rise in cytoplasmic Ca^{++}.

The data concerned with Ca^{++}, PTH, H^+, and renal gluconeogenesis have been interpreted to mean that either a change in external Ca^{++} or the addition of PTH causes an increase in intracellular Ca^{++} and/or H^+, which leads to an activation of PEP carboxykinase and an inhibition of pyruvate kinase (Fig. 13). This interpretation is consistent with the observations of Borle (1969b) that both PTH and an increase in external Ca^{++} will cause a rise in intracellular Ca^{++} in the tissue culture cells derived from kidney. The data obtained on the isolated tubules add the important point that a part of this extra calcium has important metabolic effects within the cell.

The other important conclusion is that in the absence of Ca^{++}, the PTH-induced rise in 3',5'-AMP is not an effective second messenger, at least insofar as the control of renal gluconeogenesis is concerned. It is not yet possible to resolve the question as to whether adenyl cyclase activation and a change in calcium permeability are simultaneous events. The results of studies with dibutyryl 3',5'-AMP would argue in favor of an effect of 3',5'-AMP on Ca^{++} permeability if the only effect of dibutyryl 3',5'-AMP is that of replacing 3',5'-AMP at the proper site within the cell. At present it is by no means clear that the effects of dibutyryl 3',5'-AMP are confined this precisely.

In summary, the present weight of experimental evidence leads to the conclusion that a major effect of parathyroid hormone is upon cellular calcium influx and the level of calcium and possibly hydrogen ion activity within the cell. The immediate questions that these data and this hypothesis raise are (1) can a change in intracellular calcium explain the major metabolic and physiologic effects of parathyroid hormone? and (2) if so, by what mechanism does CT influence bone cell function?

E. The Relative Importance of 3′,5′-AMP and Ca^{++} as Second Messengers

Before turning to these questions it is worth bringing out a particularly interesting aspect of the general relationship between 3′,5′-AMP, Ca^{++}, and the enzymes, adenyl cyclase and phosphodiesterase. In contrast to adenyl cyclase, phosphodiesterase is present in the cytosol. If this enzyme is present in high enough concentration and active, very little 3′,5′-AMP would be expected to diffuse far from its site of synthesis in the membrane. Hence, by regulating the ratios of the activities of these two enzymes in particular cells, the extent of 3′,5′-AMP diffusion, and thus its role as a direct intracellular messenger could be regulated. On the other hand, a change in Ca^{++} permeability concomitant to adenyl cyclase activation would lead to increased calcium entry and this Ca^{++} would represent a second messenger that is not readily transformed as it diffuses into the cell. For this reason, it may be that Ca^{++} is a more important second messenger than 3′,5′-AMP in certain cells.

F. Intracellular Calcium and the Effects of PTH on Bone

1. Calcium and Bone Cell Function

The major effects of parathyroid hormone on bone are four in number: (1) an inhibition of collagen synthesis in active osteoblasts (Vaes and Nichols, 1962); (2) an enhancement of osteocytic osteolysis (Belanger and Rasmussen, 1968; Talmage, 1967); (3) an enhancement of osteoclastic osteolysis (Heller *et al.*, 1950); and (4) a probable increase in the rate of maturation of precursor cells into both osteoblasts and osteoclasts, Talmage, 1967). As shown by Park and Talmage (1968), increasing extracellular calcium will mimic effects 1 and 4, but not 2 and 3. In regard to effect 4, it has also been shown by Perris and Whitfield (1967) that Ca^{++} increases the mitotic rate in some types of cells, and that PTH has a similar effect. However, at present there is no evidence that increased extracellular calcium will enhance osteocytic osteolysis. In fact the data of Rasmussen *et al.* (1967b) suggest the contrary. Nonetheless, this may not be an appropriate criterion because of the difference in the composition of the bulk extracellular fluids and those in bone. A particular difficulty is that of understanding how a net movement of calcium from osteocytic lacunae to blood can be brought about by cells with no obvious structural polarity. This difficulty can be overcome, if one assumes that the lysosomes in bone cells are an important aspect of their ability to induce osteolysis (Vaes, 1965, 1966), and further, that their enzymes are released into the lacunar spaces. In this view, the secretion of these enzymes would be similar to the mechanism by which insulin, for example, is released from β-cells. In this latter case it is known that Ca^{++} and 3',5'-AMP are involved (Milner and Hales, 1967; Malaisse *et al.*, 1967). Hence a logical model for PTH action on bone is that the increased intracellular 3',5'-AMP and calcium are responsible for the release of lysosomal enzymes as well as for the metabolic changes, i.e., increased citrate production. The release of these enzymes would induce bone destruction and lead to an increased concentration of calcium outside the cell (in the bone extracellular fluid compartment), which would thus establish a gradient of calcium from lacunar fluid to blood, and a movement of the calcium toward blood. This movement would involve the activity of the membrane-bound calcium-activated ATPase of osteocytes and osteoblasts.

In the light of the previous discussion concerning the relationship between intracellular Ca^{++} and H^+ (see Section IV,D), it is possible to understand how an increased acid production could be brought about by PTH, and how this might be an additional important determinant of the total process of bone resorption; and account for the long-established fact that sites of active bone resorption are associated with low pH (5.5–6.5) (Cretin, 1951; Schartum and Nichols, 1962).

Note should also be made of the fact that the major metabolic effects of parathyroid hormone, an increase in citrate and lactate production, can be accounted for by this model. From the work of Nagata and Rasmussen (1968), it seems clear that an increased cell calcium leads to an inhibition of citrate oxidation. Also from the work of Namm *et al.* (1968), in the heart, the activation of glycolysis involves both Ca^{++} and 3',5'-AMP. A similar requirement in bone cells could be the basis of increased lactate production after PTH administration.

This model would account for one of the most interesting, but unexplained effects of parathyroid hormone, first observed by Copp (1965). He noted that the administration of highly purified PTH into young experimental animals was followed by an immediate and transient hypocalcemia before the expected rise in plasma calcium was seen (Fig. 16). In the converse situation, he has also noted that cessation of PTH infusion

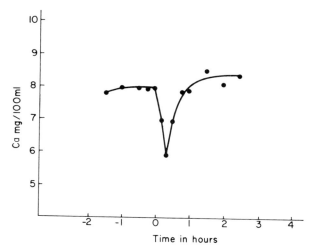

FIG. 16. The change in plasma calcium concentration in a young sheep receiving an infusion of PTH at time 0. Figure kindly supplied by Prof. D. H. Copp. See Copp (1969).

in the absence of the thyroid glands led to an increase in plasma calcium that may last an hour or more even though PTH has a half-life in plasma of less than 20 minutes. Both of these changes could be accounted for by a PTH-induced uptake of calcium into cells (Copp, 1969).

The other aspect of PTH action upon bone cell function could also be accommodated by this theory. This is the inhibition of collagen synthesis seen after PTH administration. Park and Talmage (1968) have noted that either Ca^{++} or PTH infusion into a parathyroidectomized animal leads to an inhibition of ^{14}C-proline incorporation into collagen. These results could be explained by assuming that both infusions led to an increase in intracellular calcium in active osteoblasts. However, if this is the case then an immediate question is why these cells do not become osteolytic. Two factors can be suggested as to why this does not happen. First, these cells do not have the characteristic lysosomes seen in osteocytes or osteoclasts. Thus, a rise in intracellular calcium does not trigger the release of hydrolases. Also, it would be expected that at sites of active bone formation, the calcium content of the extracellular fluids on the bone side of the osteoblastic curtain is lower than on the plasma side because of the uncalcified and partially calcified matrix, which acts as an ion sink or site of mineral crystal nucleation and growth. Hence a PTH-induced rise in intracellular calcium would probably lead to a shift of calcium into the bone rather than out of it, and may well contribute to the transient initial hypocalcemia following PTH administration, and the converse hypercalcemia seen after PTH infusion is stopped.

2. Role of Pyrophosphate in Bone Resorption

A completely different suggestion as to the biochemical mechanisms regulating bone resorption and formation has been made by Fleisch (1964). He has proposed that pyrophosphate plays a key role in regulating bone crystal growth and bone crystal dissolution by acting as a crystal poison. It is clear that PP_i has such effects upon crystal growth and dissolution *in vitro*, but whether these phenomena are of physiologic significance *in vivo* is quite difficult to prove. The thesis requires that PTH somehow enhances the activity of extracellular pyrophosphatase, which in turn leads to an increased breakdown of surface bound pyrophosphate with an increase in bone mineral crystal dissolution. The difficulties with this theory are several: (1) the association between pyrophosphatase and bone resorption is not clear; (2) the enzyme pyrophosphatase is strongly inhibited by Ca^{++}, hence as soon as significant mineral dissolution occurred further enzymatic activity would be inhibited; and (3) the theory does not in any way account for the changes in matrix breakdown, which is always seen with PTH administration. In fact, in fully calcified bone, the mineral is diffusion-locked, and thus not readily accessible to the enzyme or other components of the surrounding fluids. In order for significant osteolysis to occur it appears necessary that a concerted attack upon matrix as well as mineral is required. On these grounds alone the Fleisch theory is incomplete.

Nevertheless, DeLong and his colleagues (1970) have found that pyrophosphate infusion leads to an inhibition of PTH-induced bone resorption, which is what would be predicted by the Fleisch theory. However, DeLong *et al.* believe that the explanation of the pyrophosphate effect is quite different from the proposed by Fleisch, and is related to its effect upon the adenyl cyclase system. When adenyl cyclase converts ATP to 3',5'-AMP there is a second product PP (Fig. 5),

$$ATP \rightleftharpoons PP + 3',5'\text{-AMP}$$

Furthermore, Greengard *et al.* (1969) have shown that this reaction is readily reversible *in vitro*. Thus, an increase in PP in the intracellular fluids could cause an inhibition or reversal of the adenyl cyclase reaction, and block PTH action in this way. DeLong *et al.* (1970) have shown that this reversal can occur in PTH-treated animals *in vivo*. This evidence raises serious doubts as to the importance of pyrophosphate as a direct regulator of bone mineral exchange, and suggests that PP effects may best be accounted for in terms of the present model.

3. *Phosphate, Bone Cell Function, and PTH Action*

Another ion that has been shown to have significant effects upon bone cell function is inorganic phosphate. The work of Feinblatt, Belanger, and Rasmussen (1969), Rasmussen *et al.* (1969), and of Pechet *et al.* (1967) has clearly shown that the simultaneous administration of phosphate to thyroparathyroidectomized animals receiving parathyroid hormone does not inhibit bone resorption but leads to stimulation of both bone formation and bone mineralization. This effect of phosphate can also be demonstrated in monkey and man (Nichols and Flanagan, 1969), and has been shown *in vitro* in bone organ cultures (Raisz, 1969). These results imply that its effects are opposite to those of the parathyroid hormone on the function of active osteoblasts without having a significant effect upon the function of osteocytes or osteoclasts. The immediate question is how or whether this effect of phosphate can be explained satisfactorily in terms of the present model.

It has long been known that there is an intimate relationship between calcium and phosphate transport (Rasmussen, 1968), and that under some circumstances there is an apparent reciprocal relationship between the concentration of phosphate and calcium in blood plasma. However, it is now quite clear that calcium and phosphate exchange in bone is regulated by the activity of the various bone cells, and that under just as many circumstances there is no clear reciprocal change in the concentration of one of these ions when the other does change. In fact, at the level of cellular and subcellular transport systems, the overwhelming evidence indicates an associated movement of calcium and phosphate across the cell or membrane. The only exception is the renal tubule, where there is a clear separation of calcium and phosphate fluxes.

In the intestine the transport of both ions is increased by vitamin D, growth hormone, and parathyroid hormone. Two facts of particular interest are (1) the site along the intestine where maximal gradients of phosphate are achieved differs, being in the midgut, from the site of maximal calcium absorption, the duodenum; and (2) the transport of calcium *in vitro* does not require the presence of phosphate, but phosphate transport, even in the midgut, requires the presence of calcium (H. E. Harrison and Harrison, 1963).

The situation in isolated mitochondria is similar (Rasmussen, 1966). Calcium transport is primary, can occur in the absence of phosphate, but when phosphate is present it is accumulated with the calcium. However, in this situation the calcium and phosphate are accumulated within the mitochondria to a considerable extent in a nonosmotic or nonionic form. It is also clear that phosphate can be taken up as a counter ion to both

K^+, a monovalent cation, and Mg^{++}, a divalent cation. In fact, in the mitochondrial system it is possible to set up conditions, by changing the ionic environment in which the mitochondria are incubated, so that parathyroid hormone will cause an uptake of Mg^{++}, K^+, and phosphate into, and a release of Ca^{++} from the mitochondria. By a slight change in conditions, an uptake of Ca^{++}, Mg^{++}, and phosphate with little change in K^+ can be seen after hormone addition (Rasmussen *et al.*, 1967a). The importance of these studies cannot be overemphasized. They show that the interrelationship between a membrane and the ionic environments on its two sides is very complex. On the one hand, the membrane by its activity brings about an asymmetrical distribution of ions on its two surfaces, and on the other, the nature of the ionic environment in which the membrane resides influences its function and its response to stimuli. Furthermore, because of the differences in permeabilities of different anions and cations, a change in the flux of one cation, e.g., Ca^{++}, leads to a redistribution of the other cations and anions across the membrane. The magnitude of these changes will depend upon many factors.

In terms of transcellular transport where at least two membranes are involved, the same relationships prevail, so that the result of calcium change in the ionic composition of the fluids bathing one side of the cell will influence the activity of the cell, and the composition of the fluid upon the other side of the cell differently, depending upon the initial environmental conditions on the two cell surfaces. In the case of the bone, as already indicated, the composition of the fluids on the bone side of the curtain of active osteoblasts is undoubtedly different from the composition of the fluids surrounding osteocytes. The main determinant of this difference is the uncalcified and partially calcified matrix on the bone side of the active osteoblasts. Available evidence favors the view that phosphate is a primary determinant of mineralization (Krane *et al.*, 1965). Hence, the limiting factor in mineralization after parathyroid hormone administration could be relative lack of phosphate at this site, an increased concentration of calcium and an inhibition of further matrix formation. This would represent a very simple control system coordinating matrix formation and mineralization. In this view, the administration of phosphate would increase mineralization, lower calcium content in both bone extracellular fluid and bone cell intracellular fluid, and stimulate thereby both mineralization and matrix synthesis.

On the other hand, increasing the phosphate content of the bulk extracellular fluids might have little effect upon the activity of osteocytes being stimulated by PTH. In this case the gradient of both calcium and phosphate is from bone extracellular fluid to blood, and the small rise in plasma phosphate is accompanied by a fall in plasma calcium, hence the net result might be very little change in the total ionic gradient. This model would also account for the observation of Rasmussen *et al.* (1967b), in which lowering the plasma calcium concentration in thyroparathyroidectomized rats receiving a constant infusion of PTH leads to an increase in the rate of mobilization of hydroxyproline, i.e., presumably increases the rate of resorption by enhancing the bulk transfer of calcium from bone extracellular fluid to bulk extracellular fluid.

The one immediately apparent difficulty with this model is that of explaining how matrix synthesis continues in animals with phosphate depletion or vitamin D deficiency, both conditions with low plasma phosphate. The situation in phosphate deficiency can be explained relatively easily. When plasma phosphate falls to very low levels, plasma calcium rises, PTH production falls. In this circumstance, then, plasma calcium would be normal, but intracellular calcium would be low due to the low levels of circulating PTH. This would allow normal rates of matrix synthesis to continue even though mineralization would be impaired by a lack of phosphate.

In the case of vitamin D deficiency, the situation is much more complex. Here initially one would expect a decreased rate of bone formation because of low plasma phosphate, and high levels of PTH with nearly normal concentrations of calcium in plasma. However, when marked hypocalcemia develops, synthesis might well return to normal rates in spite of continuing hypersecretion of PTH, because cell calcium would fall as extracellular calcium declined.

It is obviously not possible, at present, to extend a discussion of this model to all the cases of changes in bone metabolism, because of a lack of critical evidence concerning the effect of these states upon cell calcium and cell metabolism. However, one additional situation is worthy of note. Vitamin D administration is characteristically followed by a rise in blood citrate, which in part at least, comes from bone. In addition, citrate oxidation is inhibited in kidney, one of the major organs involved in the metabolism of blood citrate. The simultaneous administration of cortisol will prevent this rise in blood citrate without, however, blocking the effects of the vitamin on calcium metabolism (H. C. Harrison *et al.*, 1957). The recent studies of Nagata and Rasmussen (1968) give a basis for these results without fully accounting for them. They showed that when PTH is infused into a thyroparathyroidectomized rat there was a significant rise in isocitrate and citrate, but a fall in α-ketoglutarate concentrations in renal cortex. They interpreted this as an inhibition of isocitric dehydrogenase. When similar rats were pretreated with cortisol, or made vitamin D deficient, PTH no longer produced these effects, although it continued to exert a significant metabolic effect upon the cell, interpreted as an inhibition of pyruvate kinase.

One possible interpretation of these results is that in all instances, PTH produced an increase in intracellular calcium, which in the control animal was distributed to both the mitochondrial and cytoplasmic compartments of the cell, but in both cortisol-treated and vitamin D-deficient animals, the major change occurred in the cytosol. That this interpretation may well be correct is supported by the evidence that vitamin D deficiency or cortisol excess leads to changes in the ability of isolated kidney mitochondria to accumulate calcium, and alters the activity of calcium sensitive enzymes within them. It is of particular note that Nagata and Rasmussen found the same elevation of 3',5'-AMP after PTH in control, vitamin D-deficient, and cortisol-treated animals (Fig. 7), so that the observed metabolic differences cannot be accounted for by differences in the degree of adenyl cyclase activation.

G. PTH, Ca^{++}, and Renal Function

The second major target organ for PTH action is the kidney. As discussed, much of the key data upon which the present discussion is based was obtained in studies of carbohydrate metabolism in isolated tubules prepared from this organ. However, under physiologic conditions the effect of the hormone upon renal function is quite complex. It increases the tubular reabsorption of Ca^{++} and Mg^{++}, enhances both K^+ and phosphate excretion, and decreases H^+ ion excretion. By far the most striking of these is the phosphaturia. There is no known relationship between this change in physiologic function and the changes in carbohydrate metabolism. Thus, it might seem at this point that the data on the effects of PTH and calcium on renal gluconeogenesis are academic, and of little relevance to the major physiologic effect of the hormone. However, recent studies by Eisenberg (1965) in hypoparathyroid humans have shown that calcium infusion after some period of time leads to a marked phosphaturia. These observations led him to the postulate that either transtubular calcium transport or intracellular calcium were important determinants of phosphate excretion. The one difficulty with these studies is that most of these patients had normal thyroid glands, and may well have produced CT in response to a rise in plasma calcium. In view of the present controversy concerning a possible direct action of CT on renal function and particularly phosphate reabsorption, the validity of Eisenberg's conclusion is not certain. Nevertheless, a simple model to account for the renal phosphate handling is to propose that tubular reabsorption of phosphate is controlled by the level of plasma phosphate, the intracellular pH, and the intracellular Ca^{++} concentration. Thus increased cellular uptake of calcium may be involved in the mechanism by which

PTH influences renal phosphate excretion. Clearly more definitive information is required to determine the true nature of this relationship and more information is needed before one can decide whether Ca^{++} infusion produces any of the other characteristic effects of PTH upon renal function.

This is particularly important in view of the multiple changes in renal function produced by PTH (Hellman *et al.*, 1965; Arnaud *et al.*, 1966; Pechet *et al.*, 1967). In a particularly interesting and important study, Hellman and co-workers (1965) showed that PTH infusion leads to an increased excretion of HCO$_3^-$, and a decreased excretion of H$^+$, NH$_4^+$, and titrable acidity, and that this change occurred very soon after hormone administration (Fig. 17). As discussed in a preceeding section (Section IV,B), *in vitro* evidence suggests that PTH may cause an increase in intracellular H$^+$. This might be expected to increase H$^+$ excretion in the urine, but the opposite is observed. Hellman *et al.* suggested that

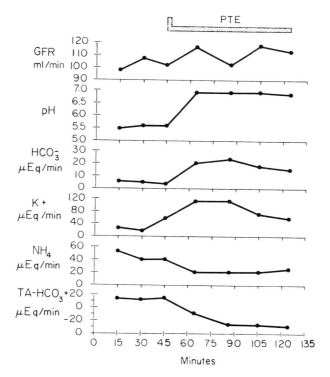

Fig. 17. The effect of the intravenous infusion of PTE (parathyroid extract) upon glomerular filtration rate, urinary pH, and the urinary excretion of HCO$_3^-$, K$^+$, NH$_4^+$, and TA-HCO$_3$ in the dog. Plotted from the data of Hellman *et al.* (1965).

PTH blocked Na^+–H^+ exchange, but did not suggest how this might be brought about. In the light of the many effects of Ca^{++} on membrane properties, it is conceivable that an increase in intracellular Ca^{++} could alter the properties of the membrane lining the renal tubular lumen. However, at present there is no evidence to support this suggestion.

V. MODE OF ACTION OF CALCITONIN

The one well-established effect of calcitonin is that of inhibiting bone resorption, both osteocytic and osteoclastic (Gudmundsson *et al.*, 1966; Aliapoulios, 1966; Rasmussen and Tenenhouse, 1967, Pechet *et al.*, 1967; Friedman and Raisz, 1965; Anast *et al.*, 1967; Foster *et al.*, 1966; MacIntyre and Parsons, 1966; Milhaud and Job, 1966; Hirsch *et al.*, 1964). This inhibition leads to a fall in the concentration of both plasma and urinary calcium, and plasma phosphate as well as decreased excretion of urinary hydroxyproline. CT blocks the enhanced resorption induced either by PTH or vitamin D infusion, but is effective in both the D-deficient and parathyroidectomized animal, or in animals treated with actinomycin D, an inhibitor of RNA synthesis, which blocks the action of vitamin D, and some of the actions of PTH on bone resorption (see review by Tenenhouse *et al.*, 1968; Foster, 1968; Pechet *et al.*, 1967; Copp, 1969).

Two other possible effects of CT remain a matter of continuing exploration. The first is that of enhancing bone mineralization and bone formation. Conflicting evidence exists on this point. One argument has been that since CT appears to produce opposite effects to those of PTH, it should enhance bone formation. In the context of the present model of PTH action, this would mean that CT should cause a decrease in cellular calcium and an increase in bone formation. However, the work of Feinblatt *et al.* (1969) and of Pechet *et al.* (1967) shows quite clearly that phosphate causes an enhanced rate of bone formation. A common feature of the action of both CT and PTH is a fall in plasma phosphate with a predicted decrease in rate of bone formation. This change might well override any direct countereffect produced by CT on cellular calcium.

The second possible additional action of CT is upon renal function. Under appropriate experimental conditions, CT infusion leads to enhanced phosphate excretion at a time when plasma phosphate is falling (Rasmussen *et al.*, 1967b; Clark and Kenny, 1969; Robinson *et al.*,

1966). Several workers have proposed that this is due to a direct para-thyroid hormonelike effect of CT upon renal tubular function. However, direct infusion of CT into the renal artery does not cause phosphaturia (Clark and Kenny, 1969), in contrast to the case with PTH, and the phosphaturia may be a consequence of the fall in plasma calcium result-ing from an inhibition of bone resorption. Thus, the available physiologic evidence is clear only in so far as establishing a role of CT in regulating bone resorption is concerned. It is equally clear that the inhibition of bone resorption is not due to a direct antagonism of PTH action on bone cells.

Evidence is available at the chemical or biochemical level as to the mechanism by which CT acts. This evidence, although by no means complete, supports the hypothesis that CT has a direct role in regulating cellular calcium exchange and does not act via the adenyl cyclase system.

Before turning to a discussion of these data, a particular aspect of CT action requires comment. Munson and Hirsch (1967) have shown that the simultaneous administration of phosphate with CT greatly enhances the hypocalcemic effect of the hormone. From this observation, one could propose that CT might act by influencing phosphate transport into cells. However, a careful analysis of phosphate and CT effects upon bone show quite clearly that their major effects are upon different cells and different parameters of bone metabolism although they both bring about a fall in plasma calcium concentration and in this way act synergistically. Phosphate produces this change primarily by an increase in mineral deposition into bone, and CT by a decrease in mineral removal from bone (Pechet *et al.*, 1967; Rasmussen and Tenenhouse, 1967).

Returning to the biochemical evidence, shortly after Chase and Aur-bach (1967) reported an increase in urinary 3',5'-AMP following PTH infusion, Rasmussen *et al.* (1968) observed PTH-like effects upon both bone resorption and renal function upon the infusion of dibutyryl 3',5'-AMP. Furthermore, CT was able to inhibit the bone resorption produced by either dibutyryl 3',5'-AMP or PTH infusion (Fig. 6). These experi-ments were interpreted to mean that CT did not act either by blocking adenyl cyclase and thereby 3',5'-AMP formation, or by enhancing phos-phodiesterase activity and thereby 3',5'-AMP hydrolysis. This interpre-tation has received direct experimental verification. Chase *et al.* (1969) have found a rise in 3',5'-AMP in mouse calvaria (bone) treated with PTH *in vitro*, and no change in this PTH-induced rise in 3',5'-AMP when CT is also added to the incubation medium, even though it had previ-ously been well established that CT blocks the PTH-induced increase in bone resorption in this *in vitro* system (Friedman and Raisz, 1965; Aliapoulios, 1966). All of this evidence clearly shows that CT does not influence the adenyl cyclase–phosphodiesterase system directly, but must act by blocking some later and/or different aspect of the cellular response to PTH. The question is: what is the nature of this effect?

In the context of our present model of PTH action, this action could be an effect upon cellular calcium exchange that would cause a decrease in cellular calcium content. In other words, CT could either inhibit the PTH-induced increase in calcium influx, or stimulate the Ca^{++}-activated ATPase and thereby calcium efflux. Two kinds of evidence suggest that CT influences the PTH-induced changes in cellular calcium. The one is morphological. In this case, CT administration leads to an apparent decrease in cellular calcium in bone cells (Baylink *et al.*, 1968). The other is biochemical. Nisbet and Nordin (1968) have shown that CT inhibits the rise in citrate production caused by PTH, and the weight of present evidence is consistent with the notion that this PTH-induced rise in citrate production is a consequence of increased intracellular calcium (Nagata and Rasmussen, 1968).

Accepting this inadequate evidence for the sake of further discussion, one is still left with the two alternative mechanisms for CT action. Two different kinds of experimental evidence favor the notion that CT acts by enhancing the activity of the calcium pump or ATPase rather than by decreasing calcium entry. By far the most direct is the fact that CT has

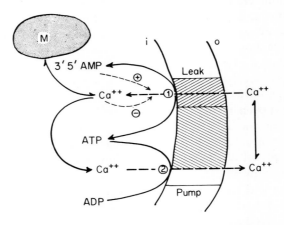

Both leak and pump carrier mediated
① PTH↑Leak
② TCT↑Pump

Fig. 18. A model of the relationship between Ca^{++} pump, Ca^{++} leak, adenyl cyclase, and the actions of PTH and TCT at the cell membrane of hormonally responsive bone cells.

been reported to enhance the activity of the Ca^{++}-activated ATPase of isolated red blood cell ghosts (Parkinson and Radde, 1969). The other more indirect evidence is that showing that the effect of CT can be overcome by continued PTH infusion, clearly implying that PTH can eventually overcome the inhibitory action of CT.

In summary: it is proposed that CT acts by altering cellular calcium exchange by a direct activation of the calcium pump or ATPase (Fig. 18). A prediction from this model is that immediately after CT infusion is begun one should observe a transient hypercalcemia before the usual hypocalcemia ensues.

VI. PTH, VITAMIN D, AND INTRACELLULAR Ca^{++}

The final relationship, which will be discussed briefly in the light of the present model, is that between vitamin D and parathyroid hormone. This relationship is discussed more fully in the chapter written by DeLuca and Melancon, Volume 2. However, in the present context we wish to present a somewhat different interpretation of the role of vitamin D. The salient features upon which this is based are (1) vitamin D, or more correctly, its metabolites, induce the synthesis of new protein(s) required as a component of the membrane, or for the synthesis of new membrane, e.g., phospholipid and other components, or for both; (2) in the intestine the major effect of vitamin D is at the brush border, i.e., vitamin D treatment leads to an enhanced rate of calcium entry into the mucosal cell; (3) the situation in bone is more complex, but here the vitamin appears to be required for the bulk transfer of calcium, but there is no obvious structural polarity in the osteocytes, nor is there evidence that vitamin D is required for osteocytic osteolysis. However, osteoclasts show definite polarity and possess a brush border, and there is good evidence that vitamin D is required for osteoclastic resorption (Arnaud *et al.,* 1966). Furthermore, the presently available data are consistent with the notion that at the unique surfaces of each of these two cell types, osteoclasts and intestinal epithelia cells, vitamin D regulates the active uptake of Ca^{++}. The simplest explanation of vitamin D action is that it directs the synthesis of a calcium activated ATPase, which is required for the bulk transport of calcium across the brush borders of these cells, i.e., intestinal mucosal cells and osteoclasts. This ATPase must be different from the one acted on by CT since CT works in D-deficient animals. In all likelihood its action is not confined to the induction of a single specific protein, but probably involves the regulation of the synthesis of new brush border membrane (Adams *et al.*, 1969). This latter likelihood must await further experimentation before being accepted as fact.

VII. SUMMARY AND CONCLUSIONS

This review has been an attempt to bring together data of many different kinds into a logical model to account for the action of the three major hormones involved in calcium homeostasis. The model proposes that all three regulate extracellular calcium homeostasis by primary effects upon cellular calcium exchange: PTH by increasing passive calcium influx; CT by increasing the activity of the Ca^{++}-activated ATPase involved in calcium efflux; and vitamin D by regulating the synthesis of a special Ca^{++}-activated ATPase involved in calcium entry across the brush border intestinal epithelial cells and osteoclasts, and possibly by regulating the synthesis of the special brush border membranes in which this ATPase is found. This model accounts for many previously unexplained experimental observations.

One special feature of this model is the relationship between PTH-induced activation and adenyl cyclase, and the increased calcium influx. Of particular note are the many other systems in which $3',5'$-AMP and Ca^{++} appear to be necessary components of the physiologic response to a specific stimulus. In all of these systems, including those regulated by PTH, it is not yet clear whether a change in Ca^{++} permeability and in adenyl cyclase activity are simultaneous and independent events resulting from the initial hormone–receptor interaction, or whether the increased $3',5'$-AMP resulting from adenyl cyclase activation is responsible for the changes in Ca^{++} permeability. Furthermore, it is not clear whether in addition to the change in intracellular calcium, which has definite metabolic effects within the cell, the rise in $3',5'$-AMP in all these systems has effects independent of those produced by calcium, but in some it is clear this is the case, e.g., epinephrine and the heart (Namm *et al.*, 1968).

Stated in another way, present data are insufficient to establish that the changes in intracellular calcium, produced in the specific cells by these different hormones, are the only or major control of intracellular events or whether the calcium is only one of several intracellular messengers involved in integrating the changes in cell function induced by specific hormonal stimuli.

ACKNOWLEDGMENTS

The work described from the author's laboratories has been supported by grants from the U. S. Atomic Energy Commission [AT(30-1)3489], the U. S. Public Health Service (AM 09650), and the Medical Research Council of Canada (MA-3205).

REFERENCES

Abe, K., Butcher, R. W., Nicholson, W. E., Baird, C. E., Liddle, R. A., and Liddle, G. W. (1969). *Endocrinology* 84, 362.

Adams, T. H., Wong, R. G., and Normon, A. W. (1969). *Federation Proc.* 28, 2799a.

Adelman, W. J., and Moore, J. W. (1961). *J. Gen. Physiol.* 45, 93.

Aliapoulios, M. A., Goldhaber, P., and Munson, P. L. (1966). *Science* 151, 330.

Alleyne, G. A. O. (1968). *Nature* 217, 847.

Alleyne, G. A. O., and Scullard, G. H. (1969). *J. Clin. Invest.* 48, 364.

Anast, C., Arnaud, C. D., Rasmussen, H., and Tenenhouse, A. (1967). *J. Clin. Invest.* 46, 57.

Arnaud, C. D., Rasmussen, H., and Anast, C. (1966). *J. Clin. Invest.* 45, 1955.

Arnaud, C. D., Tenenhouse, A., and Rasmussen, H. (1967). *Ann. Rev. Physiol.* 29, 349.

Baker, P. F., Blaustein, M. P., Manil, J., and Steinhardt, R. A. (1967). *J. Physiol. (London)* 191, 100P.

Baker, P. F., Blaustein, M. P., Hodgkin, A. L., and Steinhardt, R. A. (1969). *J. Physiol. (London)* 200, 431.

Baylink, D., Morey, E., and Rich, C. (1968). *In* "Parathyroid Hormone and Thyrocalcitonin" (R. V. Talmage and L. F. Belanger, eds.), p. 196. Excerpta Med. Found., Amsterdam.

Bdolah, A., and Schramm, M. (1965). *Biochem. Biophys. Res. Commun.* 18, 452.

Bélanger, L. F., and Rasmussen, H. (1968). *In* "Parathyroid Hormone and Thyrocalcitonin" (R. V. Talmage and L. F. Belanger, eds.), p. 156. Excerpta Med. Found., Amsterdam.

Bianchi, C. P. (1961). *Circulation* 24, 518.

Bianchi, C. P. (1968). *Federation Proc.* 27, 126.

Birmingham, M. K., Elliott, F. H., and Valere, P. (1953). *Endocrinology* 53, 687.

Borle, A. B. (1967). *Clin. Orthopaed.* 52, 267.

Borle, A. B. (1968a). *J. Cell. Biol.* 36, 567.

Borle, A. B. (1968b). *Endocrinology* 83, 1316.

Borle, A. B. (1969a). *J. Gen. Physiol.* 53, 43.

Borle, A. B. (1969b). *J. Gen. Physiol.* 53, 57.

Cameron, D. A., Paschall, H. A., and Robinson, R. A. (1967). *J. Cell Biol.* 33, 1.

Castañeda, M., and Tyler, A. (1968). *Biochem. Biophys. Res. Commun.* 33, 782.

Chance, B. (1965). *J. Biol. Chem.* 240, 2729.

Chase, L. R., and Aurbach, G. D. (1967). *Proc. Natl. Acad. Sci. U. S.* 58, 518.

Chase, L. R., Fedak, S. A., and Aurbach, G. D. (1969). *Endocrinology* 84, 761.

Cheung, W. Y., and Williamson, J. R. (1965). *Nature* **207**, 979.

Clark, J. D., and Kenny, A. D. (1969). *Endocrinology* **84**, 1199.

Copp, D. H. (1965). "The Parathyroid Glands," p. 73. Univ. of Chicago Press, Chicago, Illinois.

Copp, D. H. (1969). *Ann. Rev. Pharmacol.* **9**, 327.

Cretin, A. (1951). *Presse Med.* **59**, 1240.

Csapo, A. (1959). *Ann. N. Y. Acad. Sci.* **75**, 790.

Curran, P. F., and Gill, J. R., Jr. (1962). *J. Gen. Physiol.* **45**, 625.

Daniels, A. E., Severs, W. B., and Buckley, J. P. (1967). *Life Sci.* **6**, 545.

Dean, P. M., and Matthews, E. K. (1968). *Nature* **219**, 389.

DeLong, A., Feinblatt, J., and Rasmussen, H. (1970), in preparation.

DeRobertis, E. Arnaiz, G. R. D., Albrecht, M., Butcher, R. W., and Sutherland, E. W. (1967). *J. Biol. Chem.* **242**, 3487.

Dikstein, S., Weller, C. P., and Sulman, F. G. (1963). *Nature* **200**, 1106.

Douglas, W. W., and Poisner, A. M. (1962). *Nature* **196**, 379.

Douglas, W. W., and Rubin, R. P. (1961). *J. Physiol.* (*London*) **159**, 40.

Ebashi, S., and Endo, M. (1969). *Progr. Biophys. Mol. Biol.* **18**, 123.

Eccles, J. C. (1964). "The Physiology of Synapses." Academic Press, New York.

Eisenberg, E. (1965). *J. Clin. Invest.* **44**, 942.

Feinblatt, J., Belanger, L. F., and Rasmussen, H. (1969). *Am. J. Physiol.* (in press).

Fleisch, H. (1964). *Clin. Orthopaed.* **32**, 170.

Foster, G. V. (1968). *New Engl. J. Med.* **279**, 349.

Foster, G. V., Doyle, F. H., Bordier, P., and Matrajt, H. (1966). *Lancet* **II**, 1428.

Friedman, J., and Raisz, L. G. (1965). *Science* **150**, 1465.

Friedmann, N., and Park, C. R. (1968). *Proc. Natl. Acad. Sci. U. S.* **61**, 504.

Gilbert, D. L., and Fenn, W. O. (1957). *J. Gen. Physiol.* **40**, 393.

Gilman, A. G., and Rall, T. W. (1966). *Federation Proc.* **25**, 617.

Gingell, D., and Garrod, D. R. (1969). *Nature* **221**, 192.

Goodman, A. D., Fuesz, R. E., and Cahill, G. (1966). *J. Clin. Invest.* **45**, 612.

Goodman, D. B. P., and Rasmussen, H. (1968). *Biochim. Biophys. Acta* **153**, 749.

Goorno, W. E., and Rector, F. C., Jr. (1967). *Am. J. Physiol.* **213**, 969.

Greengard, P., Hayaishi, O., and Colowick, S. P. (1969). *Federation Proc.* **28**, 1171a.

Grodsky, G. M., and Bennett, L. L. (1966). *Diabetes* **15**, 910.

Gudmundsson, T. V., MacIntyre, I., and Soliman, H. A. (1966). *Proc. Roy. Soc.* **B164**, 460.

Hagiwara, S., and Nakajima, S. (1966). *J. Gen. Physiol.* **49**, 807.

Hales, C. N., and Milner, R. D. G. (1968). *J. Physiol.* (*London*) **194**, 725.

Harrison, H. C., Harrison, H. E., and Park, E. A. (1957). *Proc. Soc. Exptl. Biol. Med.* **96**, 768.

Harrison, H. E., and Harrison, H. C. (1963). *Am. J. Physiol.* **205**, 107.

Hasselbach, W. (1957). *Biochim. Biophys. Acta* **25**, 562.

Hasselbach, W. (1964). "Progress in Biophysics," p. 167. Macmillan, New York.

Haynes, R. C., Jr., Sutherland, E. W., and Rall, T. W. (1960). *Recent Progr. Hormone Res.* **16**, 121.

Heller, M., McLean, F. C., and Bloom, W. (1950). *Am. J. Anat.* **87**, 315.

Hellman, D. E., Au, W. Y. W., and Bartter, F. C. (1965). *Am. J. Physiol.* **209**, 643.

Herrera, F. C., and Curran, P. F. (1963). *J. Gen. Physiol.* **46**, 999.

Hirsch, P. F., Voelkel, E. F., and Munson, P. L. (1964). *Science* **146**, 412.

Hodgkin, A. L., and Keynes, R. D. (1955). *J. Physiol.* (*London*) **128**, 28.

Hodgkin, A. L., and Keynes, R. D. (1957). *J. Physiol.* (*London*) **138**, 253.

Hokin, L. (1966). *Biochim. Biophys. Acta* **115**, 219.

Howell, D. S., Rita, J. C., Marquez, J. F., and Madruga, J. E. (1968). *J. Clin. Invest.* **47**, 1121.

Ishikawa, H. (1969). Personal communication.

Kashiwa, H. K. (1968). *In* "Parathyroid Hormone and Thyrocalcitonin" (R. V. Talmage and L. F. Belanger, eds.), p. 198. Excerpta Med. Found. Amsterdam.

Keynes, R. D., and Lewis, P. R. (1956). *J. Physiol. (London)* **134**, 399.

Konijn, T. M., van de Meene, J. G. C., Bonner, J. T., and Barkley, D. S. (1967). *Proc. Natl. Acad. Sci. U. S.* **58**, 1152.

Krahl, M. E. (1961). "The Action of Insulin on Cells." Academic Press, New York.

Krane, S., Stone, M. J., and Glimcher, M. J. (1965). *Biochim. Biophys. Acta* **97**, 77.

Levine, R. (1966). *Am. J. Med.* **40**, 691.

Lowenstein, W. R., Nakao, M., and Socolar, S. J. (1967). *J. Gen. Physiol.* **50**, 1865.

MacIntyre, I., and Parsons, J. A. (1966). *J. Physiol. (London)* **183**, 31.

Maizels, M. (1956). *J. Physiol. (London)* **132**, 414.

Malaisse, W. J., Malaisse-Lagae, F., and Mayhew, D. (1967). *J. Clin. Invest.* **46**, 1724.

Manery, J. F. (1966). *Federation Proc.* **25**, 1804.

Marchesi, V. T., and Steers, E., Jr. (1968). *Science* **159**, 203.

Marchesi, V. T., and Palade, G. E. (1967). *J. Cell Biol.* **35**, 385.

Matthews, E. K., and Saffran, M. (1968). *Nature* **219**, 1369.

Mela, L. (1968). *Arch. Biochem. Biophys.* **123**, 286.

Meyer, W. L., Fischer, E. H., and Krebs, E. G. (1964). *Biochemistry* **3**, 1033.

Milhaud, G., and Job, J. C. (1966). *Science* **154**, 794.

Milner, R. D. G., and Hales, C. N. (1967). *Diabetologia* **3**, 478.

Munson, P. L., and Hirsch, P. F. (1967). *Am. J. Med.* **43**, 678.

Nagata, N., and Rasmussen, H. (1969). Unpublished studies.

Nagata, N., and Rasmussen, H. (1968). *Biochemistry* **7**, 3728.

Nagata, N., and Rasmussen, H. (1970). *Proc. Natl. Acad. Sci. U. S.* **65**, #2.

Nakao, M., Nakao, T., and Yamazoe, S. (1960). *Nature* **187**, 945.

Nakao, M., Nakao, T., Yamazoe, S., and Yoshikawa, H. (1961). *J. Biochem.* **45**, 487.

Namm, D. H., Mayer, S. E., and Maltbie, M. (1968). *Mol. Pharmacol.* **4**, 522.

Nanninga, L. B. (1961). *Biochim. Biophys. Acta* **54**, 338.

Neuman, W. F., and Neuman, M. W. (1958). "The Chemical Dynamics of Bone Mineral." Univ. of Chicago Press, Chicago, Illinois.

Nichols, G., Jr. (1963). "Mechanisms of Hard Tissue Destruction," Chapter 21, p. 557.

Nichols, G., Jr., and Flanagan, B. (1969). *J. Clin. Invest.* **48**, 595.

Nisbet, J., and Nordin, B. E. C. (1968). *In* "Calcitonin," p. 230. Heineman, London.

Ohnishi, T. (1962). *J. Biochem. (Tokyo)* **52**, 307.

Olson, E. J., and Cazort, R. J. (1969). *J. Gen. Physiol.* **53**, 311.

Orloff, J., and Handler, J. S. (1962). *J. Clin. Invest.* **41**, 702.

Ozawa, E., and Ebashi, S. (1967). *J. Biochem.* **62**, 285.

Papahadjapoulos, D., and Ohki, S. (1969). *Science* **164**, 1075.

Park, H. Z., and Talmage, R. V. (1968). *In* "Parathyroid Hormone and Thyrocalcitonin, (R. V. Talmage and L. F. Belanger, eds.), p. 203. Excerpta Med. Found., Amsterdam.

Parkinson, E. K., and Raddie, I. (1969). Abstract of the Am. Ped. Research Soc. Atlantic City, May 1969, p. 51.

Pechet, M., Bobadilla, E., Carroll, E. L., and Hesse, R. H. (1967). *Am. J. Med.* **43**, 696.

Perris, A. D., and Whitfield, J. F. (1967). *Nature* **216**, 1350.

Politoff, A. L., Socolar, S. J., and Lowenstein, W. R. (1969). *J. Gen. Physiol.* **53**, 498.

Portzehl, H., Caldwell, P. C., and Ruegg, J. C. (1964). *Biochim. Biophys. Acta* **79**, 581.

Rabinowitz, M., Desalles, L., Heisler, J., and Lorand, L. (1965). *Biochim. Biophys. Acta* **97**, 29.

Raisz, L. G. (1969). *Federation Proc.* (in press).

Rasmussen, H. (1961). *Am. J. Med.* **30**, 112.

Rasmussen, H. (1966). *Federation Proc.* **25**, 903.

Rasmussen, H. (1968). *In* "Williams Textbook of Endocrinology," Chapter 11, p. 847. Saunders, Philadelphia, Pennsylvania.

Rasmussen, H., and Nagata, N. (1969). *Brit. J. Pharmacol.* (submitted for publication).

Rasmussen, H., and Tenenhouse, A. (1967). *Am. J. Med.* **43**, 711.

Rasmussen, H., and Tenenhouse, A. (1968). *Proc. Natl. Acad. Sci. U. S.* **59**, 1364.

Rasmussen, H., Shirasu, H., Ogata, E., and Hawker, C. D. (1967a). *J. Biol. Chem.* **242**, 4669.

Rasmussen, H., Anast, C., and Arnaud, C. D. (1967b). *J. Clin. Invest.* **46**, 746.

Rasmussen, H., Pechet, M., and Fast, D. (1968). *J. Clin. Invest.* **47**, 1843.

Rasmussen, H., Feinblatt, J., Nagata, N., and Pechet, M. (1970). *Federation Proc.* (in press).

Robinson, C. J., Martin, T. J., and MacIntyre, I. (1966). *Lancet* **II**, 83.

Rutman, J. Z., Meltzer, L. E., Kitchell, J. R., Rutman, R. G., and George, P. (1965). *Am. J. Physiol.* **208**, 841.

Samli, M. H., and Geschwind, I. I. (1968). *Endocrinology* **82**, 225.

Schartum, S., and Nichols, G., Jr. (1962). *J. Clin. Invest.* **41**, 1163.

Schatzmann, H. J. (1966). *Experientia* **22**, 365.

Schoffeniels, E. (1963). *In* "Handbuch der experimentellen Pharmakolosie" (O. Gichler, and A. Farah, eds.), Vol. 17, Part I, Chapter 5, p. 114. Springer, Berlin.

Schofield, J. G. (1967). *Nature* **215**, 1382.

Schwartz, I. L., and Hechter, O. (1966). *Am. J. Med.* **40**, 765.

Schwartz, I. L., and Walter, R. (1968). *In* "Protein and Polypeptide Hormones," Part 1, p. 264. Excerpta Med. Found., Amsterdam.

Simpson, D. P. (1967). *J. Clin. Invest.* **46**, 225.

Sutherland, E. W., Oyi, I., and Butcher, R. W. (1965). *Recent Progr. Hormone Res.* **21**, 623.

Talmage, R. V. (1967). *Clin. Orthopaed.* **54**, 163.

Tenenhouse, A., Rasmussen, H., Hawker, C. D., and Arnaud, C. D. (1968). *Ann. Rev. Pharmacol.* **8**, 319.

Thorn, N. A. (1961). *Acta Endocrinol.* **38**, 563.

Turtle, J. R., Littleton, G. K., and Kipnis, D. M. (1967). *Nature* **213**, 727.

Vaes, G. (1965). *Exptl. Cell Res.* **39**, 470.

Vaes, G. (1966). *Biochem. J.* **97**, 393.

Vaes, G., and Nichols, G., Jr. (1962). *Endocrinology* **70**, 546.

Vale, W., and Guillemin, R. (1967). *Experientia* **23**, 855.

Vale, W., Burgus, R., and Guillemin, R. (1967). *Experientia* **23**, 853.

Wallach, S., Reizenstein, D. L., and Bellavia, J. V. (1966). *J. Gen. Physiol.* **49**, 743.

Weber, A. (1966). *Current Topics Bioenerget.* **1,** 203.
Weed, R. I., La Celle, P. L., and Merrill, E. W. (1969). *J. Clin. Invest.* **48,** 795.
Wells, H., and Lloyd, W. (1967). *Endocrinology* **81,** 139.
Wins, P., and Schoffeniels, A. L. (1966a). *Biochim. Biophys. Acta* **120,** 341.
Wins, P., and Schoffeniels, E. (1966b). *Arch. Intern. Physiol. Biochim.* **74,** 812.
Woodin, A. M., and Wieneke, A. A. (1964). *Biochem. J.* **90,** 498.
Zor, U., Lowe, I. P., Bloom, G., and Field, J. B. (1968). *Biochem. Biophys. Res. Commun.* **33,** 649.

CHAPTER 10

Mechanism of
Action of Thyrotropin

E. Schell-Frederick and J. E. Dumont

I. INTRODUCTION*

At the present time two complementary theories of hormone action underlie the experimental efforts in this field. One is the theory of specific hormone receptors in responsive tissues. The other is the theory that each hormone has a single primary action which accounts for all subsequent effects. Schwartz and Hechter have expanded on these theories, postulating that at its site of action the interaction of hormone and receptor serves not only as a discriminator for environmental signals but also as a signal generator (Schwartz and Hechter, 1966). In this model one views the cell functionally, with the spatially separated units of the cell involved in transport, biosynthesis, repair, and bioenergetics coupled by intracellular signals as well as coupled energetically.

During the last decade a large body of evidence has been presented which favors the hypothesis that the effects of many hormones are mediated by intracellular cyclic 3',5'-AMP (Robison et al., 1968). The enzymatic formation and destruction of cyclic AMP, the sensitivity of the enzymes to various hormones and pharmacological agents, and the known actions of cAMP in the cell have been thoroughly discussed in recent reviews (Robison et al., 1968; Sutherland et al., 1965). A model of the role of cyclic AMP in the mechanism of action of thyrotropin is presented in Fig. 1. This model postulates that TSH binds to a specific receptor in the thyroid follicular cell plasma membrane. The result of this interaction is the activation within the membrane of the enzyme adenyl cyclase which catalyzes the formation of cyclic 3',5'-AMP from ATP. Intracellular cAMP, called by Sutherland the secondary messenger, activates enzyme systems which are involved more or less directly in the observed biological effects of TSH.

In this review we shall examine the evidence for this model of thyrotropin action. The model predicts that the TSH unit hormone discriminator–signal generator, in the parlance of Schwartz and Hechter, exists both in a structural and functional sense in the thyroid plasma membrane. In simplest functional terms the hormone receptor-effector unit can be thought of as consisting of an interrelated hormone recognition subunit and an adenyl cyclase catalytic subunit. The model further predicts that

---

* *Abbreviations* used: Pi, inorganic phosphate; cAMP, cyclic 3',5'-adenosine monophosphate; DB-cAMP, N^6-2'-O-dibutyryl cyclic 3',5'-adenosine monophosphate; glucose carbon-1 oxidation, radioactive yield of $^{14}CO_2$ produced by thyroid tissue preparations from glucose-1-^{14}C; AIB, α-aminoisobutyrate; PGE$_1$, prostaglandin E$_1$; TSH, thyroid-stimulating hormone = thyrotropin.

all TSH effects may be accounted for by the initial interaction with this unit, i.e., the binding of TSH to the plasma membrane and resultant stimulation of adenyl cyclase. The cyclic AMP thus formed is the intracellular signal which couples the spatially separated units of the cell.

In attempting a critical evaluation of this model we have limited the discussion of thyrotropin to two topics. In the first section the specific binding of thyrotropin to thyroid cellular components will be discussed. In the second, the evidence that stimulation of adenyl cyclase and changes in the intracellular level of cyclic AMP can account for all the observed effects of TSH will be evaluated. The reader is referred to several recent reviews for a discussion of other aspects of thyrotropin action (Dumont, 1968; Field, 1968).

II. THE SPECIFIC INTERACTION OF THYROTROPIN WITH THYROID CELLULAR COMPONENTS

A. INTRODUCTION

1. Definition of Hormone Receptor

The experiments on thyrotropin localization and binding which will be discussed in this section may be summarized as a search for the receptor. Until now, the hormone receptor has been "a conceptual molecule" (Hechter and Halkerston, 1964), not an experimentally demonstrated one. A hormone receptor may be defined as a cellular molecule whose specific physicochemical interaction with hormone initiates the primary biological effect of the hormone (for a discussion of receptor theory, see Bush, 1965; Hechter and Halkerston, 1964). The essence of this concept, as discussed by Bush (1965), is the necessity of a combination of hormone and cellular component to produce the biological effects. The observed degree of molecular specificity of the hormone implies that the receptor will also possess molecular specificity. In addition, since minute quantities of hormone are biologically effective and the dose response curve reaches a maximum at low hormone concentration, the number of tissue receptors must be limited.

This definition is useful because it outlines experimental criteria for the identification of a cellular hormone receptor. (1) Hormone–cellular receptor interaction should be demonstrable with physiological concentrations of hormone. (2) Binding should be specific for substances with the particular hormonal action. (3) Cells not known to be responsive to the hormone should not demonstrate the interaction. (4) The formation

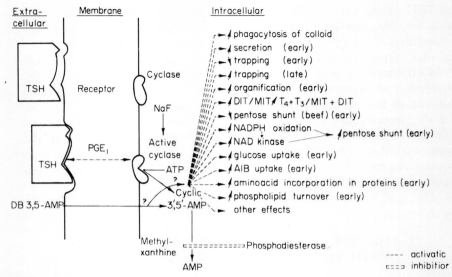

FIG. 1. Mechanism of action of thyrotropin on the thyroid cell: application of the Sutherland, Rall, and Butcher model to the thyroid. DB 3′,5′-AMP = DB-cAMP.

of hormone–receptor complex should have a limited maximum. (5) The interaction must be demonstrated to be linked to the primary biological effect.

It is obvious that the last of these criteria is at the same time the crucial criterion and the one most difficult to satisfy. At the time of writing there is no hormone for which the primary biological effect is known. Indeed it is a subject of continuing debate whether there is a single primary effect for each hormone, "the one from which all others may be logically and experimentally derived" (Hechter and Halkerston, 1964). But whether there is a single primary event, or more than one, the key to understanding the primary mechanism(s) of action of hormones at the molecular level is the experimental demonstration of a physicochemical interaction between hormone and cellular molecule which is directly related to a biological effect.

2. Characteristics of Hormone Binding

The specific binding of a hormone to a cellular component may be involved not only in initiating the primary hormonal effect, i.e., the hormone–receptor interaction, but also in other physiologically related steps in hormonal action: (1) the recognition of hormone by the responsive tissue or cell; (2) the transport of hormone into and within the cell. It is not possible to predict a priori the number of specific binding activities which will be found for any hormone as one molecule may serve more than one of these related functions, or conversely several molecules may be necessary for a single function. Several of the criteria for the identification of receptor binding, i.e, binding at physiological concentrations, and specificity for hormone and responsive cell type, are also valid for the identification of recognition and transport binding. Other specific cellular hormone-binding activities are also possible, such as the binding of hormone to enzymes involved in hormone metabolism. The general characteristics one would like to know for hormonal binding, as for any biological binding system, are outlined in Table I.

The general statements made about hormone receptors and the role of cellular binding in hormone action emphasize the features common to all hormones. No less striking are the differences between them, physicochemical differences particularly obvious between steroid and protein hormones, but differences perhaps as significant between protein and glycoprotein hormones. Thus one expects that the proposed hormone receptors, the hormone carriers, and the hormone recognition elements, when isolated and characterized, may differ widely one from the other, expressing the diversity of hormones and cells rather than their similarity.

In this section the data on thyrotropin association with thyroid cellular components will be analyzed with the aid of the characteristics of binding outlined in Table I and the criteria for evaluating the functional significance of binding. As a working model, we suggest that thyrotropin will be found to bind uniquely at the plasma membrane to a molecule which serves both as the recognition element and the receptor. Entry into the cell is therefore not necessary for the action of the hormone. If the hormone does penetrate the cell any intracellular binding will be to enzymes involved in the metabolism of the hormone.

TABLE I

CHARACTERIZATION OF A BIOLOGICAL BINDING ACTIVITY

1. Cellular location
2. Specificity
   (a) Ligand
   (b) Tissue
3. Number of types of binding sites, number of sites of each type
4. Characteristics of the binding reaction
   (a) Kinetics, e.g., time course, reversibility, affinity, effect of temperature, etc.
   (b) Nature of the link
5. Physicochemical characteristics of the binding site
6. Relationship to biological effects

B. Localization of Thyrotropin in the Thyroid

The earliest approach to the problem of TSH–cellular binding has been to detect the localization in the thyroid of injected TSH. It must always be kept in mind that the localization of hormone is not synonymous with the identification of its site of action. Mancini *et al.* (1961) observed that 5 minutes after intravenous injection of thyrotropin labeled with lissamine rhodamine B, fluorescence was present in the thyroid capillary lumina and walls, and in the basement membrane of follicular cells. This fluorescence began to disappear at 10 minutes and was absent 30 minutes following injection. Fluorescence was rarely observed over the cytoplasm. When labeled denatured TSH was injected, fluorescence was confined to the thyroid capillary lumina. The large dosage and crudeness of the TSH preparation used, the possible effect of the labeling procedure on the biological activity and therefore the binding characteristics of the hormone, and the uncertainty whether label observed in the tissue is still associated with hormone, make the significance of these results uncertain.

Attempts to localize TSH in the thyroid by the double antibody technique have yielded conflicting results. Greenspan and Hargadine (1965) detected the TSH–TSH antiserum–fluorescein antiglobulin complex in the nuclei of thyroid cells 15 minutes after injection of partially purified hormone. Nuclear fluorescence was also observed in the retro-orbital fat and the kidney. *In vitro* studies in which thyroid slices were exposed to hormone for 40 minutes and subsequently to the antibodies confirmed the *in vivo* observations (Blum *et al.*, 1967). In contrast, *in vitro* studies using the same technique, reported by Vanhaelst and Nève (1969), showed fluorescence over the cytoplasm with conspicuous sparing of the nuclei. The TSH used was highly purified and incubation with hormone was for 20 minutes. No tissues other than the thyroid were examined. In the studies of both groups frozen, unfixed sections of less than 10 μ thickness were used. Under these conditions a large percentage of the cells to be exposed either *in vitro* to TSH and antibodies or to antibodies following *in vivo* hormone injection would be expected to be broken, thus disrupting normal cell barriers and relationships. The times of exposure to the reagents and of the washing were sufficient to allow nonspecific relocation of hormone. Therefore the location of the TSH–antibody complex in the cytoplasm and/or nucleus may have been artifactual.

It seems clear from all the localization studies that TSH associates specifically with the thyroid, perhaps also with adipose tissue, but the sites of specific interaction are not clear. Isolated thyroid cell preparations should offer a better system for the direct *in vitro* evaluation of thyrotropin localization. These cells appear intact under the electron microscope, retain the metabolic properties of intact thyroid tissue, and are highly responsive to TSH (Nève *et al.*, 1968; Rodesch and Dumont, 1967; Tong, 1964). Suspensions of living cells could be incubated with varying concentrations of ^{125}I-labeled TSH for various periods of time, suitably washed, and studied as whole cells and sections by autoradiography with light and electron microscopy. The advantages of this system are the use of intact functioning cells and the direct detection of hormone. The most serious disadvantage is the use of ^{125}I-labeled hormone, as one cannot prove definitively that the labeled hormone acts in an identical way to native hormone. However, with the use of an electrochemical procedure (Rosa *et al.*, 1964, 1967) for labeling TSH at relatively low specific activity this danger can be minimized.

C. Evidence for Functionally Significant Binding of Thyrotropin to Thyroid Cells

Pastan *et al.* (1966), have attempted to demonstrate direct binding of TSH in dog thyroid slices. The slices were incubated for 15 minutes at 1°C with TSH-[131]I (20 mCi/mg) in the presence of unlabeled TSH 15 mU/ml and bovine fraction V 5 mg/ml. Control incubations contained labeled albumin or γ-globulin in place of TSH. The results, expressed as the ratio of counts in the tissue to counts in the medium, showed no difference between TSH and the other proteins either directly after incubation or after serial washings. There are several possible reasons for this failure to detect specific TSH binding. One does not like to think that the explanation is that specific binding does not occur. The authors state that "depletion of hormone from the medium by exposure to tissue is negligible." Thus specific thyrotropin binding, if present, must have involved a very small percentage of the total TSH molecules present. The addition of 15 mU/ml unlabeled TSH would be expected to reduce the specific activity of the TSH to a level where limited binding would not be detectable. In addition, in their experiments the half-maximal response to TSH, in terms of stimulation of glucose-1-^{14}C oxidation, was observed with concentrations slightly greater than 4 mU/ml. The use of supramaximal concentrations of TSH would favor nonspecific adsorption and obscure specific binding.

However, in the same paper Pastan and his colleagues present indirect evidence that thyrotropin interacts at the cell surface and that this interaction is required for the stimulation of glucose-1-^{14}C oxidation, one of thyrotropin's known effects. They measured the persistent effects of TSH on glucose carbon-1 oxidation in dog thyroid slices sequentially exposed to bovine TSH at 1°C, washed thoroughly in hormone-free medium, and incubated with glucose-1-^{14}C at 37°C in the absence of hormone. The maximal effect on glucose oxidation was obtained by 2 minutes of preincubation with 100 mU/ml TSH and did not change with preincubations as long as 60 minutes. Exposure of the preincubated, washed tissue to antibovine TSH serum before incubation with labeled glucose reversed the persistent hormone effect without altering the basal rate of $^{14}CO_2$ production or the reactivity of the treated cells to added human TSH. If the preincubation of the slices in the presence of TSH was prolonged beyond 15 minutes, a great part of the subsequent TSH effect became nonsuppressible by antibody. Trypsin at a concentration of 100 μg/ml similarly inhibited the TSH stimulation of glucose-1-^{14}C oxidation. The results of Pastan et $al.$ indicate that TSH is very rapidly "bound" in thyroid slices to sites accessible to anti-TSH antibody and trypsin. Thus one site of TSH interaction with the cell is presumably the cell surface, and such prior association is required for the stimulation of glucose C-1 oxidation. The possibility of intracellular sites of interaction in addition is raised by these experiments because of the failure of antibody to reverse the effects of more prolonged preincubation with hormone. As pointed out by Pastan, these results could also be explained if the hormone were in an altered form on the cell surface, or had initiated reactions whose subsequent course is independent of the continued presence of the hormone. Similar results, using stimulation of ^{32}P into phospholipids as an assay, have been reported by Burke (1968a).

In a subsequent paper Macchia and Pastan (1967) reported that preincubation of dog thyroid slices with an enzyme from the growth medium of $Clostridia$ $perfringens$ also abolished the subsequent TSH stimulation of glucose-1-^{14}C oxidation. Such inhibition had previously been observed with preparations of phospholipase C (Dumont and Burelle, 1964). The $Clostridia$ enzyme, which appeared also to be phospholipase C, did not alter the baseline rate of $^{14}CO_2$ production, nor the stimulation of glucose C-1 oxidation by acetylcholine. Added phospholipid protected the slices from the phospholipase effect. These experiments suggest that phospholipase C, by disruption of the membrane binding sites, interferes with TSH binding at the cell surface. However, one cannot rule out an alternative explanation, i.e., that the enzyme results in loss of elements (e.g., substrates and enzymes) necessary for TSH action, but that hormone binding is not necessarily impaired. The experimental results have been confirmed by Burke (1969a) using stimulation of phospholipogenesis as the indicator.

The authors suggest that, "if TSH binding were impaired, but without complete destruction of the binding sites, a response to TSH might have been observed when the TSH concentration was increased 40-fold." In their experiment thyroids that were unresponsive to 25 mU/ml did not respond to concentrations as high as 1000 mU/ml. The concentration of phospholipase used was not noted. It seems important to clarify this hypothesis. One would only expect to observe an effect of high TSH concentration if the result of phospholipase C action on the membrane were a decrease in the *affinity* of the hormone receptor for TSH. To test this hypothesis adequately one must carefully select a concentration of phospholipase C which does not totally destroy the membrane binding sites, i.e., which does not completely inhibit the subsequent TSH effect. Only under these conditions can an effect of high concentrations of TSH be detectable.

The papers of Pastan and his colleagues present indirect evidence which supports but does not prove the existence of specific plasma membrane TSH receptors. The method chosen to study binding has both advantages and disadvantages. By choosing an assay which depends on a subsequent metabolic effect of the hormone an element of specificity and a criterion of function are introduced, i.e., one has selected for an *effective* hormone–receptor interaction. However, glucose C-1 oxidation is an indirect effect of TSH and multiple factors must come into play between the proposed TSH binding to the cell surface and the production of $^{14}CO_2$ from glucose-1-^{14}C. In addition, the use of tissue slices introduces difficulties in interpretation, despite the precautions taken to obtain slices of uniform thickness and to have an effective washing procedure. In short-term incubations the time required for TSH diffusion may be an important factor.

Studies of the effect of TSH on adenyl cyclase, to be discussed in detail below, also indicate that at least one site of TSH–cellular interaction is the plasma membrane. Adenyl cyclase is believed to be located uniquely in plasma membranes (Sutherland *et al.*, 1962). TSH has been shown to activate this enzyme in particulate preparations, slices, and homogenates of thyroid tissue (Klainer *et al.*, 1962; Gilman and Rall, 1968a; Pastan and Katzen, 1967). If it could be shown that all the effects of TSH on the thyroid are mediated by adenyl cyclase activity, or by other plasma membrane constituents, there would be no necessity to postulate intracellular sites of action of TSH.

Although several lines of evidence suggest that TSH binds at the cell surface, a direct *in vitro* demonstration of binding to the thyroid plasma membrane is essential for the proof. One possible approach to this problem is outlined below. Isolated thyroid cells offer several advantages as substrate. The cells are intact and seem to retain their membranal and intracellular organization and compartmentalization. If binding can be demonstrated in isolated cells one can proceed with subcellular fractionation in order to isolate and further characterize the sites, using the binding to whole cells as a reference. The possible effects on binding of the cell isolation procedure must be kept in mind. Binding may be measured by direct assay of ^{125}I-TSH association with the cells. The difficulties inherent in the use of iodine-labeled hormones as biological tracers have already been mentioned (see Section II,B). The essence of the direct demonstration of binding is the proof of specificity. Use of very low concentrations of labeled TSH without unlabeled carrier should favor specific binding. With isolated cells in suspension the TSH concentration per cell is the physiologically important parameter, rather than the concentration per milliliter (Rodesch, 1968). If the binding is reversible, one may differentiate specific from nonspecific association by the addition of a large excess of unlabeled TSH after a preliminary incubation of cells with the labeled hormone. The percentage of radioactivity associated with the cells which can be displaced by unlabeled TSH, but not by unrelated hormones or other proteins, may be considered to be specifically bound. As a further measure of specificity, thyrotropin binding to cells isolated from other tissues by the same methods must be measured.

Preliminary results in our laboratory suggest that after incubation of isolated bovine thyroid cells with 5–10 μU/10^6 cells ^{125}I-TSH (0.025–0.05 mU/ml) for 15 minutes at 37°C there is association of label with the cells. Addition of 1000-fold excess of cold TSH at 15 minutes with further incubation for 10 minutes displaces approximately half of the counts. Addition of a 1000-fold excess of prolactin results in no displacement of radioactivity. Cell-associated radioactivity appears to be maximal within 5 minutes of addition of hormone. These very early experiments appear to be a direct demonstration of TSH binding sites in the thyroid plasma membrane which have at least some specificity for the hormone. Experiments are in progress to further characterize the binding, to establish whether it satisfies the biological criteria of a receptor, as already outlined, and to investigate the relationship between the binding and the stimulation of adenyl cyclase and the other metabolic effects of TSH.

D. Evidence from Other Systems for Hormone Binding and Action at the Plasma Membrane

In view of the paucity of data on the binding of TSH to cellular sites, one is forced to consider results from other systems which may shed light on the problem.

1. Use of Protein Hormones Bound to Insoluble Substrates

We have suggested the possibility that TSH binds selectively to the plasma membrane and exerts its action without entering the cell. Recent experiments of Schimmer *et al.* (1968) offer support for this view in the action of ACTH on the adrenal. In these experiments ACTH or the active eicosapeptide analog was diazotized to the large insoluble molecule *p*-aminobenzoyl cellulose, thus rendering the hormone unable to penetrate the cell. Such hormone complexes, like the unmodified hormone, stimulated the steroid production of adrenal cell cultures. The filtrate of the eicosapeptide–cellulose complex showed no biological activity when compared to β-naphthol cellulose alone. The ACTH–cellulose filtrate contained a small amount of residual stimulating activity. The activity of the hormone–cellulose complex therefore does not appear to be attributable to undiazotized hormone which may have penetrated the cell. Few details of the diazotization procedure are given and the ratio of ACTH or eicosapeptide to cellulose in the final product is not clear. Comparing the response of the adrenal cells to the given amounts of unmodified and modified hormone one must conclude either that the diazotization is very incomplete, or that the process markedly reduces the steroid-stimulating activity of the reacted hormone. The latter might be only a physical effect of the large cellulose molecule, preventing complexed but normally active ACTH molecules from interaction with adrenal cells.

Similar experiments with TSH and isolated thyroid cells would be of great interest. In the absence of precise knowledge as to what TSH effect(s) may be primary and direct, it is important to assay as many hormone effects as possible. The demonstration that effects occurring both early (e.g., iodide organification and decreased iodide trapping) and late after hormone administration (e.g., increased iodide trapping) were stimulated by cellulose-linked TSH would affirm the independence of TSH action and hormone entry into the cell.

2. The Long-Acting Thyroid Stimulator (LATS)

Mammalian thyroids may be stimulated by the long-acting thyroid stimulator (LATS) of thyrotoxic sera as well as by thyrotropin. Investigations have been carried out on the purification, chemical nature, production, and biological activity of this substance and the results compared with those of TSH. The extensive literature has been well summarized in several recent reviews (Burke, 1968b; McKenzie, 1967, 1968).

It is clear now that TSH and LATS are physicochemically and immunologically different, that LATS is neither an altered nor conjugated form of thyrotropin. Yet despite their distinctiveness the pattern of response of the thyroid to the two substances is qualitively the same with no definite exceptions. Quantitative differences in their effects have been noted (Field *et al.*, 1968; Scott *et al.*, 1966). Some effects which have been established for TSH, e.g., the stimulation of cAMP production *in vitro*, have yet to be definitely demonstrated for LATS. But the essential identity of their stimulatory effects on the thyroid has suggested that TSH and LATS may bind and act at the same site.

A number of groups have reported that incubation of LATS-containing sera or LATS-IgG with preparations of human thyroid glands results in a decrease in the *in vivo* stimulating activity of the postincubation supernatants (Beall and Solomon, 1966a; Dorrington *et al.*, 1966; El Kabir *et al.*, 1966; Kriss *et al.*, 1964; Sharard and Adams, 1965). There is now convincing evidence that this represents a specific interaction of LATS with a thyroid cell component, and is not due to enzymatic destruction of LATS (Beall and Solomon, 1966b, 1967) or entirely to nonspecific adsorption of γ-globulin (Benhamou-Glynn *et al.*, 1969; Burke, 1967).

Several observations support the hypothesis that LATS binding *in vivo* occurs on the plasma membrane and that the binding constituent demonstrated *in vitro* is of plasma membrane origin. (1) Antibodies do not normally enter into living cells except by endocytosis. Although LATS has not been proved to function as antibody, it is an immunoglobulin by physicochemical criteria. If LATS does function as an antibody, the antigen would be likely to be available on the plasma membrane (Benhamou-Glynn *et al.*, 1969). (2) LATS initiates endocytosis at the basal margin of thyroid follicular cells (see Benhamou-Glynn *et al.*, 1969). After injection of LATS-IgG and IgG conjugated with ferritin into mice, one observes the formation of ferritin-containing vesicles at the base of the thyroid cells. This is direct demonstration of an effect of LATS on the plasma membrane. It does not necessarily indicate that thyroid recognition of LATS as a thyroid stimulator occurs at these sites. There may be more than one type of LATS binding site on the cell surface. (3) Burke has measured the persistent effects of LATS (and TSH) on ^{32}P incorporation into phospholipids in sheep thyroid slices (Burke, 1968a) in experiments entirely analogous to those of Pastan *et al.* (1966). The stimulation of ^{32}P incorporation, observed maximally after 5 minutes of preincubation with LATS, is abolished by antihuman IgG antibody. However, in contrast to the results with TSH, antibody abolishes the subsequent LATS effect after preincubation for as long as 60 minutes. Also in analogy to the work of Macchia and Pastan (1967), Burke has demonstrated that phospholipase C inhibits LATS and TSH stimulation of phospholipogenesis (Burke, 1969a). (4) Preliminary *in vivo* experiments suggest that LATS stimulates adenyl cyclase activity in the thyroid (Bastomsky and McKenzie, 1968). This observation remains to be confirmed *in vitro*. (5) LATS-binding activity has been found in all thyroid subcellular fractions. Some groups report the microsomes to be most active (Beall and Solomon, 1966a; Dorrington *et al.,* 1966), others the cell sap (Berumen *et al.,* 1967). The subcellular fractions have been prepared by homogenization and differential centrifugation although the exact conditions have varied from study to study. In several systems, the subcellular distribution of enzymes has been demonstrated to depend on the homogenizing conditions (Wallach, 1967). The plasma membrane breaks up into fragments whose size and therefore sedimentation properties depend on the shear forces applied. The greater the shear the greater the fraction which is expected to be recovered in the microsomes. Thus the heterogeneity of location of LATS absorption activity, and its preponderance in the microsomes of many preparations, hints at its original location in the membrane. One must keep in mind the possibility of more than one type of binding substance originating in different cellular loci. (6) Beall *et al.* (1969) have reported that the distribution of LATS-absorbing activity in microsomes and soluble fractions parallels the distribution of 5′-nucleotidase activity in these fractions. 5′-Nucleotidase has been proposed as a plasma membrane marker (Bodansky and Schwartz, 1968; Bosmann *et al.,* 1968). Its validity as a marker in thyroid cells has not been proved.

It would be of great interest to assay LATS-absorbing fractions for adenyl cyclase activity. In all mammalian cells so far tested, the enzyme has been shown to be located in the plasma membrane (Sutherland *et al.,* 1962). When subcellular fractions of turkey erythrocytes are prepared by gentle techniques no adenyl cyclase activity is associated with the microsomes. Following more vigorous homogenization a large percentage of the activity sediments at 78,000g (Davoren and Sutherland, 1963). Active enzyme has not been measurable in significant quantities in soluble fractions. The demonstration of parallelism of adenyl cyclase activity and LATS-absorbing activity in the microsomal particles would endorse the hypothesis that the LATS binding material is a plasma membrane constituent. It would be consistent with the idea, but not proof, that adenyl cyclase is an integral component of the LATS binding site. Subsequent assay of the hormonal sensitivity of the enzyme would further test these ideas. It has been shown that the specific hormonal sensitivity of adenyl cyclase is more easily destroyed than the nonspecific stimulation of the enzyme by sodium fluoride (Robison *et al.,* 1968). If LATS can be shown to stimulate adenyl cyclase in homogenates or thyroid slices but fails to stimulate the activity in the microsomal preparations, one must reason that some degree of membranal organization is required for hormonal sensitivity of the enzyme. Such a result would also imply a LATS receptor site independent of the adenyl cyclase molecule or containing more elements than the adenyl cyclase enzyme alone. If, however, LATS stimulates adenyl cyclase activity in the microsomes, the intimate association of recognition and catalytic subunits of adenyl cyclase in a binding site is still a possibility. The microsomal stimulating activity of TSH and unrelated hormones such as ACTH should also be tested.

A variety of bits of evidence suggest that LATS binds and acts at the plasma membrane. But for LATS, as for TSH, there is not yet sufficient direct proof. Similarly, one cannot answer definitively the question of whether LATS and TSH bind at the same site. TSH apparently does not associate specifically with the LATS-binding material of thyroid homogenates, microsomes, or soluble fractions (Beall and Solomon, 1966a; Benhamou-Glynn *et al.*, 1969; Burke, 1967; Dorrington *et al.*, 1966; El Kabir *et al.*, 1966). But the interaction of TSH with these preparations has not been sufficiently studied. The data are fragmentary, coming from studies whose main object is the elucidation of the LATS–cellular interaction. The report of Benhamou-Glynn *et al.* (1969) is the only one in which more than one concentration of tissue was tested. They incubated TSH 0.5 mU/ml with increasing amounts of lyophilized thyroid homogenate and measured the percent decrease in TSH activity in the McKenzie assay (McKenzie, 1958). TSH activity was 78% of control when 1 gram equivalent of homogenate per milliliter was added. With 3.4 gEq/ml tissue the TSH response was nearly the same, 75% of control. Figure 2 compares the binding of LATS and TSH to increasing concentrations of thyroid and kidney homogenate. In contrast to LATS, only a small percentage of TSH activity was absorbed by thyroid homogenate, and this percentage changed very little with increasing amounts of tissue. Nevertheless, it is perhaps premature to conclude conclusively that TSH does not bind to the LATS-binding material. The specific LATS-binding molecule or several different binding molecules must represent a very small percentage of the total preparations, homogenate, microsomes, or cell sap. It is possible that only one binding activity is identical for LATS and TSH and this will only be demonstrable after extensive purification of the cellular subfractions.

Lepp and Oliner (1967) have reported that in a chick bioassay system no LATS activity was demonstrable in samples of LATS serum or LATS IgG which were strongly positive in the mouse. Bovine and human TSH were reproducibly measured in the chick assay. Thus in the chick, and perhaps in other nonmammalian species as well, a binding site for TSH

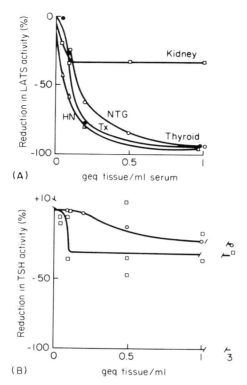

Fig. 2. A. Reduction in LATS activity of thyrotoxic serum after absorption with human thyroid and kidney homogenates. NTG, nontoxic colloid goiter; Tx, thyrotoxic thyroid; HN, hyperfunctioning nodule. B. Effect of absorption with thyroid and kidney homogenate upon activity of pituitary TSH. ○, thyroid; □, kidney (from Benhamou-Glynn *et al.*, 1969, with permission of the authors and publisher).

may be postulated which will not react with LATS. The question remains open whether in mammals a TSH-binding site has evolved in a way now also allowing LATS binding, or whether an independent specific LATS-binding site has developed.

E. Conclusion

The data on the specific interaction of thyrotropin with thyroid cellular components are clearly very incomplete. Both direct and indirect experiments indicate that TSH binds at the cell surface, but other intracellular binding sites have not been ruled out. Preliminary results suggest that this binding is hormone specific. Direct studies of binding in other tissues are largely lacking. Surface binding appears to be reversible but this is the only information available on the characteristics of binding. The nature of the binding site or sites is completely unknown. The relation of TSH binding to the plasma membrane and TSH stimulation of adenyl cyclase activity, presumably also taking place in the plasma membrane, also remains to be elucidated. This coincidence of effects is the best clue at present to a physicochemical interaction leading to biological effect and thus to the primary mechanism of action of thyrotropin.

III. CYCLIC 3′,5′-AMP AS THE INTRACELLULAR MEDIATOR OF THYROTROPIN ACTION ON THE THYROID

A. Introduction: Earlier Arguments on the Sutherland, Rall, Butcher Model

In this part of the review, we shall analyze the evidence which has been presented in favor or against the applicability of the Sutherland, Rall, and Butcher model of hormone action to thyroid and thyrotropin. The principal features of the model are schematized in Fig. 1. As applied to thyrotropin (TSH) and thyroid, this model postulates that TSH binds to a specific receptor on the outer side of the follicular cell plasma membrane. This binding activates adenyl cyclase at the inner side of the membrane. Adenyl cyclase catalyzes ATP transformation to cyclic 3′,5′-AMP (cAMP). Intracellular cAMP activates various enzymes and thus elicits, more or less directly, the hormonal effects. In all the tissues in which this system has been demonstrated, NaF greatly enhances adenyl cyclase activity in disrupted cell preparations, homogenates, or particulate fractions. cAMP is hydrolyzed to 5′-AMP by a specific phosphodiesterase. cAMP phosphodiesterase is inhibited by methylxanthines (theophylline, caffeine, etc.).

As early as 1961, Rall and Sutherland suggested that adenyl cyclase and cAMP were involved in the mechanism of action of TSH. However, in 1966, this model was still little considered (Dumont, 1965, 1966; Field, 1965; Pastan, 1966a; Rosenberg and Bastomsky, 1965). Direct evidence in favor of the Rall and Sutherland hypothesis was available, i.e., the stimulation by TSH of cAMP formation by a sheep thyroid particulate preparation (Klainer *et al.*, 1962). However, in this preliminary study, the TSH concentration was high (500 to 1000 mU/ml), only crude hormone was used, the effect was weak (25 to 30% stimulation), and no attempt had been made to confirm the identity of the product cAMP. Although they were not originally interpreted in this way, additional experimental results were also suggestive of an involvement of cAMP in TSH action:

1. TSH, like epinephrine, ACTH, and glucagon, stimulates lipolysis and its metabolic concomitants in rat adipose tissue (Freinkel, 1961); this effect appears to be mediated by cAMP (Robison *et al.*, 1968).

2. NaF mimics some effects of TSH on thyroid tissue, i.e., the stimulation of glucose carbon-1 and glucose carbon-6 oxidation in thyroid slices (Dumont and Burelle, 1964; O'Malley and Field, 1964).

3. The substitution of K^+ for Na^+ in the incubation medium of sheep thyroid slices produces a TSH-like stimulation of the pentose phosphate pathway (Dumont and Van Sande, 1965) and of the incorporation of ^{32}Pi into phospholipids. Such a substitution leads to an increased intracellular content of cyclic 3′,5′-AMP in several tissues (Robison *et al.*, 1968).

4. Intravenous injection of caffeine in the dog has been reported to stimulate thyroid hormone secretion (Amviagova, 1962).

5. Known intracellular effects of cyclic 3′,5′-AMP (Sutherland and Robison, 1966) could account for several effects of TSH on thyroid tissue: decrease of ^{14}C-glucose incorporation into glycogen (Merlevelde *et al.*, 1963; Dumont and Tondeur-Montenez, 1965) and in the fatty acids of lipids, stimulation of glycolysis (Dumont and Tondeur-Montenez, 1965), and increased iodide exit (Halmi *et al.*, 1960; Isaacs and Rosenberg, 1967).

The fact that cAMP itself did not mimic the effects of TSH on glucose metabolism in beef thyroid slices (Field *et al.*, 1961; Merlevelde *et al.*, 1963) and did not activate the pentose phosphate pathway in sheep thyroid homogenate (Dumont, 1965) cast doubt on the applicability of the model of Sutherland to the thyroid. However, this negative evidence could certainly be explained in several other ways, first of all by a choice of unsuitable experimental conditions. For example, as noted by the authors, the inactivity of extracellular cAMP could be due to its poor penetration and immediate hydrolysis in the cells. Since 1966, the validity of the model of Sutherland for TSH action on the thyroid has been more carefully analyzed.

B. CRITERIA FOR ASSESSING THE VALIDITY OF A POSTULATED MECHANISM OF ACTION OF A HORMONE

A model of the mechanism of action of a hormone may be considered, in a simplified way, as a postulated sequence of causal relationships between the biochemical phenomena which result from the first inter-action of the hormone with the target tissue (Fig. 1). The term bio-chemical phenomenon should be considered in a broad sense; it may represent changes in rate of biochemical reactions as well as of transport or diffusion processes, changes in concentration, availability, or activity of involved biochemical components, etc. To evaluate a model, criteria should be set up which must be fulfilled if the model is not to be rejected. Such criteria may include (Dumont, 1965):

1. Each of the phenomena of the sequence should be evidenced and the kinetics of these phenomena should be consistent with the model.

2. Each of the causal relationships should be demonstrated.

3. Any agent which causes one of the phenomena of the sequence should also produce the consequent phenomena, provided it does not interfere at a distal point of the sequence.

4. The inhibition or suppression of any phenomenon of the sequence should cause the inhibition or suppression of the phenomena which follow.

5. If a reaction or a pathway is activated by an agent, the activation should take place at the level of the rate-limiting factor(s) of the reaction or the rate-limiting step(s) of the pathway.

If these general criteria are met, the model should further be tested quantitatively. For instance, the hormone dose–response curve for each of the phenomena of the sequence, as well as the order of potency of hormone analogs in eliciting the different effects, should be consistent with the model. These qualitative and quantitative criteria have been verified to some extent for the model of TSH action through activation of thyroid adenyl cyclase.

In evaluating the significance of experimental results it should be kept in mind that there are marked species differences in the metabolism of thyroid tissue. For example, TSH at low concentrations decreases glucose carbon-1 oxidation (Dumont, 1964; Gilman and Rall, 1968b; Merlevelde et al., 1963) in beef thyroid slices but increases it in dog thyroid slices. Iodide activates the pentose phosphate pathway in thyroid slices from sheep but not in other species (Dumont, 1961a; Jarrett and Field, 1964). The pattern of thyroid metabolic response to TSH may therefore vary from one species to another. It is also conceivable that identical hormone effects may be brought about by different mechanisms in different species. This would be more likely for effects which represent the end result of various metabolic processes. For instance, any process which increases the ATP consumption in the cell will activate mitochondrial and therefore cell respiration (Lamy et al., 1967); also, any process which increases the supply of $NADP^+$ in the thyroid cell will activate the pentose phos-phate pathway (Dumont, 1961b, 1966). The stimulation of either of these two variables may therefore result from entirely different mechanisms in different conditions.

C. FIRST AND SECOND CRITERIA: THYROTROPIN ENHANCES THE ACCUMULATION OF cAMP IN THYROID TISSUE BY ACTIVATING ADENYL CYCLASE

TSH *in vitro* causes an increase in the cAMP content of bovine thyroid slices (Fig. 3) (Gilman and Rall, 1968a). This effect is potentiated by addition of theophylline 1 mM to the incubation medium. It is present at the first measurement, i.e., 3 minutes after the beginning of the incubation, and is maximal after 3 to 6 minutes. The cAMP content of the slices returns slowly toward control values after this early peak. The maximum cellular cAMP level is observed at about the same time or earlier than the earliest *in vivo* and *in vitro* effects of TSH (Dumont and Rocmans, 1965). In beef thyroid slices, depression by TSH of glucose carbon-1 oxidation begins 15 minutes after the beginning of the incubation (Gilman and Rall, 1968b). So far as it has been tested, the increased cAMP content in the thyroid is specific for TSH. It is obtained with TSH preparations of various purities, and is not caused by other polypeptide hormones (ACTH, LH, FSH, GH, human chorionic gonadotropin, prolactin). Epinephrine is the only compound tested which has a similar although weaker and shorter effect in beef thyroid slices (Gilman and Rall, 1968a). The Rall-Sutherland model of TSH action therefore satisfies to a large extent the first criterion: TSH specifically increases thyroid cAMP content, and this effect occurs earlier than other known effects.

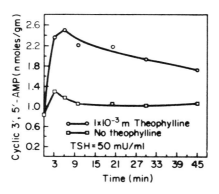

FIG. 3. Time course of cAMP content of bovine thyroid slices following addition of 50 mU/ml of TSH. Incubations were performed in the presence or absence of 1 mM theophylline as indicated (from Gilman and Rall, 1968a, with permission of the authors and publisher).

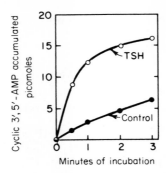

Fig. 4. Time course of the effect of TSH on the accumulation of cAMP in beef thyroid homogenates. Each reaction mixture contained 0.67 mg of thyroid homogenate protein and, where indicated 20 mU of TSH (from Pastan and Katzen, 1967, with permission of the authors and publisher).

TSH could increase the cAMP content of thyroid tissue by increasing its synthesis or by decreasing its hydrolysis. The experiments of Klainer *et al.* (1962) already suggested the possibility of an activation of thyroid adenyl cyclase by TSH. Pastan and Katzen (1967) have shown that TSH enhances the accumulation of cAMP in beef and dog thyroid homogenates within 30 seconds (Fig. 4). This effect is obtained with purified TSH but not with other polypeptide hormones. Although the cAMP formed has not been biologically characterized, it has been identified by paper chromatography in several systems. In beef thyroid homogenates, TSH does not decrease the hydrolysis of cAMP to 5'-AMP (Pastan and Katzen, 1967), i.e., phosphodiesterase activity. An objection has been raised that the latter experiments would not demonstrate any ATP-dependent destruction of the cyclic nucleotide (Gilman and Rall, 1968a). Nevertheless, there is no evidence of an effect of TSH on cAMP catabolism and there seems to be little doubt that TSH increases the intracellular cAMP level in thyroid by activating thyroid adenyl cyclase. Whether the activation of thyroid adenyl cyclase by TSH accounts for each of the effects of the hormone (criterion 2) must now be examined in detail.

D. SECOND CRITERION: EVIDENCE ON THE POSSIBLE MEDIATION BY cAMP OF THE VARIOUS EFFECTS OF THYROTROPIN

1. Interpretation of the Results of Tests Used to Assess if a Hormonal Effect Is Mediated by cAMP

Three types of experiments have been proposed to test the hypothesis that a given effect of TSH is secondary to increased formation of cAMP in thyroid cells:

1. The effect is mimicked by cAMP itself in intact cells.

2. The effect is mimicked by DB-cAMP, a less polar derivative of cAMP.

3. The effect is reproduced or enhanced by inhibitors of cAMP phosphodiesterase, the methylxanthines, theophylline and caffeine.

In experiments which are on the whole animal one should, of course, always take into account the possibility that factors affecting cAMP metabolism may modify thyroid function by acting at other levels than the thyroid. For instance, cAMP has been implicated in the stimulation of pituitary hormone secretion (Gagliardino and Martin, 1968; Jutisz and Llosa, 1969). Besides this general drawback of *in vivo* experiments, each of the proposed tests may give false negative and false positive results.

a. Reproduction of the Effect by cAMP. The reproduction by extracellular cAMP of a hormone effect mediated by intracellular cAMP obviously depends on the penetration and rate of intracellular degradation of the nucleotide, and on the sensitivity of the target system, i.e., in part on the basal level of cAMP intracellular concentration and of organ metabolic activity. These factors may vary with the species and with the pretreatment of the animal as well as with the nature of the experimental system. For instance, whereas TSH, cAMP, and dibutyryl cyclic 3′,5′-AMP (DB-cAMP) enhance the organic binding of iodide in the thyroids of rats pretreated with thyroxine and low doses of TSH, only TSH does so in untreated animals (Ahn and Rosenberg, 1968). In tissues with high phosphodiesterase activity, the small amounts of cAMP penetrating the cells would be rapidly hydrolyzed and thus hormonelike activity would not be expected to be observed unless phosphodiesterase activity is inhibited. Optimal conditions for reproducing TSH effects with extracellular cAMP would therefore seem to be the use of relatively high concentrations of the nucleotide, effective concentrations of methylxanthines and resting thyroids from pretreated animals (Rodesch *et al.*, 1969).

If the effect of cAMP on the thyroid has any specificity, one should not expect other nucleotides to mimic this effect. However, the addition of adenine nucleotides or adenosine to the incubation medium of brain slices results in an increased intracellular concentration of cAMP (Kakiuchi *et al.*, 1969). There is evidence that *in vivo* adenine nucleotides penetrate the thyroid cells: Intraperitoneal injections of ATP markedly enhance the ATP content of rat thyroid (Maayan and Rosenberg, 1968); no evidence of such a penetration was obtained in sheep thyroid slices *in vitro* (Tyler, *et al.*, 1968). Reproduction in the thyroid of cAMP effects by other adenine nucleotides or adenosine could be caused by increase of the cellular cAMP content and therefore does not necessarily bear against the significance of hormone mimicry by cAMP. Another factor in the interpretation of such data is the fact that methylxanthines inhibit in brain slices the enhancement of cyclic 3′,5′-AMP content caused by extracellular adenine nucleotides (Kakiuchi *et al.*, 1969). In the presence of methylxanthines, absence of enhancement of a thyroid function by adenine nucleotides other than cAMP may give therefore no indication on the effects of these adenine nucleotides in the absence of methylxanthines. However, the stimulation of a thyroid function by cAMP and methylxanthines, but not by other adenine nucleotides and methylxanthines, suggests the specificity of cAMP effect. Indeed, inhibition by methylxanthines of an adenine nucleotide effect but not of a cAMP effect would indicate either that the inhibition takes place proximal to cAMP in a sequence involving cAMP or that it occurs in a sequence which does not involve cAMP.

b. *Reproduction of the Effect by DB-cAMP.* In many systems, acyl derivatives of cyclic 3′,5′-AMP such as dibutyryl cyclic 3′,5′-AMP mimic the effects of the hormones on intact cells while cAMP itself is inactive. The effectiveness of DB-cAMP has been attributed to two of its characteristics: (1) Acyl derivatives of cAMP are more resistant to the action of phosphodiesterase than the parent compound. (2) These derivatives were synthesized with the hope that being more lipophilic they would penetrate more rapidly into intact cells (Posternak *et al.*, 1962; Robison *et al.*, 1968); this assumption has not yet been verified experimentally. An effect of DB-cAMP on a system of an intact cell depends on the penetration and the intracellular degradation of the nucleotide, like cAMP, and on the activity of its intracellular derivatives. Intracellular activity probably requires the removal of at least one of the butyryl moieties (Gilman and Rall, 1968b; Robison *et al.*, 1968). Failure of DB-cAMP to reproduce qualitatively or quantitatively TSH effects in intact cells may therefore be due to low rates of penetration or deacylation, to high phosphodiesterase activity or to low intrinsic activity of the acyl derivatives on the target enzymes systems. Acyl derivatives of cAMP might even compete in the cell with cAMP itself for allosteric sites of enzymes and therefore when used with the hormone partially inhibit the hormonal effects. This hypothesis would explain the partial inhibition of TSH stimulation of ^{32}P incorporation into phospholipids by DB-cAMP reported by Burke (1968c).

If the effect of DB-cAMP on the intact tissue is by the same mechanism as the action of cAMP, one would expect this effect not to be produced by butyrate. This should be carefully controlled as it is known that fatty acids alter profoundly the metabolism of thyroid tissue (Freinkel, 1965). Mimicry by adenine nucleotides of DB-cAMP effects does not necessarily bear against the significance of these effects, as these nucleotides may also, as discussed previously (Section III,D,1,a), raise the intracellular concentration of cAMP.

c. Reproduction and Enhancement of the Effect by Methylxanthines. The third way of attempting to increase the intracellular cAMP concentration has been to block its catabolism by phosphodiesterase. The mimicry or potentiation by methylxanthines of hormonal effects mediated by cAMP requires that:

1. The methylxanthines penetrate the cell in sufficient concentrations.
2. Basal phosphodiesterase activity is relatively high.
3. Most of cAMP catabolism occurs by way of the methylxanthine-inhibited cAMP phosphodiesterase; the existence in toad bladder of another catabolic pathway has been suggested (Gulyassi, 1968).
4. Further increases in intracellular cAMP levels can enhance the effect; no potentiation by methylxanthines would be expected at hormone concentrations at which the effect is already maximal.
5. Methylxanthines do not inhibit cAMP formation as theophylline does in brain slices (Kakiuchi *et al.,* 1969).
6. Other unrelated effects of the methylxanthines on cellular metabolism, such as the probable stimulation by theophylline of phosphorylase A phosphatase activity (Hess *et al.,* 1963) or the inhibition of glucose oxidation in fat cells (Zor *et al.,* 1969), do not interfere with the action of intracellular cAMP. Such interference could perhaps be demonstrated by testing inhibition of the TSH effect on the intact cell at concentrations of hormones corresponding to the inflection point of the concentration–effect curve.

Failure to meet any one of these requirements may represent a false negative result, i.e., a negative finding which does not invalidate the model. The fact that methylxanthines may have other effects in intact cells than inhibition of phosphodiesterase, of course, raises the alternative possibility that observed positive, i.e., hormonelike or hormone-potentiating effects, may be unrelated to cyclic 3′,5′-AMP.

In evaluating evidence on methylxanthines, it is important to distinguish between hormone mimicry and hormone potentiation: The first suggests that intracellular cAMP can reproduce a hormonal effect, while the second is the only evidence suggesting that cAMP actually mediates the hormonal effect.

Some information is available on the inhibition of thyroid cAMP phosphodiesterase by theophylline. In beef thyroid homogenates, 1 mM theophylline inhibits phosphodiesterase activity 80–85% (Pastan and Katzen, 1967). A similar concentration considerably increases the effect of TSH on intracellular cAMP accumulation in beef thyroid slices (Gilman and Rall, 1968a). In fact, in the absence of theophylline, the effect of

TSH is small. In this system one would therefore also expect theophylline to potentiate very markedly the subsequent effects of TSH. However, the true potentiation by theophylline of the stimulation of cAMP formation may have been overevaluated in these experiments. In the absence of methylxanthine in the cells, rapid hydrolysis of cAMP between the end of the incubation and the chemical inactivation of phosphodiesterase may considerably decrease the observed values of cAMP content in the slices.

d. *Evidence that a Hormonal Effect Is Not Mediated by cAMP.* The best evidence that a given effect of TSH is not mediated by cAMP would be that agents which mimic other TSH effects by way of the cAMP system do not reproduce the effect in question. However, such a refutation of the model must include compatible data on the concentration–response and time–effect relationships for all the effects, both with TSH and the other agents. There are few data available on the concentration–response relationship. Even high concentrations of cAMP and DB-cAMP may only correspond to very small concentrations of TSH. For instance, as evaluated from their respective effects on glucose C-1 oxidation by thyroid slices of pretreated dogs, concentrations of 5 mM cAMP (in the presence of caffeine), and of 0.075 mM DB-cAMP would be less active than concentrations of 1 mU/ml of bovine TSH (Willems and Dumont, 1969). With the same tissue and variable, Zor *et al.* (1968) obtained lower effects with DB-cAMP 0.75 mM than with TSH 1 mU/ml. In beef thyroid slices, DB-cAMP 1 mM has a similar or slightly lower effect than 2 mU/ml TSH on glucose carbon-1 oxidation and glycolysis (Gilman and Rall, 1968b). In mouse thyroids *in vitro* (Ensor and Munro, 1969), cAMP 10 mM and human TSH 0.66 mU/ml (MRC Human Thyrotrophin Research Standard A) have similar effects on ^{131}I release. It will be seen in the following part of the review that in most negative experiments on hormone mimicry, cAMP, DB-cAMP, and methylxanthines have been compared to concentrations of TSH much higher than their "equipotent" concentration. It is of course hardly possible to increase further the concentrations of cAMP, DB-cAMP, and methylxanthines used, for fear of introducing new artifacts, but the effects of lower TSH concentrations should be explored. Time–effect relationships should also be checked, as Gross and Gafni (1968) have shown that for the TSH-induced intracellular colloid droplet formation this relation varies greatly with the concentration of the hormone. Even with compatible data on concentration–response and time–effect relationships, in the evaluation of negative evidence for one TSH effect, one should take into account the possibilities that DB-cAMP and its derivatives may not act like cAMP on some target enzyme systems, that methylxanthines may inhibit some effects of cAMP, and perhaps that exogenous substances may not get equal access to all intracellular sites.

In conclusion, positive evidence that cAMP, DB-cAMP, or methyl-xanthines mimic an effect of TSH thus suggests that intracellular cAMP could account for a TSH effect and therefore that cAMP is involved in this effect. Potentiation of a TSH effect by a methylxanthine further suggests that the effect of TSH is mediated by cAMP. On the contrary, negative evidence, i.e., the failure to mimic or potentiate a TSH effect, should not be considered to bear against this hypothesis unless other obvious alternative explanations have been ruled out.

2. *Effects of Thyrotropin on Iodine Metabolism*

The possible involvement of cyclic 3′,5′-AMP in the action of TSH on the iodine metabolism in the thyroid has been much investigated *in vivo* and *in vitro*.

a. Early Decrease of Iodide Trapping. In the first hours after its *in vivo* injection, TSH decreases the trapping of iodide by the thyroid (Halmi *et al.*, 1960). This effect is caused by an increase in the iodide exit rate from the thyroid, which is ascribed to greater cell permeability (Halmi *et al.*, 1960; Isaacs and Rosenberg, 1967). A similar effect of TSH has been observed in isolated beef thyroid cells. This hormonal effect was mimicked by DB-cAMP but not by AMP, ATP, or cAMP itself (Wilson *et al.*, 1968). The absence of a cAMP effect is probably explained by the concentrations used: TSH 100 mU/ml, DB-cAMP 3 mM, cAMP 3 mM (see Section III,D,1,d). The evidence is therefore compatible with a mediation of this effect by cAMP.

b. Delayed Stimulation of Iodide Trapping. In the delayed phase of its action, TSH enhances iodide trapping by the thyroid by activating its transport (Halmi *et al.*, 1960). In rats, this effect of TSH was observed with doses of TSH and theophylline, which are inactive when adminis-tered separately (Bastomsky and McKenzie, 1967). In isolated beef thyroid cells, enhancement of iodide trapping was induced by DB-cAMP as well as by TSH, but not by other adenine nucleotides or by cAMP itself (Wilson *et al.*, 1968). Some reservations are necessary in the inter-pretation of both types of experiments: *In vivo* experiments do not demonstrate a direct effect of theophylline on the thyroid, and the in-creased iodide uptake in isolated cells might be related to a structural reorganization of the cells (aggregation, formation of intracellular fol-licular lumina, etc.) rather than to an activation of iodide transport (Nève *et al.*, 1968). Nevertheless the combination of these two types of results suggests the involvement of cAMP in the TSH stimulation of iodide transport in the thyroid.

c. Enhancement of Iodide Organification and of Iodothyronine Synthesis. TSH *in vivo* stimulates very rapidly the binding of iodide to thyroid proteins, i.e., iodide organification (Rosenberg *et al.*, 1965).

DB-cAMP, as well as cAMP, other adenine nucleotides, and theophylline also stimulated iodide organification in rat thyroid *in vivo* (Ahn and Rosenberg, 1968). For cyclic 3',5'-AMP, this effect has been reproduced in hypophysectomized animals, suggesting that it is direct. This conclusion is supported by the observation that DB-cAMP as well as TSH stimulates iodide organification in various *in vitro* preparations: thyroid slices from pig (Kerkof and Tata, 1969) and dog (Rodesch *et al.*, 1969), and isolated cells from beef (Wilson *et al.*, 1968), and sheep (Rodesch *et al.*, 1969) (Fig. 5). No similar effects were obtained with adenine nucleotides or with butyrate (Rodesch *et al.*, 1969). Under suitable conditions, i.e., in thyroids slices of animals pretreated with thyroid extract and in the presence of caffeine 1 mM, cAMP also stimulated iodide organification. In these slices, the effect of low concentration of TSH was potentiated by caffeine 1 mM, which by itself had no effect (Fig. 6) (Rodesch *et al.*, 1969). In isolated beef thyroid cells, TSH, like DB-cAMP, enhanced the incorporation of iodide preferentially into thyroglobulin (Wilson *et al.*, 1968). These data therefore strongly sup-

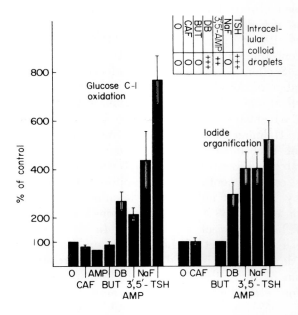

FIG. 5. Effects of TSH, cAMP, and DB-cAMP on iodide organification, glucose carbon-1 oxidation, and intracellular colloid droplet formation in dog thyroid slices. CAF, caffeine 1 mM; AMP, 5'-AMP 7 mM + caffeine 1 mM; BUT, butyrate 0.6 mM; DB, DB-cAMP 0.3 mM; 3',5'-AMP, cAMP 7 mM + caffeine 1 mM; NaF, 3 mM; TSH, 100 mU/ml. Incubation times: 45 minutes and 1 hour (Rodesch *et al.*, 1969).

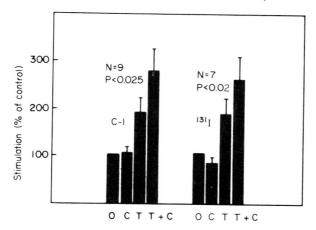

F<small>IG.</small> 6. Potentiation of thyrotropin stimulation of iodide organification and glucose carbon-1 oxidation in dog thyroid slices by caffeine 1 mM (Rodesch *et al.*, 1969). C-1, glucose carbon-1 oxidation; ^{131}I, iodide organification; O, controls; C, caffeine 1 mM; T, TSH 0.5 mU/ml; T + C, TSH 0.5 mU/ml + caffeine 1 mM. Significance of the results calculated on paired data (Dumont, 1964).

port the hypothesis that the stimulation of iodide organification by TSH is mediated by cAMP.

The iodination of MIT to DIT, as well as the oxidative coupling of iodotyrosines to iodothyronines is a function of the activity of the thyroid iodinating system (DeGroot, 1965). TSH injection increased the ratio DIT-^{131}I to MIT-^{131}I and the radioiodine labeling of iodothyronines in rat thyroid *in vivo*. This effect was mimicked by cAMP, other adenine nucleotides, and theophylline (Ahn and Rosenberg, 1968). In mice, doses of TSH and theophylline, which by themselves were ineffective, increased the ratio DIT/MIT and enhanced the synthesis of iodothyronines (Bastomsky and McKenzie, 1967). These effects appear to be direct as they were also obtained *in vitro*, with DB-cAMP in isolated beef thyroid cells (Wilson *et al.*, 1968), and in the case of iodothyronine synthesis, with cyclic 3′,5′-AMP, caffeine, and theophylline but not with other adenine nucleotides, also in mouse thyroids prelabeled *in vivo* (Ensor and Munro, 1969). In the latter experiments cAMP stimulated less the formation of iodothyronines than iodine secretion, in comparison to TSH. In the absence of kinetic data, it is not possible to infer a real discrepancy; TSH may have a more sustained effect than the rapidly hydrolyzed cAMP and iodothyronine formation may depend more closely than secretion on a continuous increase of intracellular cAMP level. Like the stimulation of iodide organification, the effects of TSH on thyroid DIT/MIT ratio and iodothyronine synthesis seem therefore to be mediated by intracellular cAMP.

Increased iodide trapping and iodide organification probably account for the higher uptake of iodide by thyroids of mice treated with TSH for 3 days (Bastomsky and McKenzie, 1967). Increased iodide uptake was also demonstrated with theophylline, and with doses of TSH and theophylline that were ineffective by themselves.

It seems, therefore, probable that cAMP mediates the action of TSH on the anabolism of thyroid hormones in the thyroid, i.e., iodide trapping, iodide organification, and iodothyronine synthesis.

3. Stimulation of Thyroid Secretion by Thyrotropin

The secretion of thyroid hormones by the thyroid involves at least two consecutive processes: the endocytosis of colloid by phagocytosis resulting in the formation of intracellular colloid droplets, and the digestion of colloid thyroglobulin by lysosomal enzymes with the release of thyroid hormone (Nadler et al., 1962; Wetzel et al., 1965).

a. Induction of Endocytosis. As the endocytosis of colloid or other material by thyroid cells has not yet been studied directly, the information available on endocytosis is mainly derived from studies on the formation of apical pseudopods or intracellular colloid droplets in stimulated thyroid tissue. Pseudopod formation is difficult to quantitate, and therefore the frequency of intracellular colloid droplets (number of droplets per cell) has been taken as a measure of the activity of the endocytic process. In interpreting these experiments, one must keep in mind that (1) Light microscope examination may fail to reveal small or less-colored droplets; (2) the frequency of droplets does not necessarily reflect the amount of colloid present in the cells as the size of the droplets varies; (3) the amount of colloid present in a cell at a given time is not a function only of the rate of endocytosis, but a function of the equilibrium between the two processes, endocytosis and colloid digestion.

TSH in vitro causes the formation of colloid droplets in follicular cells of thyroid slices from guinea pig (Junqueira, 1947), dog (Dumont, 1965; Pastan and Wollman, 1967), and rat (Pastan and Macchia, 1967). This effect was mimicked in dog thyroid slices by DB-cAMP (Pastan and Wollman, 1967; Rodesch et al., 1969), and by 10 times higher concentrations of cAMP in the presence of caffeine (Rodesch et al., 1969), but not with concentrations of cAMP equivalent to those of DB-cAMP or in the absence of caffeine (Pastan and Wollman, 1967); these observations have been confirmed by electron microscopy (Nève and Dumont, 1969). The effect was not mimicked by other adenine nucleotides (Pastan and Wollman, 1967; Rodesch et al., 1969), caffeine, or by butyrate (Rodesch *et al.*, 1969). In rat thyroid slices DB-cAMP did not mimic this effect of TSH (Pastan and Macchia, 1967); however, in these experiments, DB-cAMP also failed to reproduce the TSH stimulation of glucose oxidation. As discussed earlier, there are many possible explanations for such a discrepancy, the most obvious one being that DB-cAMP 0.38 mM is too low a concentration to mimic TSH 50 mU/ml. The available evidence is therefore very suggestive of an involvement of cAMP in the induction of colloid phagocytosis in thyroid cells. It would be of great interest to investigate the possible role of cAMP on phagocytosis in other cells.

b. Enhancement of Iodine Secretion. TSH rapidly stimulates the secretion of thyroid iodine (Söderberg, 1959). In mice *in vivo* this effect is mimicked by DB-cAMP (Burke, 1968c), by theophylline, by cAMP and adenine nucleotides, but not by other nucleotides. Doses of TSH and theophylline, which are inactive by themselves, considerably enhance the secretion when they are combined. The latter phenomenon is also observed in rat *in vivo* (Bastomsky and McKenzie, 1967). The stimulation of thyroid iodine secretion by TSH has been reproduced *in vitro* with prelabeled intact mouse thyroids. The effect of TSH was mimicked by theophylline, caffeine, and cAMP but not by other adenine nucleotides. However, in the case of methylxanthines, a large part of the radioiodine release was represented by proteins (Ensor and Munro, 1969). This peculiarity may suggest that this effect of methylxanthines does not correspond to the physiological secretion, or that methylxanthines inhibit the hydrolysis of thyroglobulin. Combinations of maximally effective concentrations of TSH and theophylline, TSH and cAMP, or of cAMP and theophylline produced no increase over the plateau effect of each of these compounds acting separately. The level of these plateaus differed only slightly. These observations are compatible with the hypothesis of a final common pathway in the mechanism of action of these agents. Concentrations of theophylline which gave minimal responses potentiated the effects of lower than maximal concentrations of cAMP and of TSH (Ensor and Munro, 1969). There is therefore very good evidence that the secretory effect of TSH is mediated by cAMP.

4. Effects of Thyrotropin on Glucose and Energy Metabolism

a. Increase of Sugar Uptake. TSH stimulation profoundly alters the pattern of energy and glucose metabolism in the thyroid *in vitro*. It has been reported to increase the distribution space of some stereospecific sugars in calf thyroid slices. This effect was mimicked by cAMP but not by 5′-AMP (Tarui *et al.*, 1963). These observations have suggested that TSH activates stereospecific sugar transport and that this effect may be mediated by cAMP. TSH enhances glucose uptake in sheep and dog thyroid slices (Dumont, 1964; Field *et al.*, 1960; Freinkel, 1960). In beef thyroid slices, this effect was obtained only for large concentrations of TSH and was not mimicked by DB-cAMP (Gilman and Rall, 1968b). However, the concentration of nucleotide used (1 mM) corresponds to low concentrations of TSH (≤ 2 mU/ml) when the relative potency of the two compounds on other aspects of glucose metabolism is compared. It is therefore quite possible that the effect of TSH on glucose and sugar uptake is mediated by cAMP, but the physiological meaning of this effect has been questioned.

   b. *Decrease of Glucose Incorporation into Glycogenlike Material.* TSH decreases the incorporation of glucose-^{14}C into glycogenlike material in beef and dog thyroid slices (Merlevelde *et al.*, 1963; Dumont and Tondeur-Montenez, 1965). F. R. Butcher and Serif (1968) have reported that TSH rapidly elevates phosphorylase A levels in dog thyroid slices. This effect was qualitatively mimicked by DB-cAMP and carbamylcholine. The interpretation of these results has been questioned (Gilman and Rall, 1968b). It assumes that thyroid phosphorylase is of the muscle type. On the contrary, in beef thyroid homogenate, phosphorylase activity is fourfold greater in the presence of ATP, Mg^{++}, and fluoride, than in the presence of 5'-AMP alone, which rather indicates the existence of phosphorylase kinase activity and liver-type phosphorylase. TSH at various concentrations and for various incubation times did not modify significantly phosphorylase activity (Gilman and Rall, 1968b). Gilman and Rall (1968b) have suggested that dog thyroid phosphorylase is also of the liver type and not, as assumed by F. R. Butcher and Serif (1968), of the muscle type. They point out that stimulation by 5'-AMP does not constitute evidence for the presence of a muscle-type phosphorylase, as 10 to 15% of total enzyme activity is expressed when liver phosphorylase is exposed to 5'-AMP as compared to less than 3% in its absence. The finding of increased phosphorylase activity in stimulated dog thyroid slices could therefore merely reflect increases in 5'-AMP tissue level. This hypothesis is quite consistent with the shift toward less phosphorylated nucleotides observed in stimulated thyroid slices (Lamy *et al.*, 1967). It would also explain the decreased activity of phosphorylase in slices incubated in the presence of glucose, and the increased activity in carbamylcholine treated slices. Indeed, glucose would tend to increase AMP phosphorylation while carbamylcholine would favor ATP consumption. Catabolism of DB-cAMP could also, of course, increase the supply of 5'-AMP. There is therefore, at the present time, no evidence that TSH activates glycogenolysis in thyroid tissue. Decreased incorporation of glucose into glycogen may therefore result from inhibition of glycogen synthesis which could, as in the liver (Larner, 1966), be mediated by cyclic 3',5'-AMP.

c. *Enhancement of Glycolysis.* TSH stimulates the formation of lactate in thyroid slices from sheep, dog (Dumont, 1964), and beef (Gilman and Rall, 1968b). In sheep thyroid slices this effect could be explained by the increased uptake of glucose (Dumont and Eloy, 1966). In beef thyroid slices this effect is obtained for concentrations of TSH which do not influence the uptake of glucose; it is quantitatively reproduced by DB-cAMP (Gilman and Rall, 1968b). This observation is in keeping with the known role of cAMP as an allosteric activator of phosphofructokinase (Robison *et al.*, 1968). Conversion of fructose-6-phosphate to fructose-1,6-diphosphate by phosphofructokinase is a rate-limiting step in glycolysis in many tissues (Scrutton and Utter, 1968). The evidence available is therefore compatible with the hypothesis of cAMP-mediated TSH stimulation of glycolysis in the thyroid.

d. *Inhibition by Low Concentrations of Thyrotropin of the Activity of the Pentose Phosphate Pathway in Beef Thyroid.* At low concentrations (≤ 1 mU/ml), TSH decreases the oxidation of glucose carbon 1 in beef thyroid slices (Merlevelde *et al.*, 1963). This effect reflects a decrease of the activity of the pentose phosphate pathway; it occurred in the same range of TSH concentration as the stimulation of cAMP accumulation; it is mimicked by DB-cAMP and theophylline (Gilman and Rall, 1968b), but not by relatively high concentrations of cAMP (Gilman and Rall, 1968b; Merlevelde *et al.*, 1963). However, no evidence on the eventual penetration of cAMP in the cells is available. Contrary to previous observations (Merlevelde *et al.*, 1963), 5'-AMP has been reported to decrease glucose carbon-1 oxidation by beef thyroid slices (Gilman and Rall, 1968b). However, the effect of 5'-AMP appears to be of a different nature than the effect of dibutyryl cyclic 3',5'-AMP as it involves both glucose carbon-1 and carbon-6 oxidation, whereas TSH and DB-cAMP only decrease glucose carbon-1 oxidation. The inhibition of the pentose phosphate pathway by low concentrations of TSH is potentiated by theophylline (Gilman and Rall, 1968b). There is therefore good evidence that this effect of TSH is mediated by cAMP.

e. *Activation of the Pentose Phosphate Pathway.* TSH enhances the oxidation of glucose carbon 1 by thyroid slices, over a wide range of hormone concentrations in some species, e.g., dog (0.06 to 256 mU/ml) (Dumont, 1964), but only at high TSH concentrations in other species, e.g., beef (> 1 mU/ml) (Merlevelde *et al.*, 1963). This effect reflects an activation of the pentose phosphate pathway (Dumont, 1961b; Dumont and Tondeur-Montenez, 1965; Merlevelde *et al.*, 1963). The activity of this pathway is limited, in the thyroid as in many tissues, by the supply of $NADP^+$ (Dumont, 1961b). Stimulation of this pathway may therefore result from the activation of several different processes. For the TSH effect, two such processes have been identified: the oxidation of

NADPH (Dumont and Eloy, 1966) and the synthesis of NADP+ (Pastan *et al.*, 1963). However, enhanced NADP+ synthesis may be at least partly secondary to the activation of NADPH oxidation (Dumont and Eloy, 1966; Oka and Field, 1967).

The stimulation by TSH of glucose carbon-1 oxidation by dog thyroid slices was qualitatively reproduced by DB-cAMP but not by noncyclic adenine nucleotides (Burke, 1968c; Pastan, 1966b; Pastan and Macchia, 1967; Rodesch *et al.*, 1969; Zor *et al.*, 1968), butyrate, caffeine (Rodesch *et al.*, 1969), or theophylline (Zor *et al.*, 1969). In dog the highest concentrations of DB-cAMP used (1 mM) gave responses lower than TSH 5 mU/ml (Willems and Dumont, 1969). This effect was also mimicked by cAMP (3 to 7 mM) itself in the presence of caffeine (1 mM) (Rodesch *et al.*, 1969). The absence of an effect of cAMP reported by other authors (Burke, 1968c; Pastan, 1966b; Zor *et al.*, 1969) can probably be explained by lack of pretreatment of the animals, absence of methylxanthine protection, and the low concentration of nucleotide (<1.5 mM) used. Caffeine 1 mM, although inactive by itself, enhanced the stimulation of glucose carbon-1 oxidation by low, but not by high, concentrations of TSH (> 2 mU/ml) (Rodesch *et al.*, 1969). There is therefore good evidence that this effect is mediated by cAMP. In pig thyroid slices, theophylline (50 μM) failed to enhance the activation of glucose carbon-1 oxidation by low concentrations of TSH (0.5 to 10 mU/ml). This negative evidence seems to bear against the role of cAMP (Zor *et al.*, 1969) but, as discussed earlier, there are many possible explanations for such negative findings, e.g., the use of an ineffective concentration of theophylline.

There is no good evidence that the stimulation of the pentose phosphate pathway by high concentrations of TSH (> 10 mU/ml) is mediated by cAMP. DB-cAMP (up to 1 mM), cAMP and methylxanthines (1 mM) failed to reproduce this effect in beef thyroid slices (Gilman and Rall, 1968b), or to mimic it quantitatively in dog thyroid slices (Pastan, 1966b; Pastan and Macchia, 1967; Rodesch *et al.*, 1969). In the latter system DB-cAMP reproduced, of course, the weaker effects of low concentrations of TSH. Similarly DB-cAMP (up to 0.45 mM), and cAMP failed to stimulate, like high concentrations of TSH, glucose carbon-1 oxidation by sheep (500 mU/ml TSH) (Burke, 1968c) and rat (50 mU/ml TSH) (Pastan and Macchia, 1967) thyroid slices. However, this evidence does not disprove the hypothesis of an involvement of cAMP in this effect as the concentrations of DB-cAMP and cAMP may not be comparable to the concentrations of TSH. The stimulation of glucose carbon-1 oxidation by large concentrations of TSH was not potentiated by methylxanthines in beef, sheep, or dog thyroid slices

(Burke, 1968c; Gilman and Rall, 1968b; Rodesch *et al.*, 1969). Furthermore, above 10 mU/ml, increasing the concentration of TSH further enhanced glucose carbon-1 oxidation but not cAMP accumulation by beef thyroid slices (Gilman and Rall, 1968a,b). However, increasing doses of TSH, while not increasing the measurable tissue level of cAMP after 10 minutes, may sustain this level, thus producing a greater overall effect on glucose carbon-1 oxidation which was measured at 45 minutes. Although none of these negative evidences is therefore conclusive, it seems possible that the stimulation by high concentrations of TSH of the pentose phosphate pathway in thyroid is not mediated by cAMP as is the effect of low concentrations.

f. Enhancement of Pyruvate Oxidation. TSH stimulates the oxidation of pyruvate to CO_2 by the thyroid. The effect is more pronounced for pyruvate carbon 3 which shows a true activation of the oxidation of exogenous pyruvate by the Krebs cycle (Dumont and Tondeur-Montenez, 1965). In beef thyroid slices, a significant effect is only obtained for concentrations of TSH (20 mU/ml) higher than those required for enhancing glycolysis and decreasing glucose carbon-1 oxidation (2 mU/ml). It is therefore not surprising that this effect was not mimicked by DB-cAMP (Gilman and Rall, 1968b) at a concentration (1 mM) corresponding to less than 2 mU/ml TSH. Theophylline (1 mM) mimicked and potentiated the effect of TSH on pyruvate oxidation (Gilman and Rall, 1968b). On the other hand, increasing the concentration of TSH above 10 mU/ml further enhanced pyruvate oxidation, while it did not further increase the tissue concentration of cAMP after 10 minutes' incubation. The evidence on the possible mediation by cAMP of the TSH stimulation of pyruvate oxidation is therefore not conclusive. The stimulation of pyruvate oxidation in thyroid slices probably reflects, like the increased Q_{O_2}, an activation of mitochondrial respiration (Dumont, 1965). We have not observed any modification of the respiration, oxidative phosphorylation, or respiratory control of isolated thyroid mitochondria in the presence of various concentrations of cAMP (Mockel and Dumont, 1969). Even if it is mediated by cAMP, increased mitochondrial respiration in stimulated thyroid tissue seems therefore, as previously suggested, to be caused by an increased ADP supply, i.e., to result from all the endergonic effects of TSH (Lamy *et al.*, 1967).

5. Effects of Thyrotropin on Phospholipid Metabolism

a. Enhancement of Precursor Incorporation into Phospholipids. TSH rapidly stimulates *in vitro* and *in vivo* the incorporation of various precursors (^{32}Pi, inositol-^{14}C, etc.) into thyroid phospholipids, particularly into some classes of phospholipids (e.g., phosphoinositides) (Freinkel,

1964). In sheep thyroid slices the stimulation by TSH of ^{32}P incorporation into phospholipids was mimicked by DB-cAMP, cAMP, and theophylline 0.3 mM. In addition, concentrations of theophylline and of cAMP, AMP, ADP, and ATP, but not of CTP, GTP, or UTP, which are individually ineffective, stimulate phospholipogenesis when added together (Burke, 1968c, 1969b). However theophylline, at concentrations either stimulatory (0.3 mM) or inactive (30 μM), did not potentiate the effect of TSH or LATS (Burke, 1969b). This negative finding may perhaps be explained by an action of theophylline on phospholipid metabolism unrelated to the inhibition of phosphodiesterase: In these experiments it is apparent that theophylline inhibited the effects of maximal concentrations of TSH and LATS. For other species, the role of cAMP seems conflicting. In beef thyroid slices, DB-cAMP, 0.15 to 0.3 mM, increased ^{32}P incorporation into phospholipids in 6 of 12 experiments whereas TSH 100 mU/ml was always active. This discrepancy was unexplained (Pastan and Macchia, 1967). However, as discussed previously, the concentrations of DB-cAMP used corresponded to less than 2 mU/ml of TSH and could not therefore be expected to mimic effects of 100 mU/ml TSH. In dog thyroid slices, DB-cAMP but not cAMP reproduced the TSH stimulation of [32]Pi incorporation into phospholipids (Pastan, 1966b). In a later paper Pastan and Macchia (1967) failed to reproduce the effect of DB-cAMP. No comment was made on this discrepany with their previous results. DB-cAMP did not mimic the TSH stimulation of inositol-^{3}H incorporation into phospholipids either. However, the concentrations of TSH (100 mU/ml) and DB-cAMP (less than 0.4 mM) used in the latter experiments are not comparable. Burke (1968c) has confirmed the effect of DB-cAMP on ^{32}P incorporation into dog thyroid phospholipids and obtained a similar effect with higher concentrations of cAMP but not with 5'-AMP. Differences in tissue sensitivities may account for the discordant results of the two groups. In pig thyroid slices, DB-cAMP, but not cAMP, stimulated, like TSH, the incorporation of [32]Pi into phospholipids (Kerkof and Tata, 1969). Theophylline 50 μM did not potentiate the effect of TSH (Zor et al., 1969); but, as recognized by the authors, it is doubtful whether the concentration used was sufficient to inhibit phosphodiesterase activity significantly. In conclusion, the available evidence strongly supports the hypothesis that cAMP, like TSH, stimulates the incorporation of [32]Pi into thyroid phospholipids and suggests that the TSH stimulation is mediated by cAMP. Of course, overall incorporation of ^{32}P into phospholipids is a complex variable and it would be of interest to obtain information on the pattern of labeling of the different thyroid phospholipids in tissues treated with TSH and cAMP and its analogs.

   b. Phospholipogenesis. In pig thyroid slices DB-cAMP, like TSH, stimulates the incorporation of ^{32}Pi into phospholipids. However, when this incorporation was corrected for the increased uptake of ^{32}Pi, the increase in phospholipid labeling, although still observable with TSH, was no longer apparent in the DB-cAMP stimulated slices. From these experiments, it has been concluded that if DB-cAMP enhances the incorporation of phosphate into phospholipids in thyroid slices, it does not mimic the stimulation of phospholipid synthesis (Kerkof and Tata, 1969). This interpretation is subject to some reservations. A parallel increase in the radioactivity of the precursor pool and in the radioactivity of the product cannot be taken as evidence of increased synthesis, but it does not exclude it. If the precursor pools were enlarged, such data would indeed demonstrate an increased synthesis. In this regard, cAMP and even its acylated derivatives could dilute the specific activity of the adenine nucleotides and even of the phosphate pool. Furthermore, the concentrations of TSH (130 mU/ml) and DB-cAMP (0.30 mM) used in these experiments were not truly comparable, and it is quite possible that lower concentrations of TSH would have given results similar to those obtained with DB-cAMP, i.e., parallel increases of radioctivity of precursors and phospholipids. The fact that in these experiments DB-cAMP quantitatively mimicked the stimulation by TSH of iodide organification does not bear against this argument as this TSH effect reaches a plateau for low concentrations of TSH (Rodesch *et al.*, 1969). Whether cAMP mediates the TSH stimulation of phospholipid synthesis in the thyroid remains, therefore, an open question.

6. *Effects of Thyrotropin on RNA and Protein Synthesis*

a. Stimulation of RNA Synthesis. TSH *in vitro* and *in vivo* stimulates the incorporation of precursors into thyroid RNA (Dumont, 1968). DB-cAMP, but not cAMP or 5'-AMP, qualitatively mimicked the stimulation by TSH of ^{32}Pi incorporation into the RNA of pig thyroid slices. The stimulatory effect of DB-cAMP was no longer apparent when the data were corrected for the uptake of ^{32}Pi. These data suggested that the action of TSH on RNA biosynthesis was not mediated by cAMP (Kerkof and Tata, 1969). However, as discussed previously for the effect of TSH on phospholipid synthesis, this interpretation may not be valid, as it assumes that the size of precursor pools was constant in the different conditions, and that the concentrations of TSH and DB-cAMP used were comparable. It is therefore still quite possible that cAMP mediates the stimulation by TSH of RNA synthesis.

b. Increase of AIB Uptake. TSH stimulates the uptake of α-aminoisobutyrate (AIB)-^{14}C into thyroid slices and isolated thyroid cells (Debons and Pittman, 1962; Tong, 1964). This effect of TSH on isolated cells was

mimicked by DB-cAMP (Wilson *et al.*, 1968). The functional significance
of these data is not clear, as the effect of TSH is specific for α-amino-
isobutyrate and does not reflect a general stimulation of amino acid uptake (Segal *et al.*, 1966).

c. *Enhancement of Amino Acid Incorporation into Proteins.* TSH
stimulates the synthesis of proteins in the thyroid. This effect has been
difficult to demonstrate, probably because of the dilution of intracellular
pools of aminoacids by thyroglobulin hydrolysis *in vivo* or *in vitro* in
short-term experiments. It was quite apparent 12 hours after TSH
injection *in vivo* (Raghupathy *et al.*, 1963). In isolated thyroid cells,
which are devoid of large thyroglobulin stores (Nève *et al.*, 1968), TSH
stimulates the incorporation of leucine-^{14}C into proteins. This effect was
mimicked by DB-cAMP, but not by cAMP or ATP, which suggests the
involvement of cAMP in the TSH effect (Wilson *et al.*, 1968). Whether
this effect truly represents an activation of protein synthesis must be
examined in detail, in view of the suggestion of Kerkof and Tata (1969)
that cAMP may be involved in membrane or transport phenomena but
not in the stimulation of biosyntheses. The main argument in favor of
the hypothesis that increased amino acid incorporation into proteins in
TSH-stimulated isolated cells represents increased protein synthesis,
rather than enhanced uptake of amino acids, has been that deoxyglucose
completely inhibited the stimulation of amino acid incorporation while
it inhibited only partially the stimulation of AIB uptake (Tong, 1967).
This argument is not conclusive. Even if increased incorporation is
secondary to increased uptake, deoxyglucose may very well suppress
stimulation of incorporation by inhibition at the level of protein synthesis. Furthermore, AIB uptake is not a good index of the uptake of
other amino acids by the thyroid (Segal *et al.*, 1966). A better argument
in favor of Tong's hypothesis is the the fact that Segal *et al.* (1966) did
not observe any stimulatory effect of TSH on the uptake of other amino
acids by beef thyroid slices. However, in these negative experiments,
only one very high concentration of TSH (500 mU/ml) was used. In
conclusion, TSH stimulates the incorporation of amino acids into the
proteins of isolated thyroid cells by a mechanism which could involve
cAMP, but it is still uncertain whether this effect reflects a true stimulation
of protein synthesis.

There are other arguments in favor of the hypothesis of a cAMP-
mediated TSH effect on protein synthesis in the thyroid. In sheep
thyroid slices, TSH induced a shift in the ribosome pattern from monosomes to polysomes (Lecocq and Dumont, 1967). A quantitatively
greater shift was obtained in thyroid slices from pretreated dogs with
TSH, DB-cAMP, and cAMP (Lecocq and Dumont, 1969). Such a shift

generally accompanies an activation of protein synthesis (Tata, 1966). Preliminary experiments on aminoacid incorporation into proteins carried out with slices incubated in the presence of saturating concentrations of amino acids indeed indicate such an activation (Lecocq and Dumont, 1969). These data, though incomplete, also suggest a stimulation by TSH of protein synthesis in the thyroid which could be reproduced by enhanced cAMP accumulation. Another suggestive piece of evidence is the activation by cAMP of amino acid incorporation in a thyroid cell-free system (Lissitzky *et al.*, 1969). However, the significance of this effect remains doubtful. It required very large concentrations of cAMP (0.1 mM, i.e., 10^5-fold higher than expected intracellular concentrations) and it was also obtained in liver cell-free systems, although hormones acting on liver adenyl cyclase do not appear to increase the overall protein synthesis in intact liver (Wicks, 1969). In conclusion, although none of the arguments is conclusive, several independent lines of evidence suggest that TSH stimulates through cAMP the synthesis of proteins in thyroid.

E. Third Criterion: Effects on Thyroid Metabolism of Agents Which Enhance cAMP Accumulation

If an effect of TSH is mediated by cAMP, any agent which increases the intracellular concentration of this nucleotide in the thyroid should reproduce the hormonal effect, unless the agent independently inhibits a more distal step in the cause–effect sequence.

1. Epinephrine

Epinephrine has been reported to enhance cAMP accumulation in beef thyroid slices. This effect was inhibited by a β-receptor inhibitor (dichloroisoproterenol), but not by an α-inhibitor (phenoxybenzamine) (Gilman and Rall, 1968a). However, Pastan and Katzen (1967) did not observe any stimulation of adenyl cyclase activity by epinephrine in beef thyroid homogenate. Epinephrine reproduces two effects of TSH, the stimulation of glucose carbon-1 oxidation by thyroid slices, and of the organification of iodide by isolated calf thyroid cells, but neither of them seems mediated by cAMP in the case of epinephrine. The first effect is caused by the catalytic oxidation of NADPH by adrenochrome in the thyroid cells (Pastan *et al.*, 1962; Hupka and Dumont, 1963) and the second is inhibited by α-(α-phentolamine) but not by β-(propanolol) inhibitors (Maayan and Ingbar, 1968). No effect of epinephrine which could be attributed to cAMP accumulation has therefore been demonstrated in thyroid.

2. Prostaglandin E_1

Prostaglandin E_1 (PGE_1) inhibits the activation of adenyl cyclase by several hormones in fat cells, but enhances the accumulation of cAMP in numerous tissues, e.g., lung, spleen, diaphragm, testis, etc. (R. W. Butcher and Baird, 1968). If PGE_1 increases cAMP accumulation in thyroid tissue, it should mimic the cAMP-mediated TSH effects. Indeed PGE_1 activated iodide organification (Rodesch et al., 1969), glucose carbon-1 oxidation (Rodesch et al., 1969; Zor et al., 1969), and contrary to a previous report (Rodesch et al., 1969), intracellular colloid droplet formation in dog thyroid slices (Fig. 7) (Rocmans et al., 1969). The latter result has been confirmed by electron microscopy, which showed in addition that PGE_1, like TSH, induces the formation of numerous pseudopods at the apex of the follicular cells (Nève and Dumont, 1969).

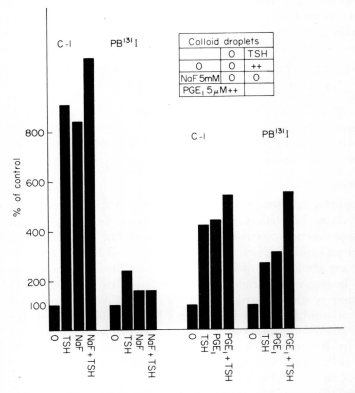

FIG. 7. Effects of fluoride and prostaglandin E_1 on glucose carbon-1 oxidation, iodide organification, and intracellular colloid droplet formation in dog thyroid slices. NaF, 5 mM; PGE_1, 5 μM; TSH, 1 mU/ml.

PGE$_1$ failed to mimic the TSH stimulation of ^{32}Pi incorporation into the phospholipids of dog thyroid slices (Zor *et al.*, 1969). However, the concentration of PGE$_1$ used stimulated glucose carbon-1 oxidation to the same extent as TSH 0.5 mU/ml, and the results suggest that such a concentration of TSH would also have little effect on phospholipid turnover. The available evidence therefore suggests that PGE$_1$ enhances cAMP accumulation in dog thyroid slices and by this mechanism mimics the effects of TSH on glucose carbon-1 oxidation, iodide organification, and colloid phagocytosis.

3. Fluoride

Fluoride is the most potent activator of adenyl cyclase in homogenates of thyroid (Pastan and Katzen, 1967) and of other tissues. It is reported not to act in intact cells presumably because of its poor penetration (Sutherland *et al.*, 1968). However, in relatively high concentrations (10 m*M*) fluoride inhibited glycolysis in sheep thyroid slices as in other tissues (Dumont, 1966), which demonstrates its penetration into the cells. Fluoride should therefore mimic the cAMP-mediated TSH effects that it does not inhibit by different mechanisms. Indeed, fluoride activated glucose carbon-1 oxidation in sheep (Dumont and Burelle, 1964), beef (Pastan *et al.*, 1968), and dog (O'Malley and Field, 1964; Rodesch *et al.*, 1969) thyroid slices, glucose carbon-6 oxidation in sheep and beef thyroid slices (Dumont, 1966; Pastan *et al.*, 1968), iodide organification in dog thyroid slices (Rodesch *et al.*, 1969), and ^{32}Pi incorporation into phospholipids in beef thyroid slices (Pastan and Macchia, 1967).

Fluoride is not a specific agent. Besides its action on adenyl cyclase, it inhibits many enzymes, e.g., enolase, tributyrinase, mitochondrial ATP-ase, etc. It is therefore not surprising that the actions of TSH and NaF on the thyroid *in vitro* differ in several respects. At high concentrations, NaF ($>$ 9 m*M*) enhanced more glucose carbon-6 than glucose carbon-1 oxidation (Dumont, 1966; Pastan *et al.*, 1968). This has been interpreted as evidence that at such concentrations fluoride does not affect enolase (Pastan *et al.*, 1968). This argument is not valid, as glucose carbon-6 oxidation is not a good index of glycolysis, but measures the amount of glucose which is completely oxidized through the Embden-Meyerhof pathway and the Krebs cycle, i.e., only a small proportion of the glucose metabolized through the Embden-Meyerhof pathway (Dumont and Tondeur-Montenez, 1965). In fact, NaF 50 m*M* greatly inhibited the Embden-Meyerhof pathway and mitochondrial activity, as shown by reductions in lactate formation of 78%, glucose uptake of 33%, and oxygen uptake of 27%. Nevertheless, it still increased glucose carbon-6 oxidation by 101%, presumably by increasing considerably the proportion of pyruvate that is completely oxidized (Dumont, 1966). The action of NaF on glucose oxidation seems therefore to reflect two effects: the activation of the pentose phosphate pathway and the inhibition of glycolysis. The latter effect becomes more prevalent at high concentrations. Another difference between the actions of TSH and NaF on the thyroid is the failure of NaF to induce the formation of colloid droplets in the follicular cells of dog thyroid slices (Pastan *et al.*, 1968; Rodesch *et al.*, 1969). This discrepancy would bear against the hypothesis that NaF activates thyroid adenyl cyclase, if, as reported by Pastan *et al.*, (1968), NaF by itself did not inhibit the formation of intracellular colloid droplets induced by TSH. However, in our preparation, with concentrations of NaF (5 m*M*) giving reproducible stimulations of glucose carbon-1 oxidation, and concentrations of TSH equal to or lower than the concentration giving a maximal effect on colloid droplet formation (1 mU/ml), NaF completely inhibited the effect of TSH on colloid droplet formation (Rocmans *et al.*, 1969). As NaF per se appears to inhibit colloid droplet formation, it is not surprising that it fails to elicit this response. In the experiments of Pastan *et al.* (1968), the inhibitory effect of NaF may have been masked because a supramaximal concentration of TSH was used (50 mU/ml). In conclusion, the available data are compatible with the hypothesis that NaF activates adenyl cyclase in intact thyroid cells and in this way mimics the cAMP-mediated TSH effects that it does not inhibit by another mechanism.

F. Fourth Criterion: Effects of Agents Which Decrease cAMP Accumulation

If effects of TSH are mediated by cAMP, inhibition of TSH action at the level of adenyl cyclase, or inhibition of cAMP accumulation should depress these effects.

1. α-and β-Adrenergic Inhibitors

Phentolamine and *d,l*-propanolol, α- and β-adrenergic inhibitors, respectively, inhibited the activation by TSH of adenyl cyclase in dog and in beef thyroid homogenates (Levey *et al.*, 1969). The observation that the effect of *d,l*-propanolol was reproduced by *d*-propanolol and phentolamine suggested that it was not a specific β-adrenergic blockade. These compounds did not act on cAMP phosphodiesterase (Levey *et al.*, 1969). In intact cells inhibitors acting at the adenyl cyclase level should inhibit cAMP-mediated TSH effects but not the action of DB-cAMP or of cAMP. Phentolamine suppressed the stimulation by TSH of glucose carbon-1 oxidation in dog thyroid slices, at concentrations lower (0.3 m*M*) than those which have been shown to abolish nearly completely the TSH stimulation of adenyl cyclase activity (0.75 mM) (Levey *et al.*, 1969). However, the published data suggest that phentolamine also decreased the basal level of glucose oxidation and inhibited its activation by DB-cAMP. *d,l*-Propanolol (0.15–0.3 mM) largely reduced the stimulation by TSH of glucose carbon-1 oxidation in dog thyroid slices (Levey *et al.*, 1969; Zor *et al.*, 1969). While Levey *et al.* (1969) observed only a slight decrease and often no inhibition of the DB-cAMP effect, Zor *et al.* (1969) observed equal inhibition of the TSH, DB-cAMP, and carbamyl-choline effects. It is therefore doubtful that these effects of *d,l*-propanolol are specific and bear only on adenyl cyclase. When slices were incubated with *d,l*-propanolol and then washed, in a subsequent incubation, glucose carbon-1 oxidation could still be activated by DB-cAMP but not by TSH (Levey *et al.*, 1969). Under such conditions, *d,l*-propanolol seems to act at the level of adenyl cyclase. These data, therefore, further suggest that the TSH stimulation of glucose carbon-1 oxidation in dog thyroid slices is mediated by cAMP. On the other hand, concentrations of propanolol which inhibited beef thyroid adenyl cyclase failed to modify the enhancement of glucose carbon-1 oxidation in beef thyroid slices incubated in the presence of high concentrations of TSH (Levey *et al.*, 1969). These data cast some further doubt about the hypothesis that cAMP may mediate the latter effect of TSH.

2. Activators of cAMP Phosphodiesterase

If an effect of TSH is mediated through cAMP, enhancement of cAMP hydrolysis should inhibit this effect of TSH. Little information is available on this topic. Nicotinic acid, which activates phosphodiesterase in other tissues (Robison *et al.*, 1968), was reported not to inhibit the stimulation by TSH of glucose carbon-1 oxidation in dog thyroid slices (Field *et al.*, 1963). In our dog thyroid slice preparations, imidazole 5 mM, which is also reported to activate phosphodiesterase (Robison *et al.*, 1968), did not inhibit the stimulation by TSH of glucose carbon-1 oxidation or iodide organification (Willems and Dumont, 1969). In the absence of any evidence that these compounds actually activated cAMP hydrolysis in the intact cells, interpretation of such data is impossible.

G. Fifth Criterion: Identification of Rate-Limiting Steps and Factors

Little is known on the rate-limiting steps of the metabolic pathways which are activated by TSH in thyroid. Mitochondrial respiration appears to be regulated mainly by ADP supply, i.e., ATP consumption in thyroid as in other tissues. The stimulation of this respiration by TSH may therefore result from the activation of many endergonic processes by the hormone (Lamy *et al.*, 1967), including the synthesis of cAMP. This information gives therefore no clue as to a possible metabolic point of action of cAMP. The pentose phosphate pathway is limited by $NADP^+$ supply in thyroid as in other tissues (Dumont, 1961b; Field *et al.*, 1961). Increased $NADP^+$ supply in the stimulated dog thyroid, and therefore activation of the pentose phosphate pathway, is caused by increased NADPH oxidation (Dumont and Eloy, 1966), and by increased $NADP^+$ synthesis (Pastan *et al.*, 1963), the former mechanism probably preceding the latter (Oka and Field, 1967). How cAMP may affect NADPH oxidation in thyroid is not known. Recent data of Meldolesi and Macchia (1968) suggest that cAMP may activate thyroid NAD kinase, which would be in keeping with the increasing evidence relating cAMP role and its effects on various kinases (Robison *et al.*, 1968). It will be of great interest to learn the respective roles of cAMP activation of thyroid NAD kinase and of the increased $NADP^+$ ($NADP^+ + NADPH$) ratio (Dumont and Eloy, 1966; Oka and Field, 1967) in the stimulation of NADP synthesis by TSH.

H. Possible Involvement of cAMP in the Delayed Growth-Promoting Action of Thyrotropin

We have often emphasized the differences between the early effects of TSH, which occur within the first two hours after the beginning of stimulation, and the delayed effects (Dumont and Rocmans, 1965; Dumont, 1965, 1968). The early effects are related to secretion and are not dependent on new protein and/or RNA synthesis; the delayed effects, which are generally not observed in conventional *in vitro* preparations, are generally related to tissue growth and require such new syntheses. In this review it has been shown that most of the early effects of TSH can probably be accounted for by the primary activation of thyroid adenyl cyclase. Little is known about the possible involvement of cAMP in the delayed effects of the hormone. Kerkof and Tata (1969) have proposed the provocative hypothesis that cAMP may mediate only the rapid effects on cellular permeability and modulation of enzyme activities, but that cAMP does not exert a direct influence on the slower biosynthetic responses to the hormone. The evidence in favor of this concept, i.e., the failure of DB-cAMP to mimic the TSH stimulation of phospholipid and RNA synthesis is certainly not conclusive (Section III,D,5 and 6). Moreover, there are indications of cAMP action on protein synthesis in the thyroid, e.g., stimulation of the incorporation of amino acids by DB-cAMP in isolated beef thyroid cells (Wilson *et al.*, 1968), activation of amino acid incorporation into proteins by cAMP in thyroid acellular systems (Lissitzy *et al.*, 1969), induction by cAMP and DB-cAMP of a shift in the ribosome profile toward polysomes in thyroid slices (Lecocq and Dumont, 1969). Available evidence supports the hypothesis that the stimulation by TSH of iodide uptake is mediated by cAMP. This delayed effect of TSH appears to require *de novo* synthesis of RNA and proteins, i.e., it was inhibited by actinomycin and puromycin (Wilson *et al.*, 1968). Evidence from other systems also seems to bear against the general concept of Kerkof and Tata (1969). cAMP activates protein synthesis in bacteria, at the transcriptional level (Perlman *et al.*, 1969) and at the translational level (Pastan and Perlman, 1969). It appears to mediate the induction in the liver of tyrosine-α-ketoglutarate transaminase and soluble phosphoenolpyruvate carboxykinase by glucagon (Wicks, 1969). Epinephrine and isoproterenol, which are believed to act on the salivary gland by way of the β-receptor and adenyl cyclase, stimulate the growth of this organ. The stimulation by isoproterenol of the synthesis of DNA in the gland is potentiated by theophylline (Malamud, 1969). There are some indications that cAMP may mediate the growth-promoting action of ACTH on the adrenal (Robison *et al.*, 1968). A mechanism for an action of cAMP at the transcriptional level is even suggested by the activation of histone phosphorylation by cAMP (Langan, 1968). However, cAMP has also been shown to inhibit the growth of HeLa cells and strain L cells in culture (Ryan and Heidrick, 1968). This type of evidence is therefore not conclusive. In our opinion, the very challenging concept of Kerkof and Tata does not seem to apply to thyrotropin and thyroid, nor possibly to the action of trophic hormones. It deserves, however, further careful analysis.

If cAMP mediates all the effects, early and delayed, of TSH, very different mechanisms of action of cAMP will certainly apply to these effects. The time–response relationship of the hormonal effects should provide clues to the mechanisms. With continuous TSH stimulation, the increase in the cellular level of cAMP occurs early and is rather short lived (Gilman and Rall, 1968a). Hormonal effects having these same characteristics will be more likely to be caused by a direct activation of the involved enzyme systems by cAMP and should be so investigated. The fact that stimulation of iodide organification by cAMP *in vivo* is very short lived (Ahn and Rosenberg, 1968) suggests a close dependence of this effect on the intracellular cAMP concentration. The activation of metabolic pathways by increased phosphorylation of one of the key components, such as the histones in RNA synthesis, could account for

Cascade effects in TSH action

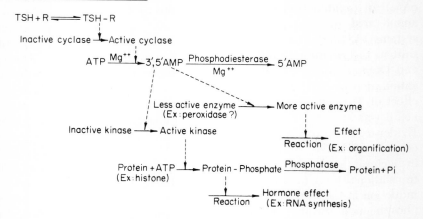

FIG. 8. Application of the cascade concept to the mediation by cAMP of TSH action: proposed working hypothesis; →, known chemical changes; ‒‒→, connect chemical agents and the changes they are known to influence or catalyze.

more delayed and sustained hormonal actions. The cascade concept (Bowness, 1966) has been proposed to explain the great amplification, from stimulus to action, which characterizes the mediation of hormonal action by cAMP. This concept might also explain the wide range of time–response relationships in hormonal action. The application of the cascade concept to the mechanism of action of thyrotropin (Fig. 8) could provide a useful conceptual frame-work for the design of experimental and theoretical studies.

I. Conclusion

Thyrotropin activates thyroid adenyl cyclase and thereby causes the accumulation of cyclic 3′,5′-AMP in the thyroid. There is strong evidence that the TSH stimulation of iodide trapping, iodide organification, iodothyronine synthesis, iodine secretion, phospholipid turnover, and glucose carbon-1 oxidation in dog thyroid, and the TSH inhibition of glucose carbon-1 oxidation in beef thyroid are mediated by increased intracellular cAMP. Thus there is strong support for the hypothesis that TSH exerts these effects by the stimulation of thyroidal adenyl cyclase. Nevertheless, even for these effects, all five criteria proposed to assess the validity of a mechanism of hormonal action have not yet been fulfilled. For only one TSH effect, i.e., the stimulation of the pentose phosphate pathway by high concentrations of hormone, are there indications that cAMP may not be involved; whether this hormonal effect is of physiological significance is doubtful. For all the other effects of TSH tested, the available evidence is compatible with the hypothesis of cAMP mediation of the hormonal effect. The question of non–cAMP-mediated physiological TSH effects deserves further study, particularly among the delayed hormonal effects. The mechanisms of action of cAMP in the thyroid cell must now begin to be investigated at the enzymatic level.

ACKNOWLEDGMENTS

The investigations referred to from this laboratory have been carried out under Contract Euratom, University of Brussels, University of Pisa (026-63-4 BIAC), and aided by grants of the Fonds National de la Recherche Scientifique, and Fonds de la Recherche Scientifique Médicale (Belgium).

E. Schell-Frederick is an advanced Fellow of the Belgian American Educational Foundation.

REFERENCES

Ahn, C. S., and Rosenberg, I. N. (1968). *Proc. Natl. Acad. Sci. U. S.* **60**, 830.

Amviagova, M. C. (1962). *Byul. Eksperim. Biol. i Med.* **54**, 54.

Bastomsky, C. H., and McKenzie, J. M. (1967). *Am. J. Physiol.* **213**, 753.

Bastomsky, C. H., and McKenzie, J. M. (1968). *Endocrinology* **83**, 309.

Beall, G. N., and Solomon, D. H. (1966a). *J. Clin. Invest.* **45**, 552.

Beall, G. N., and Solomon, D. H. (1966b). *J. Clin. Endocrinol. Metab.* **26**, 1382.

Beall, G. N., and Solomon, D. H. (1967). *Biochim. Biophys. Acta* **148**, 495.

Beall, G., Doniach, D., Roitt, I., and El Kabir, D. (1969). *J. Lab. Clin. Med.* **73**, 988.

Benhamou-Glynn, N., El Kabir, D. J., Roitt, I. M., and Doniach, D. (1969). *Immunology* **16**, 187.

Berumen, F. O., Lobsenz, I. L., and Utiger, R. D. (1967). *J. Lab. Clin. Med.* **70**, 640.

Blum, A. S., Greenspan, F. S., Hargadine, J. R., and Lowenstein, J. M. (1967). *Metab., Clin. Exptl.* **16**, 960.

Bodansky, O., and Schwartz, M. K. (1968). *Advan. Clin. Chem.* **11**, 277.

Bosmann, H. B., Hagopian, A., and Eylar, E. H. (1968). *Arch. Biochem. Biophys.* **128**, 51.

Bowness, J. M. (1966). *Science* **152**, 1370.

Burke, G. (1967). *J. Clin. Endocrinol.* **27**, 1095.

Burke, G. (1968a). *Endocrinology* **83**, 1210.

Burke, G. (1968b). *Am. J. Med.* **45**, 435.

Burke, G. (1968c). *J. Clin. Endocrinol. Metab.* **28**, 1816.

Burke, G. (1969a). *Metab. Clin. Exptl.* **18**, 720.

Burke, G. (1969b). *Endocrinology* **84**, 1055.

460   E. Schell-Frederick and J. E. Dumont

Bush, I. E. (1965). *Proc. 2nd Intern. Congr. Endocrinol., London, 1964* Intern. Congr. Ser. No. 83, p. 1324. Excerpta Med. Found., Amsterdam.
Butcher, F. R., and Serif, G. S. (1968). *Biochim. Biophys. Acta* **156**, 59.
Butcher, R. W., and Baird, C. E. (1968). *J. Biol. Chem.* **243**, 1713.
Davoren, P. R., and Sutherland, E. W. (1963). *J. Biol. Chem.* **238**, 3016.
Debons, A. F., and Pittman, J. A. (1962). *Endocrinology* **70**, 937.
DeGroot, L. J. (1965). *New Engl. J. Med.* **272**, 243.
Dorrington, K. J., Carneiro, L., and Munro, D. S. (1966). *J. Endocrinol.* **34**, 133.
Dumont, J. E. (1961a). *Compt. Rend. Soc. Biol.* **155**, 2225.
Dumont, J. E. (1961b). *Biochim. Biophys. Acta* **50**, 506.
Dumont, J. E. (1964). *Bull. Soc. Chim. Biol.* **46**, 1131.
Dumont, J. E. (1965). *Ann. Soc. Roy. Sci. Med. Nat. Bruxelles* **18**, 111.
Dumont, J. E. (1966). *Bull. Soc. Chim. Biol.* **48**, 419.
Dumont, J. E. (1968). *Bull. Soc. Chim. Biol.* **50**, 2401.
Dumont, J. E., and Burelle, R. (1964). *Compt. Rend. Soc. Biol.* **158**, 2500.
Dumont, J. E., and Eloy, J. (1966). *Bull. Soc. Chim. Biol.* **48**, 155.
Dumont, J. E., and Rocmans, P. (1965). *Proc. 2nd Intern. Congr. Endocrinol., London, 1964* Intern. Congr. Ser. No. 83, pp. 81 and 86. Excerpta Med. Found., Amsterdam.
Dumont, J. E., and Tondeur-Montenez, T. (1965). *Biochim. Biophys. Acta* **111**, 258.
Dumont, J. E., and Van Sande, J. (1965). *Bull. Soc. Chim. Biol.* **47**, 321.
El Kabir, D. J., Benhamou-Glynn, N., Doniach, D., and Roitt, I. M. (1966). *Nature* **210**, 319.
Ensor, J. M., and Munro, D. S. (1969). *J. Endocrinol.* **43**, 477.
Field, J. B. (1965). *Proc. 5th Intern. Thyroid Conf., Rome, 1965* pp. 581–584. Academic Press, New York.
Field, J. B. (1968). *Metab., Clin. Exptl.* **17**, 226.
Field, J. B., Pastan, I., Johnson, P., and Herring, B. (1960). *J. Biol. Chem.* **235**, 1863.
Field, J. B., Pastan, I., Herring, B., and Johnson, P. (1961). *Biochim. Biophys. Acta* **50**, 513.
Field, J. B., Johnson, P., Kendig, E., and Pastan, I. (1963). *J. Biol. Chem.* **238**, 1189.
Field, J. B., Remer, A., Bloom, G., and Kriss, J. P. (1968). *J. Clin. Invest.* **47**, 1553.
Freinkel, N. (1960). *Endocrinology* **66**, 851.
Frienkel, N. (1961). *J. Clin. Invest.* **40**, 476.
Frienkel, N. (1964). *In* "The Thyroid Gland" (R. Pitt-Rivers and W. R. Trotter, eds.), Vol. I, p. 131–162. Butterworth, London and Washington, D. C.
Freinkel, N. (1965). *In* "Metabolism and Physiological Significance of Lipids" (R. M. C. Dawson and D. N. Rhodes, eds.), p. 455. Wiley, New York.
Gagliardino, J. J., and Martin, J. M. (1968). *Acta Endocrinol.* **59**, 390.
Gilman, A. G., and Rall, T. W. (1968a). *J. Biol. Chem.* **243**, 5867.
Gilman, A. G., and Rall, T. W. (1968b). *J. Biol. Chem.* **243**, 5872.
Greenspan, F. S., and Hargadine, J. R. (1965). *J. Cell Biol.* **26**, 177.
Gross, J., and Gafni, M. (1968). *Proc. 3rd Intern. Congr. Endocrinol., Mexico City, 1968* Abstr. 37. Excerpta Med. Found., Amsterdam.
Gulyassi, P. F. (1968). *J. Clin. Invest.* **47**, 2548.
Halmi, N. S., Granner, D. K., Doughman, D. J., Peters, B. H., and Muller, G. (1960). *Endocrinology* **67**, 70.

Hechter, O., and Halkerston, I. D. K. (1964). *In* "The Hormones" (G. Pincus, K. V. Thimann, and E. B. Astwood, eds.), Vol. 5, pp. 697–825. Academic Press, New York.

Hess, M. E., Hottenstein, D., Shanfeld, J., and Haugaard, N. (1963). *J. Pharm. Exptl. Therap.* **141**, 274.

Hupka, S., and Dumont, J. E. (1963). *Biochem. Pharmacol.* **12**, 1023.

Isaacs, G. H., and Rosenberg, I. N. (1967). *Endocrinology* **81**, 981.

Jarrett, R. J., and Field, J. B. (1964). *Endocrinology* **75**, 711.

Junqueira, L. C. (1947). *Endocrinology* **40**, 286.

Jutisz, M., and Llosa, P. M. (1969). *Compt. Rend.* **268**, 1636.

Kakiuchi, S., Rall, T. W., and McIlwain, H. (1969). *J. Neurochem.* **16**, 485.

Kerkof, P. R., and Tata, J. R. (1969). *Biochem. J.* **112**, 729.

Klainer, L. M., Chi, Y. M., Freidberg, S. L., Rall, T. W., and Sutherland, E. W. (1962). *J. Biol. Chem.* **237**, 1239.

Kriss, J. P., Pleshakov, V., and Chien, J. R. (1964). *J. Clin. Endocrinol. Metab.* **24**, 1005.

Lamy, F. M., Rodesch, F. R., and Dumont, J. E. (1967). *Exptl. Cell. Res.* **46**, 518.

Langan, T. A. (1968). *Science* **162**, 579.

Larner, J. (1966). *Trans. N. Y. Acad. Sci.* [2] **29**, 192.

Lecocq, R. E., and Dumont, J. E. (1967). *Biochem. J.* **104**, 13C.

Lecocq, R. E., and Dumont, J. E. (1969). Unpublished data.

Lepp, A., and Oliner, L. (1967). *Endocrinology* **80**, 369.

Levey, G. S., Roth, J., and Pastan, I. (1969). *Endocrinology* **84**, 1009.

Lissitzky, S., Manté, S., Attali, J. C., and Cartouzou, G. (1969). *Biochem. Biophys. Res. Commun.* **35**, 437.

Maayan, M. L., and Ingbar, S. H. (1968). *Science* **162**, 124.

Maayan, M. L., and Rosenberg, I. N. (1968). *Endocrinology* **82**, 1223.

Macchia, V., and Pastan, I. (1967). *J. Biol. Chem.* **242**, 1864.

McKenzie, J. M. (1958). *Endocrinology* **63**, 372.

McKenzie, J. M. (1967). *Recent Progr. Hormone Res.* **23**, 1.

McKenzie, J. M. (1968). *Physiol. Rev.* **48**, 252.

Malamud, D. (1969). *Biochem. Biophys. Res. Commun.* **35**, 754.

Mancini, R. E., Vilar, O., Dellacha, J. M., Davidson, O. W., and Castro, A. (1961). *J. Histochem. Cytochem.* **9**, 271.

Meldolesi, M. F., and Macchia, V. (1968). *Proc. 2nd Meeting European Thyroid Assoc., Marseille, 1968* Abstr. 8.

Merlevelde, W., Weaver, G., and Landau, B. R. (1963). *J. Clin. Invest.* **42**, 1160.

Mockel, J., and Dumont, J. E. (1969). Unpublished results.

Nadler, N. J., Sarkar, S. K., and Leblond, C. P. (1962). *Endocrinology* **71**, 120.

Nève, P., and Dumont, J. E. (1969). Unpublished results.

Nève, P., Rodesch, F. R., and Dumont, J. E. (1968). *Exptl. Cell. Res.* **51**, 68.

Oka, H., and Field, J. B. (1967). *Endocrinology* **81**, 1291.

O'Malley, B. W., and Field, J. B. (1964). *Biochim. Biophys. Acta* **90**, 349.

Pastan, I. (1966a). *Ann. Rev. Biochem.* **35**, 369.

Pastan, I. (1966b). *Biochem. Biophys. Res. Commun.* **25**, 14.

Pastan, I., and Katzen, R. (1967). *Biochem. Biophys. Res. Commun.* **29**, 792.

Pastan, I., and Macchia, V. (1967). *J. Biol. Chem.* **242**, 5757.

Pastan, I., and Perlman, R. L. (1969). *J. Biol. Chem.* **244**, 2226.

Pastan, I., and Wollman, S. H. (1967). *J. Cell Biol.* **35**, 262.

Pastan, I., Herring, B., Johnson, P., and Field, J. B. (1962). *J. Biol. Chem.* **237**, 287.

Pastan, I., Johnson, P., Kendig, E., and Field, J. B. (1963). *J. Biol. Chem.* **238**, 3366.

Pastan, I., Roth, J., and Macchia, V. (1966). *Proc. Natl. Acad. Sci. U. S.* **56**, 1802.

Pastan, I., Macchia, V., and Katzen, R. (1968). *Endocrinology* **83**, 157.

Perlman, R. L., De Crombrugghe, B., and Pastan, I. (1969). *Nature* **223**, 910.

Posternak, T., Sutherland, E. W., and Henion, W. F. (1962). *Biochim. Biophys. Acta* **65**, 558.

Raghupathy, E., Tong, W., and Chaikoff, I. L. (1963). *Endocrinology* **72**, 620.

Rall, T. W., and Sutherland, E. W. (1961). *Cold Spring Harbor Symp. Quant. Biol.* **26**, 347.

Robison, G. A., Butcher, R. W., and Sutherland, E. W. (1968). *Ann. Rev. Biochem.* **37**, 149.

Rocmans, P., Willems, C., and Dumont, J. E. (1969). Unpublished results.

Rodesch, F. R. (1968). Unpublished results.

Rodesch, F., and Dumont, J. E. (1967). *Exptl. Cell Res.* **47**, 386.

Rodesch, F. R., Nève, P., Willems, C., and Dumont, J. E. (1969). *European J. Biochem.* **8**, 26.

Rosa, U., Scassellati, G. A., Pennisi, F., Riccioni, N., Giugnone, P., and Giordani, R. (1964). *Biochim. Biophys. Acta* **86**, 519.

Rosa, U., Pennisi, F., Bianchi, R., Federighi, G., and Donato, L. (1967). *Biochim. Biophys. Acta* **133**, 486.

Rosenberg, I. N., and Bastomsky, C. H. (1965). *Ann. Rev. Physiol.* **27**, 71.

Rosenberg, I. N., Athans, J. C., and Isaacs, G. H. (1965). *Recent Progr. Hormone Res.* **21**, 33.

Ryan, W. L., and Heidrick, M. L. (1968). *Science* **162**, 1484.

Schimmer, B. P., Ueda, K., and Sato, G. H. (1968). *Biochem. Biophys. Res. Commun.* **32**, 806.

Schwartz, I. L., and Hechter, O. (1966). *Am. J. Med.* **40**, 765.

Scott, T. W., Good, B. F., and Ferguson, K. A. (1966). *Endocrinology* **79**, 949.

Scrutton, M. C., and Utter, M. F. (1968). *Ann. Rev. Biochem.* **37**, 249.

Segal, S., Roth, H., Blair, A., and Bertoli, D. (1966). *Endocrinology* **79**, 675.

Sharard, A., and Adams, D. D. (1965). *Proc. Univ. Otago Med. School* **43**, 25.

Söderberg, V. (1959). *Physiol. Rev.* **39**, 777.

Sutherland, E. W., and Robison, G. A. (1966). *Pharmacol. Rev.* **18**, 145.

Sutherland, E. W., Rall, T. W., and Menon, T. (1962). *J. Biol. Chem.* **237**, 1220.

Sutherland, E. W., Øye, I., and Butcher, R. W. (1965). *Recent Progr. Hormone Res.* **21**, 623.

Sutherland, E. W., Robison, G. A., and Butcher, R. W. (1968). *Circulation* **37**, 279.

Tarui, S., Nonaka, K., Ikura, Y., and Shima, K. (1963). *Biochem. Biophys. Res. Commun.* **13**, 329.

Tata, J. R. (1966). *Progr. Nucleic Acid Res. Mol. Biol.* **5**, 191.

Tong, W. (1964). *Endocrinology* **75**, 527.

Tong, W. (1967). *Endocrinology* **80**, 1101.

Tyler, D. D., Gonze, J., Lamy, F., and Dumont, J. E. (1968). *Biochem. J.* **106**, 123.

Vanhaelst, L., and Nève, P. (1969). *Z. Ges. Exptl. Med.* **150**, 1.

Wallach, D. F. H. (1967). *In* "The Specificity of Cell Surfaces" (B. D. Davis and L. Warren, eds.), pp. 129–163. Prentice-Hall, Englewood Cliffs, New Jersey.

Wetzel, B. K., Spicer, S. S., and Wollman, S. H. (1965). *J. Cell Biol.* **25**, 593.

Wicks, W. D. (1969). *J. Biol. Chem.* **244**, 3941.

Willems, C., and Dumont, J. E. (1969). Unpublished results.

Wilson, B., Raghupathy, E., Tonoue, T., and Tong, W. (1968). *Endocrinology* **83**, 877.

Zor, U., Lowe, I. P. Bloom, G., and Field, J. B. (1968). *Biochem. Biophys. Res. Commun.* **33**, 649.

Zor, U., Bloom, G., Lowe, I. P., and Field, J. B. (1969). *Endocrinology* **84**, 1082.

CHAPTER 11

The Thymus
as an Endocrine Gland:
Hormones and Their Actions

Allan L. Goldstein and Abraham White

I. INTRODUCTION

The thymus is among the newest additions to the list of endocrine glands. Although this structure has long been of interest to biologists and clinicians, definitive evidence for humoral roles of the thymus has appeared only within recent years. The thymus formerly had been assigned a role of dubious significance in normal physiology and in the etiology of two clinical syndromes, namely, myasthenia gravis and autoimmune thyroiditis. However, within modern times the thymus has become the focus of major studies that have led to the conclusion that this gland is of prime importance in the normal development and maintenance of host immunological competence. The latter encompasses normal lymphoid tissue structure and function, organ and tissue transplantation, autoimmune disorders, immunological deficiency states and certain specific malignant processes.

In this chapter we shall not consider at length the historical aspects of the thymus, since these and other facets of thymic biology have been treated adequately in a number of recent monographs and reviews (Good and Gabrielson, 1964; Seidel *et al.*, 1965; Metcalf, 1966; Miller and Osoba, 1967; Hess, 1968; White and Goldstein, 1968, 1970). Rather, we shall restrict this presentation primarily to those studies that have appeared within the last two decades. It is during this period that the diverse types of thymic extracts and their actions have been described that establish an endocrine role for the thymus gland.

II. MODERN CONCEPTS OF THE THYMUS AS AN ENDOCRINE GLAND

EFFECTS OF EXTIRPATION OF THE THYMUS

One postulate that must be fulfilled experimentally for establishing an endocrine role for a given anatomical structure is evidence that physiological and biochemical deficiencies ensue following extirpation of the organ or tissue in question. Although investigators have sought such evidence in studies of experimental thymectomy over a period of more than 100 years (cf. White and Goldstein, 1968), the results and their interpretations have been controversial. It is only within the last decade that unequivocal evidence has been provided for the deleterious results that ensue as a consequence of removal of the thymus. The severity of the results depend upon the age at which thymectomy is done.

A series of observations of major significance were made practically simultaneously in a number of laboratories (Archer and Pierce, 1961; Fichtelius *et al.*, 1961; Miller, 1961; Arnason *et al.*, 1962; Good *et al.*, 1962; Jankovic *et al.*, 1962) which initiated an explosive growth of interest and publications concerned with the thymus and marked what has been termed "the beginning of the golden age of thymology" (Miller, 1967). These studies established the essential role of the thymus for the development of host immunological competence in neonatal animals. The description of the effects of thymectomy in mice included (1) the development of a syndrome described as a "wasting disease" in the sense that in the operated mice there was a failure to grow at a normal rate, the development of atrophic symptoms, and death of the animals within a few months postoperatively; (2) a deficiency in lymphocyte populations of the blood and the lymphoid tissue; (3) a loss of the ability of the operated animals to elicit cell-mediated immune responses, e.g., the homograft reaction; and (4) a decreased capacity to produce circulating antibodies in response to the administration of some antigens.

It is now established that in many animals, including mice, rabbits, rats, guinea pigs, hamsters, opossums, dogs, and, clinically in the human, removal or failure of the thymus to develop normally in the newborn will produce a diminished population of lymphocytes in lymphoid tissue, as well as in the blood. In addition, host immunological competence either fails to develop normally or is markedly depressed. More recently, it has been recognized that thymectomy in older animals may lead to a slow diminution of lymphocyte populations, with accompanying alteration of phenomena that are dependent on normal numbers and functions of these cells.

The demonstration that thymic tissue enclosed in cell-impermeable Millipore diffusion chambers, as well as thymic grafts or thymocytes, could prevent wasting disease and restore immunological responsiveness in neonatally thymectomized animals of several species (cf. Miller and Osoba, 1967) rekindled interest in a possible humoral function of the thymus (cf. White and Goldstein, 1968). Lymphocytopoietic activity and partial alleviation of some of the deficiencies of neonatally thymectomized mice with cell-free thymic extracts have been reported by several laboratories (cf. Miller and Osoba, 1967; White and Goldstein, 1968, 1970). Additional recent evidence for the secretion by the thymus of a humoral factor influencing host immunological competence has been provided by Stutman *et al.* (1968). These investigators demonstrated that a chemically induced nonlymphoid thymoma, placed in a Millipore chamber in neonatally thymectomized mice, promoted lymphoid tissue growth and restored allograft and graft vs host capacities of the operated animals.

Although reports in the older literature had periodically suggested a relationship of the thymus to the functioning of other endocrine glands, this aspect of interest in the thymus has been revived only relatively recently. This has been due to the recognition of (1) the role of the thymus in influencing lymphoid tissue structure and function, and (2) the long established regulatory actions of at least three additional hormonal secretions viz., growth hormone, the adrenocorticotropic–adrenal corticosteroid secretory axis, and the thyrotropic–thyroid mechanism, on lymphoid tissue proliferation and involution (Dougherty, 1952). It is presently indicated that not only do thymic–adenohypophyseal endocrine secretions alter lymphoid tissue structure and function, but balanced interrelationships among these hormonal factors may comprise homeostatic mechanisms for modulating the functions of the lymphoid system. In view of the significant roles of the latter in host immunological competence, the endocrine roles of the thymus have been the focus of extensive and intensive recent study, including a wide diversity of immunological disorders ranging from the inability to synthesize antibody to autoimmune diseases, to a variety of malignant disorders, both lymphoid and nonlymphoid in origin. Because it is in these areas of biology that an endocrine role for the thymus is more strongly supported, we shall limit our considerations here primarily to reported thymic factors with activities relevant to these topics or whose occurrence has been limited to the thymus or other lymphoid organs. Thus, the presence in thymic tissue of certain basic peptides with, for example, antimycobacterial activity (Dubos and Hirsch, 1954; Hirsch and Dubos, 1954) is not considered relevant to the present survey inasmuch as similar products could be obtained from other organs. Although it is true that a hormone may be present in more than one tissue, e.g., glucagon and calcitonin, the possible immunobiological functions of the thymus seem best established at the present time. It is these features of thymus biology to which this presentation will be primarily limited.

III. CHEMISTRY AND ACTIONS OF THYMIC FRACTIONS

Consideration of the chemistry of the multitude of thymic fractions with reported biological activities is made difficult not only because of the vast diversity of substances of thymic origin that have been described but also because of the enormous range of biological effects claimed. This confused state of the literature can be ascribed in part to several factors: (1) the crude nature of the extracts employed; (2) the embryological development of the thymus, which relates to origins similar to those of the thyroid and the parathyroid glands and, in some species, to the ultimobranchial body; (3) the interrelationships between the thymus and the other endocrine glands, notably the adenohypophysis, thus complicating interpretations of reported assay systems for thymic factors; (4) the constant exchange of the population of the thymus with immigrating cell types of origins other than the thymus; and (5) the possible presence in crude thymic extracts of substances derived from blood and lymph,

TABLE I
SOME REPORTED NONPOLAR FRACTIONS OF THYMIC TISSUE

Type of thymic fraction	Reported biological effects	Bibliographic reference
Lipid extract of calf thymus (thymohormon)	Diabetogenic in rats, guinea pigs, and rabbits; leukocytosis in rats	Bomskov and Brachet, (1940); Bomskov and Sladovic (1940); Bomskov (1941)
Ether soluble–acetone insoluble lipid-rich extract of calf thymus	Blood lymphocytosis in young rabbits	Nakamato (1957)
Rat thymic lipid, lipoprotein, or lipo-soluble components	Lymphocytopoiesis in neonatally thymectomized rats and improved immunological responsiveness of delayed-hypersensitivity type	Jankovic et al. (1965)
CHCl₃-soluble material from calf thymic tissue previously extracted with acetone and anhydrous ether	Decrease in inorganic phosphate and increase in ATP content of skeletal muscle of young, thymectomized rabbits	Potop et al. (1966)
Lipid fraction from calf thymus	Stimulation of growth of Ehrlich ascites tumor in mice	Potop et al. (1967)
Lipid and lipoprotein fractions from calf thymus	Antitumorigenic and inhibitory of cell proliferation	Potop (1966)

including viral agents. One example of the unusual claims made for thymic functions is the long-recognized and frequently reported effects of thymectomy on skeletal growth and maturation (cf. Park and McClure, 1919) and on calcium and phosphate metabolism (Bracci, 1905; Schwartz et al., 1953; Potop et al., 1966). This aspect of thymic action now appears to be somewhat clarified by the recent demonstration of the presence of calcitonin in the human thymus (Galente et al., 1968).

For purposes of convenience, we have assembled in Tables I and II some of the extracts and substances that have been described from thymic tissue and for which diverse biological activities have been claimed. Our compilation has been generally limited to thymic preparations that have been tested in assay systems reflecting an aspect of lymphoid tissue structure and function, or reported to function in metabolism wholly or in part *in lieu* of the thymus in a thymectomized animal. Certain of the properties and biological activities of these preparations will be discussed, with consideration given primarily to reports that have appeared in the past three decades.

TABLE II

SOME REPORTED POLAR FRACTIONS OF THYMIC TISSUE

Type of thymic fraction	Reported biological effects	Bibliographic reference
Lipid and protein free, aqueous, soluble extract of calf thymus (thymocresin)	Growth promotion in young rats	Nowinski (1930, 1932)
Ethanol insoluble fraction of a saline extract of calf thymus	Stimulation of lymphocytopoiesis and increased lymphoid tissue size in adult rats	Roberts and White (1949)
Extract of thymus of irradiated pigs	Production of hyperplastic changes in regional lymph nodes of rats	Gregoire and Duchateau (1956)
Heat labile, nondialyzable saline extracts of thymic tissue	Blood lymphocytosis in young mice	Metcalf (1956, 1966)
Acetic acid extract of calf thymus	Blood lymphocytosis in young rabbits	Nakamoto (1957)
Aqueous–$CHCl_3$–methanol extract of thymus, other organs and human urine (promine, retine, and sterilizing factor)	Stimulation or inhibition of cellular proliferation	Szent-Györgyi et al. (1962, 1967); Hegyeli et al. (1963)
Heat labile thymic protein factor	Lymphocytosis in baby rats subjected to small doses of whole body radiation	Camblin and Bridges (1964)
Saline homogenate of thymi of neonatal mice	Protection of mouse skin against carcinogenic action of 20-methylcholanthrene	Maisin (1964)
Aqueous–acetone or acid–alcohol extracts of AKR mouse thymus	Hypoglycemic activity in AKR mice	Pansky et al. (1965)
Partially purified protein from calf thymus (thymosin)	Stimulation of lymphocytopoiesis and lymphoid tissue growth in either normal, neonatally thymectomized, germ-free, x-irradiated, or adrenal ectomized mice; prevention of wasting disease and restoration of cellular immunity in neonatally thymectomized mice; acceleration of allograft rejection in normal mice; an antithymosin serum	Klein et al. (1965, 1966); A. L. Goldstein et al. (1966); Hardy et al. (1968, 1969); Law et al. (1968); White and Goldstein (1968, 1970); Asanuma et al. (1970); A. L. Goldstein et al. (1970a,b,c)

TABLE II (*continued*)

Type of thymic fraction	Reported biological effects	Bibliographic reference
	suppresses allograft rejection; thymosin either potentiates or negates immunosuppressive effects of antilymphocyte serum	
Purified glycopeptide from veal thymus; molecular weight 3000	Prevention of endocrine imbalances consequent to thymectomy in young guinea pigs and rats	Bernardi and Comsa (1965); Comsa (1965, 1966)
Protein extract from thymus (thymin)	Causes myositis and myasthenia neuromuscularlike block in guinea pigs and inhibition of transmission at the neuromyal synapse in rats	G. Goldstein (1966, 1968)
Cell-free aqueous extract of sheep, calf, or rabbit thymus; 20–40% $(NH_4)_2SO_4$ fraction; properties of a heat labile protein	Stimulation of lymphopoiesis and prevention of wasting in neonatally thymectomized mice; repair of damaged immune responses in neonatally thymectomized mice or in adult thymectomized mice; restoration of cellular and humoral immunity in neonatally thymectomized mice	Trainin *et al.* (1966, 1967, 1968); Trainin and Linker-Israeli (1967)
Sucrose–CaCl$_2$ extract of young rat thymocytes	Prolongation of homograft survival in rats	Brunkhorst and Herranen (1967)
"Crystalline" basic protein from $(NH_4)_2SO_4$ and methanol fractionation of an aqueous extract of calf thymus (lymphocyte-stimulating hormone)	Increase in lymphocyte/polymorphonuclear leukocyte ratios in neonatal mice	Hand *et al.* (1967)
Aqueous or aqueous–acetone extracts of thymus	Neuromuscular blocking activity in rat sciatic nerve-tibialis anterior preparation	Parkes and McKinna (1967)
Purified calcitonin fraction from human thymus	Lowering of blood calcium in normal rats	Galante *et al.* (1968)

In general, two broad classes of biologically active fractions have been described from thymic tissue: those soluble in nonpolar media (Table I), and appearing to be lipoidal in nature, and those soluble in polar solvents (Table II).

A. Thymic Factors Soluble in Nonpolar Solvents (Table I)

Four laboratories have reported biological activity extractable from thymic tissue with nonpolar solvents. In each instance, some care was taken to dehydrate the tissue prior to its exposure to the nonpolar solvents thus giving some assurance that the reported soluble activity was not a result of solubility in an aqueous–organic medium due to residual water in the thymic tissue. Bomskov and co-workers (Bomskov, 1941; Bomskov and Brachet, 1940; Bomskov and Sladovic, 1940) prepared a total lipid extract of calf thymic tissue that provoked hyperglycemia and leukocytosis when injected in rats, guinea pigs, and rabbits. This "diabetogenic agent" was termed "thymohormon." Wells *et al.* (1942) were not able to reproduce the activity of this fraction in young rats, chicks, or pigeons. It may be noted at this point that an insulinlike activity has been described for an acetone-insoluble fraction from thymic tissue of AKR mice (Pansky *et al.*, 1965), although this could not be confirmed in another laboratory (Solomon *et al.*, 1967). In view of the possible interrelationships among the thymus and the adenohypophysis, the question of a possible direct influence of the thymus on parameters of carbohydrate metabolism should be regarded as unanswered at the present time.

Nakamoto (1957) reported that a lipid-rich extract of cow thymus produced a lymphocytosis when injected into young rabbits. This observation was confirmed and extended recently by Jankovic and co-workers (1965) to include additional biological activities on which the thymus has been reported to exert an influence. These investigators prepared a hot chloroform–methanol extract of the residue obtained by lyophilization of a saline homogenate of thymic tissue of young rats. A similar lipid fraction was prepared from rat central nervous tissue and used as one type of control. The emulsified lipid fractions were administered to neonatally thymectomized rats in a total of eleven injections, beginning at 21 days of age and continuing until 58 days of age, each injection being 2.5 mg of thymic (or nervous tissue) lipid. Animals receiving the thymic lipid, in contrast to rats receiving either the lipid from nervous tissue or a third group receiving no treatment, showed normal body weight gain, and a partial restoration of the total number of blood lymphocytes and lymphoid cells in lymph nodes and spleen. In addition, these rats exhibited some restoration of immunological competence as reflected in a delayed hypersensitivity response to bovine serum albumin. The authors suggest that a thymic lipid, lipoprotein or lipid-soluble component, by restoring partially the numbers of tissue and blood lymphocytes, can influence favorably an impaired immunological deficiency of neonatally thymectomized animals.

A series of publications has appeared describing the preparation and effects of lipid fractions from thymic tissue on malignant growth as well as on normal metabolism. These data have been reviewed recently by a member of this group of investigators (Potop, 1966). Both nonpolar and polar fractions were obtained from veal thymus. Lipid fractions were reported to affect a number of metabolic parameters of tumor tissue, e.g., respiration and glycolysis, as well as to retard the rate of growth of several types of experimentally induced tumors. Subsequently, this same laboratory (Potop *et al.*, 1967) described the preparation from thymic tissue of a lipid fraction that accelerated the development and growth of the Ehrlich ascites tumor of mice.

In addition to these reports, Potop and co-workers (1966) have described yet another biological activity for a nonpolar fraction of thymus. A cold chloroform extract was prepared from thymic tissue previously extracted with cold acetone and anhydrous ether. The crude chloroform-soluble fraction, dissolved in olive oil, was administered to young thymectomized rabbits and produced an increase to above-normal values of the depressed level of ATP in the skeletal muscle of the operated animals. In the same experiments, the elevated muscle inorganic phosphate concentrations observed in the operated control rabbits were reduced by injection of the lipid fraction.

B. THYMIC FACTORS SOLUBLE IN POLAR SOLVENTS (TABLE II)

Of the thymic fractions extractable with aqueous, aqueous–acetone, or aqueous–alcohol mixtures, only those described by Nowinski (1930, 1932) and by Szent-Györgyi and co-workers (1962, 1967; Hegyeli *et al.*, 1963) appeared to have biological activity in a fraction devoid of protein. In all other reports of thymic fractions soluble in aqueous media, biological activity has been associated with products having the characteristics of a protein. However, these publications show some variation regarding some of the properties of these protein fractions. Unfortunately, there is a lack in some instances, of suitable criteria of purity and of homogeneity, as well as the use of differing indices for assessment of biological activity. These variables make difficult a comparison of the thymic fractions described by various investigators.

The first reported preparation of an aqueous, cell-free fraction from thymic tissue capable of producing lymphocytosis and lymphoid tissue growth in experimental animals was described by Roberts and White

(1949). These authors fractionated saline extracts of calf thymic tissue by the cold ethanol procedure of Cohn *et al.* (1946). Of the fractions obtained, one was particularly effective in augmenting lymphocytopoiesis when injected daily for 10 days into adult rats. Subsequently, Gregoire and Duchateau (1956) obtained from rat thymic tissue exposed to a lethal dose of x-irradiation, a cell-free fraction that, when administered to normal animals, produced a lymphocytosis and a proliferation of lymphoid tissue. In the same year, Metcalf (1956) described the preparation of an aqueous extract of thymic tissue that, when injected into newborn mice, produced a lymphocytosis. The substance responsible for this activity was termed by Metcalf the lymphocyte stimulating factor (LSF). This same investigator has also reported (Metcalf, 1966) that this factor could be demonstrated in various types of leukemic sera, and that the plasma lymphocytosis factor is of thymic origin.

Supplementing these above observations, many additional reports utilizing crude, cell-free thymic extracts have appeared which support the concept of the production by the thymic cells of a humoral agent that stimulates lymphocytopoiesis and is capable, under appropriate experimental conditions, of replacing thymic function in thymectomized animals (cf. White and Goldstein, 1968, 1970).

The extraction with polar solvents and further purification of crude cell-free thymic extracts with diverse biological effects has been reported by several laboratories. Beginning in 1938, Comsa initiated studies of the effects of thymic extracts in thymectomized-thyroidectomized guinea pigs. These studies stemmed from interests centered on the interrelationships of the thymus to other endocrine organs, notably the thyroid, adrenals, and gonads. In a series of papers over a period of approximately 30 years, Comsa and his co-workers have reported isolation of a polypeptide that in their assay systems, replaces to a significant degree the functions that their laboratory has assigned to the thymus (Comsa, 1957, 1965, 1966; Bezssonoff and Comsa, 1958; Comsa and Bezssonoff, 1958).

Comsa and his co-workers used an initial extraction of fresh calf or sheep thymus with $0.5 M$ H_2SO_4. This extract was neutralized with NH_4OH and fractionated with $(NH_4)_2SO_4$. After removal of material insoluble at a concentration of 35% $(NH_4)_2SO_4$, the biological activity precipitated when $(NH_4)_2SO_4$ was added to saturation. This precipitate was then dissolved in $0.03 M$ HCl, brought to pH 6.2 with NH_3 ($0.15 M$ in ethanol) and the concentration of alcohol raised to 66% by volume. The precipitate that formed was dissolved in $0.03 M$ HCl and brought to pH 7.0 with NH_3 ($0.15 M$ in ethanol). The concentration of ethanol was raised to 20% by volume; this precipitate was discarded. The biologically active fraction in the supernatant was then precipitated from solution by addition of absolute ethanol at a pH 6.2. The precipitated fraction was subjected to successive chromatography on an hydroxyapatite column, using 0.5 M phosphate buffer, and on a G-25 Sephadex column equilibrated with 0.001 M phosphate buffer (pH 6.8). The final biologically active product exhibited apparent homogeneity in the ultracentrifuge. On the basis of gel chromatography, the molecular weight of the product was estimated to be about 3000. The presence of carbohydrate indicated that the isolated fraction was a glycopeptide. Further chemical characterization of this product as well as confirmation of its biological properties are awaited with interest.

A second laboratory has reported (Hand *et al.*, 1967), in a preliminary communication, the isolation from calf thymus of a crystalline, basic protein with the properties of a histone. The product had a molecular weight of approximately 17,000, was heat labile, and was designated as the lymphocyte stimulating hormone (LSH). The assessment of the biological activity of the various fractions, as well as of the final product, was based on the average ratio of lymphocytes to polymorphonuclear leukocytes in the peripheral blood of groups of five neonatal mice used for each assay. The animals were injected intraperitoneally and the blood counts made 6 days later. Unfortunately, in the absence of data for the total numbers of leukocytes, it is not possible to assign significance to ratios of white cell types as an index of an absolute lymphocytopoietic effect. The latter can be assessed only in terms of absolute numbers of total circulating lymphocytes. Metcalf (1966) has presented in detail the difficulties inherent in standardizing assay procedures based on determination of blood lymphocyte levels. It may be anticipated that the protein isolated by Hand and co-workers will be examined in additional biological systems more critically designed to assess lymphocytopoiesis and other functions that have been attributed to the thymus.

Several papers have appeared from the laboratory of Szent-Györgyi and his co-workers, concerned with studies of naturally occurring growth-stimulating and growth-inhibiting substances. In initial publications (Szent-Györgyi *et al.*, 1962; Hegyeli *et al.*, 1963), these investigators described the preparation from calf thymus initially, and later from other biological sources, of several low molecular weight fractions with diverse biological activities. One of these fractions inhibited the growth of a transplantable adenocarcinoma, and was designated as retine. A second fraction, which accelerated growth in this assay system, was named promine. A third fraction was reported to induce a sterile state when administered to mice.

In subsequent years, the Szent-Györgyi group appears to have concentrated their efforts on the isolation and characterization of retine

(Szent-Györgyi *et al.*, 1967). Inasmuch as the data suggest that the low molecular weight products obtained by Szent-Györgyi and his colleagues are not limited to the thymus in their occurrence, and do not as yet have a discernible significance for the control of lymphoid tissue structure and function, they will not be considered further in our discussion of reported thymic hormones. We do recognize, however, that the production of a humoral agent need not be necessarily limited to a single organ or tissue, and that the "purified" products reported by others as being present in the thymus and having significant biological activities could well be contaminated by the presence of low molecular weight aldoketones of the type postulated by Szent-Györgyi *et al.* (1967) as being of prime significance in the regulation of cell division. It may be noted that Dalmasso *et al.* (1963) have reported that in their experiments, a preparation of promine provided by Szent-Györgyi's laboratory was ineffective in preventing wasting disease or restoring immune responses after neonatal thymectomy.

Trainin and his collaborators (1966, 1967, 1968; Trainin and Linker-Israeli, 1967) have also pursued recently the purification from the thymus of what they have termed the thymic humoral factor (THF). Starting with fresh calf or sheep thymus, the initial steps were those described previously from our own laboratory (Klein *et al.*, 1965, 1966; A. L. Goldstein *et al.*, 1966). A homogenate of thymic tissue was prepared with 0.1 M phosphate buffer, pH 7.4. The supernatant fraction obtained by high speed centrifugation (105,000g) for 1 hour was freed of insoluble lipid by passing through gauze. Trainin and his co-workers then introduced fractionation with $(NH_4)_2SO_4$. The precipitate that formed in the 20–40% $(NH_4)_2SO_4$ fraction was redissolved in phosphate buffer and refractionated at least twice by the same procedure until no further precipitate was obtained at $(NH_4)_2SO_4$ concentrations less than 20% of saturation. Purification of the thymic humoral factor was assessed by a bioassay procedure identical to that described by our laboratory (Klein *et al.*, 1965, 1966; A. L. Goldstein *et al.*, 1966) except that adult thymectomized, rather than adult normal, mice were employed. Trainin and his group reported that thymectomy diminishes the degree of nonspecific proliferation of lymphoid tissue seen in normal mice following administration of antigenic substances and thus increases the specificity of the assay. However, our own data (Unpublished results) show that adult CBA/W mice, 1 to 2 months post-thymectomy, still respond with nonspecific lymphoid tissue proliferation to the larger quantities of nonthymic protein used by Trainin and co-workers.

Characterization of the chemical properties of the active THF obtained in the 20–40% $(NH_4)_2SO_4$ fraction led Trainin and his associates (1968) to conclude that biological activity was associated with a heat labile, nondialyzable macromolecule. Activity was destroyed by boiling for 5 minutes as judged by assay of the fraction remaining in solution after this heat treatment. Also, some activity appeared to be lost on dialysis at pH 5.7, due to formation of an insoluble precipitate, and was almost completely destroyed by incubation with pronase. The most active fraction showed four major bands on acrylamide gel electrophoresis in Tris-glycine buffer, pH 8.3. When this same fraction was subjected to ultra-centrifugation, four sedimenting bands were seen with reported s_{20} values of 19, 13, 6.5, and 3. Their relative concentrations were, respectively, approximately 15%, 15%, 40%, and 30%.

Our interest in the hypothesis that the thymus might secrete a humoral factor developed from a series of studies a number of years ago in collaboration with Dr. T. F. Dougherty. These experiments demonstrated that lymphoid cells are a prime target cell of the action of the 11-oxygenated adrenal cortical steroids (Dougherty and White 1945; White, 1947–1948; Dougherty, 1952). The dramatic dissolution of lymphoid tissue produced by these steroid hormones, considered in the light of the known "feed-back" action of target tissue steroid hormones on the secretory activity of the adenohypophysis, led us to postulate that lymphoid tissue might produce one or more factors that could repress or modulate adreno-corticotropic–adrenal cortical secretory levels. As an initial test of this hypothesis, lymphoid tissue extracts were tested for their ability to induce changes characteristic of adrenal cortical suppression, i.e., a state of hypoadrenalcorticalism or of "functional adrenalectomy." This led us to prepare a protein fraction from calf thymus (Roberts and White, 1949), which when administered to normal rats over a 10-day period, stimulated lymphocytopoiesis.

The resurgence of interest in the thymus within the past decade and the evidence for an endocrine role for the gland (cf. Miller and Osoba, 1967; White and Goldstein, 1968, 1970) rekindled our interest in thymic hormones, their nature, functions, and mode of action. These studies have led to the partial purification of a thymic lymphocytopoietic factor, which we have designated as thymosin (A. L. Goldstein *et al.*, 1966). In our recent studies, we utilized initially syngeneic mouse thymic tissue. As the need for larger quantities of tissue developed, we turned to rat thymus and, subsequently, to the calf as a source of thymic tissue for fractionation studies. The fractionation procedure to be described has been developed with calf thymus but is equally applicable to the isolation of thymosin-containing fractions from the thymic tissue of other animals.

All procedures are carried out at 5°C except where indicated. The calf thymic tissue is homogenized with 0.15 M NaCl, followed by a low-speed centrifugation that removes insoluble cellular debris. The supernatant fraction is then centrifuged at 105,000g for approximately 60 minutes; the clear supernatant solution obtained exhibits lymphocytopoietic activity when administered daily to adult CBA/W mice or Swiss-Webster CD-1 mice (Klein *et al.*, 1965, 1966). The treated mice show an increase in lymph node weight expressed as milligrams per gram of body weight, and an increase in the numbers of circulating lymphocytes. The active soluble component of this crude thymic fraction was subsequently further purified (A. L. Goldstein *et al.*, 1966).

Thymosin also stimulates incorporation of precursors of DNA, RNA, and protein into lymph nodes of injected mice, reflecting at a biochemical level the gross increases in lymph node weight seen following thymosin administration to adult mice. The stimulatory action of a thymosin fraction on the incorporation of a labeled precursor into a macromolecular component of mouse lymphoid cells is depicted in Fig. 1. On the basis of these findings, we have developed an *in vivo* assay for use in the purification of thymosin (A. L. Goldstein *et al.*, 1966, Unpublished results).

For the assay of lymphocytopoietic activity, adult CBA/W mice from our own colony are generally used. The animals are injected subcutaneously daily for three days with the material to be assayed. Twenty-two

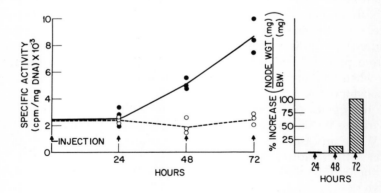

Fɪɢ. 1. Lymph node weights and the incorporation *in vivo* of ³H-thymidine (10 µCi per animal) into the total DNA of pooled axillary, brachial, and inguinal lymph nodes of adult Swiss-Webster CD-1 mice after daily injections (indicated by arrows) of ●——● a calf thymic fraction (fraction 1A) equivalent to 2.4 mg protein (each injection) dissolved in 0.25 ml 0.15 *M* NaCl, and ○ - - - - ○ 0.15 *M* NaCl, 0.25 ml. Animals sacrificed 24 hours after the last injection; each animal received the dose of tritiated thymidine 1.5 hours prior to sacrifice. Each point in the figure represents the value for the pooled lymph nodes of four mice. (From A. L. Goldstein *et al.*, 1966.)

and one-half hours following the third injection of the test preparation, each mouse receives an intraperitoneal injection of 10 μCi of ^{3}H-thymidine. The mice are sacrificed 1½ hours later by cervical fracture, the axillary, inguinal, and brachial lymph nodes rapidly dissected out, transferred to cold 7% perchloric acid and weighed. Pooled nodes from several (generally three or four) mice are then used for extraction of the total DNA. Aliquots of the extract are used for quantitation of the DNA content and for determination of total radioactivity by liquid scintillation spectrometry. A unit of thymosin is arbitrarily defined as the total quantity of protein that, when injected daily for 3 days, produces a 100% increase in incorporation of ^{3}H-thymidine into lymph node DNA.

In the assay of lymphocytopoietic activity, data reflecting a stimulatory action of thymic fractions on lymphocytopoiesis in normal immunologically competent animals must be interpreted with some caution (A. L. Goldstein et al., 1970b). Injection of preparations with a high content of foreign protein into test animals may induce a proliferation of lymphoid tissue characteristic of the response to any antigenic stimulus. We have indeed found this to be the case on injection into adult CBA/W mice of thymic fractions other than those from syngeneic donors. The degree of antigenicity of such fractions is influenced by the quantity of protein administered and the immunological competence of the recipient animal. Thus, the more highly purified thymosin fractions, when administered in microgram quantities (<25 μg), induce lymphoid tissue proliferation not only in normal mice (vida infra) but also in mice whose immunological responsivity has been depressed by prior exposure to x-irradiation (Unpublished results) as well as in either adrenalectomized (Unpublished results), germ-free Swiss (Unpublished results), or neonatally thymectomized (Asanuma et al., 1970) mice. However, at higher doses, the most active preparations of thymosin presently available, and that have the properties of a protein, are antigenic (Hardy et al., 1968, 1969). Antigenic activity, however, can be dissociated from certain of the other biological activities of thymosin to be considered below.

The procedure presently in use in our laboratory for the extraction and purification of thymosin includes several modifications of that described previously (A. L. Goldstein et al., 1966). The thymosin activity in the high speed supernatant fraction (105,000g) described previously is remarkably heat stable, in contrast to the heat lability of the lymphocyte stimulating factor described by Camblin and Bridges (1964), Metcalf (1966), and Trainin et al. (1967, 1968). The relative heat stability of our preparation permits subjecting the previously described high-speed supernatant fraction to a heat step (>80°C for 15 minutes), which precipitates approximately 85% of the contaminating proteins. The latter are removed by high speed centrifugation ($>$20,000g), and the thymosin activity in the supernatant solution precipitated by slowly pouring the latter with stirring into 10 volumes of cold acetone ($-30°C$). The precipitate is collected by filtration and fractionated with (NH_4)$_2SO_4$ (Unpublished results). The most active fraction, which is insoluble in 25–50% saturation with (NH_4)$_2SO_4$, is dialyzed free of salt and further purified by successive column chromatography on DEAE-cellulose and Sephadex G-100. The most highly purified preparation available at this time represents an approximately 200-fold purification in comparison with the activity, per milligram of protein, of the initial high speed supernatant. The fraction obtained from the Sephadex G-100 chromatography step will produce a significant increase in the incorporation of tritiated thymidine into lymph node DNA when injected in a concentration of $<$25 μg protein/day for 3 days in our *in vivo* assay. Preliminary evidence suggests that during the described fractionation of thymosin, an inhibitor of lymphocytopoiesis is removed. This is being explored further.

Chemical studies of the purified thymosin fraction have yielded the following data (Unpublished results). Polyacrylamide gel electrophoresis in Tris-glycine buffer, pH 8.3, reveals one major and two minor components, all migrating toward the anode. On the basis of calibrated Sephadex gel chromatography, the active component appears to have a molecular weight of less than 100,000 and exhibits some tendency to aggregate. The preparation has less than 1% carbohydrate and a trace of lipid, which is not essential for biological activity. This activity is either identical to, or closely associated with, a protein. The preparation at this stage appears to have nothing unusual in its amino acid composition. The purified material, as described also for the early fractions, is relatively heat stable and does not contain nucleic acid. Activity is unchanged after incubation with either RNase or DNase, but is destroyed by digestion with proteolytic enzymes.

Thymosin lymphocytopoietic activity has also been demonstrated in thymic tissue of a variety of animals, including rat, rabbit, guinea pig, hog, and the human. It may also be of interest to report that although it has been generally accepted that the functional roles of the thymus are important primarily for the newborn and for younger animals prior to puberty, we have found that the quantity of thymosin that can be isolated, per gram of thymus, is as great or greater in the thymus of older animals, e.g., old cows and steers, than of young calves (Unpublished results). These observations are in harmony with data suggesting that the humoral agent of the thymus is not elaborated by the mature thymocyte but probably by the epithelial cells. In the thymus of the older animal, the relative proportion of epithelial cells to mature thymocytes is higher than in the thymus of the younger animal. Also, these observations are relevant for the developing concept of a functional role for the thymus in the adult animal (Metcalf, 1965; Miller, 1965; Taylor, 1965).

Similar stimulation of incorporation into lymph node RNA occurs with a precursor such as ^{3}H-uridine, and into the total protein of pooled lymph nodes with either leucine or phenylalanine as labeled precursor, following administration of thymosin for 3 days to mice, as described previously.

In closing this section on the chemistry of thymic fractions, it may be worthwhile to comment briefly on the heat lability of the thymic lymphocytopoietic factor reported by several laboratories (Metcalf, 1956, 1966; Camblin and Bridges, 1964; Trainin et al., 1967, 1968), and the relative heat stability of our lymphocytopoietic factor, thymosin (A. L. Goldstein et al., 1966; White and Goldstein, 1968, 1970). Evidence of heat lability has been based generally on studies in which aqueous solutions of active lymphocytopoietic fractions were subjected to varying degrees of heat treatment, the heat coagulated proteins removed by centrifugation, and the lymphocytopoietic activity of the supernatant fraction assessed by injection into either normal (Metcalf, 1956, 1966; Camblin and Bridges, 1964) or thymectomized (Trainin et al., 1967) mice. It should be emphasized that injection of a wide variety of materials into animals with intact adenohypophyseal–adrenal cortical systems produces a release of endogenous adrenal cortical steroids (Dougherty and White, 1947; White, 1949). Lymphoid cells are end target cells that are exquisitely sensitive to the actions of these steroids, of which one of the most characteristic is an antiproliferative effect based on inhibition of mitosis (Dougherty and White, 1945). Thus, in assessing the possible proliferative activity on lymphoid tissue of a crude supernatant extract that may contain microscopically dispersed particulate material, the test animal may also be receiving an injection that can cause nonspecific release of "antiproliferative" adrenal cortical steroids. In our own experience (unpublished results), solutions to be assayed for possible lymphoid tissue proliferative activity should be first subjected to high speed centrifugation ($>20,000g$) for at least 20 minutes and then passed through a Millipore filter. Thus, an active solution of thymosin subjected to heat treatment and assayed under appropriate precautionary conditions, still exhibits lymphocytopoietic activity. In contrast, if a heated solution of thymosin is centrifuged only at low speed, and the supernatant fraction, which contains discernible, finely dispersed particulate material, is then assayed in our standard 3-day lymphocytopoietic procedure, little biological activity is detectable.

We do not wish to imply that the foregoing comments may explain completely the disparate claims regarding the relative heat stability of the various reported thymic lymphocytopoietic factors. Prior to the time when each of the various preparations is available in chemically pure form, comparisons of properties will not be possible. Also, at that later time, it will be possible to answer more precisely the question of whether there is a single thymic humoral factor that is responsible for the diverse biological effects considered in the following sections, or whether multiple hormonal agents may be synthesized and secreted by the thymus.

IV. BIOLOGICAL EFFECTS OF THYMIC EXTRACTS

As is evident from Tables I and II, a great diversity of biological activities have been attributed to thymic extracts and factors prepared from thymic tissue. We have chosen arbitrarily to restrict our comments in this section primarily to studies of the past decade with cell-free preparations. It was during this period (Miller, 1967; Miller and Osoba, 1967; White and Goldstein, 1968, 1970), as mentioned previously, that unequivocal evidence developed for the role of the thymus in host immunological competence and in the regulation of lymphoid tissue structure and function. These areas encompass tissue and organ transplantation, autoimmune diseases, and host reaction to foreign cell invasions, in addition to myasthenia gravis, in which the thymus has long been implicated.

A. In Nonthymectomized Animals

An enormous diversity of biological activities has been reported for thymic extracts in nonthymectomized animals (Tables I and II). Although our prime considerations in this presentation have been the possible endocrine role of the thymus in the regulation of lymphoid tissue structure and function, including host immunological competence, brief mention should be made of the myriad metabolic effects reported for thymic preparations. In the case of many of these data, as is true generally for the metabolic actions of hormones, it is not always clear which responses reflect those of a true target cell of the administered hormonal preparation, i.e., primary effects, and which are secondary consequences modulated or mediated via some other endocrine organ or, indeed, nonendocrine structure such as the liver. Thus, the diabetogenic (Bomskov, 1941; Bomskov and Brachet, 1940; Bomskov and

Sladovic, 1940) and antidiabetogenic (Pansky *et al.*, 1965) actions reported for thymic fractions could be secondary to effects mediated, for example, by the liver, pancreas, or adenohypophysis. It seems evident that this last endocrine organ, which influences lymphoid tissue structure and function (White, 1949; Dougherty, 1952), may have interrelationships with similar activities now attributable to the thymus and thymic fractions. Comsa (1966), in particular, has presented many data that elucidate certain of these interrelationships, which have also been reviewed by Seidel *et al.* (1965) and Metcalf (1966). Dougherty and his colleagues (1961) have provided evidence for the interesting hypothesis that the thymus may have an important interrelationship with the effects of adrenal cortical steroids by functioning as an important site for the inactivation of cortisol. With this point of view, the thymus could play a role in regulating the circulating levels of effective adrenal cortical steroids. On the other hand, the stimulatory action of thyroxine on the lymphatic system in guinea pigs is not dependent on the presence of the thymus (Ernström, 1965). This is in contrast to the interrelationships of the thymus and thyroid hormone proposed by Comsa (1966). However, the immunological deficiency and hypotrophic thymus and lymphoid tissue of hypopituitary dwarf mice can be restored to normal by treatment with somatotropic (growth) hormone and thyroxine (Pierpaoli *et al.*, 1969). These more recent findings reemphasize the importance of a thymus–hypophyseal relationship.

The long-suspected clinical relationship of the thymus to myasthenia gravis lends additional interest to the reports by G. Goldstein (1966, 1968) that aqueous or aqueous–acetone crude extracts of the thymus can block neuromuscular activity as reflected in the response of a sciatic nerve preparation from normal rats injected with this fraction. The latter thymic humoral factor has been designated as thymin. Additional recent data by G. Goldstein and Hofmann (1969) with normal rats and with rats thymectomized shortly following birth and given multiple isogeneic thymic grafts support the existence of thymin and its possible role in myasthenia gravis and in autoimmune thyroiditis. The method of preparation of the thymin fraction is similar to the early steps in our fractionation procedure for obtaining thymosin, i.e., an initial saline homogenization followed by high speed centrifugation and $(NH_4)_2SO_4$ fractionation. Thymin has also been found to be relatively heat stable (up to 70°C).

If the reported actions of thymic extracts on calcium and phosphate metabolism (Bracci, 1905; Schwartz *et al.*, 1953; Potop *et al.*, 1966) can now find explanation in the recently discovered presence of calcitonin in the human thymus (Galante *et al.*, 1968) and if certain other reported actions of thymic fractions are a result of an indirect influence of other endocrine glands and organs, then the majority of the diverse biological actions of thymic factors (Table I and Table II) can be classified as reflecting alterations in host resistance. The latter may, in turn, be manifested in several ways because of the numerous functions of the lymphoid system. It is in this latter area that the last two decades of research activity have provided experimental evidence for a possible humoral role of the thymus in the normal adult animal. Thus, thymectomy in older animals has been found to lead to a slow diminution of lymphocyte populations with attendant alterations of phenomena that are dependent on normal numbers and functions of these cells (Metcalf, 1965; Miller, 1965; Taylor, 1965).

Our own studies on adult animals have, as mentioned earlier, led to an *in vivo* assay for thymic extracts based on their lymphocytopoietic activity (Klein *et al.*, 1965, 1966; A. L. Goldstein *et al.*, 1966). A detailed histological study has been made in collaboration with Dr. T. F. Dougherty of the University of Utah School of Medicine of the tissues of adult CBA/W mice injected subcutaneously daily with 3 mg of a thymosin fraction for 7 days and sacrified 24 hours following the last injection (Unpublished results). Dr. Dougherty has reported (Personal communication) extensive changes in the cellular populations of both the lymph nodes and spleens in animals treated with these active extracts. There was a marked proliferation of lymphoid cells in the lymph nodes; many of the cells were in active mitosis. Indeed, rather surprising mitotic activity was observed in single free lymphocytes in the loose connective tissue. In the spleen of thymosin-treated animals there was extensive replacement of the erythroid elements by lymphoid cell populations.

As indicated previously, any foreign antigen will promote proliferation of lymphoid tissue in a normal animal and that thymosin activity is identical to, or closely associated with, a protein which itself may be antigenic (Hardy *et al.*, 1968, 1969). Nonetheless, we have demonstrated in properly controlled studies that the administration of thymosin enhances lymphocytopoiesis in normal mice (Klein *et al.*, 1965, 1966; A. L. Goldstein *et al.*, 1966), rats and guinea pigs (Unpublished results), adrenalectomized mice (Unpublished results), germ-free mice (Unpublished results), x-irradiated mice (A. L. Goldstein *et al.*, 1970b), and neonatally thymectomized mice (Asanuma *et al.*, 1970).

We have also demonstrated (Hardy *et al.*, 1968) that in normal mice thymosin administration accelerated first- and second-set skin allograft rejection (Figs. 2 and 3). These data support the concept that thymosin increases the cell-mediated responsiveness of the host animals receiving the allografts. Moreover, injection of an antithymosin serum, prepared in rabbits, into normal mice delayed the rejection of first- and second-

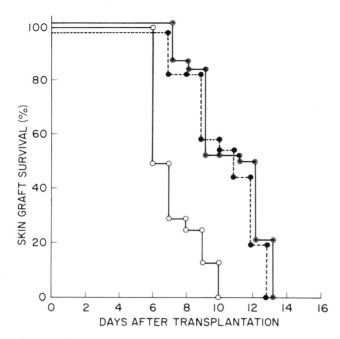

FIG. 2. Effect of thymosin on first-set skin grafts. Adult $B_{10}D_2/Sn$ mice were used as recipients of grafts, and C57Bl/6 mice as donors. Prospective recipients were injected daily with 4.0 mg of thymosin (○—○), saline (●--●), or 4.0 mg of liver extract (⊙—⊙) beginning at 7 days prior to receiving the skin transplant, and injections were continued daily for the duration of the experiment. Beginning at 6 days after transplantation, each animal was examined and evaluations were made of the percent of the skin area transplanted that had survived (ordinate). Each point is the average value for a group of fifteen animals. (From Hardy *et al.*, 1968.)

set skin allografts (Figs. 4 and 5). Of considerable interest and potential practical significance is the recent demonstration by Quint *et al.* (1969) that thymosin may either potentiate or negate the immunosuppressive effects of antilymphocyte serum, depending upon the dosage and time relationships of administration of each of these two agents.

In contrast to our described data for the influence of thymosin on cell-mediated immune phenomena, our attempts to demonstrate an effect of this thymic fraction on humoral antibody responses have been essentially negative. Thus, administration of thymosin to either normal or x-irradiated mice immunized with sheep erythrocytes did not alter the level of their hemagglutinin titers, as compared with similar mice receiving saline as controls (A. L. Goldstein *et al.*, 1970a). Also, thymosin injection in adult thymectomized, lethally x-irradiated, bone-marrow-

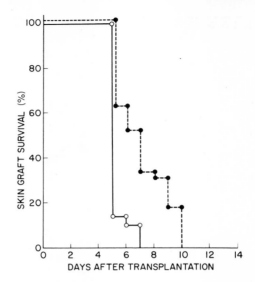

FIG. 3. Effect of thymosin on second-set skin grafts; $B_{10}D_2/Sn$ mice that had rejected a first-set skin graft from C57Bl/6 mice were utilized as recipients of a second C57Bl/6 skin graft. Treatment, evaluation, and number of animals same as in Fig. 2, except that only one control group, which received saline injections (●---●), is presented; thymosin-treated animals (○—○). (From Hardy et al., 1968.)

restored mice immunized with sheep erythrocytes did not elevate significantly the number of antibody forming cells in the spleen (A. L. Goldstein et al., 1970a), as assessed by the Jerne plaque assay (Jerne and Nordin, 1963). These observations suggest that the humoral immune response, in contrast to cell-mediated immune responses, is not, on the basis of presently available data, influenced significantly by the administration of thymosin.

In summary of this section on the biological effects of thymic extracts in normal animals, three conclusions appear warranted:

(1) Thymosin injection augments the rate of lymphoid tissue proliferation in lymphoid organs, as well as in selected individual lymphocytes.

(2) Cell-mediated immune phenomena are augmented in animals treated with thymosin. In contrast, humoral immune responses do not appear to be altered significantly by thymosin administration.

(3) Several laboratories have isolated thymic fractions that, when administered to normal animals, affect metabolic parameters ranging from neuromuscular transmission and modulation of calcium and phosphate metabolism to alterations of blood glucose levels.

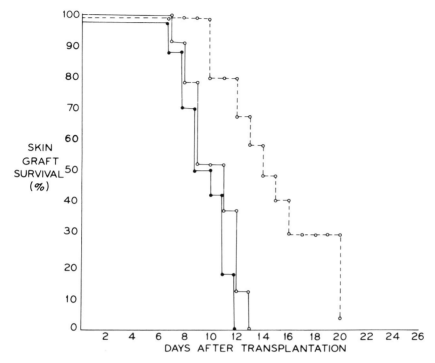

FIG. 4. Effect of a rabbit antithymosin serum on first-set C57Bl/6 skin grafts on A/J mice. Other details as in Fig. 2, except that groups of recipient mice either were not treated (○—○) or received either 0.15 ml normal rabbit serum (●—●) or 0.15 ml antithymosin serum (○ - - - ○) daily for 7 days prior to the allogeneic transplant and daily thereafter. (From Hardy *et al.*, 1968.)

B. In Thymectomized Animals: Replacement Therapy

Several laboratories have provided some evidence that cell-free preparations of thymic tissue may function *in lieu* of the thymus in experimental designs in which obvious deleterious consequences result from absence of the thymus. This approach of replacement therapy is one of the classical means of establishing a possible endocrine role for an extirpated anatomical structure.

Trainin and co-workers (1966, 1967, 1968) have reported that their partially purified fraction of thymic tissue (see Table II) prevents the development of, or ameliorates in part, certain of the deleterious consequences of neonatal thymectomy. Thus, an initial, relatively crude fraction from thymus was reported (Trainin *et al.*, 1966) to prevent

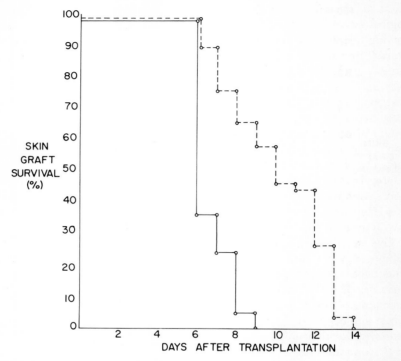

FIG. 5. Effect of a rabbit antithymosin serum on second-set skin grafts. Other details as in Fig. 4 except that recipient A/J mice used had rejected a first-set skin graft and only two groups of animals are presented, one injected with 0.15 ml antithymosin serum daily (○ - - - ○) and the other injected with 0.15 ml normal rabbit serum daily (○—○). (From Hardy *et al.*, 1968.)

partially the lymphoid cell depletion and the wasting disease character-istic of neonatally thymectomized mice. These observations with a crude thymic fraction confirmed the earlier report of DeSomer *et al.* (1963) but are in conflict with the reports of Dalmasso *et al.* (1963) and Miller (1964), who found no beneficial effects of saline extracts of thymus on the wasting syndrome or immunological competence of thymectomized animals.

Shortly after the initial report from their laboratory, Trainin and Linker-Israeli (1967) presented suggestive evidence in support of the claim that their thymic humoral factor restored in part the impaired immune response seen following either neonatal thymectomy or thymectomy combined with sublethal radiation (550 R) in adult mice. The most recent report available from Trainin's laboratory (Trainin *et al.*, 1968), utilizing a refractionated $(NH_4)_2SO_4$ precipitate from calf thymic

extracts, described activity of the thymic humoral factor in several biological systems. Restoration of immunologic reactivity was observed following injection of the thymic fraction in neonatally thymectomized mice,
as reflected in the capacity of the treated animals to reject an allogeneic
tumor graft. In several variations of the graft vs host reaction assay
system, these authors also reported that administration of their thymic
fraction restored partially the immunological competence of spleen cells
from neonatally thymectomized mice.

Our own experience with replacement therapy by thymic fractions,
using a partially purified thymosin preparation, has also been in experiments with neonatally thymectomized mice. In addition, we have used
adult, thymectomized mice subjected to whole body lethal x-irradiation
and maintained with syngeneic bone marrow cells. This latter procedure
has been established as useful in studies of the role of the thymus in
host immunological competence (cf. Miller and Osoba, 1967).

One of our early studies was concerned with whether thymosin could
replace thymic function in the neonatally thymectomized mouse, and
thus moderate the severity of symptoms developing in such operated
animals. These studies have been conducted in collaboration with Dr.
Asanuma of our department (Asanuma *et al.*, 1970). Our CBA/W mice,
when subjected to thymectomy within 24 hours after birth, have a high
mortality incidence; this reaches 75% by 9 weeks postoperatively. The 25%
of the operated animals that survive 63 days or longer look quite normal,
although their body weight is less than normal. These survivors have been
shown to be immunologically impaired and are highly susceptible to
infections. Wasting disease begins to be discernable shortly after weaning, generally about 30 days post-thymectomy, and progresses as the
mice age.

Neonatally thymectomized CBA/W mice were divided into three
groups. Each animal received, beginning 3 days post-thymectomy, an
intraperitoneal injection three times a week during the first week of either
saline, 0.5 mg of bovine serum albumin (BSA), or 0.5 mg of a thymosin
preparation. During the second to the ninth weeks, the dose of protein
was doubled, i.e., each animal received either saline, 1.0 mg of BSA, or
1.0 mg of thymosin three times a week. Injections during these latter
weeks were made subcutaneously.

The data plotted in Fig. 6 illustrate the percent cumulative mortality of
the animals. The results suggest that the rate at which the mice suc-
cumbed was significantly lower in those animals that received thymosin
than in animals that received either saline or BSA. Additional data
obtained in this study are presented in Table III. The thymosin-
treated mice, in contrast to those injected either with saline or with BSA,

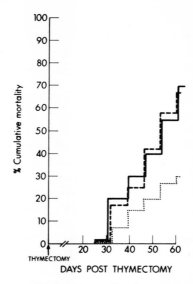

FIG. 6. Cumulative mortality in neonatally thymectomized CBA/W mice. ———, animals injected with saline; - - - - - - -, animals injected with BSA; ...., animals injected with thymosin (Fraction 3; A. L. Goldstein *et al.*, 1966). (From Asanuma *et al.*, 1970.)

have a markedly increased rate of survival and a significantly better rate of increase of body weight. The total leukocyte counts (WBC) in the thymosin-treated mice (7983/mm³) although higher than in the saline- (5476/mm³) or BSA-(6420/mm³) injected animals, still do not return to normal (10,469/mm³) values under these experimental conditions. This is also reflected in the numbers of absolute lymphocytes (LMC),

TABLE III

EFFECT OF THYMOSIN ON NEONATALLY THYMECTOMIZED CBA/W MICE
TREATED UNTIL 9 WEEKS OF AGE

Treatment[a]	Average body weight at 63 days	WBC/mm³	LMC/mm³	Polys/mm³	Survival (No. %)	
Sham-operated (14)[b]	19.5	10469	7577	2892	14	100
Saline (24)	12.7	5476	1429	4047	8	33
BSA (20)	13.5	6420	1650	4770	6	30
Thymosin (40)	16.5	7983	3258	4725	28	70

[a] First week: 0.50 mg protein, three times a week; second to ninth weeks: 1.0 mg protein, three times a week.

[b] Numbers in parentheses are number of animals in each group (Asanuma *et al.*, 1970).

which, although higher in the thymosin treated animals ($3258/mm^3$) than in the saline- ($1429/mm^3$) or BSA- ($1650/mm^3$) injected mice, did not reach normal ($7577/mm^3$) levels. Histological examination of the lymph nodes and spleens of the thymosin-treated mice also showed significant restoration of lymphoid cell populations, particularly in the cortical ("thymic-dependent") areas of lymph nodes and spleens (Figs. 7 and 8).

Figure 9 is a photograph of two neonatally thymectomized mice from the foregoing experiment, 9 weeks postoperatively. The animal on the left was treated with thymosin three times a week, the one on the right, which shows wasting, received a similar quantity of BSA. Once wasting begins, the animal does not survive more than 2–3 weeks.

These data obtained with neonatally thymectomized mice support previous evidence in mice from a number of laboratories (cf. Miller and Osoba, 1967) that a neonatally thymectomized mouse does not grow at a normal rate, shows depletion of its lymphoid cells, and dies prematurely as a consequence of infection. This has led us to examine two aspects of the role of the thymus in host immunological competence, namely, its influence on cell-mediated immune processes as reflected in the homo-graft response, and humoral antibody production as revealed by the capacity to synthesize 19 S antibody. These studies have been conducted in collaboration with Drs. M. A. Hardy and J. Quint of our Department of Surgery and Dr. J. R. Battisto of our Department of Microbiology and Immunology (A. L. Goldstein *et al.*, 1970a).

CBA/W mice were thymectomized within 24 hours after birth, divided into groups, and treated as indicated in Table IV. Animals surviving at 9 weeks of age received at that time an allograft of skin from A/J strain

TABLE IV

INFLUENCE OF THYMOSIN ON ALLOGRAFT SURVIVAL IN NEONATALLY
THYMECTOMIZED CBA/W MICE[a]

Group	No. of mice per group	Allograft survival[b] 32 days post-grafting
Thymectomized + saline	10	7
Thymectomized + BSA[c]	4	2
Thymectomized + spleen fraction[c]	4	4
Thymectomized + thymosin[c]	22	1
Sham-thymectomized	14	0

[a] Thymectomy within 24 hours of birth.

[b] A/J strain skin.

[c] First week: 0.50 mg protein, three times per week; second to ninth weeks: 1.0 mg protein, three times per week. (From A. L. Goldstein *et al.*, 1970a.)

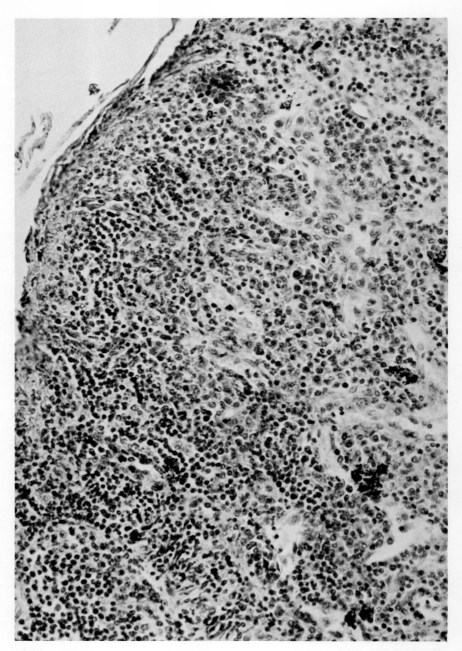

FIG. 7. Section of lymph node taken from saline-treated, neonatally thymectomized CBA/W mouse 9 weeks postoperatively. Note depletion of small lymphocytes, general "washed out" appearance, absence of follicular development, and hyperplasia of reticular epithelial elements. (From Asanuma *et al.*, 1970.)

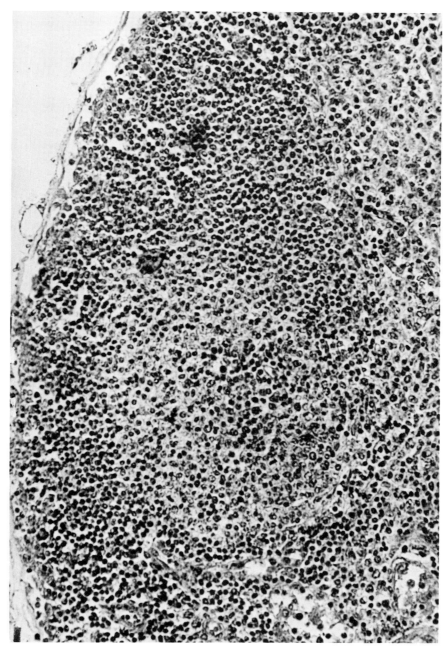

Fig. 8. Section of lymph node taken from thymosin-treated, neonatally thymecto-mized CBA/W mouse 9 weeks postoperatively. Note increased population of lymphocytes, well developed follicle with evident germinal center, and numerous small lymphocytes in paracortical region. (From Asanuma et al., 1970.)

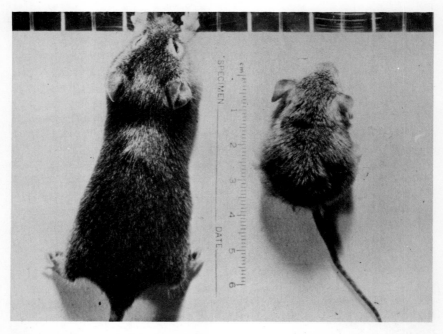

FIG. 9. Photograph of neonatally thymectomized CBA/W mice at 9 weeks of age. On left, thymosin-treated; on right BSA-treated. (From Asanuma *et al.*, 1970.)

mice. The data show the number of allografts that survived 32 days after the skin graft, that is, until the mice were 95 days of age. At 91 days of age, each animal received an intraperitoneal injection of 1 ml of a 2.5% suspension of sheep erythrocytes (SRBC). Four days later the animals were sacrificed and the number of antibody forming cells per spleen determined using the Jerne assay (Jerne and Nordin, 1963). The data in Table IV show that neonatally thymectomized animals treated either with saline, BSA, or a calf spleen fraction do not reject allografts readily. A normal rejection time by CBA/W mice of an A/J allograft is approximately 14 days. In the saline-, BSA-, and spleen fraction-treated groups, most of the grafts were still intact at 32 days post-grafting, with evidence of normal hair growth. The several mice that did reject their grafts, did so much later than sham-thymectomized controls, i.e., between days 20 and 28. In striking contrast, only one of the twenty-two animals treated with thymosin retained the allograft for 32 days post-grafting. Most of the thymosin-treated mice rejected their grafts within 16 days. Figure 10 shows two animals from the group providing the data in Table IV; the photograph was taken at 95 days of age. These results support the suggestion that in this experimental design, a thymosin preparation did indeed function *in lieu* of the thymus in the thymectomized animal in endowing the host with specific capacity to reject a skin allograft.

The number of antibody-producing cells within a single experimental group, as measured by the Jerne plaque assay, showed a wide degree of variability. This variability has also been encountered routinely by other investigators. Despite this, the plaque assay has utility in detecting antibody production at an early time prior to appearance of measurable circulating titers. The data plotted in Fig. 11 indicate that the number of antibody-producing cells per spleen in the neonatally thymectomized control animals treated either with saline or with BSA are in the low range, as reported previously by others. Although the mean number of antibody-producing cells in the plaque assays for the animals treated with thymosin (3399) is slightly elevated above these values for the saline- (845) or the BSA- (892) injected mice, the wide variability within each group prevents the data from having significance with the number of animals used. These studies are being repeated with both larger numbers of animals and doses of thymosin.

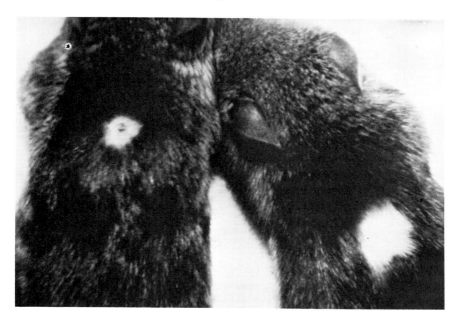

Fig. 10. Photograph of two neonatally thymectomized CBA/W 95-day-old mice grafted with A/J skin 32 days previously. On left, thymosin treated; note total rejection of allograft with scar tissue remaining. On right, saline treated; note allograft survival with obvious hair growth. (From A. L. Goldstein *et al.*, 1970.)

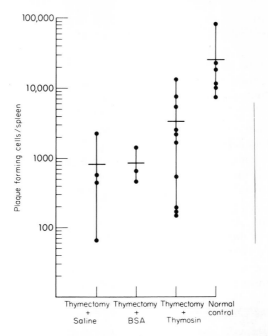

Plaque forming cells/spleen

Thymectomy + Saline   Thymectomy + BSA   Thymectomy + Thymosin   Normal control

FIG. 11. Individual values of 19 S antibody-producing cells (plaque forming) in spleens of neonatally thymectomized CBA/W mice treated either with saline, BSA, or thymosin. (From A. L. Goldstein *et al.*, 1970a.)

At present, therefore, it may be concluded from these data that at a time when the ability of the neonatally thymectomized, thymosin-treated mice appears to be relatively normal with regard to their capacity to reject an histoincompatible skin graft, their response to an antigenic challenge of SRBC does not appear to be significantly restored. Whether or not there is an influence of thymosin on 19 S antibody production remains to be established. In additional studies using adult thymectomized, lethally x-irradiated mice given syngeneic bone marrow cells, we have similarly not succeeded in demonstrating a marked influence of thymosin on the formation of 19 S antibody (A. L. Goldstein *et al.*, 1970a).

In a collaborative study with Dr. Lloyd Law of the National Cancer Institute, neonatally thymectomized mice have also been used to examine the influence of thymosin on another cell-mediated immune phenomenon, viz., the sensitive graft vs host reaction (Law *et al.*, 1968). Some of the data obtained are presented in Table V. It is evident that

TABLE V

EFFECT OF THYMOSIN (FRACTION 3) AND A SPLEEN EXTRACT ON GRAFT VS
HOST REACTION[a]

Spleen cells from C57Bl/KaLw donors	No. of BALB/c recipients	No. of graft vs host reactions	Average time of death after injection, in days (range)
Control, intact	20	18 (90%)	15.8 (13–30)
Thymectomized, new born	66	0	—
Thymectomized + 1 mg thymosin 3 times a week for 4 weeks	63	48 (76%)	17.8 (9–37)
Thymectomized + 1 mg spleen preparation 3 times a week for 4 weeks	41	0	—

[a] After Law et al. (1968).

thymosin administration to neonatally thymectomized mice restored to
the spleen cells of these animals their immunological competence as
reflected in the capacity of these cells to elicit a normal graft vs host
reaction when injected into newborn mice of an allogenic mouse strain.
In contrast, an extract prepared from spleen (Table V) or other tissue
extracts (Unpublished results) does not restore the immunological competence of spleen cells of the neonatally thymectomized animals.

In summary of this section, which has considered biological effects of
thymic extracts in thymectomized animals, the following conclusions
appear warranted on the basis of the experimental evidence that has
been reviewed:

1. Partially purified, cell-free extracts of thymic tissue from several
species, notably bovine and ovine, have been prepared which exhibit
some capacity to replace certain of the functions attributed to the thymus
in the newborn animal. These include growth stimulation, certain
manifestations of host immunological competence, and prevention of
the appearance of wasting disease. The body of available evidence obtained in these studies supports the concept that the thymus normally
secretes one or more humoral factors.

2. Initial studies with both neonatally thymectomized and adult thymectomized, lethally x-irradiated mice indicate that the available preparations of thymic fractions influence significantly parameters based upon
cell-mediated immune phenomena but are less effective in modulating
humoral immune responses.

TABLE VI

INFLUENCE OF THYMOSIN ON LYMPHOID TISSUE STRUCTURE AND FUNCTION

A. Enhances lymphocytopoiesis in:

   1. Normal mice, rats and guinea pigs
   2. Adrenalectomized mice
   3. Germ-free mice
   4. X-irradiated mice

B. In neonatally thymectomized mice:

   1. Reduces wasting and mortality
   2. Increases body weight gain
   3. Increases absolute numbers of blood lymphocytes
   4. Increases lymphoid organ size
   5. Partially restores lymph node and spleen morphology

C. On humoral antibody response:

   1. Slight to sheep erythrocytes in neonatally thymectomized mice (plaque assay)
   2. Slight to sheep erythrocytes in adult thymectomized, lethally x-irradiated, bone marrow restored mice (plaque assay)
   3. None to sheep erythrocytes in normal or x-irradiated mice (hemagglutinin titers)

D. On cell-mediated immune response:

   1. In normal mice:
     (a) accelerates first- and second-set skin allograft rejection
     (b) an antithymosin serum delays first- and second-set skin allograft rejection
     (c) potentiates or negates effects of antilymphocyte serum
   2. In neonatally thymectomized mice:
     (a) restores ability to reject skin allografts
     (b) restores to spleen cells their capacity to elicit a graft vs host reaction

The presently established biological activities of thymosin, a cell-free preparation from calf thymus prepared in our laboratory, are summarized in Table VI. Some of the activities listed are based on results of as yet unpublished studies. It remains to reexamine all of the responses listed in Table VI with a chemically pure preparation of thymosin, when this becomes available. Until this has been done, it will not be possible to decide whether these diverse biological properties are those of a single thymic humoral principle or a reflection of the presence in the thymus of multiple hormonal factors. At that time also, it may be anticipated that a more rational approach to the possible clinical applications of thymic preparations could be initiated. For the present, it can be concluded that the thymus is an endocrine gland, and that its humoral roles are of prime significance in the regulation of host resistance.

V. SUMMARY

In this chapter we have presented evidence from the literature as well as from our own laboratory in support of the conclusion that the thymus is an endocrine gland. The vital roles of the thymus, both cellular and endocrine, in the normal development and homeostasis of the lymphoid system have only recently been revealed. In addition to its influence on lymphoid tissue per se, the thymus has been implicated in a number of clinical disorders ranging from autoimmune diseases, such as myasthenia gravis, to malignant growth.

Although the mechanisms by which the thymus and its secretory products exert their actions are only beginning to be understood, it is now evident that in some of its roles, the thymus functions as a typical endocrine gland.

The isolation of a number of nonpolar and polar fractions from thymic tissue of several species is described, as well as their reported biological activities. The latter include (1) partial replacement of the functions of the thymus in neonatally thymectomized mice; (2) stimulation of lymphocytopoiesis under several types of experimental conditions; and (3) regulation of specific phenomena that reflect cell-mediated immune processes.

The isolation and purification from calf thymic tissue of thymosin in our laboratory is described. This partially purified fraction prevents wasting disease and restores cell-mediated host immunity of neonatally thymectomized mice. These findings suggest possible future applications for thymic preparations in the treatment of immunological deficiency disorders.

In view of the many reported "thymic factors," it remains to be determined whether the endocrine function of the thymus residues in the secretion of a single hormone or whether the thymus secretes a multiplicity of factors that act to modulate lymphoid tissue structure and function.

ACKNOWLEDGMENTS

Data referred to in this paper from our own laboratory have been obtained in studies supported by grants from the American Cancer Society (P-68), the National Science Foundation (GB-6616X), the Damon Runyon Fund for Cancer Research (DRG-920), and the National Cancer Institute, National Institutes of Health, USPHS (CA-07470). Grateful acknowledgement is also made of the helpful financial and technical support of Merck Sharp and Dohme Research Laboratories.

Allan L. Goldstein is a recipient of a Career Scientist Award of the Health Research Council of the City of New York under contract I-519.

REFERENCES

Archer, O. K., and Pierce, J. C. (1961). *Federation Proc.* **20**, 26.

Arnason, B. G., Jankovic, B. D., Waksman, B. H., and Wennersten, C. (1962). *J. Exptl. Med.* **116**, 177.

Asanuma, Y., Goldstein, A. L., and White, A. (1970). *Endocrinol.* **86**, 600.

Bernardi, G., and Comsa, J. (1965). *Experientia* **21**, 416.

Bezssonoff, N. A., and Comsa, J. (1958). *Ann. Endocrinol. (Paris)* **19**, 222.

Bomskov, C. (1941). *Deut. Med. Wochschr.* **67**, 148.

Bomskov, C., and Brachet, F. (1940). *Endokronologie* **23**, 145.

Bomskov, C., and Sladovic, L. (1940). *Deut. Med. Wochschr.* **66**, 589.

Bracci, C. (1905). *Rev. Clin. Pediat.* **3**, 572.

Brunkhorst, W., and Herranen, A. (1967). *Nature* **214**, 181.

Camblin, J. G., and Bridges, J. B. (1964). *Transplantation* **2**, 785.

Cohn, E. J., Strong, L. E., Hughes, W. L., Jr., Mulford, D. J., Ashworth, J. N., Melin, M., and Taylor, H. L. (1946). *J. Am. Chem. Soc.* **68**, 459.

Comsa, J. (1938). *Compt. Rend. Soc. Biol.* **127**, 903.

Comsa, J. (1957). *Acta Endocrinol.* **26**, 361.

Comsa, J. (1965). *Am. J. Med. Sci.* **250**, 79.

Comsa, J. (1966). *Arzneimittel-Forsch.* **16**, 18.

Comsa, J., and Bezssonoff, N. A. (1958). *Acta Endocrinol.* **29**, 257.

Dalmasso, A. P., Martinez, C., Sjodin, K., and Good, R. A. (1963). *J. Exptl. Med.* **118**, 1089.

DeSomer, P., Denys, P., and Leyten, R. (1963). *Life Sci.* **11**, 810.

Dougherty, T. F. (1952). *Physiol. Rev.* **32**, 379.

Dougherty, T. F., and White, A. (1945). *Am. J. Anat.* **77**, 81.

Dougherty, T. F., and White, A. (1947). *J. Lab. Clin. Med.* **32**, 584.

Dougherty, T. F., Berliner, D. L., and Berliner, M. L. (1961). *Metab., Clin. Exptl.* **10**, 966.

Dubos, R. J., and Hirsch, J. G. (1954). *J. Exptl. Med.* **99**, 55.

Ernström, U. I., (1965). *Acta Pathol. Microbiol. Scand.* **65**, 192.

Fichtelius, K. E., Laurell, G., and Phillipsson, L. (1961). *Acta Pathol. Microbiol. Scand.* **51**, 81.

Galante, L., Gudmundsson, T. V., Mathews, E. W., Tse, A., Williams, E. D., Woodhouse, N. J. Y., and MacIntyre, I. (1968). *Lancet* **II**, 537.

Goldstein, A. L., Slater, F. D., and White, A. (1966). *Proc. Natl. Acad. Sci. U. S.* **56**, 1010.

Goldstein, A. L., Asanuma, Y., Battisto, J. R., Hardy, M. A., Quint, J., and White, A. (1970a). *J. Immunol.* **104**, 359.

Goldstein, A. L., Banerjee, S., Schneebeli, G. L., Dougherty, T. F., and White, A. (1970b). *Radiation Res.* **41**, 359.

Goldstein, A. L., Asanuma, Y., and White, A. (1970c). *Recent Progr. Hormone Res.* **26**, In press.

Goldstein, G. (1966). *Lancet* **II**, 1164.

Goldstein, G. (1968). *Lancet* **II**, 119.

Goldstein, G., and Hofmann, W. W. (1969). *Clin. Exptl. Immunol.* **4**, 181.

Good, R. A., and Gabrielson, A. E., eds. (1964). "The Thymus in Immunobiology." Harper (Hoeber), New York.

Good, R. A., Dalmasso, A. P., Martinez, C., Archer, O. K., Pierce, J. C., and Papermaster, B. W. (1962). *J. Exptl. Med.* 116, 773.

Gregoire, C., and Duchateau, G. (1956). *Arch. Biol. (Liège)* 67, 269.

Hand, T., Caster, P., and Luckey, T. D. (1967). *Biochem. Biophys. Res. Commun.* 26, 18.

Hardy, M. A., Quint, J., Goldstein, A. L., State, D., and White, A. (1968). *Proc. Natl. Acad. Sci. U. S.* 61, 875.

Hardy, M. A., Quint, J., Goldstein, A. L., White, A., State, D., and Battisto, J. R. (1969). *Proc. Soc. Exptl. Biol. Med.* 130, 214.

Hegyeli, A., McLaughlin, J. A., and Szent-Györgyi, A. (1963). *Proc. Natl. Acad. Sci. U. S.* 49, 230.

Hess, M. W. (1968). "Experimental Thymectomy. Possibilities and Limitations." Springer, Berlin.

Hirsch, J. G., and Dubos, R. J. (1954). *J. Exptl. Med.* 99, 65.

Jankovic, B. D., Waksman, B. H., and Arnason, B. G. (1962). *J. Exptl. Med.* 116, 159.

Jankovic, B. D., Isakovic, K., and Horvat, J. (1965). *Nature* 208, 356.

Jerne, H. K., and Nordin, A. A. (1963). *Science* 140, 105.

Klein, J. J., Goldstein, A. L., and White, A. (1965). *Proc. Natl. Acad. Sci. U. S.* 53, 812.

Klein, J. J., Goldstein, A. L., and White, A. (1966). *Ann. N. Y. Acad. Sci.* 135, 485.

Law, L. W., Goldstein, A. L., and White, A. (1968). *Nature* 219, 1391.

Maisin, J. (1964). *Nature* 204, 1211.

Metcalf, D. (1956). *Brit. J. Cancer Res.* 10, 442.

Metcalf, D. (1965). *Nature* 208, 1336.

Metcalf, D. (1966). *Recent Results Cancer Res.* 5, 1.

Miller, J. F. A. P. (1961). *Lancet* II, 748.

Miller, J. F. A. P. (1964). *In* "The Thymus in Immunobiology" (R. A. Good and A. E. Gabrielsen, eds.), pp. 436–464. Harper (Hoeber), New York.

Miller, J. F. A. P. (1965). *Nature* 208, 1337.

Miller, J. F. A. P. (1967). *Lancet* II, 1299.

Miller, J. F. A. P., and Osoba, D. (1967). *Physiol. Rev.* 47, 437.

Nakamoto, A. (1957). *Acta Haematol. Japon.* 20, 187.

Nowinski, W. W. (1930). *Biochem. Z.* 226, 415.

Nowinski, W. W. (1932). *Biochem. Z.* 248, 421.

Pansky, B., House, E. L., and Cone, L. A. (1965). *Diabetes* 14, 325.

Park, E. A., and McClure, R. D. (1919). *Am. J. Diseases Children* 18, 317.

Parkes, J. D., and McKinna, J. A. (1967). *Nature* 214, 1116.

Pierpaoli, W., Baroni, C., Fabris, N., and Sorkin, E. (1969). *Immunology* 16, 217.

Potop, I. (1966). *Rev. Roumaine Endocrinol.* 3, 185.

Potop, I., Boeru, V., and Mreană, G. (1966). *Biochem. J.* 101, 454.

Potop, I., Juvina, E., Mreană, G., and Boeru, V. (1967). *Arch. Geschwulstforsch.* 30, 190.

Quint, J., Hardy, M. A., and Monaco, A. P. (1969). *Surgical Forum* 20, 252.

Roberts, S., and White, A. (1949). *J. Biol. Chem.* 178, 151.

Schwartz, H., Price, M., and Odell, C. A. (1953). *Metab., Clin. Exptl.* 2, 261.

Seidel, K., Felsch, G., and Bosseckert, H. (1965). *Muenchen Med. Wochschr.* 107, 2384.

Solomon, S. S., Poffenbarger, P. L., Heep, D., Fenster, L. F., Ensinck, J. W., and Williams, R. H. (1967). *Endocrinology* **81**, 213.

Stutman, O., Yunis, E. J., and Good, R. A. (1968). *J. Natl. Cancer Inst.* **41**, 1431.

Szent-Györgyi, A., Hegyeli, A., and McLaughlin, J. A. (1962). *Proc. Natl. Acad. Sci. U. S.* **49**, 230.

Szent-Györgyi, A., Együd, L. G., and McLaughlin, J. A. (1967). *Science* **155**, 539.

Taylor, R. B. (1965). *Nature* **208**, 1334.

Trainin, N., and Linker-Israeli, M. (1967). *Cancer Res.* **27**, 309.

Trainin, N., Bejerano, A., Strahilevitch, M., Goldring, D., and Small, M. (1966). *Israel J. Med. Sci.* **2**, 549.

Trainin, N., Burger, M., and Kaye, A. M. (1967). *Biochem. Pharmacol.* **16**, 711.

Trainin, N., Burger, M., and Linker-Israeli, M. (1968). *In* "Advance in Transplantation" (J. Dausset, J. Hamburger, and E. Mathe, eds.), pp. 91–95. Williams & Wilkins, Baltimore, Maryland.

Wells, B. B., Riddle, O., and Marvin, H. N. (1942). *Proc. Soc. Exptl. Biol. Med.* **49**, 473.

White, A. (1947–1948). *Harvey Lectures* **43**, 43.

White, A. (1949). *Ann. Rev. Physiol.* **11**, 355.

White, A., and Goldstein, A. L. (1968). *Perspectives Biol. Med.* **11**, 475.

White, A., and Goldstein, A. L. (1970). *In* "Control Processes in Multicellular Organisms," Ciba Found. Symp. (G. E. W. Wolstenholme and J. Knight, eds.), pp. 210–237. Churchill, London.

CHAPTER 12

Plant Hormones

Carlos O. Miller

I. INTRODUCTION

In current practice, five types of chemically known compounds often are classified as plant hormones. All occur naturally and presumably play roles in growth and development. In this discussion, the auxins, gibberellins, and cytokinins will receive most attention and abscisic acid and ethylene rather brief mention.

II. AUXINS

A. EFFECTIVE STRUCTURES

The auxin most frequently detected in a wide variety of plant species appears to be indole-3-acetic acid (I).

(I)

Even most of the exceptions are closely related to (I) and are capable of yielding the latter under the influence of certain plant tissues. A great number of synthetic compounds active in auxin bioassays share with (I) a ring structure having unsaturation next to a side chain that is termi- nated by a carboxyl group. There have been some apparent exceptions to the generalization, however. A universal property of active molecules seems to be the presence of a negative charge (at the carboxyl group) separated from a partial positive charge by a distance of 5.5 Å (Porter, 1962; Thimann, 1963). This characteristic fits a concept developed in earlier years by investigators of auxin structures and growth kinetics (Foster *et al.*, 1952, 1955). The concept implied that an auxin, when active, attaches or interacts at two points. To date, we do not know the nature of either attachment. Nevertheless, the concept should be kept in mind in attempts to explain auxin actions.

B. ALTERATION OF CELL WALLS

Of the many phenomena controlled by auxin, one of the simplest morphologically is the promotion of cell enlargement. Enhancement by auxin has been observed in many plant species and a wide variety of tissues and parts, and several assay systems for auxins are based on the effect. Since enlargement can be detected quickly and easily in these systems, they have been utilized very frequently in biochemical studies of auxin action. A loosening of the cell wall seems to be required for the enlargement resulting from auxin application (literature summary by Cleland, 1968a). Considerable attention has been focused, therefore, on the changes in elasticity and plasticity of the cell walls. Investigators have not agreed on the relative importance of the two properties (see discus- sion by Morré and Eisinger, 1968). Masuda (1969) recently stated that in oat coleoptiles the change in elasticity occurs first and is better correlated with at least the early growth promotion by auxin.

Even aside from the question of auxin intervention, the basis for wall loosening really is not clear. The alteration in physical properties could be effected by synthesis of new materials as well as by modification of preformed wall materials. In 1934, Bonner demonstrated that cell wall synthesis is increased in oat coleoptiles when elongation is promoted by auxin. More recently, Ray (1962, 1967) and Baker and Ray (1965) have offered evidence that the incorporation of new material into the wall contributes to expansion and perhaps is important in the auxin promotion. Ray and Abdul-Baki (1968) believe that the increased wall synthesis is due to an enhanced uptake of sugar from the incubation medium after induction of elongation by auxin and to internal changes that permit more rapid polysaccharide synthesis. In particular, these authors suggest that auxin affects transport within the cell in some manner that increases the access of hexokinase to glucose; this results in a greater rate of glucose-6-phosphate formation. M. A. Hall and Ordin (1968) have prepared a particulate enzyme system from oat coleoptiles which synthesizes considerable cellulose and smaller amounts of mixed β-1,4 and β-1,3 glucan. Auxins had no effect on this enzyme system *in vitro* but did increase activity if applied to intact tissue before preparation of the system. The authors believe that growth promoting activity of the auxins may be due in part to increased production of cellulose synthetase and, therefore, increased cellulose formation. At the present time, however, it is not certain that the polysaccharide synthesis is essential to enhancement of enlargement by auxin even though such synthesis results from auxin treatment. In fact, Baker and Ray (1965) have shown that the "direct" effect of auxin on rate of wall synthesis in oat coleoptiles begins *after* the auxin promotion of elongation is apparent.

Neither is the role for wall material modification very clear. If auxin enhancement of cell elongation results from some enzymatic degradation of polysaccharides in the wall, direct application of the proper enzyme might cause the cells to elongate much as they would if treated with auxin. Thus, Masuda and Wada (1967) and Masuda (1968) observed that a β-1,3-glucanase preparation quickly promoted pea stem elongation and wall extensibility much as auxin. Cleland (1968a), however, failed in attempts to confirm this. The possibility that auxin in some manner enhances activity of a polysaccharide hydrolase also has received considerable attention recently. Fan and MacLachlan (1966) observed that (I) caused synthesis of large amounts and increased specific activity of cellulase when applied to decapitated pea seedlings. MacLachlan *et al.* (1968) confirmed this and extended the observations to bean and maize seedlings. Whereas the specific activity and amount of β-1,4-glucanase was correlated with auxin effects on growth, the enhancement of β-1,3-glucanase was not. The activity of the latter was correlated, however, with the general increase of total protein. Perhaps running counter to this line of evidence, Cleland (1968a,b) found that the auxin-induced increase of wall plasticity was reversed in the presence of respiratory inhibitors and he cast doubt on the idea that wall loosening is mediated by degradative enzymes such as cellulase or other glucanases. Rather, he favored the idea of a special enzyme or enzymatic complex that reversibly cleaves some wall polymer when an as yet unidentified reactant (produced by respiration) is sufficiently available. Cleland's hypothesis further suggests that auxin does not act directly on this cleaving reaction but in some manner makes more of the enzyme available at the site of the reaction. Morré and Eisinger (1968), on the other hand, feel that auxin may serve as a cofactor for an enzyme acting at the cell wall.

The mechanism by which wall loosening occurs, its true role in enlargement, and its relationship to the prime action of auxin obviously remain unexplained. If one is willing to assume that a single prime action of auxin initiates all auxin effects, then direct action of the hormone on the wall or on known hydrolases seems unlikely. More intricate and indirect mechanisms may be plausible.

C. SYNTHESIS OF RIBONUCLEIC ACID AND PROTEINS

Generally, growth-promoting concentrations of auxins increase synthesis of ribonucleic acid (RNA) and protein in numerous plant species and supraoptimal concentrations diminish synthesis (review and comments by Key, 1969). Although the stimulation of RNA and protein synthesis may be detected in some material only after cell elongation has reached a maximum rate (Trewavas, 1968a,b), the promotion of RNA synthesis may occur even though cell enlargement is prevented by incubating the tissue on mannitol solutions (Masuda et al., 1967); the stimulation of synthesis therefore seems not to result from enlargement. At least some synthesis seems necessary for substantial auxin promotion of growth since inhibitors of both RNA and protein formation prevent or greatly reduce the magnitude of responses to auxins in several test systems (Noodén and Thimann, 1963, 1966; Key, 1964). The unanswered questions still are how, and at what point, the control of protein synthesis comes about and whether the initial action of auxin is on the RNA and protein synthetic systems.

Several investigators have particularly looked at the auxin stimulation of RNA synthesis. Much of the increase often is in the ribosomal RNA fraction, but soluble RNA and species of RNA rich in adenine also increase (review by Key, 1969). The adenine-rich RNA from soybean has many properties of messenger RNA (Key and Ingle, 1968), and, in oat coleoptiles, (I) stimulated the formation of what was probably messenger RNA (Masuda *et al.*, 1967). The adenine-rich RNA seems to be the most essential to auxin action. Thus, the auxin-induced increases in ribosomal and soluble RNA were largely prevented by 5-fluorouracil whereas the auxin-induced growth was almost unaffected. Furthermore, the synthesis of adenine-rich RNA was stimulated by auxin in the presence of the inhibitor. On the other hand, actinomycin D severely reduced both the synthesis of the adenine-rich RNA and growth; synthesis and growth were correlated quite well (Key and Ingle, 1968). Much the same conclusions have been reached in experiments with oat coleoptiles (Masuda *et al.*, 1966).

There have been failures to completely eliminate auxin effects with actinomycin D. The inhibitor apparently was unable to prevent a small increment of growth elicited by auxin in pea stem segments (Penny and Galston, 1966). The compound, although greatly reducing RNA synthesis and growth in oat coleoptile tissue, did not prevent the auxin-induced increase of wall plasticity in experiments by Cleland (1965) but did block wall loosening in experiments by Coartney *et al.* (1967). Masuda and Wada (1966) observed that only after a fairly long pretreatment was actinomycin D capable of eliminating elongation and extensibility changes due to auxin. One possibility for explaining the conflicting results is that actinomycin D simply is not as fully effective in eliminating RNA synthesis in some setups as it is in others. Another possibility is that auxin action can depend on preformed RNA although the stability and amount of such RNA may vary with plant materials.

Some reports that auxin stimulates RNA synthesis in isolated nuclei have appeared but these seem to need more elaborate confirmation. Roychoudhurry *et al.* (1965) made such an observation with nuclei from coconut milk. Matthysse (1968) has claimed that RNA synthesis was increased by auxin in isolated pea-bud nuclei and also in nuclei from tobacco or soybean tissue, provided the auxin was present during the isolation process. The investigator reported such effects on isolated chromatin and suggested that proteinaceous factors necessary for the auxin action are easily lost during the isolation of the nuclei.

Contrary to the disagreements concerning the role of RNA synthesis in auxin effects, there seems to be rather good agreement as to the necessity for protein synthesis (see next paragraph, however). Examination

of *in vitro* protein synthesizing systems with respect to auxin action
might therefore be instructive. Recently, Davies and MacLachlan (1969)
have made such studies by following the synthesis of cellulase by pea
microsomes. Treatment of the pea tissue with (I) before homogenization
increased the ability of the microsome preparation to synthesize cellulase.
The control preparations formed considerable protein but (I) preferentially favored the appearance of new cellulase activity. Although the
in vitro system was sensitive to cycloheximide, puromycin, and ribonuclease, it was not affected by adding actinomycin D, streptomycin, or
(I). The authors concluded that (I) had no *in vitro* effects but, rather,
caused an *in vivo* induction of polyribosomes able to synthesize cellulase.
This, of course, is consistent with the emphasis by others on the formation
of messenger RNA but also with the conclusion by Trewavas (1968b)
that increased polyribosome formation may be due to enhanced ribosome
production rather than increased messenger RNA synthesis. Other
interesting examples of auxin stimulation of induction or synthesis of
particular enzymes include an *in vitro* stimulation of the synthesis of
isocitrate lyase in potato tuber (Datta *et al.*, 1965) and the induction
of enzymes that catalyze the formation of complexes between (I) or other
acids and aspartic acid (Sudi, 1964; Venis, 1964). Perhaps of equal
interest is the inhibition of development of invertase activity in Jerusalem
artichoke (Edelman and Hall, 1964).

The role of RNA and protein synthesis with respect to auxin action
recently has been strongly questioned. Early work by Köhler (1956) and
Ray and Ruesink (1962) demonstrated that auxin-induced growth is
measurable in just a few minutes. Evans and Ray (1969), using delicate
optical equipment to measure elongation of a stack of oat coleoptile
sections, have detected a growth promotion by auxin in about 10 minutes
and this has been further reduced to much less than 5 minutes by use of a
methyl ester of (I) (Evans *et al.*, 1968). The time required for onset of
the promotion of elongation was not extended by either RNA or protein
synthesis inhibitors although the rate of subsequent growth was lessened;
cycloheximide even seemed to shorten the lag period somewhat. This
can be used to argue against the initial action of auxin being a direct
stimulation of RNA synthesis (Evans and Ray, 1969). When one considers
the logistics for such an action, the time available seems too short. Consider that movement of the hormone through the tissue to the nuclei (or
mitochondria or plastids) in rather large cells, synthesis of the RNA,
movement of the RNA to the sites of protein synthesis, synthesis of the
protein, movement of the protein to a point where it could influence
physical properties of the cell wall in some manner, and then the actual

enlargement itself must occur. Evans and Ray (1969) feel that auxin may possibly act at the translational level in the synthesis of structural rather than enzymatic protein but warn that the evidence for this is not really good. The idea is consistent with the observations by Evans and Hokanson (1969) on the timing of response of maize coleoptiles to the application and withdrawal of auxins. In this study, the response of the tissue to auxin was quite rapidly diminished after removal of the supply of auxin. The reduction was so rapid that if an enzymatic protein were responsible for the auxin effect, the enzyme half-life would have to be extremely and unusually short. Utilization of structural protein in the growth process, however, could account for the reduction. Perhaps contrary to the foregoing discussion is the observation by Masuda and Kamisaka (1969) that auxin enhancement of RNA synthesis in oat coleoptiles may be detected in as little as ten minutes. Thus, it is still possible that both transcription and translation are involved.

There can be no doubt that auxin in some way may quickly influence RNA and protein production and that prevention of either synthesis eliminates large and continued effects by auxin. However, an absolute requirement for RNA and protein synthesis in the chain of reactions leading to auxin effects still is open to question.

D. OTHER POSSIBILITIES

Although current emphasis is on the relationship between RNA and protein synthesis and auxin action, other possibilities should not be ignored. The timing experiments mentioned may be pointing away not only from the first auxin action being on RNA synthesis but also away from a direct effect on protein production. Early reports claiming that auxins influence quite quickly the rates of respiration continue to be supported. Van Hove and Carlier (1968) recently detected stimulation of the glycolysis-Krebs cycle pathway in mung bean tissue by auxin and believe the action is on some step between the formation of pyruvate and the decarboxylation of oxalsuccinate. It is possible that control of a step of respiration is so closely coupled to some aspects of nucleic acid or protein synthesis as to make it appear that auxin is having rather direct effects on all the processes. Of course, the effects on respiration may be completely secondary. Even other effects such as those of auxin on permeability, other membrane properties, and cyclosis could represent prime control points. In fact, promotion of protoplasmic streaming has been observed to occur in less than 1 minute (Thimann and Sweeney,

1937); this is so fast that it might at least reflect the initial action of auxin. Dahlhelm (1969) has shown that heavy water (D_2O) prevents growth, RNA synthesis, and the auxin-induced alteration of a protein band in material from pea plants. The author suggests that (I) causes allosteric changes in protein structure. This is consistent with the suggestion by Sarkissian (1968) that auxin acts as an allosteric effector of citrate synthetase.

III. GIBBERELLINS

A. ACTIVE STRUCTURES

At the time this article was written, at least 24 compounds having gibberellin activity had been studied as to chemical structures (see Binks *et al.*, 1969). All bear a close relationship to gibberellic acid (II), which is also known as GA$_3$.

(II)

No generalizations drawn from the studies of structures have as yet pointed to modes of action. (II) is the most readily available of the compounds and has been used for most of the biochemical studies.

B. ENZYMES AND NUCLEIC ACIDS

The morphological effects of gibberellins are many and varied but these have not been investigated extensively in a biochemical sense. Instead, a rather unique response has received most of the attention. When a barley grain is germinating, the starch in the endosperm becomes hydrolyzed. This is due to the action of α-amylase, which is synthesized by the aleurone layer surrounding the endosperm. The aleurone layer is stimulated to form α-amylase and other hydrolytic enzymes such as proteases and ribonuclease by gibberellins given off by the germinating embryo. Aleurone layers isolated from the grain produce these enzymes if supplied with gibberellins. That the increase in α-amylase activity really represents *de novo* protein synthesis has been demonstrated in buoyant density comparisons of enzymes formed in the presence or absence of ^{18}O-labeled amino acids (Filner and Varner, 1967). In similar experiments, evidence has been obtained that the proteases also are formed from amino acids as a result of gibberellin stimulation (Jacobsen and Varner, 1967).

Production of the α-amylase by the aleurone layers can be prevented by inhibitors of oxidative phosphorylation, of protein synthesis, or of RNA synthesis. Apparently, the gibberellin stimulation requires both RNA and protein formation (review, Varner and Johri, 1968). Whether or not the gibberellin directly controls such synthesis is a critical question. Investigations with isolated pea nuclei at least suggest that this may be so. In such nuclei, (II) increased the specific activity of RNA associated with DNA and of that which tightly bound on a methylated-albumin-kieselguhr column. The RNA resulting from gibberellin treatment had a higher average molecular weight than that synthesized by control nuclei and was different in composition. The gibberellin was effective only if present during the isolation procedure. No stimulation by the compound was detected when it was added to completely isolated nuclei (Johri and Varner, 1968). This may mean that stimulation by (II) is dependent upon some factor that may be lost during isolation of the nuclei. (II) conceivably could prevent this loss or an interaction between the factor and gibberellin could yield a product which is retained by the nuclei. Further fitting the idea that gibberellins act through a stimulation of RNA synthesis is the fact that α-amylase appears in aleurone layers only after a considerable lag following gibberellin treatment. Continued presence of gibberellin is required for continued production of the enzyme (Chrispeels and Varner, 1967); so any particular RNA whose synthesis is promoted by gibberellins must therefore be rather short-lived. This seems to be contrary to the long lag observed.

IV. CYTOKININS

A. STRUCTURES

Cytokinins are characterized primarily by their ability to greatly promote cell division in certain standard tissue systems. In such systems, the most active cytokinins are adenine derivatives in which a fat-soluble constituent is added to the amino group of the adenine. Probably zeatin (III) (Letham *et al.*, 1964) is the most effective compound at very low concentrations in the cell-division assays with N^6-(Δ^2-isopentenyl)adenine (IV) being a little less effective.

(III), including its ribonucleoside and ribonucleotide derivatives, thus far is the only fully characterized cytokinin isolated from higher plant tissues and also has been isolated from the fungus *Rhizopogon roseolus* (Miller, 1967, 1968). (IV) is known to be produced by a plant pathogen, *Corynebacterium fascians* (Klämbt *et al.*, 1966; Helgeson and Leonard, 1966), and is also a widely occurring constituent of certain transfer ribonucleic acid (tRNA) molecules. Cytokinin activity may be elicited by various modified molecules; for example, a replacement of the number 8 carbon by nitrogen in the purine ring lessens but does not eliminate activity. Blockage of the number 1 position by addition of a substituent, however, seems to destroy the ability to act as a cytokinin. The same may be true of the number 3 position (Skoog *et al.*, 1967). An interchange of the 8-carbon and the 9-nitrogen eliminates activity (Strong, 1958). The side chain may be a simple alkyl group; for example, 6-methylaminopurine has activity although longer chains are more effective. Or the side chain may contain branched or ring structures. Adenine itself shows a little activity at quite high concentrations (Miller, 1968). Since a wide variety of chemically differing side groups may be used, it is likely that some physical property determines effectiveness. Substituted ureas such as *sym*-diphenylurea (V) (Steward and Shantz, 1955; Bruce *et al.*, 1965) also exhibit activity, although the concentrations required are high when compared with those needed with the purine compounds.

(V)

If one assumes that all these molecules act through the same mechanism (in bioassays that seem to be quite specific), then a functioning by direct incorporation into a specific complex by covalent bonding is perhaps hard to imagine; some less demanding physical interaction might be easier to visualize (Miller, 1968). On the other hand, there are reasons to believe that some of the most active purine cytokinins can become parts of certain nucleic acids. It could be that the less effective compounds such as (V) or adenine act as cytokinins only indirectly; that is, after some intermediate reactions.

B. RNA METABOLISM

The fact that most active cytokinins are adenine derivatives has long suggested that the compounds are involved in an adeninelike role. Some possible function in ribonucleic acid metabolism has been seriously considered especially since Lang and Richmond (1957) found that kinetin (the first identified cytokinin, 6-furfurylaminopurine) helped to maintain high levels of protein, RNA, and chlorophyll in detached leaves; this work has since been extended to many species by numerous investigators. In the same year Guttman (1957) reported that kinetin caused an increase of RNA content in onion root tips. The line of work springing from or related to the findings is unique in that the most promising approach thus far has been in actually looking at the incorporation or occurrence of the cytokinin units in more complex molecules. Fox (1966) first offered evidence that labeled cytokinins supplied to plant tissues get incorporated into certain fractions containing soluble RNA. This fits the findings that (IV) is a part of yeast tRNA (R. H. Hall *et al.*, 1966; Robbins *et al.*, 1967) and that some serine (Zachau *et al.*, 1966) and tyrosine (Madison *et al.*, 1967) tRNA's contain (IV). Cytokinin activity has been detected in hydrolyzed tRNA from several plant species but has not been detected in ribosomal RNA (Skoog *et al.*, 1966; Matsubara *et al.*, 1968). In serine tRNA (Zachau *et al.*, 1966), (IV) is known to be specifically located next to the anticodon and therefore seems to be in a good position to play some crucial role. Modification of (IV) in serine tRNA by addition of iodine across the side chain double bond does not interfere with acceptance of the amino acid but does decrease the degree of attachment of the tRNA to the messenger RNA (Fittler and Hall, 1966). It is clear that certain critical units when separated from the tRNA may exhibit cytokinin activity. The question still remains, however, whether or not cytokinins actually function by becoming incorporated into larger molecules such as transfer RNA. Cytokinin units in some organisms may be formed from adenine *after* incorporation of the adenine into the nucleic acid (Peterkofsky, 1968). For cytokinins to act as part of tRNA of higher plants, incorporation of the preformed odd base would be necessary. Although some evidence has been offered that this is so, the proof is not yet firm enough to know that it really happens. However, even if the cytokinins do not act by being incorporated into certain tRNA's, they still might interact in some manner with those RNA's that contain similar units.

C. Another Approach

Another approach to biochemical action of cytokinins seems to be available. Tissues of several species of plants respond to certain plant hormones by altered synthesis of various phenolic compounds (discussion, Miller, 1969). Aseptically cultured soybean tissue, which is often used for cytokinin assay, responds to the presence of cytokinin in a deficient medium (lacking components necessary for growth) by synthesizing considerable quantities of daidzin (a deoxyisoflavone glucoside) and related compounds. These compounds are easily detected in crude extracts by optical density readings. In liquid culture, the response is fairly quick but shows a time lag (Miller, 1969a). The response requires aeration and is inhibited by *p*-fluorophenylalanine, chloramphenicol, cycloheximide, actinomycin D, and *aza*-guanine. Apparently both RNA and protein synthesis are required for the response even though the tissue had been making small amounts of the daidzin before being transferred from a complete to the deficient medium. The involvement of cell division in this response is unlikely since the production of related phenolic compounds is stimulated by kinetin and reduced by the foregoing inhibitors even when the cells are placed in sucrose or mannitol solutions that cause plasmolysis of the soybean cells (Miller, 1969b).

V. ABSCISIC ACID

A. Structure

Abscisic acid (VI) was previously known as abscisin II and also as dormin. Because it is of fairly recent discovery, little information concerning necessary structural characteristics is available.

(VI)

B. BIOCHEMICAL ROLE

The observed effects of (VI) have been mainly inhibitory ones. Several of these inhibitions are reversed by gibberellins and others by cytokinins. This, however, does not very much increase our understanding of the biochemical action of (VI). Perhaps it will when more is known about the roles of the gibberellins and cytokinins. Conditioned by present emphases, one looks for some role in nucleic acid or protein metabolism. Inhibition of deoxyribonucleic acid synthesis in *Lemna* by (VI) was antagonized by cytokinins (Van Overbeek *et al.*, 1967), whereas inhibition of α-amylase synthesis in barley grains was antagonized by gibberellins (Chrispeels and Varner, 1967; Thomas *et al.*, 1965). Pearson and Wareing (1969) observed that (VI) inhibited RNA synthesis in a system comprised of isolated chromatin and other ingredients. This was so only if (VI) was added before isolation of the chromatin was complete. This is, of course, very analogous to the results obtained with auxins and gibberellins (Sections II,C and III,B) and makes one wonder if these three plant hormones work in similar fashions.

VI. ETHYLENE

A. STRUCTURAL REQUIREMENTS

Burg and Burg (1967) have concluded that for the ethylene type of biological activity several properties are important. Activity requires an unsaturated bond next to a terminal carbon atom, is inversely related to molecule size, and is dependent upon a high electron density in the unsaturated position. For several reasons, including the fact that carbon monoxide at very low concentrations produces ethylene-type effects, these authors believe that ethylene binds to a metal-containing receptor. Carbon dioxide is considered to compete with ethylene for the binding site thereby lessening the developmental effects of ethylene as observed. Oxygen is necessary for the binding of ethylene and it is also necessary for the developmental effects. The nature of the receptor or its role once bound to ethylene is unknown. Studying abscission of leaves, Abeles and Gahagan (1968) generally agreed with the molecular requirements but did not agree with the role of oxygen.

B. Various Possibilities

Several possibilities for the molecular action of ethylene have been proposed and are discussed by Pratt and Goeschl (1969). No single biochemical role seems to have been especially emphasized as yet, however.

REFERENCES

Abeles, F. B., and Gahagan, H. E. (1968). *Plant Physiol.* **43**, 1255.

Baker, D. B., and Ray, P. M. (1965). *Plant Physiol.* **40**, 360.

Binks, R., MacMillan, J., and Pryce, R. J. (1969). *Phytochemistry* **8**, 271.

Bonner, J. (1934). *Proc. Natl. Acad. Sci. U. S.* **20**, 393.

Bruce, M. L., Zwar, J. A., and Kefford, N. P. (1965). *Life Sci.* **4**, 461.

Burg, S. P., and Burg, E. A. (1967). *Plant Physiol.* **42**, 144.

Chrispeels, M. J., and Varner, J. E. (1967). *Plant Physiol.* **42**, 1008.

Cleland, R. (1965). *Plant Physiol.* **40**, 595.

Cleland, R. (1968a). *Science* **160**, 192.

Cleland, R. (1968b). *In* "Biochemistry and Physiology of Plant Growth Substances" (F. Wightman and G. Setterfield, eds.), pp. 613–624. Runge Press, Ottawa.

Coartney, J. S., Morré, D. J., and Key, J. L. (1967). *Plant Physiol.* **42**, 434.

Dahlhelm, H. (1969). *Planta* **86**, 224.

Datta, A., Sen, S. P., and Datta, A. G. (1965). *Biochim. Biophys. Acta* **108**, 147.

Davies, E., and MacLachlan, G. A. (1969). *Arch. Biochem. Biophys.* **129**, 581.

Edelman, J., and Hall, M. A. (1964). *Nature* **201**, 296.

Evans, M. L., and Hokanson, R. (1969). *Planta* **85**, 85.

Evans, M. L., and Ray, P. M. (1969). *J. Gen. Physiol.* **53**, 1.

Evans, M. L., Rayle, D., and Hertel, R. (1968). Plant Research 1968. MSU/AEC Plant. Res. Lab. Michigan State Univ., East Lansing, Mich.

Fan, D. F., and MacLachlan, G. A. (1966). *Can. J. Botany* **44**, 1025.

Filner, P., and Varner, J. E. (1967). *Proc. Natl. Acad. Sci. U. S.* **58**, 1520.

Fittler, F., and Hall, R. H. (1966). *Biochem. Biophys. Res. Commun.* **25**, 441.

Foster, R. J., McRae, D. H., and Bonner, J. (1952). *Proc. Natl. Acad. Sci. U. S.* **38**, 1014.

Foster, R. J., McRae, D. H., and Bonner, J. (1955). *Plant Physiol.* **30**, 323.

Fox, J. E. (1966). *Plant Physiol.* **41**, 75.

Guttman, R. (1957). *J. Biophys. Biochem. Cytol.* **3**, 129.

Hall, M. A., and Ordin, L. (1968). *In* "Biochemistry and Physiology of Plant Growth Substances" (F. Wightman and G. Setterfield, eds.), pp. 659–671. Runge Press, Ottawa.

Hall, R. H., Robbins, M. J., Stasiuk, L., and Thedford, R. (1966). *J. Am. Chem. Soc.* **88**, 2614.

Helgeson, J. P., and Leonard, N. J. (1966). *Proc. Natl. Acad. Sci. U. S.* **56**, 60.

Jacobsen, J. V., and Varner, J. E. (1967). *Plant Physiol.* **42**, 1596.

Johri, M. M., and Varner, J. E. (1968). *Proc. Natl. Acad. Sci. U. S.* **59**, 269.

Key, J. L. (1964). *Plant Physiol.* **39**, 365.

Key, J. L. (1969). *Ann. Rev. Plant Physiol.* **20**, 449.

Key, J. L., and Ingle, J. (1968). In "Biochemistry and Physiology of Plant Growth Substances" (F. Wightman and G. Setterfield, eds.), pp. 711–722. Runge Press, Ottawa.

Klämbt, D., Thies, G., and Skoog, F. (1966). *Proc. Natl. Acad. Sci. U. S.* **56**, 52.

Köhler, D. (1956). *Planta* **47**, 159.

Lang, A., and Richmond, A. E. (1957). *Science* **125**, 650.

Letham, D. S., Shannon, J. S., and McDonald, I. R. (1964). *Proc. Chem. Soc.* **1964**, 230.

MacLachlan, G. A., Davies, E., and Fan, D. F. (1968). In "Biochemistry and Physiology of Plant Growth Substances" (F. Wightman and G. Setterfield, eds.), pp. 443–453. Runge Press, Ottawa.

Madison, J. T., Everett, G. A., and Kung, H. (1967). *J. Biol. Chem.* **242**, 1318.

Masuda, Y. (1968). *Planta* **83**, 171.

Masuda, Y. (1969). *Plant Cell Physiol.* (*Tokyo*) **10**, 1.

Masuda, Y., and Kamisaka, S. (1969). *Plant Cell Physiol.* (*Tokyo*) **10**, 79.

Masuda, Y., and Wada, S. (1966). *Physiol Plantarum* **19**, 1055.

Masuda, Y., and Wada, S. (1967). *Botan. Mag.* (*Tokyo*) **80**, 100.

Masuda, Y., Setterfield, G., and Bayley, S. T. (1966). *Plant Cell Physiol.* (*Tokyo*) **7**, 243.

Masuda, Y., Tanimoto, E., and Wada, S. (1967). *Physiol. Plantarum* **20**, 713.

Matsubara, S., Armstrong, D. J., and Skoog, F. (1968). *Plant Physiol.* **43**, 451.

Matthysse, A. G. (1968). *Plant Physiol.* **43**, S-42.

Miller, C. O. (1967). *Science* **157**, 1055.

Miller, C. O. (1968). In "Biochemistry and Physiology of Plant Growth Substances" (F. Wightman and G. Setterfield, eds.), pp. 33–45. Runge Press, Ottawa.

Miller, C. O. (1969a). *Planta* **87**, 26.

Miller, C. O. (1969b). Unpublished observations.

Morré, D. J., and Eisinger, W. R. (1968). In "Biochemistry and Physiology of Plant Growth Substances" (F. Wightman and G. Setterfield, eds.), pp. 625–645. Runge Press, Ottawa.

Noodén, L. D., and Thimann, K. V. (1963). *Proc. Natl. Acad. Sci. U. S.* **50**, 194.

Noodén, L. D., and Thimann, K. V. (1966). *Plant Physiol.* **41**, 157.

Pearson, J. A., and Wareing, P. F. (1969). *Nature* **221**, 672.

Penny, P., and Galston, A. (1966). *Am. J. Botany* **53**, 1.

Peterkofsky, A. (1968). *Biochemistry* **7**, 472.

Porter, W. L. (1962). Doctoral Thesis, Harvard University, Cambridge, Massachusetts.

Pratt, H. K., and Goeschl, J. D. (1969). *Ann. Rev. Plant Physiol.* **20**, 541.

Ray, P. M. (1962). *Am. J. Botany* **49**, 928.

Ray, P. M. (1967). *J. Cell Biol.* **35**, 659.

Ray, P. M., and Abdul-Baki, A. A. (1968). In "Biochemistry and Physiology of Plant Growth Substances" (F. Wightman and G. Setterfield, eds.), pp. 647–658. Runge Press, Ottawa.

Ray, P. M., and Ruesink, A. W. (1962). *Develop. Biol.* **4**, 377.

Robbins, M. J., Hall, R. H., and Thedford, R. (1967). *Biochemistry* **6**, 1837.

Roychoudhurry, R., Datta, A., and Sen, S. P. (1965). *Biochim. Biophys. Acta* **107**, 346.

Sarkissian, I. V. (1968). In "Biochemistry and Physiology of Plant Growth Substances" (F. Wightman and G. Setterfield, eds.), pp. 473–485. Runge Press, Ottawa.

Skoog, F., Armstrong, D. J., Cherayil, J. D., Hampel, A. E., and Bock, R. M. (1966). *Science* **154**, 1354.

Skoog, F., Hamzi, H. Q., Szweykowska, A. M., Leonard, N. J., Carraway, K. L., Fujii, T., Helgeson, J. P., and Loeppky, R. N. (1967). *Phytochemistry* **6**, 1169.

Steward, F. C., and Shantz, E. M. (1955). *J. Am. Chem. Soc.* **77**, 6351.

Strong, F. M. (1958). "Topics in Microbial Chemistry." Wiley, New York.

Sudi, J. (1964). *Nature* **201**, 1009.

Thimann, K. V. (1963). *Ann. Rev. Plant Physiol.* **14**, 1.

Thimann, K. V., and Sweeney, B. M. (1937). *J. Gen. Physiol.* **21**, 123.

Thomas, T. H., Wareing, P. F., and Robinson, P. M. (1965). *Nature* **205**, 1270.

Trewavas, A. (1968a). *Arch. Biochem. Biophys.* **123**, 324.

Trewavas, A. (1968b). *Phytochemistry* **7**, 673.

Van Hove, C., and Carlier, A. (1968). *Z. Pflanzenphysiologie* **58**, 395.

Van Overbeek, J., Loeffler, J. E., and Mason, M. I. R. (1967). *Science* **156**, 1497.

Varner, J. E., and Johri, M. M. (1968). *In* "Biochemistry and Physiology of Plant Growth Substances" (F. Wightman and G. Setterfield, eds.), pp. 793–814. Runge Press, Ottawa.

Venis, M. A. (1964). *Nature* **202**, 900.

Zachau, H. G., Dütting, D., and Feldmann, H. (1966). *Angew. Chem.* **78**, 392.

AUTHOR INDEX

Numbers in italic refer to the pages on which the complete references are listed.

SUBJECT INDEX

A

Abscisic acid, 514
Acetabulariae, 153
Acetate, incorporation into protein, 282
Acetoacetate, 352
Acetylcholine, 192, 422
Acetyl CoA, 352
N-Acetyl-D-glucosamine, 168
N-Acetylserotonin, 138, 141, 142
Acidity, tissue, 31
Acidosis and renal gluconeogenesis, 392
Acid phosphatase, 21, *see also* Phosphatase
Acid proteases, 32
Acinar cells, 20
   during anuran metamorphosis, 39
ACTH, 60–61, 105–106, 124, 127, 137, 192, 194, 210, 377, 425
   eicosapeptide analog of, 425
   secretion, cyclic pituitary, 137
Actin, 304
Actinomycin D, 28–29, 34–35, 38, 58–59, 64–65, 68, 70, 76–78, 99, 105–107, 174–176, 182–183, 186, 190–191, 303, 331, 345, 404, 457, 507–508, 514
   sodium transport and, 332
Actomyosin, 176
Adenine, 29
   incorporation, 303
   nucleotide pool, 303
   nucleotides, intracellular cyclic AMP, 435
Adenosine, 28–29
S-Adenosylmethionine, 141
Adenyl cyclase, 38, 126–128, 370, 374, 395, 405–406, 451
   activation by fluoride, 453
   calcium ion and, 370
   catalytic subunit, 416
   in cell membrane, 312
   integral component of LATS binding site, 427
   parathyroid hormone sensitive membrane bound, 381

red cell, 38
   in sarcoplasmic reticulum of muscle cells, 375
   stimulation of, 424
      by LATS, 427
      by parathyroid hormone, 381
AIB (Aminoisobutyric acid), 170–171, 175, 185, 187, 193, 195–196, 198
   stimulation by TSH, 449
   transport of, 173
   uptake, 176–168, 183, 187
Adrenal atrophy, 61
Adrenal cortex, 60, 73
   stage of function, 57
Adrenal differentiation, pituitary control, 61
Adrenal hormones, 19
Adrenal insufficiency, 248
Adrenal medulla, 73
Adrenal organogenesis, 60
Adrenal-pituitary axis, 20, *see also* Pituitary-adrenal axis
Adrenal steroidogenic enzymes, 127
Adrenal steroid secretion, 146
Adrenalectomy, 65, 69, 72–73, 78, 143, 146–147, 248, 348
   at birth, 59, 65
   maternal, 61
   movements of sodium and, 323
   plasma
      amino-nitrogen levels, 178
      chloride, 322
      magnesium, 322
      potassium, 322
      sodium, 322
Adrenaline, 126, 168, *see also* Epinephrine
Adrenergic inhibitors, 454
Adrenochrome, 451
Adrenocortical hormones, 73
Adrenocorticoid-thyroid relationship, 249
Affinity constants, 227
   determined by equilibrium dialysis, 251
β-Alanine, 283, 288
Alanine aminotransferase, 72–73